Critical Concepts to
Providing Compassionate Cancer Care

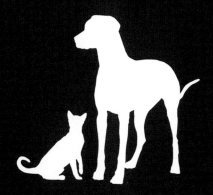

Gregory K. Ogilvie
DVM, Diplomate ACVIM
(Specialties of Internal Medicine and Oncology)
Diplomate ECVIM-CA (Oncology)
Director, Angel Care Cancer Center
California Veterinary Specialists
Carlsbad Research Center
2310 Faraday Avenue
Carlsbad, California, 92008 USA

Professor and Program Director of Veterinary Oncology
University of California San Diego
Department of Radiation Medicine and Applied Sciences
3855 Health Sciences Drive
La Jolla, CA 92037

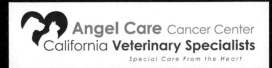

UC San Diego Health

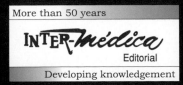

www.intermedica.com.ar

XXI – 2017
Buenos Aires – República Argentina

Critical concepts to providing compassionate cancer care

Deposit was made under the law 11.723
ISBN N° 978-950-555-xxx-x

NOTICE

Veterinary Medicine is an ever-changing field. Standard safety precautions must be followed, but as new research and clinical experience broaden our knowledge, changes in treatment and drug therapy may became necessary or appropriate. Readers are advised to check the most current product information provided by the manufacturer of each drug to be administrated to verify the recommended dose, the method and duration of administration, and contraindications. It is the responsibility of the treating veterinarian, relying on experience and knowledge of the patient, to determine dosages and the best treatment for each individual animal. Neither the publisher nor the editor assumens anuy liability for any injury and/or damage to animals or property arising fron this publication.

© 2017 – by Editorial Inter-Médica S.A.I.C.I.
   Junín 917 – Piso 1º "A" – C1113AAC
   Ciudad Autónoma de Buenos Aires - República Argentina
   Tels.: (54-11) 4961-7249 / 4961-9234 / 4962-3145
   FAX: (54-11) 4961-5572
   E-mail: info@inter-medica.com.ar
   E-mail: ventas@inter-medica.com.ar
   http://www.inter-medica. com.ar
   www.seleccionesveterinarias. com.ar

Ogilvie, Gregory K.
   Critical concepts to providing compassionate cancer care. - 1a ed. - Ciudad Autónoma de Buenos Aires : Inter-Médica, 2017.
   472 p. : il. ; 28x20 cm.

   ISBN 978-950-555-xxx-x

   1. Oncología. 2. Medicina Veterinaria. I. Título
   CDD 636.089

Author

Dr. Ogilvie is director of the Angel Care Cancer Center at California Veterinary Specialists and Professor and Division Director of Veterinary Oncology, Department of Radiation Medicine and Applied Sciences, University of California-San Diego, Moores Cancer Center. At the Angel Care Cancer Center, he cares for patients, their families, and teaches interns, residents, veterinary students, and has an active cancer research program.

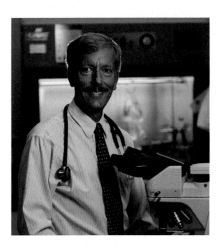

Prior to his move to Southern California, Greg was a full tenured professor, internist, head of medical oncology and director of the Medical Oncology Research Laboratory, Animal Cancer Center at Colorado State University from 1987 until 2003. During this 16-year period at CSU, Greg also spent one year on sabbatical teaching and developing new, innovative cancer therapies at the medical school and the Laboratoire Nutrition, Croisance et Cancer at the Université François Rabelais in Tours France. Dr. Ogilvie lectures to thousands of veterinary students, physicians, graduate veterinarians and scientists each year about compassionate care for pets and people.

Dr. Ogilvie received his DVM from Colorado State University and was in private practice in Connecticut before completing a residency at Tufts University/Angell Memorial Animal Hospital. From there he joined the faculty as a professor at the University of Illinois before moving on to his professorship in Colorado. Dr. Ogilvie is board certified in both the specialties of internal medicine and oncology by the American College of Veterinary Internal Medicine and in oncology and is a Diplomate of the European College of Veterinary Internal Medicine-Companion Animals, Specialty of Oncology.

He is co author with Dr. Antony Moore of three books, *Managing the Veterinary Cancer Patient* (Veterinary Learning Systems, 1995, in English, French and Japanese), *Feline Oncology: Compassionate Care for Cats with Cancer* (Veterinary Learning Systems, 2001 in English and Japanese) and *Managing the Canine Cancer Patient: A Practical Guide to Compassionate Care* (Veterinary Learning Systems, 2006 in English, Spanish and Japanese). He has written over 200 scientific articles and chapters, as well as over 120 scientific abstracts and posters. He has been awarded two international patents, over 10 million dollars in research grants and endowments as a principal or co-investigator, and is the recipient of many awards including: the Arnold O. Beckman Research Award, the Beecham Research Award, the Purina Small Animal Research Award, the Scheidy Memorial Research Award and the AVMA/American Kennel Club Award.

Dr. Ogilvie has lectured in scores of countries to many thousands of students, veterinarians, physicians and scientists in Africa, Australia, New Zealand, Asia, Europe, the Middle East, South America, and North America by shares his love of the practice of veterinary medicine and oncology. Dr. Ogilvie's teaching skills have also been frequently recognized. He is the recipient of the Outstanding Teachers Award; two Norden Distinguished Teacher Awards; the MSD Agvet Award for Creativity in Teaching; the SCAVMA Award for "Dedication to Students and the Profession", and was named Outstanding Companion Animal Speaker for 1999 at the North American Veterinary Conference.

Greg has also been recognized with: the American Veterinary Medical Association's "Veterinarian of the Year-1995"; the American Animal Hospital Association's "Veterinarian of the Year-1996"; the Colorado Veterinary Medical Association Outstanding Faculty Award-1996; and the 1999 SHARE Human Animal Bond Companion Animal Award. Greg was awarded the World Small Animal Veterinary Association Hills Award for Excellence in Veterinary Healthcare for the year 2001.

When not caring for pets and people, Greg is a certified ski instructor and enjoys camping, SCUBA and long distance cycling. He has volunteered as a counselor at the Sky High Hope Camp for children who have cancer for 15 years and is on the board of directors for Angel on a Leash to benefit children with cancer. His greatest joys are his daughter, Torrie, and his wife, Karla.

Acknowledgments

This book is the fourth in a series created to keep pace with the massive advance in knowledge in the area of veterinary oncology. Extraordinary acclaim goes to the Modyeievsky family who has done more than single group or family to empower veterinarians internationally with information to provide compassionate care for pets and their families. Special thanks to Eduardo Modyeievsky for his special friendship that I will treasure forever.

The focus of this book is on caring for pets, people, and the veterinary health care team with compassionate care. Unlike the previous three books, this effort was done without the direct involvement of friend, colleague and my personal hero, Dr. Tony Moore. Tony's indirect presence, wisdom and expertise is felt throughout the entire work. Each page of the entire book would not have been possible without the input, advice and editorial expertise of Ms. Torrie Kristen Ogilvie. Her grace, wisdom and standards of excellence have been beyond indispensable. Thanks also to Dr. Debra Channick who helped direct and enhance the impact of the first section. Her best friend, my special friend "Catch" is with us in spirit; Catch taught us all the joy and magic of living and life. Board certified specialist in emergency and critical care, Dr. Amy Carr deserves high acclaim for providing guidance and direction for the second section of the book on urgent problems associated with the cancer patient. Similarly, board certified medical and board certified radiation oncologist, Dr. David Proulx, board certified surgeons Dr. Sarit Dhupa and Christian Osmond and the veterinary oncology nurses infused the entire work with their insight and experience. Each member of the Angel Care Cancer Center at California Veterinary Specialists and the Special Care Foundation cannot be thanked enough for making each aspect of the book what it is today. Finally, thanks to my lifelong friend, mate and friend, Karla Ogilvie who, flanked by Luna-Tuna and Mia-Papaya gave me the support to create this book.

Dedication

Torrie Kristen Ogilvie
Editor, Angel, Mentor and Friend

Content

Section 4: Clinical briefing for busy practitioners

Appendix

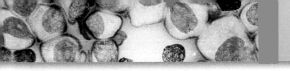

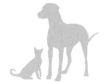

Chapter I

Introduction to: a practical guide to compassionate cancer care

"Your pet has cancer." Such dreaded words often evoke images of pain, discomfort, baldness, nausea, vomiting, cachexia and anorexia. Indeed, the client who hears the diagnosis of cancer often equates it with a death sentence. It is the veterinarian who must dispel the myths and fears that accompany such overwhelming news and provide options along with medical support for the client's beloved pet. Sadly, many members of the veterinary community, including clinicians and nurses, also share the belief that cancer is a torturous and fatal disease. In reality, that assumption is just not true. Few responsibly treated patients ever suffer from these adverse effects and many can even be cured. In fact, compared with heart and renal disease, cancer is the most curable of all the chronic diseases. The author of this book has taken great steps to provide readers with practical, up-to-date information and personal experience in the management of malignant disorders in pets because we believe that, in short, each and every cancer patient can and should be helped. The increasing popularity of oncology can be attributed, in part, to the many improvements in veterinary cancer diagnostics and therapeutics.[2-7] Advanced cancer care used to be restricted to veterinary schools, but the dramatic increases in availability of specialized veterinary care centers now make such resources readily available. In fact, private practice specialty centers are often equipped with superior technology and information than many university veterinary hospitals. As a result, there is an increased ability to help a larger number of animals with a wide variety of malignancies. This greater accessibility has also increased awareness of veterinarians and clients alike regarding the availability of sophisticated veterinary cancer treatment. Despite the proliferation of centers that can provide advanced cancer care, oncology and surgery exist primarily because of the importance of companion animals in our society.

Key point

Cancer care is best done by empowering clients with honest, realistic, truthful balanced hope and information about their best friend's disease and its treatment.

Every practitioner wants to provide the very best care for their patients with cancer. Thus, the caring professional often asks how to make sense of newly emerging data and how to reconcile it with the proposed cancer treatment. This task can be daunting because, unlike human medicine in which conclusions are often not made unless studies have been performed on much larger data sets and then confirmed by other individuals and subsequently published in refereed journals of high integrity, in veterinary medicine, the studies are frequently small, uncontrolled and underpowered. Many veterinarians now turn to evidence-based medicine, the negotiation and synthesis of clinical experience with new scientific data.

COMPASSIONATE CANCER CARE AND THE PRACTICE OF EVIDENCE-BASED MEDICINE

Since evidence-based medicine emerged as a clinical discipline in the 1990s, it has provided an important way not only for health care professionals to make conclusions about patient care, but for veterinarians who need to assess the information at hand to make clinical judgments for patients coming into our clinics and hospitals today.[10,11] Evidence-based medicine is often defined as a conscientious, explicit and judicious discipline that formalizes the long-practiced principle of managing patients based on current scientific evidence as well as expert and personal experience.[10,11] This balanced approach to the practice of veterinary medicine and oncology in particular requires the ability to integrate individual clinical expertise with the best available external clinical evidence from systematic research all the while keeping our client's and patient's unique values and circumstances in mind. Since this type of decision making is based on the most up-to-date information available, its success is only as good as the practitioner's access to the latest information and a dedication to lifelong learning skills. In essence, the management of each patient evolves over time as the knowledge about the disease, patients, diagnostics and therapeutics evolves.

> **Key point**
>
> A balanced approach to the practice of veterinary medicine and oncology requires the integration of individual clinical expertise with the best available external clinical evidence from systematic research all the while keeping our client's and patient's unique values and circumstances in mind.

In practicing evidence-based medicine, here is a general hierarchy of information that requires analysis based on the probability of its accuracy and applicability to the population as a whole. The hierarchy from least to most reliable is as follows:

- Personal experience.
- Case reports.
- Case series.
- Retrospective studies (cross-sectional, case–control).
- Uncontrolled clinical trials.
- Nonrandomized controlled clinical trials.
- Randomized controlled clinical trials.

By meeting the medical needs of the patient and the nonmedical needs of the client through the practice of evidence-based medicine, the veterinary health care team can enhance, celebrate and enrich the relationship between animal and humans. This relationship, the human-animal bond, is the very reason why veterinary medicine and advanced veterinary cancer care exists and flourishes. Some may consider this verbiage "evangelical." Others consider the concept of caring from the heart and the science so obvious that it is unnecessary to even mention. Regardless, the human–animal bond is the foundation of the veterinary profession and worthy of note, especially in regard to cancer.

> **Key point**
>
> The human-animal bond is the very reason why veterinary medicine and advanced veterinary cancer care exists and flourishes.

Cancer care can be provided while enhancing quality of life for the vast majority of patients. To do so requires a strong commitment to the Commandments of Cancer Care. The Commandments of Cancer Care address core fears almost every client has about cancer and cancer therapy. Addressing these fears in oral and written formats is absolutely vital to begin the process of providing compassionate care.

THE COMMANDMENTS

Do not let them hurt! [1-4]

Every caregiver should know in advance that the veterinary team will not tolerate the patient suffering any pain. Provide a preemptive and ongoing pain-management/prevention program for the dog or cat with cancer. An active pain-management program reassures the client that the patient's quality of life is optimal. Management should begin with comfort care and then, when needed, be extended to include oral medications (e.g., morphine, codeine, piroxicam, carprofen), transdermal delivery systems (fentanyl patches), acupuncture or more advanced analgesic delivery systems (e.g., constant-rate intravenous infusion, epidural catheters, intrathoracic pleural analgesia). A more complete discussion about pain management can be found elsewhere in this text.

> **Key point**
>
> The single most important thing in all of veterinary medicine is compassionate care that is defined as meeting the medical needs of the patient, and the non medical needs of the client.

Do not let them vomit or have diarrhea! [1-4]

This commandment strikes at the preconceived fear that pets who undergo chemotherapy suffer from significant bouts of nausea and diarrhea. This fear is simply not true. With recent advances in cancer care, nausea, vomiting and diarrhea are no longer commonly associated with chemotherapy. Moreover, the introduction of a large number of antiemetics and antidiarrheals in clinical practice has made it possible to control these problems should they occur. Dispensing oral medication such as metoclopramide to the caregiver each and every time that a potentially nauseating drug is administered will enable the caregiver to prevent this symptom at home. To stop nausea and vomiting, the veterinarian should ensure that medications and supportive care are immediately available. Providing the caregiver with drugs such as maropitant citrate, ondansetron hydrochloride and dolasetron mesylate, although costly, will assure all members of the team that the patient is comfortable. Some oncologists believe that tylosin, metronidazole, and loperamide hydrochloride can reduce the risk of small and large-bowel diarrhea, so they often dispense these drugs to their cancer patients as a preventative. Increasing fiber intake can also be of great value in enhancing bowel health. A more comprehensive discussion about the management of nausea and vomiting can be found later in this book.

Key point

Appetite and adequate nutritional support absolutely depend on the treatment plan's success in preventing and treating discomfort and nausea.

Do not let them starve! [1-4]

This final commandment is just as fundamental as the first two. Ensuring that our patients will eat is critical to their quality of life. The reality is that appetite and adequate nutritional support absolutely depend on the treatment plan's success in preventing and treating discomfort and nausea. If the plan has not resolved the problem, then nursing care (e.g., warming food, providing aromatic foods and comfortable environments), medicinal appetite stimulants and, when needed, assisted feeding techniques such as esophagostomy, gastrostomy or jejunostomy tube placement should be employed. All of these components of nutritional care need to be available early in the course of the disease. Weight loss must not be tolerated, particularly in cats and dogs that have fewer reserves due to their size. A more extensive discussion of nutritional care can be found later in this book.

STEPS TO PROVIDE COMPASSIONATE CANCER CARE

Each member of the veterinary healthcare team plays a critical role in providing compassionate care for cancer patients. Before treatment with specific therapeutics can begin, the veterinarian needs to perform three crucial steps in order to ensure the highest quality of cancer care.[1-8] First, dispel the myths that blind almost everyone to the possibilities of providing exceptional care for the cancer patient. Second, build a team to care for the pet clients' and the patient with equal attention. Only after these first two steps have been accomplished, can the third step—true compassionate care—begin.

The following are examples of actions steps you may consider for employing the commandments:

• Make your veterinary technician/nursing team in charge of pain management.
• Make the client aware that discomfort, nausea or

anorexia is not normal and that early intervention is recommended.
• Make frequent follow-up calls to ensure that the patient is doing well.

Step one: dispel the myths

Regardless of our culture, nationality or religion, most of us are indoctrinated early on that cancer and cancer therapy are horrible. Therefore, clients, nursing staff, and even veterinarians often perceive cancer and its therapy as something frightening and hopeless. In reality, most of the fears and misconceptions about cancer and cancer care are wrong or out of proportion. These myths serve as barriers that often preclude early, decisive therapy and obscure true understanding of the disease, consequently blocking out all hope. Surgical procedures such as amputation, chest wall resection, hemipelvectomy and maxillectomy are perceived as traumatic, not only to the patient, but to the client and healthcare providers as well. We imagine that chemotherapy protocols are inevitably accompanied by horrible side effects. We fear that therapy will physically debilitate the patient and will financially devastate the client with little benefit for either patient or client. In essence, we are often paralyzed by fear and remain indecisive as we, our team, and our clients wonder, "Is it worth it?"

Key point

Most of the fears and misconceptions about cancer and cancer care are incorrect or blown out of proportion. The devastating consequence of these myths is that they serve as a barrier that often precludes early, decisive therapy from the veterinary healthcare team and client.

Do not underestimate the role that education plays in empowering both the team and the client. Identify and then dispel the misconceptions and myths existing within all members of the veterinary healthcare team, including receptionists, nurses, veterinarians and other allied team members (boxes 1-1 and 1-2). Explain how you interpret the statistics and review them with your client. Since some clients can become obsessed with numbers, it is important that they learn how to process such information in order to maintain a positive attitude; for example, many studies rely on averages of all dogs at all stages of disease. Moreover, in adhering to the guidelines and practice of evidence based medicine, many veterinary studies are limited by the lack of statistically significant data.

Remember to recite to your team, including the client, the commandments of cancer care

---

Box 1-1. Examples of ways to dispel myths of clients who have animals with cancer[8]

- Record and provide an audio transcript of actual discussions regarding the disease and its treatment.
- Give clients written "bullet points" of discussions.
- Provide information on the most common disorders and treatments.
- Keep an updated list of clients whose pets have undergone cancer treatment and who are willing to discuss realities of care and disease with others. It is best to match clients based on common diseases in their pets.
- Carefully prescreen and review Website information on diseases to ensure that your clients can obtain truthful, accurate facts about cancer and cancer care.
- Take new clients on a tour of the hospital and introduce them to the staff.
- Include the client in as much patient care as law and ethics allow.
- Encourage clients to summarize critical information.
- Call clients days to weeks after euthanasia to ensure they are doing reasonably well.

Box 1-2. Examples of ways to deliver the care[8]

- Do not prejudge client desires and capabilities; give all options regardless of cost or outcome.
- Review team philosophy for patient care with the client, nurses and others if indicated.
- Define the importance of preventing toxicity or illness and the steps to doing so.
- Outline contingency plans for when problems occur. Include plans for weekends, nights and holidays.
- Educate clients on information about disease and treatment so that, ideally, they know as much as the rest of the team.
- Listen and respond to client's needs, goals, concerns, desires, fears, time commitments, financial limitations and philosophy regarding quality and quantity of life.

---

to reassure them that enhancing quality of life always informs the decision-making process and treatment plan.

Quantitating quality of life

Key point

The somewhat vague question of how to quantitate the pet's quality of life should not be elusive, but discussed with each client as quality of life is the holy grail of cancer therapy.

Each and every veterinarian takes a personal and professional oath to alleviate the pain and suffering of animals, yet few published papers directly define and quantitate this most important and essential objective. While contributing factors of quality life for all animals are subjective, they often include a high activity level and enjoyment of relationships, mental stimulation, health, food consumption, stress and control over their environment. Since people define quality of life differently for both themselves and their pets, the veterinary healthcare team must have a clear understanding of each client's definition and standards. It is important to note the contrast between the myths of cancer care and the actual perception of clients whose pets undergo cancer treatment, which is remarkably positive. In one study that asked clients to assess the quality of their dog's life during multidrug chemotherapy to treat lymphoma, sixty-eight percent of the clients considered their dog's quality of life to be the same as before the lymphoma occurred and the rest felt that the quality of life was acceptable, albeit poorer, than before the lymphoma occurred.[7] Sixty-eight percent of the clients considered their dog's quality of life to be the same as before the lymphoma occurred and the rest felt that their dog's quality of life was acceptable, though poorer than before the lymphoma occurred. Almost all (92%) of the study participants had no regrets about treating their dog with chemotherapy.

Even though it is difficult to convert the myriad of subjective parameters into objective, numeric data for subsequent analysis and comparison in both human and veterinary medicine, several investigators have tried to enumerate parameters of toxicity and performance (Tables 5-1 and 5-2).[8] More recent efforts, especially those in enumerating parameters associated with discomfort, have employed a scale of 0 to 100. The caregiver is asked to subjectively rate parameters such as quality of life, appetite, and nausea initially and at subsequent specified time points during treatment, then to compare the subsequent assessments to the initial finding.[5] The veterinary healthcare team scores and records these assessments for later analysis. For many oncologists and clients alike, this standard is at least as important—if not more—than duration of remission.

Step two: establish the team

Establishing a dedicated, trained, cohesive caring veterinary healthcare team is essential to adequately care for cancer patients and their caregivers as well as to fight the disease. All staff members, including office personnel and nurses, must understand that they play a vital role in caring for both the cancer patients and the people who bring them to us. Everyone must be united in focus, philosophy and the ultimate goal of enhancing and improving the cancer patient's quality of life while supporting one another (figure 1-1). Each veterinarian, nurse and receptionist within a facility must be prepared to accept a role as part of the team. This team must be prepared to reach out to specialists and consultants such as pathologists, pharmacists and veterinary oncologists whenever appropriate. Finally, the most vital link to the team is the caregiver. The caregiver must feel like an active part of this team through education and support. In working as part of a team to provide ongoing day-to-day care and assessment, the client's confidence and commitment to treatment will build; perhaps most importantly, such a collaborative effort in treating the pet will empower the client. Indeed, without the client's ability to closely observe and care for the patient, optimal treatment cannot be achieved.

Cancer treatment is not easy. Inevitably, cancer arouses negative feelings in staff and colleagues that often results in a mental roadblock to hope, care and cure. It is imperative that everyone on the healthcare team acknowledge such negative feelings in order to dispel them. Ongoing support, information and care must be provided to all members of the veterinary healthcare team to prevent burnout and "compassion fatigue", thus retaining individuals who will provide quality, compassionate care on a continuous basis (see subsequent section).

Care of the cancer patient requires unique skills, knowledge, drugs, procedures and philosophies. The healthcare team must dedicate itself to an aggressive continuing education program to maximize care for their patients. Since canine and feline cancer patients usually have a dynamic course to their disease, ongoing communication is essential to maximize

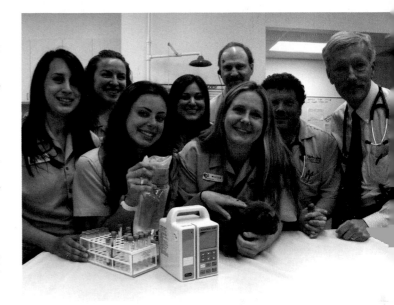

Figure 1-1: All staff members, , including office personnel and nurses, must understand that they play a vital role in caring for both the cancer patients and the people who bring them to us. Everyone must be united in focus, philosophy and the ultimate goal of enhancing and improving the cancer patient's quality of life while supporting one another.

care for both patient and caregiver. In addition to daily communication during hospitalization, continuous communication by multiple members of the veterinary healthcare team can greatly improve the patient's quality of care by providing the veterinarian with ongoing reassessments and progress reports. These and other policies and procedures regarding patient care should be established long in advance.

The caregiver is perhaps the most vital—and often most overlooked—member of the healthcare team. Once their misconceptions have been dispelled so that they can make rational, educated decisions regarding cancer care, caregivers must know that they are essential to the team. Only the client can provide quality of life assessments, administration of medication and daily (or even hourly) patient monitoring. In order to be effective, the client needs to understand the disease, its treatment, and their role as caretaker as the extension of the healthcare team at home. Emergency preparedness as well as its prevention is only possible with an informed, attentive caregiver. In fact, effective cancer treatment can make significant progress under the watchful eye of a conscientious caregiver who provides 24-hour outpatient care. Another benefit of including caregivers on the healthcare team is that it empowers them; it gives them an active responsibility in combating a disease that makes them feel helpless. Moreover, it reinforces the bond between them and their beloved pet.

The following examples demonstrate ways to create, inspire, and enhance the veterinary healthcare team[8]:

- Identify, reward and promote only the best, most compassionate people.
- Openly celebrate, review and revise mission statement and goals written by the team.
- Ensure the team participates in all interviews and assists in decisions to hire new applicants.
- Share and celebrate when a team member is recognized by clients or others.
- Meet at least weekly to listen to team members; acknowledge their input, feelings and thoughts.
- Introduce clients to the team, including nurses and receptionists, during the first visit.

Step three: deliver the care [1–8]

Compassion, the single most important term in veterinary medicine, should always define and inform every aspect of cancer care. The phases of compassionate care include: 1) defining and describing the disease and the health status of the patient through diagnostics and staging (i.e., determining the extent of the cancer in the body; see following section); 2) providing caring support by responding to the pet's needs and client's concerns through the commandments of cancer care (see another section in this book); 3) providing direct therapy for the underlying disease using the appropriate tools, such as surgery, chemotherapy or radiation therapy. These steps are interdependent and must be given equal attention. The veterinary healthcare team must work to establish a bond of trust with the client. This bond begins with communication, which requires time and open, honest discussions with all parties involved. Ideally, sufficient time should be set aside during the first visit to discuss the pet's condition, prognosis, and treatment options. Encourage the client to take notes and ask questions, or, alternatively, the veterinarian can take notes during the discussion and give them to the client. As a supplement to the oral discussion, provide preprinted, plain language information sheets that describe your practice, the patient's disease and the treatments that may be used. A summary of all major discussions with the caregiver should be either taped or written so that a copy is available for the hospital records and the client. The members of the veterinary healthcare team should recognize that most clients are so overwhelmed by emotion that they cannot make an immediate, rational decision or even completely comprehend the information provided to them during the first visit. To help the client absorb the information, a follow-up telephone call or personal conference is invaluable. Clients should not be forced to make quick or immediate decisions; allow them time to weigh the options available for their dog or cat. By presenting the client with an accurate prognosis, information regarding quality of life and duration of therapy, and treatment choices, you restore a sense of control and power to the client.

Key point

The average caregiver of a patient with cancer will visit your clinic frequently over the next year, therefore it is imperative that the entire veterinary team constantly cultivate the bond of trust with the client.

Since the average caregiver of a patient with cancer will visit your clinic frequently over the next year, it is imperative that the entire veterinary team constantly cultivate the bond of trust with the client. Cancer by itself can engender many feelings of loss and bereavement, even though treatment is a viable option and the patient's prognosis may not be guarded. Nevertheless, the emotional and physical impact of pet loss and bereavement should be discussed during the care of the cancer patient. When discussing the option of euthanasia, information about the philosophy, procedures and aftercare of the animal's body should be provided in both oral and written forms.

References

1. Ogilvie GK, Moore AS: Compassionate care of the cancer patient, in Ogilvie GK, Moore AS: *Feline Oncology: A Comprehensive Guide for Compassionate Care.* Yardley, PA, Veterinary Learning Systems, 2002, pp 1–6.
2. Ogilvie G: Préservation de la santé des animaux âgés, in *Gériatrie vétérinaire. Les Editions du Point Vétérinaire*, Nantes, France 2004, Intervet, pp 51–56.
3. Ogilvie GK: Pris en charge du cancer chez l'animal âgé, in *Gériatrie vétérinaire. Les Editions du Point Vétérinaire*. Nantes, France, Intervet, 2004, pp 61–66.
4. Ogilvie GK: The care of animals with cancer, in Dobson JM, Lascelles BDX (eds): *BSAVA Manual of Canine and Feline Oncology*, ed 2. Gloucester, UK, British Small Animal Veterinary Association, 2003, pp 68–72.
5. Mitchener KL, Ogilvie GK: Rekindling the bond. *Vet Econ* 40:30–36, 1999.
6. Mitchener KL, Ogilvie GK: Giving cancer patients hope. *Vet Econ* 40:84–88, 1999.
7. Downing R: Pets Living with Cancer: *A Pet Client's Resource.* Denver, American Animal Hospital Association, 2000, pp 1–8.
8. Ogilvie GK: Meeting the needs of patient and client through compassionate care, in Ettinger SJ, Feldman EC (eds): *Textbook of Veterinary Internal Medicine.* WB Saunders, 2005, pp 534–538.

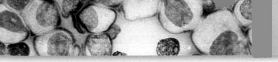

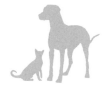

Chapter 2

Setting goals for compassionate care

Once the myths have been dispelled, the team established and the commandments initiated to enhance quality of life (see above), the goals of therapy need to be defined so that the patient can be cared for. Patient care includes providing direct therapy for the underlying disease and providing compassionate care focused at accomplishing the goals set by the client in close cooperation with the veterinary health care team. Care to fulfill these goals is provided by using the appropriate tools at hand, such as supportive care, surgery, chemotherapy or radiation therapy.

Some clients and members of the veterinary health care team think that if cure is not achievable, then "success" cannot be secured. This is simply not true, especially with the advent of more recent therapies that can control or arrest cancer for sustained periods. In addition, each client has his or her own goals for quality and length of life, as well as his or her own limits for the possibility for adverse effects and cost of care. In short, all options should be given—from the very highest level of curative and palliative therapy, supportive and hospice care and, finally, to euthanasia. Each step should be made and supported by the whole veterinary team. However, this may require that the veterinary health care team define their limits and capabilities in advance. The following are a few of the many options that may be considered for each patient.

Key point

All options for each patient with cancer should be given—from the very highest level of curative and palliative therapy, supportive and hospice care and, finally, if appropriate, euthanasia.

DEFINITIVE, CURATIVE INTENT[1–8]

To say that cancer is the most curable of all chronic diseases in human and veterinary medicine is perhaps surprising. Nevertheless, cure is the goal of every client and veterinary health care team, although it is often mistaken as the only aim. The majority of cures are accomplished through good surgical techniques combined with a clear understanding of cancer biology. Radiation therapy and chemotherapy may be essential to the realization of some of these benefits, but to a lesser degree. While the definition of "cure" is elusive since there is no absolute cutoff past which it can be guaranteed that the cancer is eradicated, some veterinary oncologists define it as living cancer free for two years while other veterinary oncologists consider it to be five years.

Key point

Cancer is the most curable of all chronic diseases in human and veterinary medicine.

The success rate of curative intent will increase by first knowing the name and extent of the disease and by planning to control or cure the cancer while maintaining quality of life.

PALLIATIVE CARE[1–8]

Palliative care endeavors to improve the patient's quality of life through treatment; it does not necessarily extend length of life. For example, coarse fraction radiation to a site of bony metastasis is primarily designed to alleviate pain. This approach to palliative care is similar to many other, nonneoplastic, chronic diseases such as osteoarthritis and chronic renal failure. Indeed, cancer is being redefined in biomedical sciences as a chronic disease. Veterinary medicine is going to have to go through a paradigm shift as molecular therapeutic agents, radiation therapy and other treatments are developed and evaluated, so that we can be pleased with the improvement of quality of life despite the fact that the length of life may not be extended.

Key point

Little difference exists between palliative and supportive care because both approaches are defined as treatment to improve quality of life without necessarily increasing length of life.

SUPPORTIVE/HOSPICE CARE [1-8]

Little difference exists between palliative and supportive care because both approaches are defined as treatment to improve quality of life without necessarily increasing length of life. Supportive care often implies treating the patient's clinical signs rather than the tumor itself and is often used in combination with palliative care. Ways to provide supportive care include administering analgesics, antiemetics, appetite stimulants and treatments for anemia and leukopenia. Hospice care is a type of supportive care that is generally administered at the end of life. Hospice care, or care to maintain quality of life, especially to maximize comfort in the terminal phases of a disease, is a defined specialty in human medical care. In veterinary medicine, this type of care is rapidly developing. Dignity and comfort until death, whether from euthanasia or natural causes, are rapidly becoming a necessity in many practices.

The most common misconceptions—and the realities—of hospice care are as follows:

- Patients have to be cared for 24 hours a day, seven days a week. With appropriate arrangements for patient care and safety, pets can be left alone for short periods.
- Hospice care is not sophisticated. The care of the animal patient in a hospice setting can be as complex as the client and the rest of the veterinary health care team wish. Oxygen cages, constant-rate infusion, nutritional support and epidural analgesia are always possible in a home environment with appropriate education and support.

- Animals who enter a hospice care environment cannot be admitted to the hospital for routine care. The level of care is totally up to the client and the veterinary health care team at all times.
- Animals who enter a hospice care situation cannot be resuscitated. Caregivers can ensure that resuscitation is possible if and when their pet has a cardiac or respiratory arrest.

EUTHANASIA [1-8]

Euthanasia is an important aspect of many levels of care, including hospice care, because it is also often employed to alleviate pain, suffering or unwanted aspects of care or the disease. The importance of doing euthanasia properly cannot be emphasized enough. More clients leave a practice as a result of an unpleasant experience over the loss of a pet than for any other reason. Managing this difficult aspect of compassionate care involves adequate preparation as well as an ongoing dialogue between the entire veterinary health care team and the caregivers both before and at the time of euthanasia and death. Since euthanasia is such an important part of veterinary medicine, a brief description of that process is included in a subsequent section.

Key point

More clients leave a practice as a result of an unpleasant experience over the loss of a pet than for any other reason.

The following are examples of ways to quantitate quality of life. The first is a simplification of the Karnofsky's performance score (Table 2-1), the second, from an adaptation of the Eastern Cooperative Oncology Group scheme (Table 2-2), the third is a document designed to pose key questions to determine quality of life (Table 2-3).

Table 2-1. Karnofsky's performance criteria (*circle grade*)	
Grade	**Criteria**
0 (normal)	Fully active; able to perform at predisease level
1 (restricted)	Activity less than predisease level, but able to function as an acceptable pet
2 (compromised)	Severely compromised activity level; ambulatory only to point of eating, sleeping, and consistently urinating and defecating in acceptable areas
3 (disabled)	Completely disabled; must be force-fed; unable to control urination and defecation

[Reprinted with permission from: Ogilvie GK, Fettman MJ, Mallinckrodt CH, et al: Effect of fish oil, arginine, and doxorubicin chemotherapy on remission and survival time for dogs with lymphoma: a double-blind, randomized placebo-controlled study. *Cancer* 2000 88(8):1916-1928, 2000.]

Table 2-2. Modified *Eastern Cooperative Oncology Group* evaluation (*completely circle appropriate boxes or strike out with "NA"*)

	0	1	2	3	4
Leukopenia					
WBC x 10^3	>5.5	3–<5.5	2–<3	1–<2	<1
Neutrophils x 10^3	>2.5	1.5–<2.5	1–<1.5	0.5–<1	<0.5
Lymphocytes x 10^3	>1.5	1–<1.5	0.5–<1	0–<0.5	0
Thrombocytopenia, Plt x 10^3	>130	90–<130	50–<90	25–<50	<25
Anemia					
Hct%	>25	20–<25	15–<20	10–<15	<10
Clinical	None	–	–	Sx	Trans
Hemorrhage	None	Min	Mod	Debil	Threat
Infection	None	No Rx	Req Rx	Debil	Threat
Urinary					
BUN mg/dl	<20	21–40	41–60	>60	Sympt
Creatinine mg/dl	<2	2.1–4	4.1–6	>6	Uremia
Proteinuria	None	1+	2+–3+	4+	
Hematuria	None	Micro	Grss	Grss-Cl	Obstr
Hepatic (x NL)					
ALT	<1.5	1.5–2	2.1–5	>5	
ALP	<1.5	1.5–2	2.1–5	>5	
Bilirubin	<1.5	1.5–2	2.1–5	>5	
Clinical	None			Precoma	Coma
Nausea and vomiting	None	Nausea	Cont vom	Intract	
Diarrhea	None	Loose	Sec dehyd	Bloody	
Pulmonary (clinical)	None	Mild	Mod	Svr	Req O_2
Cardiac	None	HR >200	Arryth	Mild CHF	Svr CHF
Neuro					
Peripheral nerves	None	Mild	Mod	Mod-Svr	Svr Seitz's sign
Central nervous system	None	Depress	Mod +/- trmr	Svr +/- coma	Coma

Table 2-3. Quality of life questionnaire

Happiness	1	2	3	4	5
My dog wants to play					
My dog responds to my presence					
My dog enjoys life					
Mental status	1	2	3	4	5
My dog has more good days than bad days					
My dog sleeps more, is awake less					
My dog seems dull or depressed, not alert					
Pain	1	2	3	4	5
My dog is in pain					
My dog pants frequently, even at rest					
My dog shakes or trembles occasionally					

The table follows in next page

Table 2-3. Quality of life questionnaire (cont.)					
Appetite	**1**	**2**	**3**	**4**	**5**
My dog eats the usual amount of food					
My dog acts nauseous or vomits					
My dog eats treats/snacks					
Hygiene	**1**	**2**	**3**	**4**	**5**
My dog keeps him/herself clean					
My dog smells like urine and has skin irritation					
My dog's fur is greasy, matted, rough looking					
Water intake (hydration)	**1**	**2**	**3**	**4**	**5**
My dog drinks adequately					
My dog has a diarrhea					
My dog is urinating a normal amount					
Mobility	**1**	**2**	**3**	**4**	**5**
My dog moves normally					
My dog lays in one place all day long					
My dog is as active as he/she has been					
General health	**1**	**2**	**3**	**4**	**5**
General health compared to last evaluation					
	Worse		**Same**		**Better**
General health compared to initial diagnosis					
	Worse		**Same**		**Better**
Current quality of life					
	Worse		**Same**		**Better**

References

1. Ogilvie GK, Moore AS: Compassionate care of the cancer patient, in Ogilvie GK, Moore AS. *Feline Oncology: A Comprehensive Guide for Compassionate Care*. Yardley, PA, Veterinary Learning Systems. 2001, pp 1–6.
2. Ogilvie GK: Préservation de la santé des animaux âgés. *Gériatrie vétérinaire*. Les Editions du point vétérinaire, Nantes, 2004, pp 51–56.
3. Ogilvie GK: Pris en charge du cancer chez l'animal âgé. *Gériatrie vétérinaire*. Les Editions du point vétérinaire, Nantes, 2004, pp 61–66.
4. Ogilvie GK: The care of animals with cancer, in Dobson JM, Lascelles BDX (eds): *BSAVA Manual of Canine and Feline Oncology*, ed 2. Gloucester, UK, British Small Animal Veterinary Association, 2003, pp 68–72.
5. Mitchener KL, Ogilvie GK: Rekindling the bond. *Vet Econ* 40:30–36, 1999.
6. Mitchener KL, Ogilvie GK: Giving cancer patients hope. *Vet Econ* 40:84–88, 1999.
7. Downing R: *Pets Living with Cancer: A Pet Client's Resource*. Denver, American Animal Hospital Association, 2000, pp 1–8.
8. Ogilvie GK: Meeting the needs of patient and client through compassionate care, in Ettinger SJ, Feldman EC (eds). *Textbook of Veterinary Internal Medicine*. Philadelphia, WB Saunders, 2005, pp 535–538.

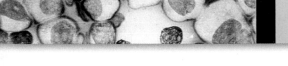

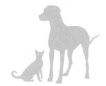

Chapter 3

Pet loss and bereavement

More people leave a veterinary practice because of a bad experience dealing with the death of their pet than any other reason. Veterinarians and veterinary nurses physically or mentally "leave" the practice of veterinary medicine over these deaths more than any other cause. Therefore, this subject is more important than almost any other in the pursuit of providing compassionate care for pets and their families.

The wisest veterinary health care teams often bring up the topic of euthanasia and the inevitable process of grieving and bereavement with their clients before it is imminent. Early discussions are a key part of preparing clients while they are still able to think clearly for this very important event. If clients consider the options facing their pet at a time when they are level-headed, then they will be able to make clearer decisions that benefit them later. It is also a good idea for caregivers to make a list of the positive aspects of their pet's life at a time before treatment has started and before the cancer is advanced. This list can be life-affirming and may also act as a "baseline" for future assessments of the impact of the cancer and treatment on quality of life.

Key point

The wisest veterinary health care teams often bring up the topic of euthanasia and the inevitable process of grieving and bereavement with their clients before it is imminent.

KNOWING WHEN "IT IS TIME"

Most clients ask how they will know when it is time to euthanize their pet. Each person bases his or her decision on their own value system, but the timing is often quite similar for most pet clients. While it is tempting to respond to the question, "What would

you do if it were your dog or cat, doc?" most clinicians believe that the veterinarian and other members of the veterinary health care team should take the role of educator and leave the ultimate decision to the client.

The veterinary health care team can assist the client by defining objective parameters for quality of life, such as appetite, normal behavioral patterns and energy level that can be monitored and assessed at home. These definitions and measured observations allow the caregiver to objectively assess their pet's quality of life and monitor changes. Unless there are extenuating circumstances, clients should be supported once they have come to the conclusion that euthanasia is the best option for them. This support can happen in a number of ways, such as validating the client's decision or assisting the client in understanding the euthanasia and bereavement processes. By supporting the caregivers and allowing them to be active decision makers, the veterinary health care team provides a sense of empowerment during a time that would otherwise be marked by feelings of helplessness and defeat.

Key point

Unless there are extenuating circumstances, clients should be supported once they have come to the conclusion that euthanasia is the best option for them and their pet.

PREPARING THE CLIENT AND STAFF

The success of the euthanasia process can be enhanced by preparing the client adequately about what will take place. Myths can be dispelled with an open, clear description of the euthanasia process and the impact that it may have on the pet client for the

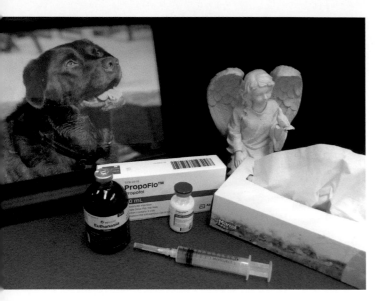

Figure 3-1: Essential supplies for euthanasia should be known by the entire veterinary health care team to ensure that the process is efficient and that the experience is meaningful for the client. A towel or blanket is often helpful, especially if there is loss of bowel or bladder control. Facial tissues should always be plentiful and easily accessible. Thiopental sodium and the euthanasia solution should be drawn up prior to euthanasia into Luer-Lock syringes to prevent accidental loss of drug at the time of injection into the patient. Thiopental relaxes the patient and prevents unwanted movements, gasps and trembles when the euthanasia solution is injected. Finally, transition objects to help grieving should also be available. A plastic bag and scissors for clipping fur and clay for making paw prints can help the family long after the euthanasia itself is complete.

months or years to come. The caregivers need to first understand how a patient is euthanized. Empowering clients with information and the ability to select details such as the timing, location and tempo of the euthanasia process can help them feel more in control. Each client will differ in his or her needs and wants, but examples include organizing the presence of family and friends, reading poetry or books, or reciting favorite stories about their beloved pet. When possible, a secluded, comfortable location in the clinic should be available with a private entrance and exit to avoid any embarrassing situations such as having the tearful client walk through a waiting room full of healthy dogs, cats and clients.

Key point

Empowering clients with information and the ability to select details such as the timing, location and tempo of the euthanasia process can help them feel more in control.

The caregiver is not the only one who will be affected by euthanasia. Indeed, each member of the veterinary health care team is likely to be impacted by the loss of the patient. Therefore, time should be set aside before and after the procedure, not only for the caregiver and his or her family, but also for the health care team to say goodbye. Finally, the health care team should ensure that the caregiver and all staff members who might be seriously affected by the loss of the pet have thought in advance of how they will get home safely.

In families with children, an open and honest discussion with the children is imperative. They should be allowed the chance to say goodbye to their pet too. Indeed, the children are often involved in the decision to perform euthanasia. It is important that children not be sheltered from the decision-making process because excluding children or making up stories (e.g., Fluffy ran away) is destructive and can cause psychological damage that can impact the way they process grief. Finally, it is very important to discuss openly, frankly and compassionately what will be done with the pet's remains. Burial, cremation and disposal by your facility are viable options. If burial or cremation is considered, a choice of coffins or urns may be important to some clients. Commercial cardboard coffins are available and affordable for most. Ideally, all of these decisions can be made early in the course of treatment, but for many clients the final details will have to wait until they are prepared to consider the choices.

!

Important point

Children not be sheltered from the decision-making process because excluding children or making up stories (e.g., Fluffy ran away) is destructive and can cause psychological damage that can impact the way they process grief.

When discussing the euthanasia process, the veterinary health care team should make the family aware about every aspect of the procedure including the fact that at their pet will likely have their eyes open and in rare circumstances may lose bladder and bowel control after death.. All paper work, the bill and options for body care (cremation, burial, disposal by the hospital, etc) should be discussed and completed openly and in private. Most veterinarians offer each client the option to be present during the procedure and even to pay for the procedure. Plans are created and followed to meet the wishes of the client to identify a comfortable, quiet location to euthanize the pet. Whenever possible, the clinical team should work to assist the client in including children, friends and other family animals and encourage full participation by everyone who wishes to be involved. All persons involved should be allowed the time to celebrate, honor and grieve before and after euthanasia is performed. Clients are encouraged to memorialize their pet in any way they prefer, such as clipping hair, making paw prints, or taking photographs at any time.

THE PROCEDURE

If given the option, most clients wish to be present during the euthanasia process. To honor this request requires that the staff be trained and prepared for this emotional time, but it does not suggest that emotion should not be shared or that sadness, crying or tears are ever unprofessional. If a client decides not to be present, that decision should be supported as well.

In order to expedite the process, a catheter is often preplaced within the distal extremity. This reduces the need to acquire vascular access in a pet at a time when the client's expectations and tensions are highest. Some teams find that placement in the medial saphenous vein allows good access to a vein often not used for previous therapy. When the euthanasia solution is delivered, clients should to not be restrained or discouraged from comforting or holding the pet, nor should they have to observe the needle and syringe.

As discussed above, the veterinarian and the health care team should review the process with the caregiver regarding what to expect before, during and after euthanasia. While euthanasia can be performed with a number of different drugs, many veterinarians are comfortable administering propofol (6 mg/kg IV over 10-30 seconds) followed immediately by pentobarbital (88 mg/kg IV over 10 seconds), which results in a smooth, effortless transition to a state of death. Some veterinarians believe it is ideal to premedicate certain patients with a tranquilizer before catheter placement. A towel or other absorbent object may be placed under the pet to capture any bodily excretions as well as a towel to cover the rear end to prevent the client from seeing any elimination that might occur.

Key point

Many veterinarians are comfortable administering propofol (6 mg/kg IV over 10-30 seconds) followed immediately by pentobarbital (88 mg/kg IV over 10 seconds), which results in a smooth, effortless transition to a state of death.

After the process is reviewed with the client, the catheter is placed, the location, setting, and rituals are designed, and the time for euthanasia arrives. While every veterinarian has his or her own style and procedures, many feel it is important for other team members to be present or at least to say their goodbyes. The process may be reviewed briefly one

more time before the catheter is checked for patency and the drugs are injected. It is very important for the attending veterinarian to listen to the heart for an appropriate period and then indicate when the heart has stopped and that the beloved dog or cat has passed on. A gentle touch and an offer of facial tissues are appropriate, affirmative, supportive gestures. They tell a client that a display of emotion is accepted by everyone, including the attending clinician. At this point, client and friends and family may wish to spend time alone with their pet. Many veterinarians do not have clients deal with paying bills at this time but prefer instead to mail them the charges.

Key point

Clients, clinicians and other members of the veterinary team often go through different phases of grief, although not necessarily in a sequential order.

Clients, clinicians and other members of the veterinary team often go through different phases of grief, although not necessarily in a sequential order. These phases may even begin before the pet has died, in anticipation of the loss. Sometimes the death of a pet can re-initiate grief for another pet or person who has died. The phases of grief were initially illustrated by Kubler-Ross and used for decades thereafter. Understanding these phases and that it is a normal, healthy process is important.

Denial

"She cannot be dead., "I know you are lying to me."
Denial is often temporary and is either a conscious or unconscious refusal to accept the truth. This is likely a temporary defense for the individual that can be prolonged in some individuals.

Anger

"This is your fault!." "I paid good money and all you have done is give me back my dead pet."
When anger sets in, it means that the client has passed the denial stage. This anger can be toward the veterinary health care team, the client themselves, or to other family members. The anger does make it difficult to care for the individual. It is important to remain detached and nonjudgmental when dealing with a person experiencing anger from grief.

Bargaining

"I will go to church faithfully if you bring her back to me." " I will give my life savings if..."
The third stage revolves around offering to do something for someone or in response for postponement or reversal of death. This is an attempt to delay making final decisions.

Depression

"I'm so sad, I don't want to talk to anyone", "My pet was everything, the only one who loved me, therefore I have no reason to live."

During the fourth stage, the client begins to understand the truth or gravity of death or dying. The client or family member may become silent, refuse visitors and spend much of the time crying and grieving. Clients often disconnect themselves from people and situations where they are loved and cared for. The veterinary health care team should understand that this is a normal stage of grieving and is not to be "fixed." It's natural to feel sadness, regret, fear, and uncertainty when going through this stage. Feeling those emotions shows that the person has begun to accept the situation.

Acceptance

"It's going to be okay."; "I can't fight it, I may as well accept it and go on."

In this last stage, clients often begin to come to terms with their mortality, or that of a loved one, or other tragic event.

FOLLOW-UP

Follow-up communication can be very important for the client and the veterinary health care team alike. Cards, letters, or flowers sent by the staff can be important not only to the client, but for the entire team by bringing them closure as well. Adding a picture of the patient to a scrapbook or a bulletin board of beloved pets may also be of value in memorializing special patients.

There is no single way for clients or the team to work through their grief. Ideally, clients should be made aware of pet loss support groups, hotlines and local specialists who are knowledgeable about loss and receptive to helping people who have lost a beloved pet (Table 3-1)

HELPING BEREAVED CLIENTS

At the time of death, clients, their family members and, in many cases, members of the veterinary health care team are in a state of shock. Some clients may be distraught to the point of being violent (Table 3-2). The veterinary health care team can help these families by openly sharing their grief, by sharing personal stories about the patient and by celebrating what the family did to support and care for the patient that has passed away. The day after the pet's death, it is often very helpful to call the family to offer condolences and help. The key at this time is to be a good listener. Writing a condolence letter or penning a card of sympathy is often of profound importance to the family of a pet that has died. One to two months after the pet's death, another call or letter will show sincerity and sympathy and can be of great help to the family.

Clients and members of the veterinary health care team should be supported in their time of grief by doing the following:[1-5]
- Reassure everyone involved that the pain will subside and that grief over the loss of a pet is normal.
- Encourage clients to attend support groups that are sensitive to the importance of pets in the family.
- Encourage bereaved clients to talk to others about their feelings and thoughts.
- Encourage everyone involved to exercise regularly.
- Ensure that each person has time alone for reflection and recovery.

Table 3-1. Support resources for grieving pet clients
University of California-Davis Pet Loss Hotline (staffed by veterinary students)
Phone: 800-565-1526
Web: http://www.vetmed.ucdavis.edu/petloss/index.htm
Cornell University Pet Loss Support Hotline (staffed by Cornell University veterinary students)
Phone: 607-253-3932
Web: http://web.vet.cornell.edu/public/petloss/
Tufts University Pet Loss Support Hotline (staffed by Tufts University veterinary students)
Phone: 508-839-7966
Web: http://www.tufts.edu/vet/petloss
The Support for People and Pets Program at Colorado State University
Phone: 970-221-4535
Web: http://www.argusinstitute.colostate.edu/find.htm
Washington State University Pet Loss Hotline
Phone: 509-335-5704
Web: http://www.vetmed.wsu.edu/PLHL/home/index.asp
Pet Loss Support
Web: http://www.pet-loss.net/resources/CA.html

Table 3-2. Common feelings, behaviors, and symptoms that clients and veterinary health care members should be aware of after the death of a pet [1-5]

Feelings and behaviors

Hope or hopelessness

Disbelief

Relief, especially with a prolonged illness or financial restrictions

Helplessness

Yearning

Tearfulness and crying

Confusion or inability to concentrate

Waves of mental pain

Feelings of separation or longing

Anger or guilt

Fear or anxiety

Physical symptoms

Increased or decreased appetite with subsequent changes in body weight

Decreased energy, weakness

Nausea or diarrhea

Altered libido

Sleeplessness

Feeling that something is stuck in throat

Tightness in chest

Sensitivity to noise

Vivid dreams

Dry mouth

- Reassure everyone involved that it is normal to have negative feelings, and that each person's grief is unique.
- Ensure that each person is allowed to feel their loss and to grieve in their own way.

References

1. Ogilvie GK: The care of animals with cancer, in Dobson JM, Lascelles BDX (eds): *BSAVA Manual of Canine and Feline Oncology*, ed 2. Gloucester, UK, British Small Animal Veterinary Association, 2003, pp 68–72.

2. Mitchener KL, Ogilvie GK: Rekindling the bond. *Vet Econ* 40:30–36, 1999.

3. Mitchener KL, Ogilvie GK: Giving cancer patients hope. *Vet Econ* 40:84–88, 1999.

4. Ogilvie GK: Meeting the needs of patient and client through compassionate care, in: Ettinger SJ, Feldman EC (eds): *Textbook of Veterinary Internal Medicine*, ed 6. Philadelphia, WB Saunders, 2005, pp 535–538.

5. Lagoni L, Butler C, Hetts S: *The Human Animal Bond and Grief*, Philadelphia, WB Saunders, 1994.

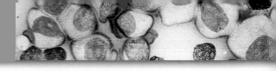

Chapter 4

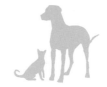

Compassion fatigue

COST OF CARING: COMPASSION FATIGUE

Providing care from the heart while relying on scientific knowledge requires the ability to express empathy, a form of sympathetic identification. While this ability is a vital aspect of cultivating a warm relationship with a client, repeated empathetic responses can lead to compassion fatigue.[1-10] When we find ourselves giving without adequately replenishing ourselves, it is only a matter of time before we experience a shortage of compassion and a sense of exhaustion. Simply put, compassion fatigue occurs when we have depleted our emotional resources as we care for others. Compassion fatigue is not a reflection of our character, professionalism or skill level, but comes from a place of strength as a caregiver. It is directly related to our willingness to be emotionally engaged with another being that is hurting. This immense capacity for compassion is what makes good veterinarians (and their teams) great at what they do. Compassion fatigue has or will strike every member of a caring health care team, including the client. The phenomenon is not limited to veterinary professionals but occurs in physicians, nurses, firemen, combat medics, and the like.[1-10] Compassion fatigue is why many caring veterinarians, nurses, receptionists and other caregivers leave the profession. Awareness and understanding of this condition is essential in its prevention and treatment and in maintaining the health of the team.

Key point

When we find ourselves giving without adequately replenishing ourselves, it is only a matter of time before we experience a shortage of compassion and a sense of exhaustion.

COMPASSION FATIGUE VERSUS BURNOUT

Compassion fatigue is perhaps the greatest threat to the health and happiness of any member of the veterinary healthcare team. Although compassion fatigue is considered to be a form of burnout,[1] the two conditions are different even though they have many of the same clinical signs. It is important to distinguish these two conditions because they have different causes and paths to recovery.

Compassion fatigue is not predictable because it results when one's internal emotional resources are depleted.[1] More specifically, members of the veterinary health care team provide so much care and compassion to clients who are experiencing an emotional moment, such as when a diagnosis of cancer is being discussed, that they find themselves depleted. Emotionally charged critical incidents often trigger compassion fatigue at a time when one's emotional resources are already exhausted. Members of the veterinary health care team often experience critical incidents when other people become emotionally distressed.

An extreme example is the experiences of those who identified or provided care to people or animals killed or injured in the September 11 World Trade Center disaster in New York City, car bombings in populated centers or the effect of wars or car crashes around the world. More commonplace examples include when a veterinarian repeatedly performs euthanasia, helps an client through the loss of a pet, informs a caregiver that his or her pet has cancer, provides terminal patient care and discusses the financial affordability of care.[1-10] Each member of the veterinary health care team must be considered unique, and the way each person deals with critical incidents differs, often based on his or her individual experiences, beliefs and values. In addition, compassion fatigue may intensify the emotional and physical symptoms in team members who are already experiencing burnout, and burnout can likewise intensify compassion fatigue.

The following feelings or thoughts are sometimes associated with compassion fatigue:[1-10]

- Avoidance of thoughts, feelings, activities or situations that remind one of a frightening experience.
- Feeling estranged from other members of the veterinary health care team or feeling that there is no one to talk to.
- Difficulty falling or staying asleep, especially when loss of sleep is related to memories or experiences being played over and over in one's mind.
- Outbursts of anger or irritability with little provocation.
- Needing to "work through" a traumatic experience associated with a patient or client to get over the event.
- Being preoccupied with a previous critical incident or with specific patients or their caregivers.
- Loss of concern about the well-being of coworkers, patients and caregivers.
- Feeling trapped, hopeless, edgy, weak, tired, rundown or depressed.
- Desire to avoid certain patients and their caregivers.
- Feeling disliked by clients and their families.
- Inability to separate work and personal life.
- Feeling like one works more for the money than for personal fulfillment.
- Feelings of failure.

Burnout is predictable and very common. It is not necessarily associated with the exhaustion of emotion or empathy but rather is a state of mental and/or physical exhaustion caused by excessive and prolonged stress. Two major causes of burnout are bureaucratic atmospheres and overwork. Burnout is not associated with the aforementioned critical incidents, but it is predictably associated with the stress of overwork, repetition or the bureaucracy of seemingly less-important tasks, such as paying bills, reviewing reports and endless paperwork without apparent value or worth.

Key point

Compassion fatigue is perhaps the greatest threat to the health and happiness of any member of the veterinary health care team.

PREVENTION AND THERAPY

Veterinarians and the entire veterinary staff must first acknowledge that we, as a profession—by the very nature of what we do and who we are—are at risk for compassion fatigue. Simply by acknowledging the condition and accepting that we are vulnerable, we can see the potential hazards, recognize likely inciting situations and hopefully prevent devastating outcomes. We also must work with all staff members to experience and then celebrate the sense of achievement in the work in which we are involved. On a daily basis, veterinary healthcare teams intervene in the lives of clients and their pets to provide high-quality medical, surgical and preventive care while offering emotional support and validating the bond that brought those pets and people to our offices. This is compassionate care; to accomplish it well requires a great deal of emotional energy from every team member. In this manner, we provide for the needs of our patients and caregivers. The act of caring is the epitome of success in our profession, regardless of the emotional nature of the situation or the medical outcome. Although compassion fatigue cannot be completely avoided, there are many strategies to help team members mitigate its impact (box 4-1):

Box 4-1. Key points in mitigating compassion fatigue

- Educate the entire veterinary healthcare team about compassionate fatigue and its consequences.
- Establish weekly debriefing sessions where the entire staff can discuss needs, concerns and cases that weigh on them.
- Establish resources about compassion fatigue, including a library for team members.
- Use relaxation techniques both within the hospital and outside the workplace.
- Take breaks during the day.
- Define and preserve a sanctuary or comfort room where team members can be alone to meditate or relax.
- Inform all team members about every case and allow them to have adequate closure at the end of any patient's life.
- Whenever possible, work out sabbatical or continuing education opportunities for personal reward and growth.
- Teach team members how to set limits and boundaries on interactions with clients and patients, especially when especially susceptible to compassion fatigue.
- Employ humor when appropriate.
- Find a friend or colleague who understands and appreciates the experience of providing empathy and compassion, and share with that person.
- Eat right and exercise.
- Get in touch with nature and the outdoors.
- Interact with children and animals.

CONCLUSION

When we employ compassion in caring for our patients, we must do so by expressing empathy, yet the act of empathizing with our clients can lead to compassion fatigue. When any member of the veterinary healthcare team finds themselves giving without allowing themselves to be replenished emotionally, it is only a matter of time before there will be a shortage of compassion. This depletion is not a reflection of the character, professionalism, or skill level of the team member. Rather, one's strength and willingness to be emotionally engaged with another being is diminished. All members of the veterinary healthcare team joined the profession to provide care, which comes from both their minds (through medical and surgical skills) and their hearts (by supporting and providing for the emotional needs of caregivers). The success of veterinary care stems from providing this level of compassionate care and supporting the individuals who provide it. By appreciating the reality of compassion fatigue and providing mechanisms to mitigate its effects, a practice can thrive by providing the finest in compassionate care.

References

1. Mitchener KL, Ogilvie GK: Understanding Compassion fatigue: Keys for the caring veterinary health care team. *JAAHA* 34(4):307–310, 2002.
2. Collins S, Long A: Too tired to care? The psychological effects of working with trauma. *Psychiatr Ment Health Nurs* 10(1):17–27, 2003.
3. Radziewicz RM: Self-care for the caregiver. *Nurs Clin North Am* 36(4):855–869, 2001.
4. Clark ML, Gioro S: Nurses, indirect trauma, and prevention. *Image J Nurs Sch* 30(1):85–87, 1998.
5. Vachon ML: Caring for the caregiver in oncology and palliative care. *Semin Oncol Nurs* 14(2):152–157, 1998.
6. Welsh DJ: Care for the caregiver: strategies for avoiding "compassion fatigue." *Clin J Oncol Nurs* 3(4):183–184, 1999.
7. Thomas RB, Wilson JP: Issues and controversies in the understanding and diagnosis of compassion fatigue, vicarious traumatization, and secondary traumatic stress disorder. *Int J Emerg Ment Health* 6(2):81–92, 2004.
8. Boscarino JA, Figley CR, Adams RE: Compassion fatigue following the September 11 terrorist attacks: A study of secondary trauma among New York City social workers. *Int J Emerg Ment Health* 6(2):57–66, 2004.
10. Radziewicz RM: Self-care for the caregiver. *Nurs Clin North Am* 36(4):855–869, 2001.

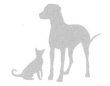

Chapter 5

Cancer prevention

Health and wellness programs for pets, especially those that focus on cancer prevention, are gaining momentum worldwide. In part, this enthusiastic interest is a result of a greater number of clients who view their pet as a family member.[1-8] Early detection and diagnosis of many diseases, including cancer, often result in enhanced cure rates. This section reveals why health care and cancer screening is so vital in all stages of the life of an animal. Included is a reminder of the reason why it is important to meet not only the medical needs of the patient, but also the nonmedical needs of the client. In addition, a brief summary is provided of a few essential points about the importance of epidemiology in guiding health and wellness programs. Finally, one example of a health and wellness program is presented, which can be freely adapted to the needs of the individual hospital or clinic.

THE PET AND THE BOND

The veterinary profession is in the middle of a renaissance, an era in which the profession is expanding in unprecedented ways along with clients concerned with issues like nutrition and disease prevention. The bond is almost indefinable, as the unique relationship between people and animals, and is described using many terms such as companionship, unconditional love, affection, and protection. The bond exists in some form between each and every caregiver and his or her pet and is at the heart of why we need to provide the best of veterinary care possible. Since cancer is the biggest healthcare concern in the hearts and minds of our clients, it is vital to include cancer screening and prevention programs in veterinary practice.

The first step for incorporating heath and wellness programs is to educate veterinary students and graduate veterinarians about the unique needs of the aging pet.[2,3] The second step is to enhance understanding of the tools, drugs, and procedures, including cancer screening, that can be used successfully to enhance health and wellness of the aging animal.[4-6] Throughout this process, it is important that the entire team acknowledge that age is a number and not a disease. Nevertheless, along with age comes a complex of disorders and diseases that increase the risk of the management of other diseases or the way drugs are handled.

Age is associated with some definable changes in body function, susceptibility, and response to diseases such as cancer. What this means is that while age itself is not a disease, when dealing with geriatric patients, conditions such as cancer, which are associated with increasing age, need to be accounted for. The following are some examples of how to initiate prevention of cancer and other diseases:[8]

- Initiate a health and wellness program for all stages of life and always include cancer screening as a vital aspect of that program.
- Recognize that aging patients have unique changes in organ function, susceptibility to complications for routine procedures, and altered metabolism of drugs and other agents.
- Identify clinically silent diseases, such as early evidence of cancer, and initiate measures to sustain health and wellness.
- Identify clinically evident diseases and initiate therapy to treat these conditions.
- Counsel clients about how to prevent cancer and other diseases associated with aging.

EPIDEMIOLOGY AND CANCER

One of the most common questions clients ask their veterinarian is, "What caused my dog or cat's cancer?" The answer to that question is difficult to answer, but as in humans, the etiopathogenesis of cancer often involves an interplay between genetics, nutrition, and environmental risk factors. Indeed, golden retrievers have recently been pointed out as having a high death rate from cancer when compared with other breeds. Similarly, exposure of pets to cigarette smoke, asbestos, and other environmental contaminants has been associated with an increased risk of developing cancer.[9] Therefore, cancer prevention is based on the identification or elimination of at-risk animals based on familial/genetic and environmental influences. Epidemiology is the science that begins to identify these genetic and environmental influences that can then be used for cancer prevention. Before venturing into the world of cancer epidemiology, a few key definitions are in order:

- *Cancer incidence*: The number of new cases of cancer occurring in an animal population at risk for this disease over a set period of time.
- *Incidence rate*: Measure of the absolute risk of a disease (in this case, cancer).
- *Annual cancer mortality rate*: The number of animals dying of cancer in 1 year per the population of animals at risk during that the set time period.
- *Odds ratio*: Statistical odds that animals with a specific cancer were exposed compared with the odds that animals without the cancer were exposed to a parameter in question. This measurement of association is determined in a case–control study.
- *Relative risk*: Ratio of the incidence or mortality rate in an exposed group to the incidence or mortality rate in an unexposed group. Relative risk is determined in prospective studies.

Key point

There is little doubt that cancer occurs more often in certain breeds and that environmental factors may influence these factors.

The identification of factors associated with an increased risk of developing cancer is in its infancy in veterinary epidemiology and oncology. Despite this early state of development, several important observations can be made.[9-26] Clients should be educated that increased risk may or may not be equated with causality; in other words, exposure to a risk factor may not have caused their pet's cancer. These factors should be included during counseling sessions. The following are a few of the many factors, including guidelines on the best ways to decrease the potential for cancer:

- *Nutrition*: A lifetime study of restricted daily intake of the same food was done with a total of 48 control-fed versus paired restricted-fed (25% less intake) Labrador retrievers that came from seven litters.[10,11] The median life span of the restricted-fed group was significantly longer. While the prevalence of cancer between groups was similar, the mean age due to cancer-related deaths was 2 years later in the dogs that received the restricted diet. The long-

chain eicosapentaenoic and docosahexaenoic acids have been shown consistently to inhibit the proliferation of breast and prostate cancer cell lines in vitro and to reduce the risk and progression of these tumors in many species.[12,13]

- Restrict daily intake to maintain a thin body weight throughout life.
- Feed a balanced diet made specifically for the dog or cat with possible consideration of the use of polyunsaturated fatty acids of the n-3 series.

Key point

The long-chain eicosapentaenoic and docosahexaenoic acids have been shown consistently to inhibit the proliferation of breast and prostate cancer cell lines in vitro and to reduce the risk and progression of these tumors in many species.

- *Ovariohysterectomy/orchiectomy*: Ovariohysterectomy has long been demonstrated to be a markedly effective method of preventing mammary tumors if it is performed before the first estrus.[13,14] Spaying is moderately effective if performed before the pet is 2½ years of age. Spaying may also be therapeutic when treating pets with mammary tumors.[16] Orchiectomy will reduce the risk of testicular tumors. Gonadectomy may not uniformly protect against all cancers. A study of Rottweilers was conducted to examine the effect of elective gonadectomy and the spontaneous development of appendicular bone sarcomas.[15] In that study, male and female Rottweilers that underwent gonadectomy before 1 year of age had an approximate one in four lifetime risk for bone sarcoma and were significantly more likely to develop bone sarcoma than dogs that were sexually intact. Have examples prevalent for cats as well.
  - Early ovariohysterectomy and orchiectomy is recommended.

- *Genetics*: There is little doubt that cancer occurs more often in certain breeds and that environmental factors may influence these factors.[9] German shepherds have been shown to have bilateral cystadenocarcinomas. Flat-coated retrievers and Bernese mountain dogs have been shown to have a high incidence of cancer, including malignant histiocytosis.[17] Scottish terriers, especially those with exposure to herbicides, have an increased risk of developing transitional cell carcinomas of the bladder.[18]
  - Encourage adoption of pets that have a low risk of cancer and that fit the family environment.

- *Environmental carcinogens*: Pets have been shown to have an increased risk of developing cancer of the respiratory tract, especially of the lung and nasal cavity, when exposed to coal and kerosene heaters and passive tobacco smoke.[19-21] Mesothelioma is more common in dogs and cats owned by people who

Table 5-1. Components of wellness program		
<1 year of age	**1–7 years of age**	**>7 years of age**
Preadoption counseling to select breeds and lines with a reduced risk of cancer and to meet the needs of the adopting family		
Behavioral counseling and suggestions regarding obedience classes		
A complete history	A complete history every 12 mo	A complete history at least every 6 mo
A complete physical examination	A complete physical examination every 12 mo	A complete physical examination at least every 6 mo
Body weight evaluation and body condition scoring	Body weight evaluation and body condition scoring	Body weight evaluation and body condition scoring
Nutritional counseling to include discussion of optimum diet, weight, and exercise	Nutritional counseling to include discussion of optimum diet, weight and exercise	Nutritional counseling to include discussion of optimum diet, weight and exercise
Select diagnostics, including complete blood count and biochemical profile	Select diagnostics, including a *minimum* of: • Complete blood count • Biochemical profile to include creatinine, potassium, serum alanine aminotransferase, and serum alkaline phosphatase • Complete urinalysis by cystocentesis • Blood pressure • Fine-needle aspiration and mapping of any masses or swelling • Counseling to reduce exposure to carcinogens such as passive smoke, industrial chemicals, direct constant sunlight, etc.	Select diagnostics, including a *minimum* of: • Complete blood count • Full biochemical profile, including electrolytes • Thyroid panel (optional) • Complete urinalysis by cystocentesis • Blood pressure • Miscellaneous diagnostic testing such as chest radiographs as needed • Fine-needle aspiration and mapping of any masses or swelling • Counseling to reduce exposure to carcinogens such as passive smoke, industrial chemicals, direct constant sunlight, etc.
Education on critical issues such as vaccination scheduling, ovariohysterectomy, orchiectomy, cancer screening, nutrition, dental screening, and obesity	Education on critical issues such as vaccination scheduling, cancer screening, nutrition, dental screening and obesity.	Education on critical issues such as vaccination schedules, cancer screening, nutrition, dental screening and obesity.

worked in the asbestos industry.[22] The use of chemicals by clients, specifically 2,4-dichlorophenoxyacetic acid, paints, asbestos or solvents, as well as radiation and electromagnetic field exposure were associated with increased risk for several types of cancer in pets.[24-26] The application of insecticides (but not in a spot-on formulation) increased the risk of bladder cancer in Scottish terriers in another study.[23]

• Eliminate exposure to environmental carcinogens such as pesticides, coal or kerosene heaters, herbicides such as 2,4-dichlorophenoxyacetic acid, passive tobacco smoke, asbestos, radiation, and strong electromagnetic field exposure. These steps may be particularly important for clients of susceptible breeds (e.g., a Scottish terrier and herbicide exposure).

Key point

Pets have been shown to have an increased risk of developing cancer of the respiratory tract, especially of the lung and nasal cavity, when exposed to coal and kerosene heaters and passive tobacco smoke.

CONCLUSION

Cancer prevention is a mainstay of human health care, and it should be the cornerstone of veterinary health care. This is not only the correct type of care for our patients, but it is also the right thing to do for our patients' human family members who are rightfully concerned about cancer in their pets and themselves. More information will become available as advances are made, and more specific recommendations will become part of the standard screening process.

References

1. Ogilvie GK, Moore AS: Compassionate care of the cancer patient, in Ogilvie GK, Moore AS. *Feline Oncology: A Comprehensive Guide for Compassionate Care.* Yardley, PA, Veterinary Learning Systems, 2002, pp 1–6.
2. Ogilvie GK: Préservation de la santé des animaux âgés. Gériatrie vétérinaire. Les Editions du point vétérinaire, Nantes, Intervet 2004, pp 51–56.
3. Ogilvie GK: Pris en charge du cancer chez l'animal âgé. Gériatrie vétérinaire. Les Editions du point vétérinaire. Nantes, Intervet 2004, 61–66.
4. Ogilvie GK: The care of animals with cancer, in Dobson JM, Lascelles BDX (eds): *BSAVA Manual of Canine and Feline Oncology,* ed 2. Gloucester, UK, British Small Animal Veterinary Association, 2003, pp 68–72.
5. Mitchener KL, Ogilvie GK: Rekindling the bond. *Vet Econ* 40:30–36, 1999.
6. Mitchener KL, Ogilvie GK: Giving cancer patients hope. *Vet Econ* 40:84–88, 1999.
7. Epstein M, Kuehn NF, Landsberg G, et al: AAHA senior care guidelines for dogs and cats. J Am Anim Hosp Assoc. 41(2):81-91, 2005.
8. Ogilvie GK: Meeting the needs of patient and client through compassionate care, in *Textbook of Veterinary Internal Medicine.* Ettinger SJ, Feldman EC, Philadelphia, WB Saunders, 2005, pp 535-537.
9. Craig LE: Cause of death in dogs according to breed: a necropsy survey of five breeds. *J Am Anim Hosp Assoc* 37(5):438–443, 2001.
10. Kealy RD, Lawler DF, Ballam JM, et al: Influence of diet restriction on life span and age-related changes in Labrador retrievers. *JAVMA* 220:1315–1320, 2002.
11. Lawler DF, Evans RH, Larson BT, et al: Influence of lifetime food restriction on causes, time and predictors of mortality of dogs. *JAVMA* 226:225-231, 2005
12. Terry PD, Rohan TE, Wolk A: Intakes of fish and marine fatty acids and the risks of cancers of the breast and prostate and of other hormone-related cancers: a review of the epidemiologic evidence. *Am J Epidemiol* 141(4):352–359, 1995.
13. Sonnenschein EG, Glickman LT, Goldschmidt MH, McKee LJ: Body conformation, diet, and risk of breast cancer in pet dogs: a case–control study. *Am J Epidemiol* 133(7):694–703, 1991.
14. Ferguson HR: Canine mammary gland tumors. *Vet Clin North Am Small Anim Pract* 15(3):501–511, 1985.
15. Cooley DM, Beranek BC, Schlittler DL, et al: Endogenous gonadal hormone exposure and bone sarcoma risk. *Cancer Epidemiol Biomarkers Prev* 11(11):1434–1440, 2002.
16. Sorenmo KU, Shofer FS, Goldschmidt MH: Effect of spaying and timing of spaying on survival of dogs with mammary carcinoma. *J Vet Intern Med* 14(3):266–270, 2000.
17. Morris JS, Bostock DE, McInnes EF, et al: Histopathological survey of neoplasms in flat-coated retrievers, 1990 to 1998. *Vet Rec* 147(11):291–295, 2000.
18. Glickman LT, Raghavan M, Knapp DW, et al: Herbicide exposure and the risk of transitional cell carcinoma of the urinary bladder in Scottish Terriers. *JAVMA* 224(8):1290–1297, 2004.
19. Bukowski JA, Wartenberg D, Goldschmidt M: Environmental causes for sinonasal cancers in pet dogs, and their usefulness as sentinels of indoor cancer risk. *J Toxicol Environ Health A* 54(7):579–591, 1998.
20. Reif JS, Bruns C, Lower KS: Cancer of the nasal cavity and paranasal sinuses and exposure to environmental tobacco smoke in pet dogs. *Am J Epidemiol* 147(5):488–492, 1998.
21. Reif JS, Dunn K, Ogilvie GK, Harris CK: Passive smoking and canine lung cancer risk. *Am J Epidemiol* 135(3):234–239, 1992.
22. Glickman LT, Domanski LM, Maguire TG, et al: Mesothelioma in pet dogs associated with exposure of their clients to asbestos. *Environ Res* 32(2):305–313, 1983.
23. Raghavan M, Knapp DW, Dawson MH, et al: Topical flea and tick pesticides and the risk of transitional cell carcinoma of the urinary bladder in Scottish terriers. *JAVMA* 225:389–394, 2004.
24. Gavazza A, Presciuttini S, Barale R, et al: Association between canine malignant lymphoma, living in industrial areas, and use of chemicals by dog clients. *J Vet Intern Med* 15(3):190–195, 2001.
25. Hayes HM, Tarone RE, Cantor KP: On the association between canine malignant lymphoma and opportunity for exposure to 2,4-dichlorophenoxyacetic acid. *Environ Res* 70(2):119–125, 1995.
26. Reif JS, Lower KS, Ogilvie GK: Residential exposure to magnetic fields and risk of canine lymphoma. *Am J Epidemiol* 141(4):352–359, 1995.

Chapter 6

Overview

Cancer creates an emergency of emotion in the hearts and minds of many people regardless of whether they themselves, or their pets, are diagnosed with cancer. As soon as a diagnosis of cancer is made, it sets in motion feelings of fear, despair, panic and urgency that spur clients to demand a rapid response to their concerns by the veterinary health care team. This heightened level of emotion is first witnessed during the initial diagnosis. The actual presence of a true medical emergency may or may not be present in the cancer patient. Regardless, many clients are unable to think, make appropriate decisions, or carry out the decision-making process. Any catastrophic change in the body as a direct or indirect effect of the cancer may be the cause of true emergencies. Some of the most common, predictable emergencies are associated with paraneoplastic syndromes. Others are a direct effect of the tumor itself. Paraneoplastic syndromes are medical conditions that are a consequence of the INDIRECT effect of cancer. These paraneoplastic syndromes are commonly the cause of an emergency presentation. Dogs and cats may hide their clinical signs until quite late in the disease process and thus are often in a debilitated state by the time cancer therapy begins; therefore, speed and decisiveness are key ingredients to successful emergency care.

It is essential that oncologic emergencies be handled with extreme medical care, but also with understanding. When an emergency or urgent situation is noted, the entire veterinary health care team should be equipped and prepared to provide timely compassionate care to meet the medical and nonmedical needs of patients and caregivers alike. In some cases, this may mean referring the patient to another facility.

There are three types of emergencies:
- True life-threatening emergencies.
- Medical problems that are perceived as life-threatening by well-meaning, concerned clients.
- Emergencies of convenience, in which the client wants the dog or cat to be evaluated immediately despite a lack of life-threatening emergencies in order to accommodate personal needs or schedule.

Regardless of the type of emergency, the following steps should be taken in rapid succession:
- Determine the primary complaint.
- Evaluate vital signs including.
  - Airway and breathing ability.
  - Heart rate, rhythm, pulse quality and character.
  - Body temperature.
  - Mucous membrane color and capillary refill time.
  - Mentation.
- Obtain a complete history, including any current or prior medical therapy treatment.
- Perform a complete physical examination.

When a dog or cat is presented in an emergency situation, the patient is assessed while permission to treat is secured and initiated (figure 6-1). In each case, oxygen should be administered as needed, blood and urine samples should be collected, and an intravenous catheter placed as soon as possible.

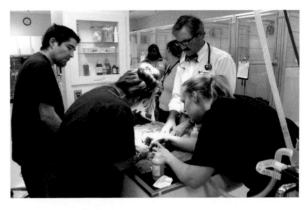

Figure 6-1: When a dog or cat is presented in an emergency situation, the patient is assessed while permission to treat is secured and initiated. In each case, oxygen should be administered as needed, blood and urine samples should be collected, and an intravenous catheter placed as soon as possible.

Blood and urine should be submitted immediately to determine pretreatment parameters based on a complete blood count, biochemical profile, activated clotting time, and urinalysis. Essential information that is rapidly obtainable and vital for initial decision-making—and that should be obtained on admission—includes urine specific gravity, packed cell volume, white blood cell count, and blood glucose.

> **Key point**
>
> When a patient is presented in an emergency situation, the team should immediately assess the patient while securing permission to diagnose and treat. First, ensure that there is a patent airway, adequate breathing, and cardiac output. Second, obtain blood and urine samples while placing an intravenous catheter. Third, ensure the medical needs of the patient and non-medical needs of the client are met.

As soon as a diagnostic and therapeutic plan is initiated, clients should be made aware of every aspect of the patient's condition. Measured, realistic information should be provided as soon as assessments are complete and the information is available. It is also important to provide a cost estimate for initial care as well as updates for ongoing supportive care. The team approach to care is vital during emergencies. The client is an integral member of the team and, once empowered with information, is supported to let them to make appropriate decisions that allow for optimal medical care of the patient while meeting the emotional needs of the caregiver and family. Ongoing communication allows for an open dialogue among team members regarding financial limitations, philosophy for continuing critical care in the face of diminishing hope, and advanced strategies for crisis situations, such as cardiac or respiratory arrest.

Oncologic emergencies, while rare, can include consequences associated with the cancer and cancer therapy. Planning for these uncommon and unwanted problems is essential for a positive outcome. It is important to recognize that the true "first step" in

handling oncologic emergencies is actually prevention. This step occurs prior to the initiation of treatment and encompasses time spent educating the caregiver about the nature of disease, the effects of each medication to be administered, and the early and often subtle signs that should be dealt with to prevent a true emergency from ever happening. Similarly, instructions about what clients can do at home to support their dogs or cats are quite helpful. Always remember, the client is perhaps the most important member of the veterinary health care team.

> **Key point**
>
> The veterinary health care team must acknowledge and respect the client's true feelings of panic, despair, and urgency and, thus, should respond appropriately while revealing the myths and misconceptions of cancer and cancer therapy and the true urgency of the situation.

The next step involves educating and empowering the entire veterinary health care team to take an active role in supporting the patient and the client. The words cancer and cancer therapy often frighten veterinary health care team members as much as they do the clients. There are emergency situations that are likely to be encountered. Developing a treatment strategy or "cookbook" approach to these situations enables the staff to intervene quickly and efficiently on behalf of the patient. In addition, providing the health care team with information that authorizes them to respond to the emotional component of the emergency on the part of the caregiver is also essential. All members of the health care team must recognize that it is this emotional component that magnifies the seriousness of almost any health problem.

References

1. Silverstein DC, Hopper K: *Small Animal Critical Care Medicine*. St. Louis, Missori, Saunders Elsevier, 2008, pp 18-20.
2. Dhaliwal RS: Tumor and tumor related complications. In: Henry CJ, Higginbotham ML (eds): *Cancer Mangement in Small Animal Practice*. St. Louis, Missori, Saunders Elsevier, 2010, pp 122-135.

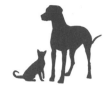

Chapter 7

Emergencies associated with hypercalcemia, hypocalcemia, hypoglycemia and hyponatremia (SIADH)

EMERGENCIES ASSOCIATED WITH HYPERCALCEMIA

Cancer is the most common cause of hypercalcemia in dogs and cats.[1-4] The condition can and often does result in an oncologic emergency. The tumors most often associated with paraneoplastic syndrome in dogs are lymphoma, anal sac adenocarcinoma (figure 7-1), multiple myeloma, and mammary gland adenocarcinoma, whereas in cats, it is lymphoma and squamous cell carcinoma, but any neoplastic process has the potential to elevate serum calcium. In 20% to 40% of dogs with lymphoma (figure 7-2 A and B) and hypercalcemia, the anterior mediastinum is involved, and a lesser percentage of cats (figure 7-2 C and D). Therefore, for dogs, thoracic radiographs are indicated whenever a persistent hypercalcemia is identified. Parathyroid adenomas have been identified as malignancy-associated causes of hypercalcemia of malignancy in dogs and cats (figure 7-3). It is not a true paraneoplastic syndrome, however.

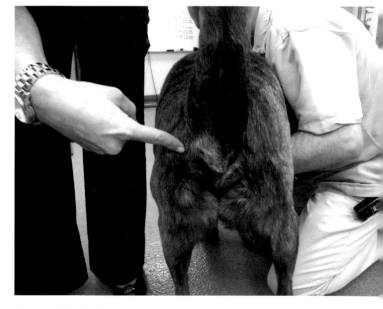

Figure 7-1: Anal sac adenocarcinoma.

> **Key point**
>
> Cancer is the most common cause of hypercalcemia in dogs or cats; the tumors most often associated with paraneoplastic syndrome in dogs are lymphoma, anal sac adenocarcinoma, multiple myeloma, and mammary gland adenocarcinoma, whereas in cats, it is lymphoma and squamous cell carcinoma.

The potential causes for hypercalcemia of malignancy include the following:[1-5]
- Direct resorption of bone by tumor cells.
- Tumor-induced production of osteoclast-activating factors (OAFs), such as interleukins, tumor necrosis factor, lymphotoxin, colony-stimulating factors, and interferon-alpha.

- Tumor-induced production of 1,25-dihydroxyvitamin D.
- Tumor-induced production of prostaglandins.
- Tumor-induced production of transforming growth factors.
- Tumor-induced production of parathyroid hormone-related peptide (PTHrP).

While all of the above named mechanisms likely play a role in hypercalcemia, the production of PTHrP is most commonly documented as the underlying mechanism. Dogs with lymphoma and anal sac adenocarcinoma most commonly develop cancer-induced hypercalcemia from production of PTHrP.[5] The cDNA of PTHrP has been cloned and found to encode a 16,000-dalton protein in which 8 of 13 amino acids are identical to parathyroid hormone.

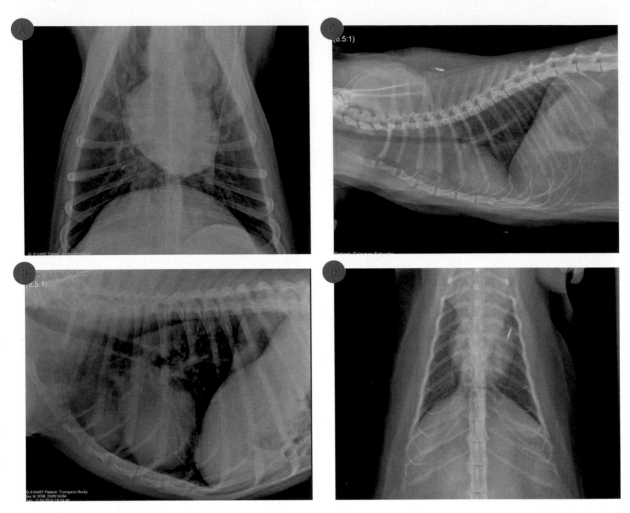

Figure 7-2: Three view chest radiographs are often indicated whenever there is a persistant, unexplained cause of hypercalcemia. This is because up to 40% of dogs with lymphoma and hypercalcemia have a mediastinal mass; a lesser percentage of cats. Ultrasound guided aspirates are often quite helpful for diagnosing the cause of the ultrasound mass.

> **Key point**
>
> Diminished renal function is the most common life threatening clinical consequence of hypercalcemia of malignancy in the veterinary patient, therefore, diagnosis and treatment of the underlying disease is critical.

Clinical presentation

Alterations in renal function including overt renal failure cause the most common clinical manifestations of hypercalcemia of malignancy in the veterinary patient.[1,4] Polyuria and nocturia in the early phases of the disease are succeeded by anorexia, nausea, fatigue, dehydration, azotemia, and coma secondary to hypercalcemia-induced renal failure. Decreased sensitivity of the distal convoluted tubules and collecting ducts to antidiuretic hormone (ADH) causes polyuria and secondary polydipsia. Vasoconstrictive properties of calcium decrease renal blood flow and glomerular filtration rate, resulting in degenerative changes, necrosis, and calcification of the renal epithelium.[1,4] Other clinical signs (e.g., constipation, muscle weakness, cardiac arrhythmias, seizures, etc.) may arise as a direct effect of the electrolyte abnormality.

Diagnosis

Clinical pathology must be combined with a good history and physical examination to rule in or out the differentials noted in box 7-1: [1,4]

It is often stated that calcium values must be interpreted in relation to serum albumin and blood pH. Clinical signs associated with hypercalcemia are intensified when the electrolyte is in the free, ionized fraction, which is increased by acidosis. A correction formula has been recommended in the veterinary literature; however, there are few if any data that validate

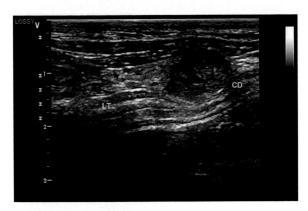

Figure 7-3: Parathyroid adenomas are a common cause of hypercalcemia. They are best identified via ultrasound as imaged here, or via magnetic resonance imaging, prior to ultrasound guided alcohol ablation or surgical removal.

this approach. Given the wide availability of in house analyzers to assess ionized calcium levels, it is always recommended that this parameter be used to validate the presence of a biologically meaningful calcium level.

Ultimately, it may be difficult to identify malignancy as the cause of hypercalcemia. Laboratory abnormalities that may accompany true hypercalcemia include an elevated serum urea nitrogen, normophosphatemia or hypophosphatemia, hypercalciuria, hyperphosphaturia, hypernatriuria, and decreased glomerular filtration rate as determined by an exogenous or endogenous creatinine clearance study. Evaluating serum phosphorus levels in hypercalcemic dogs may be helpful in pursuing a diagnosis.

Key point

Laboratory abnormalities that may accompany true hypercalcemia include an elevated serum urea nitrogen, normophosphatemia or hypophosphatemia, hypercalciuria, hyperphosphaturia, hypernatriuria, and decreased glomerular filtration rate as determined by an exogenous or endogenous creatinine clearance study.

Treatment[1-4]

Eliminating the tumor is the first and most important therapy for hypercalcemia of malignancy. Clinical signs associated with hypercalcemia of malignancy can range from very mild to a full oncologic emergency. The approach (box 7-2) to the treatment of this condition depends on the severity of the clinical signs.

In the past, it has been recommended to administer furosemide for refractory cases, however the efficacy of this therapy has not been clearly confirmed in the veterinary literature. Historically,

Box 7-1. Some of the most common differentials associated with hypercalcemia in the dog or cat

Non-Pathologic
- Young growing animals
- Laboratory error
- Spurious (lipemia)
- Hemoconcentration
- Hyperproteinemia
- Hypoadrenocorticism
- Severe hypothermia
- Idiopathic

Pathologic
- Neoplasia (e.g.: humoral hypercalcemia of malignancy)
  - Lymphoma (common)
  - Anal sac apocrine gland adenocarcinoma (common)
  - Carcinoma (uncommon)
    - Oral cavity (cats), lung, pancreas, skin, nasal cavity thyroid, mammary gland, adrenal medulla all reported
  - Thymoma (uncommon) (figure 7-4 A-C)
  - Hematologic malignancies (bone marrow osteolysis)
    - Lymphoma
    - Multiple myeloma
    - Myeloproliferative disease (uncommon)
    - Leukemia (rare)
  - Metastatic cancer of bone (uncommon)
  - Primary hyperparathyroidism
    - Adenoma (common)
    - Adenocarcinoma (uncommon)
- Chronic renal failure
- Urolithiasis (cats)
- Increased complexed fraction common (low ionized calcium)
- Tertiary hyperparathyroidism
- Hypervitaminosis D
  - Iatrogenic - oversupplementation vitamin D3
  - Plants (calcitriol glycosides)
  - Rodenticide exposure (cholecalciferol)
- Granulomatous disease
  - Blastomycosis
  - Injection site granuloma
- Parathyroid hyperplasia (uncommon)
- Acute renal failure
- Skeletal lesions (non-malignant, uncommon)
  - Bacterial or mycotic osteomyelitis
  - Hypertrophic osteodystrophy (HOD)
  - Disuse osteoporosis
- Excessive intestinal phosphate binders (uncommon)
- Excessive calcium supplementation (calcium carbonate)
- Hypervitaminosis A (uncommon)
- Mammary hyperplasia, vevere (PTHrP associated)
- Thiazide diuretics

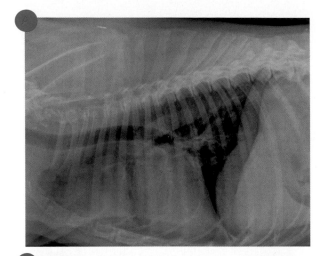

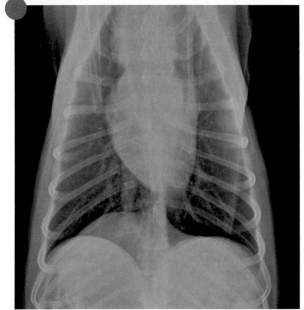

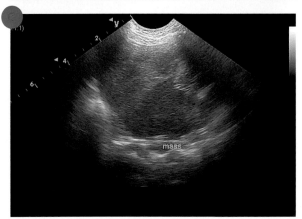

Figure 7-4: Thymomas are an uncommon cause of hypercalcemia. They can appear as an anterior mediastinal mass (A, B) like lymphoma, however ultrasound images (C) often appear cystic, septated or chambered. Cytology or histopathology is essential to diagnose the problem.

Box 7-2. Treatment of hypercalcemia depending on the severity of clinical signs

Mild hypercalcemia, minimal clinical signs

- Restore and maintain hydration and ensure calciuresis especially during anesthesia and surgery.
- Monitoring of calcium, phosphorus, and creatinine levels is indicated until the underlying cause can be identified and eliminated or until the hypercalcemia and subsequent clinical signs progress to a point requiring additional therapy.
- Avoid nephrotoxic drugs.

Moderate hypercalcemia, moderate clinical signs

More aggressive management is indicated in these patients, including:

- Administration of intravenous saline in volumes that exceed daily maintenance needs (>66 ml/kg/day) and result in urine output that exceeds 2 ml/kg/hour.
- Consider adding potassium chloride to 0.9% NaCl to prevent potassium depletion (20–30 mEq KCl/L of 0.9% NaCl) (Cautionary note, see table 7-1).
- Repeatedly assess all electrolytes, BUN and creatinine to reassess fluid rate, fluid choice, and potassium content of the fluid every 4 hours until stable, then as needed thereafter.
- Monitor patient carefully for signs of overhydration and congestive heart failure. The administration of 0.9% NaCl intravenously is effective in expanding the extracellular fluid volume, increasing glomerular filtration rate, decreasing renal tubular calcium reabsorption, and enhancing calcium and sodium excretion.

Table 7-1. IV potassium supplementation to correct hypokalemia. Warning: do not exceed 0.5 mEq KCl/kg/hr.

Serum potassium	KCl to add to each L of fluids (mEq/L)	Maximum rate of infusion (ml/kg/hr)
<2.0	80	6
2.1–2.5	60	8
2.6–3.0	40	12
3.1–3.5	28	16

furosemide (2.2–8.8 mg/kg BID IV or PO) has been administered concurrently with NaCl to well-hydrated hypercalcemic patients to prevent calcium reabsorption in the kidneys. This drug has been reported to be effective for treating many cases of anuria or oliguria. Furosemide inhibits calcium resorption at the level of the ascending loop of Henle.

Prednisone (1–2.0 mg/kg BID PO) or any other glucocorticoid inhibits osteoclast-activating factor, prostaglandins, vitamin D, and the absorption of calcium across the intestinal tract; therefore, such drugs are effective for treating hypercalcemia of malignancy. Glucocorticoids are cytotoxic to lymphoma and myeloma cells—and therefore should not be used until a histologic diagnosis of suspect tissue is made. When administered, glucocorticoids may obscure the extent of the tumor and thus may delay diagnosis of lymphoma and prevent definitive therapy. The diseases that cause hypercalcemia that appear to respond to steroid therapy include:

- Lymphoma/leukemia.
- Multiple myeloma.
- Thymoma.
- Vitamin D toxicity.
- Vitamin A toxicity.
- Granulomatous disease.
- Hypoadrenocorticism.

Severe hypercalcemia, severe clinical signs

This is considered a true oncologic emergency. Treatment is the same as for moderate hypercalcemia. In addition, other drugs are used (table 7-2).[1-4]

- Calcitonin: A dosage of 4 to 8 MRC units/kg SQ, given once, can cause a dramatic, rapid reduction in calcium levels, which may remain low for days. The authors believe this drug is very effective in most cases for normalizing elevated calcium levels for hours to days.
- Mithramycin: This drug can be used at a dosage of 25 µg/kg IV, once or twice weekly. At higher dosages, it has anticancer properties.
- Bisphosphonates: This class of agents is being explored for use in the therapy of hypercalcemia of malignancy. Didronel® (5-15 mg/kg/day) is the most commonly used member of this class in human medicine. Efficacy in dogs and cats has not been confirmed. Clodronate

Table 7-2. Treatment of hypercalcemia[1-4]

Treatment	Dosage	Suggested use
Volume expansion		
IV Saline (0.9%)	> 66 ml/kg/day to achieve urinary output of 2 mls/kg/hr	Moderate to severe hypercalcemia. Monitor serum potassium
Diuretics		
Furosemide	2-4 mg/kg BID to TID, IV, SQ, PO	Moderate to severe hypercalcemia *After* diagnosis of underlying disease
Glucocorticoids		
Prednisone	1-2 mg/kg BID PO, SQ, IV	Moderate to severe hypercalcemia
Dexamethasone	0.1-0.22 mg/kg BID IV, SQ	Moderate to severe hypercalcemia
Inhibition of bone resorption		
Calcitonin	4-6 IU/kg SQ BID to TID	Hypervitaminosis D toxicity
Bisphosphonates		
EHDP- Didronel	5-15 mg/kg Daily to BID	Moderate to severe hypercalcemia
Clodronate	20-25 mg/kg in a 4-h IV infusion	Moderate to severe hypercalcemia
Pamidronate	1-2 mg/kg in 150 ml 0.9% saline in a 2-hr IV infusion; can repeat in 1-3 weeks. Package insert suggests giving during diuresis to reduce nephrotoxicity	Moderate to severe hypercalcemia
Mithramycin	25 ug/kg IV in 5% glucose in water over 2-4 hr q2-4 wks	Severe hypercalcemia

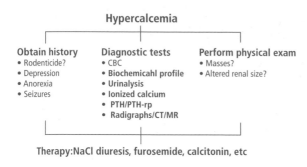

Figure 7-5: Clinical approach for hypercalcemic dogs.

(20-25 mg/kg in a 4 hour IV infusion) or pamidronate (1-2 mg/kg in 150 ml of 0.9% saline in a 2 hour IV infusion to be repeated as needed every 1-6 weeks) can both be used with success. Treatment of dogs with severe hypercalcemia and severe clinical signs suggests that pamidronate is effective in long-term control of chronic hypercalcemia. Unlike phosphates, which bind calcium in the gastrointestinal tract, biphosphonates bind to hydroxyapatite in bone and inhibit the dissolution of crystals.
- Gallium nitrate: This agent recently has been approved in human medicine for the treatment of hypercalcemia; it appears to inhibit bone resorption by binding to and reducing the solubility of hydroxyapatite crystals.
- Other things to consider include calcium-channel blockers, somatostatin congeners and calcium receptor agonists.

EMERGENCIES ASSOCIATED WITH HYPOCALCEMIA

Hypocalcemia is an unusual complication in veterinary patients. Hypocalcemia secondary to a malignancy and its treatment is much more common in human medicine.

> **Key point**
> Clinical signs of hypocalcemia are not usually seen until the total serum calcium is less than 6.5 mg/dl, or the ionized calcium less than 0.7 mmol/L, but they include seizures, twitching, weakness, arrhythmias, fever, tense or painful abdomen, and rubbing of the face.

Clinical presentation

Hypocalcemia rarely causes clinical signs but if it does, it is often dramatic and life-threatening arrhythmias may be observed. In such cases, however, partial or generalized seizures are seen. In humans with bone metastases, hypocalcemia is more common than hypercalcemia.[1,4] Clinical signs are not usually seen until the total, corrected serum calcium is less than 6.5 mg/dl, or the ionized calcium less than 0.7 mmol/L. Such signs include seizures, fever, tense or painful abdomen, and rubbing of the face. In veterinary medicine, only a few possible causes have been documented.[1,4] Causes of clinically significant hypocalcemia include primary hypoparathyroidism, surgically induced iatrogenic hypoparathyroidism, eclampsia, ethylene glycol toxicity, and administration of phosphate-containing enemas, although this rarely occurs in dogs. Another potential cause of hypocalcemia is magnesium deficiency, which can occur from prolonged intestinal drainage procedures, parenteral hyperalimentation without magnesium supplementation, cisplatin therapy, and severe liver disease.[1,4] The hypomagnesemia seems to impair the effect of parathyroid hormone on its target organs, resulting in hypocalcemia. Tumor lysis syndrome may be associated with hypocalcemia secondary to elevated phosphate levels. This is an oncologic emergency and should be addressed as such.

Treatment[1,4]

The underlying cause of hypocalcemia should be identified and treated as soon as possible. If clinical signs are present the following steps should be taken:
- Parenteral calcium should be administered slowly intravenously with ECG monitoring (10% calcium gluconate given over 10–20 minutes, 1.0–1.5 ml/kg; maintenance therapy of 2 ml/kg over 6–8 hours) followed by oral calcium supplements (i.e., calcium lactate, 400–600 mg/kg/day in 3–4 divided doses/day).
- Oral vitamin D preparations are beneficial in increasing serum calcium concentrations. Several formulations are available with different times to onset of activity and duration of action. Short acting formulations, such as calcitriol should be used for dogs and cats in which parathyroid activity may recover such as following surgical trauma. Longer acting preparations, such as dihydrotachysterol, can be initiated in those dogs and cats in which the underlying cause is not likely to be corrected. Oral calcium supplementation may be required in some dogs and cats to maximize the effect of vitamin D therapy.

EMERGENCIES ASSOCIATED WITH HYPOGLYCEMIA

> **Key point**
> Insulinoma is the most common malignancy that is associated with hypoglycemia (blood glucose <70 mg/dl) in dogs and less commonly in cats,6-12 but a wide variety of other non-islet cell tumors also have been shown to cause this condition.

Hypoglycemia can cause a wide variety of clinical signs ranging from generalized weakness to seizures and death.[1, 6-12] Insulinoma is the most common malignancy that is associated with hypoglycemia (blood glucose <70 mg/dl) in dogs and cats,[6-12] but a wide variety of other non-islet cell tumors also have been shown to cause this condition in humans, cats, and dogs by inducing ectopic hormone production.[6-12] Non-islet cell tumors that have been reported to cause hypoglycemia include hepatocellular carcinoma, hepatoma, plasmacytoid tumor, lymphoma, leiomyosarcoma, oral melanoma, hemangiosarcoma, and salivary gland adenocarcinoma.[6-12]

Insulinomas produce excessive quantities of insulin that cause very low blood glucose levels. In contrast, hypoglycemia of extrapancreatic tumors in dogs and cats has been associated with low to low-normal insulin levels.[6-11] Extrapancreatic tumors cause hypoglycemia by secretion of an insulin-like substance, accelerating the utilization of glucose by the tumor, and by failure of gluconeogenesis and/or glycogenolysis by the liver.[6-12] The most common nonmalignant causes of hypoglycemia include hyperinsulinism, hepatic dysfunction, adrenocortical insufficiency, xylitol toxicity, hypopituitarism, extrapancreatic tumors, starvation, sepsis, and laboratory error.

> **Key point**
> Subtle neurologic signs such as weakness, facial twitching, and seizures predominate in dogs and dogs or cats with hypoglycemia because carbohydrate reserve is limited in neural tissue.

Clinical signs

Neurologic signs including weakness, disorientation, behavioral changes, seizures, coma, and death predominate in dogs and cats with hypoglycemia secondary to a malignancy.[1,2,6-12] These clinical signs generally occur in dogs, cats, and ferrets when blood glucose falls below 45 mg/dl.

Catecholamines, growth hormone, glucocorticoids, and glucagon are released secondary to hypoglycemia and activate compensatory mechanisms to combat hypoglycemia by promoting glycogenolysis.

Diagnosis

Currently, it is not possible to identify the cause of hypoglycemia in many extrapancreatic tumors. Insulin-producing tumors, such as insulinomas, may be diagnosed by identifying normal to elevated insulin levels in association with low blood glucose concentrations (figure 7-6).[1,2,6-12] For accurate diagnosis, some patients require frequent evaluation of glucose and insulin concentrations during a 72-hour fast. Although very

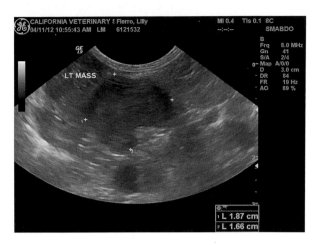

Figure 7-6: Insulinomas are generally small pancreatic masses that are best identified via abdominal ultrasound and are often associated with low serum glucose levels and associated clinical signs.

controversial, the amended insulin:glucose ratio has been advocated as a method by some to help diagnose insulin-producing tumors in pets:

$$\frac{\text{serum insulin } (\mu U/ml) \times 100}{\text{serum glucose } (mg/dl) - 30} = \text{amended insulin:glucose ratio}$$

Values above 30 are highly suggestive of an insulinoma or other insulin-producing tumors.

Treatment

Surgery is the most effective method for eliminating the underlying cause of malignancy-associated hypoglycemia, although streptozocin and tyrosine kinase inhibitors may be other adjunctive or alternate treatment options. Metastases are common in most malignant tumors associated with this condition. Therefore, surgery often is not curative. If an insulinoma is suspected, a partial pancreatectomy may be indicated. Complications include iatrogenic pancreatitis and diabetes mellitus. Medical management of the hypoglycemia is essential before, during, and after surgery because of the serious consequences of hypoglycemia and because of the high metastatic rate.[1,2,6-12] Dogs with severe cases of hypoglycemia should be treated with intravenous administration of 2.5% to 5% dextrose in parenteral fluids, such as 0.9% NaCl or Ringer's solution. Dogs that are convulsing should be given 0.5 g/kg dextrose intravenously slowly over 5 minutes. The administration of glucose containing solutions >10% is not advised.

- Prednisone (0.5–2.0 mg/kg divided BID PO) can induce hepatic gluconeogenesis and decrease peripheral utilization of glucose.

- Diazoxide (10–40 mg/kg divided BID PO), with or without hydrochlorothiazide (2–4 mg/kg daily PO), may be effective in elevating blood glucose levels by inhibiting pancreatic insulin secretion and glucose uptake by tissues, enhancing epinephrine-induced glycogenolysis, and increasing the rate of mobilization of free fatty acids. Diazoxide is expensive and difficult to obtain. Hydrochlorothiazide enhances the hyperglycemic effects of diazoxide. Limited data exist on its use in cats.
- Propranolol (0.2–1.0 mg/kg TID PO) may be effective in increasing blood glucose levels by blocking insulin release through the blockade of beta-adrenergic receptors at the level of the pancreatic beta cell, inhibiting insulin release by membrane stabilization, and altering peripheral insulin receptor affinity. Combined surgical and medical management of pancreatic tumors has been associated with remission periods of one year or more.[9,10]
- Streptozotocin (Streptozocin), a nitrosourea chemotherapeutic that is specifically toxic to beta cells and therefore specific for the treatment of insulinomas, is being used by a number of oncologists to treat canine insulinomas. Streptozocin can induce nephrotoxicity unless given with aggressive saline diuresis. The drug is also extremely emetogenic; pretreatment with butorphanol, metoclopramide, or ondansetron is required. Limited data exist on its use in cats.
- Glucagon (5 ng/kg/minute) can be used to increase gluconeogenesis. Glucagon can be used by reconstituting 1 mg of lyophilized glucagon with the diluent provided. That material can be added to one liter of 0.9% NaCl. The resulting solution will have a 1 ug/ml concentration that will allow for convenient administration rates. This treatment is most effective for the hypoglycemic crisis, but, in some cases, it may provide sustained benefits post-infusion. Few data exist on its use in cats.

Survival times for dogs with insulinomas range widely in reported studies, based on treatments selected (surgery, medical, or both) and stage of tumor. Similar data in cats is not as available. The stages are: stage 1 (pancreatic nodule only), stage 2 (regional lymph node metastasis), and stage 3 (distant metastasis, usually liver). In one study of 73 dogs,[6] stage 1 had the longest disease-free interval (no hypoglycemia-median 14 months); stage 1 and 2 had similar survivals (median of 12-18 months); and stage 3 lived on average 6 months. Five dogs lived between 24-36 months (2 stage 1, 3 stage 2). Younger dogs generally have a poorer prognosis than older dogs. Insulinomas in the cat tend to behave in the same manner as in the dog; however, surgical removal of an insulinoma in one cat did indeed result in long-term control of this disease.

Insulinomas managed surgically (+/- medical therapy post-op) generally survive longer than with medical therapy alone.[8,9-11] Debulking metastatic disease will increase survival times. The median survival with surgery in 26 dogs was 381 days, versus 70 days in 13 dogs treated with medical therapy alone.[8] In another study,[10] 31 dogs with resectable tumor/metastases had a median survival of 258 days. Dogs in that study that were hyperglycemic or normoglycemic post-op had a median survival of 680 days vs. 90 days if they were hypoglycemic. In a third study, dogs that were normoglycemic post-op (18) survived less than 435 days. Eleven dogs that were hypoglycemic post-op and treated medically survived a median of 215 days (with one dog alive more than 704 days).

EMERGENCIES ASSOCIATED WITH HYPONATREMIA

Syndrome of inappropriate secretion of antidiuretic hormone (SIADH)

Hyponatremia is the primary electrolyte defect associated with the syndrome of inappropriate secretion of antidiuretic hormone (SIADH). While SIADH is an important cause, many other etiologies exist (box 7-3). SIADH is underdiagnosed in veterinary medicine; it is one of the best characterized and most frequently encountered ectopic hormone syndromes and its associated emergencies in human medicine along with its associated emergencies.[1,4] It is likely that SIADH will be identified more frequently in dogs and cats as awareness of it grows.[1,4]

SIADH can be caused by increased expression of ADH from the pituitary gland or as a true paraneoplastic syndrome secondary to the ectopic production of ADH. In some cases, hyponatremia can cause profound clinical changes that result in life threatening situations. In addition, several drugs can indirectly cause SIADH by potentiating the release of ADH.[1,4]

Clinical signs[1,4]

Most dogs and cats SIADH are clinically normal. When sodium levels are drop to below 125 mEq/L, however, lethargy and mental dullness may be noted. When serum sodium levels drop below 120 mEq/L, more dramatic central nervous system (CNS) problems that may progress to convulsions and coma can develop. When this occurs, the animal must be treated for a medical emergency.

Diagnosis

The diagnosis of SIADH is based on the absence of hypovolemia and dehydration as well as on the following laboratory findings:[1,4]
- Hypo-osmolality.
- Hyponatremia of extracellular fluids.

Box 7-3. Causes of hyponatremia

Associated with Hypovolemia

- Excessive renal sodium loss
- Excessive external losses: diarrhea, vomiting, hemorrhage, third spacing, sweating
- Diuretics
- Renal tubular acidosis
- Hypoadrenalcorticism (secondary to cranial radiation)
- Congestive HEART FAILURE
- Nephrotic syndrome
- Malignant ascites
- Cirrhosis
- Renal failure
- Pseudohypoadrenocorticism associated with third spacing fluid in the abdomen

Associated with euvolemia

- Distal tubule diuretics
- Loop diuretics
- Hypothyroidism
- Syndrome of inappropriate secretion of antidiuretic hormone
- Cancer
- CNS Lesions
- Selected drugs including:
  - Chlorpropamide
  - Vincristine
  - Vinblastine
  - Cyclophosphamide
  - Opiates
  - Thiazide diuretics
  - Barbiturates
  - Isoproterenol
  - Mannitol
  - Morphine
  - Other diuretics
- Increased intrathoracic pressure of mediastinal tumor

Associated with hypervolemia

- Associated with hyper- and hypovolumia
- Primary polydypsia
- Excessive sodium depleted fluids
- Tap water enemas

- Urine that is less than maximally dilute.
- Absence of volume depletion.
- Sustained renal excretion of sodium.
- Normal renal, pituitary, and adrenal function.

Spurious or artifactual hyponatremia can occur in dogs with marked increases in serum lipids or serum proteins. In addition, in dogs with marked hyperglycemia, water can be drawn into the circulatory system, diluting electrolytes and causing hyponatremia.

Key point

Drugs that can cause SIADH include chlorpropamide, vincristine, vinblastine, cyclophosphamide, opiates, histamine, thiazides, barbiturates, and isoproterenol.

Treatment

The treatment of choice for patients with SIADH is to eliminate the underlying cause. The goal is to treat acute hyponatremia quickly and chronic hyponatremia slowly (<0.5 mEq/L/hr or 12 mEq/L in a day). The change in serum [Na] usually needed to alleviate the clinical signs of hyponatremia is small, usually in the order of 3-7 mEq/L. Once that change is seen, slow down further correction of serum sodium. If clinical signs warrant treatment, the following measures may be helpful:[1,4]

- *Water restriction.* This is effective for mild cases in which the animal can be watched carefully for underhydration. The objective is to raise the serum sodium level while restricting water intake to approximately 66 ml/kg/day.
- *Demeclocycline.* This drug antagonizes the actions of ADH on the kidneys and thus causes reversible nephrogenic diabetes insipidus. In humans, nausea, vomiting, skin rashes, and hypersensitivity reactions are possible side effects. Demeclocycline is effective in treating patients with mild to moderate cases of SIADH. Other drugs such as lithium carbonate and phenytoin are not as effective as demeclocycline.
- *Hypertonic sodium chloride.* This intravenous solution is generally reserved for patients that have significant clinical signs related to hyponatremia. The following formula may help to determine the approximate amount of sodium needed to correct hyponatremia:[10]

Na for replacement (mEq) = (desired serum sodium [mEq/L] – observed serum sodium [mEq/L]) × body weight (kg) × 0.6

- *Furosemide in cases of water intoxication:* Bolus 2-4 mg/kg IV or 0.1-1 mg/kg/hr while monitoring body weight and urine output. Ventilatory support may be needed in cases of severe neurologic impairment.

References

1. Dhaliwal RS: Tumor and tumor related complications. In: Henry CJ, Higginbotham ML (eds): *Cancer Mangement in Small Animal Practice*. St. Louis, Missori, Saunders Elsevier, 2010, pp 122-135.
2. Hostutler RA, Chew DJ, Jaeger JQ, et al: Uses and effectiveness of pamidronate disodium for treatment of dogs and cats with hypercalcemia. *J Vet Intern Med* 19(1): 29-33, 2005.
3. Milner RJ, Farese J. Henry CJ, et al: Bisphosphonates and cancer. *J Vet Intern Med* 18[5]: 597-604, 2004.
4. Feldman EC, Nelson RW: Hypercalcemia and primary hyperparathyroidism in dogs. in Bonagura JD (ed): *Current Veterinary Therapy XIII. Philadelphia*, WB Saunders, 2000, pp 311-348
5. Weir EC, Burtis WJ, Morris CA, et al: Isolation of a 16,000-dalton parathyroid hormone-like protein from two animal tumors causing humoral hypercalcemia of malignancy. *Endocrinology* 123: 2744–2752, 1988.
6. Caywood DD, Klausner JS, O'Leary TP, et al. Pancreatic insulin-secreting neoplasms: clinical, diagnostic, and prognostic features in 73 dogs. *J Am Anim Hosp Assoc* 24:577-584, 1987.
7. Fischer JR, Smith SA, Harkin KR. Glucagon constant-rate infusion: a novel strategy for the management of hyperinsulinemic-hypoglycemic crisis in the dog. j am anim hosp assoc 36:27-32, 2000.
8. Leifer CE, Peterson ME, Matus RE. Insulin-secreting tumor: diagnosis and medical and surgical management in 55 dogs. *J Am Vet Med Assoc* 188:60-64, 1986.
9. Steiner JM, Bruyette DS. Canine insulinoma. *Comp Cont Ed* 18:13-16, 1996.
10. Tobin RL, Nelson RW, Lucroy MD, Wooldridge JD, Feldman EC. Outcome of surgical versus medical treatment of dogs with beta cell neoplasia: 39 cases (1990-1997). *J Am Vet Med Assoc* 215:226-230, 1999.
11. Trifonidou MA, Kirpensteijn J, Robben JH. A retrospective evaluation of 51 dogs with insulinoma. *Vet Q* 20:S114-S115, 1998.
12. Moore AS, Nelson RW, Henry CJ, et al. Streptozotocin for treatment of pancreatic islet cell tumors in dogs: 17 cases (1989-1999). *J Am Vet Med Assoc* 221:811-818, 2002.
13. Cameron K, Gallagher A. Syndrome of inappropriate antidiuretic hormone secretion in a cat. *J Am Anim Hosp Assoc*. 46(6): 425-32, 2110.

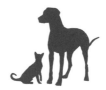

Chapter 8

Emergencies associated with hematologic manifestations of malignancy

ERYTHROCYTOSIS

An increase in the number of red blood cells (RBCs) (erythrocytosis) is relatively common in canine and less commonly in feline patients, but only a fraction of the cases can cause oncologic emergencies or be classified as true paraneoplastic syndrome.[1-7] Erythrocytosis also can be caused by dehydration and secondary volume contraction, pulmonary and cardiac disorders, venoarterial shunts, Cushing's disease, chronic corticosteroid administration, and polycythemia vera. Erythrocytosis can produce significant clinical signs resulting in a life threatening emergency as well as a diagnostic dilemma.

An elevated RBC mass secondary to malignancy most often occurs either directly by tumor production of erythropoietin or secondary due to hypoxia produced by the physical presence of a tumor that induces production of erythropoietin. Erythropoietin is normally produced by the kidney in dogs; thus, it is not surprising that kidney tumors are associated with erythrocytosis.[1-4] In addition to renal tumors, hepatic tumors and lymphoma have been associated with erythrocytosis.[1-9] When erythrocytosis is secondary to elevated erythropoietin concentrations, four possible mechanisms may be responsible:[1-7]

- Erythropoietin produced directly by the tumor.
- Erythropoietin produced either in response to tumor-initiated hypoxia or vascular obstruction.
- Erythropoietin produced by the kidney in response to a tumor-induced factor.
- Tumor-induced change in metabolism of erythropoietin.

Clinical presentation

Many dogs with erythrocytosis are asymptomatic.[1-9] Others exhibit lethargy, anorexia, polydipsia, and polyuria. If the erythrocytosis is caused by generalized hypoxia, clinical signs referable to decreased oxygenation will predominate. This decrease in oxygen saturation may cause cardiovascular decompensation, exercise intolerance, ascites, dyspnea, and cyanosis and thus may present as an emergency.

Key point

Dogs and cats with erythrocytosis of paraneoplastic origin have normal renal structure and function but show signs of extramedullary hematopoiesis and a hyperplastic erythroid series in the bone marrow.

Diagnosis

The diagnosis of erythrocytosis is based on the results of a hemogram, biochemical profile, blood gas analysis, erythropoietin levels, chest and abdominal radiographs, cardiovascular examination, renal imaging, and a splenic aspirate (tables 8-1 and 8-2).[1-3,7-9]

- Dogs and cats with erythrocytosis of paraneoplastic origin have normal renal structure and function but show signs of extramedullary hematopoiesis and a hyperplastic erythroid series in the bone marrow.
- Pets with secondary polycythemia have decreased arterial oxygen saturation or renal disease.[1-3, 7-9]
- Polycythemia vera is a myeloproliferative disorder that results from clonal proliferation of RBC precursors. The diagnosis generally is made using histology and cytology of a bone marrow core biopsy specimen and aspirate after ruling out the presence of local or systemic hypoxia. Erythropoietin concentrations are normal to decreased.

Treatment

Patients with erythrocytosis usually require no treatment unless clinical signs are significant or life threatening. Specific therapy for the underlying cause of the tissue hypoxia should be instituted in appropriate cases.[1-3, 7-9] In emergency situations, patients with relative polycythemia should be first treated with fluid therapy followed by phlebotomy, whereas patients with absolute polycythemia should be treated by phlebotomy. Phlebotomies may assist temporarily to reduce the RBC load. This procedure is performed by withdrawing approximately 20 to 40 ml/kg of blood through a large-bore needle (e.g., 12-ga) while simultaneously replacing the volume being removed with crystalloid fluids.

Table 8-1. Results of common diagnostic tests and various classifications of erythrocytosis

Erythropoietinemia classification	Erythropoietin blood levels	Blood oxygen	Bone marrow	Renal status	Extramedullary hematopoiesis
(1°) Polycythemia vera	Normal to low	Normal	Malignant	Normal	No
(2°) Paraneoplastic syndrome	Increased	Normal	Hyperplastic	Normal	Yes
(2°) Tissue hypoxia	Increased	Low	Hyperplastic	Normal	Yes
(2°) Renal disease	Increased	Normal	Hyperplastic	Abnormal	Yes

Table 8-2. Examples of cancer and non cancer related alterations in select parameters of a hemogram other than laboratory error

Hematologic parameter	Level	Cancer related etiology	Non-cancer related etiology
White blood cell count	Increase	Leukemia, Inflammatory or necrotic neoplastic process, paraneoplastic syndrome	Infection, (bacterial, mycotic, viral), inflammation (immune mediated disease, tissue trauma), physiologic leukocytosis, metabolic (stress, endogenous or exogenous steroids), responsive anemia
	Decrease	Bone marrow infiltration by cancer	Decreased production, increased consumption, phenobarbital
Red blood cells	Increase	Polycythemia	Dehydration, splenic contraction, pulmonary and cardiac disorders, venoarterial shunts, cushing's disease
	Decrease	Immune mediated hemolytic anemia as a paraneoplastic syndrome, tumor hemorrhage, vascular neoplasia inducing hemolysis, cancer induced coagulopathies and blood loss, cancer induced anemia of chronic disease, estrogen producing tumor, chemotherapy, myeloproliferative disease	Blood loss (trauma, ulcers, coagulopathies, parasites, hematuria), hemolytic anemia (microangiopathic due to dirofilariasis, vasculitis, dic, red blood cell parasites, leptospirosis, E. coli, oxidative injury via onions, kale, phenothiazenes, methylene blue), non responsive anemias (renal failure, anemia of chronic disease, endocrine disease such as hypothyroidism and hyperestrogenism, idiopathic aplastic anemia, red cell aplasia, chloramphenicol, iron deficiency, lead poisoning, infections)
Hemoglobin, hematocrit	Increase	Polycythemia	Dehydration, splenic contraction
	Decrease	Bleeding tumor, bone marrow infiltration by tumor	Hemorrhage, decreased production
Neutrophils	Increase	Tumor inflammation, chronic granulocytic leukemia	Infection (bacterial, mycotic, protozoal), inflammation (immune mediated, tissue trauma or necrosis), responsive anemia, demargination associated with endogenous/exogenous steriods

Hematologic parameter	Level	Cancer related etiology	Non-cancer related etiology
Neutrophils (cont.)	Decrease	Myelopthisis, chemotherapy	Myelofibrosis, drugs (chloramphenicol, trimethoprim sulfa, griseofulvin), idiopathic, cyclic neutropenia, immune mediated, hypersplenism, infection, endotoxemia, hypoadrenocorticism, margination
Lymphocytos	Increase	Lymphocytic leukemia	Physiologic leukocytosis, chronic antigenic stimulation
	Decrease	Chemotherapy	Stress, drugs (steriods), immunodeficiency, lymphangiectasia
Monocytes	Increase	Myelomonocytic or monocytic leukemia	Chronic inflammation, chronic infection, granulomatous disease, stress, glucocorticoids
Eosinophils	Increase	Mast cell tumor, paraneoplastic syndrome of solid tumors, eosinophilic leukemia	Allergic disease, enteritis, asthma, stomatitis, rhinitis, parasites, fungal infections, hyper-eosinophilic syndrome, hypoadrenalcorticism, pregnancy
	Decrease		Stress, hyperadrenalcorticism, exogenous steroids
Basophils	Increase	Mast cell tumors	Dirofilariasis
Platelets	Increase	Polycythemia vera	Essential thrombocytosis, rebound thrombocytosis
	Decrease	Paraneoplastic syndrome, myelopthisis	Infections, immune mediated, sequestration, hemorrhage, dic, breeds (king charles spaniels and greyhounds.

With polycythemia vera, the chemotherapeutic agent hydroxyurea (30 mg/kg/day PO for 7 days, then 15 mg/kg/day) can be used to induce reversible bone marrow suppression and reduce RBC production.[1,2,7] Alternative chemotherapeutic agents are chlorambucil, busulfan, and pipobroman. Radioactive phosphorus and alpha interferon can also be employed, but periodic phlebotomies may be equally as effective as any other therapy.

Key point

The treatment of choice for the erythropoietin-producing tumor or the tumor that induces regional or systemic hypoxia is emergency care and stabilization followed by surgical removal. Phlebotomies and hydroxyurea can be used if needed.

EMERGENCIES ASSOCIATED WITH ANEMIA

Anemia occurs frequently in veterinary cancer patients and it occasionally results in a medical emergency. The causes of anemia are obvious in many cases and may result from increased blood loss, decreased RBC production (e.g., abnormal bone marrow function), or increased RBC destruction (e.g., immune-mediated diseases).[1-6] More specific causes of malignancy-associated anemia include anemia of chronic disease, bone marrow invasion by tumor cells, marrow suppression by chemotherapy, hypersplenism, immune-mediated disease, megaloblastic anemia, vitamin and iron deficiency, microangiopathic hemolytic anemia, and pure red cell aplasia.[1-6] Anemia of any cause arising as an indirect effect of the tumor is indeed a paraneoplastic syndrome. In most patients, a clear cause of the anemia is not found and the diagnosis of "anemia of chronic disease" is made.

Blood loss anemia is seen in many types of cancer. It can occur as a direct effect of the cancer or indirectly as a result of coagulopathies linked with hemangiosarcomas, thyroid carcinomas, and inflammatory mammary carcinomas. Histamine released from canine mast cell tumors may activate parietal cells in the stomach, increasing production of hydrochloric acid and inducing gastric or duodenal ulceration and consequent blood loss. This syndrome of mast cell induced GI ulceration is rare in the cat. If anemia is secondary to blood loss, the cause

> **Key point**
>
> Vincristine can be administered in cases of life threatening thrombocytopenia to increase platelet counts after 3-4 days.

EMERGENCIES ASSOCIATED WITH LEUKOCYTOSIS

An increased WBC count attributable to either increased production, decreased loss, or decreased destruction is common in veterinary cancer patients.[1,2,12-14] Any cell line can be involved. When leukocytosis is a remote effect of underlying malignancy, the laboratory finding may be classified as a paraneoplastic syndrome. Paraneoplastic leukocytosis in dogs and cats arises from a variety of malignancies, including lymphoma and hemangiosarcoma (see table 8-2).[1,2,4,5,12-14] Although some cases of leukocytosis are caused by malignant clonal proliferation of a specific WBC line, they are not considered paraneoplastic syndromes.

Clinical presentation

Dogs and cats with paraneoplastic leukocytosis are often clinically normal. Human patients occasionally describe bone pain due to the high proliferative rate in the bone marrow.

> **Key point**
>
> The mechanism of the malignancy-associated leukocytosis may involve the direct or indirect production of hematopoietic growth factors, such as granulocyte colony-stimulating factor, granulocyte-macrophage colony-stimulating factor, or interleukin-3 or may occur as a result of tissue necrosis and granulocyte breakdown with positive feedback that increases neutrophil production.

Diagnosis

The diagnosis is based on a CBC and bone marrow examination. Occasionally, special stains may be performed by the clinical pathology laboratory to determine whether the increased number of leukocytes are from a neoplastic clone.

Treatment

The condition is not generally of clinical significance however in those patients where significant marrow pain, coaggulopathies or leukocytosis induced hyperviscosity results in confusion, thrombosis and DIC, fluid therapy and pheresis is indicated.

EMERGENCIES ASSOCIATED WITH NEUTROPENIA AND SEPSIS

> **Key point**
>
> Sepsis due to chemotherapy or cancer-related neutropenia is one of the more common emergencies handled in veterinary cancer medicine.

Sepsis due to chemotherapy or cancer-related neutropenia is one of the more common emergencies handled in canine and feline cancer medicine.[13-24] Bleeding due to thrombocytopenia is much less common. Both conditions are usually preventable by judicious monitoring and appropriate supportive care during cancer therapy. In addition, caregivers should be educated about the early clinical signs of neutropenia and thrombocytopenia induced by cancer treatment, thus empowering the client to assist in early detection and seek immediate treatment.

In humans, sepsis is a common cause of death in cancer patients, exceeding all other causes combined.[14-21] As the popularity of advanced medicine increases and the use of chemotherapy and radiation soar in private practice, this observation is likely to be repeated in canine and feline cancer medicine. Since dogs and cats may hide their symptoms until late in the disease, the condition of sepsis may be quite advanced when first recognized and requires prompt intervention by the veterinary health care team.

Neutropenia secondary to malignancy, or as a result of the myelosuppressive effects of chemotherapy or radiation therapy, is a common predisposing factor for development of sepsis in dogs and cats. Septic shock is the state of circulatory collapse that occurs secondary to overwhelming sepsis and/or endotoxemia. This syndrome is frequently fatal, with a mortality rate of 40% to 90%. The profound systemic effects of septic shock include:

- Vasoconstriction leading to multi-organ failure.
- Cardiac dysfunction, in part from lactic acidosis secondary to poor perfusion.
- Increased vascular permeability, leading to hyperviscosity and hypovolemia.
- Liver dysfunction from splanchnic vascular pooling and tissue ischemia.
- Acute renal failure.
- Worsening neutropenia and thrombocytopenia.
- Coagulopathies.
- Severe gastrointestinal damage and bacterial translocation.
- Hypocalcemia.
- Decreased insulin release.
- Initial hyperglycemia followed by hypoglycemia.

The bacteria that most commonly cause morbidity and mortality in veterinary cancer patients arise from the dog or cat's own flora.[21] The most important thing a clinician can do for the septic canine and feline cancer patient is to quickly identify the source and type of bacterial infection, and initiate therapy with broad-spectrum antibiotics as well as appropriate and aggressive supportive care. Factors such as prolonged hospitalization, the presence of urinary, venous, chest, endotracheal and other tubes or catheters, and antibiotic administration may result in increased susceptibility to increasingly resistant strains of organisms. These factors should be avoided or minimized wherever possible. Minimizing the chance for exposure to, or the opportunity for development of, resistant strains of bacteria enhances the chance for rapid recovery in response to appropriate antibiotic therapy.

Key point

The frequency and severity of infections is directly related to the severity and duration of neutropenia.

Predisposing factors

The following are predisposing factors for neutropenia-associated sepsis:[14-21]

- Defects in cellular immunity are a cause of sepsis in dogs and cats with cancer. Cellular immune dysfunction, while extraordinarily difficult to diagnose in the dog or cat, may be due to an underlying cause or the result of administration of antineoplastic agents and/or corticosteroids. These defects may result in various bacterial, mycobacterial, fungal, and viral infections. Humoral immune dysfunction is also associated with an increased prevalence of sepsis in human patients with cancer and may cause similar problems in animals. Agammaglobulinemic or hypogammaglobulinemic dogs and cats are suspected as being susceptible to infections. Multiple myeloma and chronic lymphocytic leukemia are common neoplasms associated with humoral immune dysfunction in people, and are likely causes in the dog or cat as well.

Key point

Patients with multiple myeloma and chronic lymphocytic leukemia often have humoral immune dysfunction and thus, increased succeptibility to infection, especially when receiving chemotherapy.

- The myelosuppressive effects of chemotherapy may cause neutropenia. The myelosuppressive effects of chemotherapeutic agents can be categorized as high, moderate, or mild (table 8-3). These drugs cause a nadir (lowest part of the white blood cell count) at different times after administration (table 8-4).
- Splenectomized dogs and cats are susceptible to

overwhelming sepsis when infected with a strain of encapsulated bacteria against which they have not made antibodies.

- Indwelling vascular or urinary catheters have been associated with an increased prevalence of sepsis. The longer a catheter is present, the higher the probability for infection, especially in neutropenic dogs and cats.
- Frequent acquisition of blood samples greatly increases the risk of sepsis in dogs and cats with cancer.
- Prolonged hospitalization can result in serious consequences, in part because the patient is continually exposed to bacterial strains that are resistant to the antibiotics most commonly used in that practice.
- Malnutrition is a serious cause of debilitation and decreased resistance to bacterial infection, especially in those dogs and cats with neutropenia.
- Dogs and cats with neurologic dysfunction or nonambulatory patients from any cause are at increased risk for sepsis as well.

Whenever possible, these risk factors must be avoided or minimized, and associated problems recognized and corrected early to reduce the probability of sepsis. The first approach for clinician and client is to understand the myelosuppressive effects of various drugs. The myelosuppressive effects of chemotherapeutic agents can be categorized as high, moderate, or mild (table 8-3). These drugs cause a nadir at different times after administration (table 8-4). Clients and the veterinary health care team should be encouraged to be more vigilant for the clinical signs associated with neutropenia and thrombocytopenia around the time of the nadir for the drug being used. With monitoring of CBCs at the appropriate times, especially early on in the course of chemotherapy, the veterinarian will have a general idea of how low the white blood cell count is actually dropping. If the count appears too low (less than 1000/ul), or the patient becomes even mildly symptomatic, subsequent dose reduction of that drug should be considered.

Further steps can be taken to minimize the risk of sepsis for the dog or cat with cancer. One logical step is to minimize the administration of immunosuppressive drugs, especially corticosteroids. Whenever a splenectomized dog or cat is treated for cancer, they should be watched carefully for complications, including sepsis. The risk of catheter-induced sepsis can be minimized by using aseptic technique and by placing a new catheter in a new site every 2 to 3 days. Strict aseptic procedures should be used, especially with dogs and cats that are myelosuppressed. The use of semipermanent indwelling catheters in patients with cancer may be safe if caregivers and health care professionals follow strict aseptic procedures. Proper aseptic technique and changing of catheters are especially important in dogs and cats with neurologic dysfunction, as these dogs and cats are at a much higher risk for sepsis. The duration of hospitalization should be limited whenever possible to limit exposure to resistant bacteria.

Table 8-3. Myelosuppressive effects of chemotherapeutic agents used in veterinary medicine		
Highly myelosuppressive	**Moderately myelosuppressive**	**Mildly myelosuppressive**
Doxorubicin	Melphalan	L-asparaginase
Vinblastine	Chlorambucil	Vincristine
Cyclophosphamide	5-fluorouracil	Bleomycin
CCNU	Methotrexate	Corticosteroids

Table 8-4. Myelosuppressive drugs associated with the development of pyrexia and sepsis at different times after treatment		
Delayed myelosuppression (3–4 weeks)	**Mid-range myelosuppression (7–10 days)**	**Early myelosuppression (<7 days)**
Carmustine (BCNU)	Cyclophosphamide	Taxol
Lomustine (CCNU)	Doxorubicin	
Mitomycin C	Mitoxantrone	
Carboplatin		

Key point

The incidence of sepsis significantly increases when the neutrophil count drops to less than 1000 /µl, especially when the patient has diarrhea.

Diagnosis

Dogs and cats presented with septic shock secondary to neutropenia require immediate intervention and careful client support. Diagnostic and therapeutic interventions must begin concurrently for the patient's benefit. The differential list for neutropenia is quite extensive.

The diagnosis of septic shock begins with the physical examination as a catheter is placed and blood samples are acquired for initial diagnostics. Mucous membrane color can be difficult to identify in pets, however, in some dogs and cats with septic shock, brick-red mucous membranes may be noted in early stages. In addition, some of the following signs may be identified on physical examination in dogs and cats in the hyperdynamic state of septic shock:[14-21]

- Tachycardia.
- Short capillary refill time.
- Gastrointestinal signs.
- Altered mentation.
- Decreased blood pressure .

End-stage signs reflect a hypodynamic state and include:[14-20]

- Hypothermia.
- Mucous membrane pallor.
- Marked mental depression.

- Bloody diarrhea.
- Vasodilation.
- Signs of multi-organ failure.

Thrombocytopenia and neutropenia are often identified during the course of septic shock. Hyperglycemia is an early finding that often is followed by hypoglycemia. Metabolic acidosis is commonly identified.

Cultures of urine and blood should always be obtained, even though they may be negative and require a significant amount of time for results to be available. Appropriate broad-spectrum antibiotics and combinations must be available immediately for parenteral administration. When positive, the results of cultures will guide follow-up oral antibiotic selection.

Blood and urine taken at the time of initial presentation can be very helpful for supporting a diagnosis of septic shock. At a minimum, samples should be obtained for a complete blood count (CBC), biochemical profile, and urinalysis on each cat. These clinical pathologic findings are often combined with other tests.

The absence of circulating neutrophils affects many of the commonly used clinical, laboratory and radiographic findings that may normally suggest a localized or systemic infection. For example:

- Neutropenia results in a urinalysis without pyuria, despite infection.
- Without a neutrophilic infiltrate, which otherwise would be responsible for many of the radiographic changes associated with pneumonia, thoracic radiographs often appear "normal" even in the presence of significant pneumonia.

Thus, any suspicious sites should be cultured.[21-24] This includes, but is not necessarily limited to:

- Blood cultures: Two, and preferably four, sets of blood cultures (aerobic and anaerobic) should be acquired. However, extreme care should be taken to be cognizant of the total volume of blood taken, including blood for hemograms, biochemical profiles and other tests, because these pets almost always have some degree of anemia of chronic disease. The timing of the sampling intervals is controversial, however, sampling every 20 to 30 minutes prior to initiation of antibiotic therapy may be adequate. At least 2 ml of blood should be injected into appropriate culture containers.
- Catheter cultures: If central venous catheters are present, cultures of the port should be obtained. Ideally, culture bottles that contain an antibiotic-binding resin or other antibiotic-binding substance should be included with each culture for patients on antibiotics.
- Urine culture: A cystocentesis specimen for urine culture and analysis should be acquired in each case.
- CSF culture: When neurologic signs are present, a cerebrospinal fluid (CSF) tap should be obtained and cultured appropriately. CSF should be sent for Gram stain, bacterial culture, cell count and differential, and glucose and protein determination. A cryptococcal antigen titer or India ink preparation should be performed in suspect cases. Acid-fast stains and culture are probably not indicated routinely.
- Stool cultures: For dogs and cats with diarrhea, appropriate cultures should be done for clostridial bacteria, including appropriate assays for endotoxin.
- Lung cultures: Thoracic radiographs and a transendotracheal wash should be obtained, especially when the patient shows any sign of respiratory difficulty such as increased respiratory effort or a cough.

Other diagnostic studies that should be considered include:[14-21]

- Complete blood count with differential, biochemical profile, and urinalysis.
- Thoracic and abdominal radiographs to look for signs of infection.
- Abdominal ultrasonography looking for pancreatitis, abscesses, abdominal effusion, etc.
- Echocardiography to identify the presence of valvular endocarditis.
- Bronchoscopy with bronchoalveolar lavage if pulmonary disease is suspected.
- Skin biopsy, if deep cutaneous infection is identified.
- Bone marrow aspirate or biopsy to determine the cause and severity of neutropenia.

- Percutaneous or laparascopic-guided liver biopsy or aspirate to evaluate for hepatic infection or abscessation.
- Exploratory laparotomy in select cases when other, less invasive tests are not successful, yet there is clinical evidence of disease in the abdomen.
- Blood gas analysis.

Treatment [21-24]

Treatment for septic shock should begin as soon as the condition is suspected. This is usually at the time the dog or cat is initially presented for an acute, emergency condition.

Treatment for the septic, neutropenic dog or cat is primarily directed at:

- Restoring adequate tissue perfusion.
- Improving the alterations in metabolism.
- Controlling systemic infection.

- *Restoring adequate tissue perfusion:* Standard therapy includes crystalloid or hypertonic saline or colloid solutions, pressors and antibiotics. Although the use of hypertonic solutions for the treatment of shock is being investigated, balanced electrolyte solutions are cited in most texts as "the first line of therapy." The initial infusion rate for critical dogs is 90 ml/kg IV for 1 hour, then 10 to 12 ml/kg/hour thereafter (in cats, the initial dosage that is often stated is 60 mls/kg IV then 10 ml/kg thereafter). In both species the patient is checked every 15 minutes for fluid overload and the rate of fluids is then either continued or modified. The fluid rate should then be adjusted to meet the needs of each dog or cat as determined by monitoring body weight, serum lactate concentrations, heart and respiratory rates, central venous pressure, ongoing losses (e.g., vomiting and diarrhea), and urine output. During that first hour of fluid administration, it is vitally important to monitor at 15-minute intervals for evidence of fluid overload and adjust appropriately.
- *Improving alterations in metabolism:* When choosing the type of fluids, some authorities prefer a non-lactate containing fluid; lactate must be metabolized to bicarbonate by a functional liver that may be impaired during shock and sepsis. Normosol R® and Plasmalyte® are examples of non-lactate-containing fluids with acetate and gluconate as buffers. Dextrose should be included in fluids when systemic hypoglycemia is identified during constant patient monitoring.
- *Controlling or preventing infection:* Asymptomatic dogs and cats with fewer than 1000 neutrophils/μl should be started prophylactically on antibiotics. Trimethoprim-sulfa (7.5 mg/kg BID parenterally or PO) is often recommended for prophylactic therapy in the

asymptomatic, yet neutropenic, patient. Neutropenic dogs and cats in septic shock should be started on intravenous fluids and intravenous antibiotic therapy as soon as samples for bacterial cultures are acquired (tables 8-5 and 8-6). Re-evaluation of the initial antibiotic regimen is mandatory when the identity and sensitivity patterns of the bacteria become available. For gram-negative infections, two antibiotics that are effective against the isolated organism are often recommended.

Initially, broad-spectrum antibiotic therapy, usually combinations of an aminoglycoside plus penicillin or 2nd generation cephalosporin (e.g., cefoxitin, cefamandole, cefaclor, cefuroxime, cefonicid, ceforanide, cefotetan, cefetazole), is commonly used in sepsis. If the infection doesn't respond within 24 hrs, the antibiotics should be changed. For gram-negative organisms, a different aminoglycoside, quinolone, or aztreonam may be used. Extended-spectrum penicillins (e.g., ticarcillin, carbenicillin, azlocillin, piperacillin sodium, and mezlocillin), 3rd generation cephalosporins (e.g., cefotaxime, moxalactam, cefoperazone, ceftizoxime, ceftriaxone, ceftazidime, cefixime), or imipenem with cilastatin sodium have sufficiently broad spectrums to be used alone. Dogs and cats placed on aminoglycosides, particularly gentamicin, should be monitored for nephrotoxicity via urinalysis (urine sediment should be examined for the presence of casts) and measurement of BUN and creatinine concentrations and ensure they are well-hydrated and receiving fluids.

Other treatments include:

- *Corticosteroids:* Steroids remain extremely controversial in septic shock but there is some consensus for administering steroids only in the case of septic shock after blood pressure is identified to be poorly responsive to fluid and vasopressor therapy. Recommended doses in shock are hydrocortisone at 300 mg/kg, methylprednisolone or prednisone at 10-30 mg/kg, or dexamethasone at 4-8 mg/kg. Short-term use (i.e., less than 2 days of massive doses) does not result in as many adverse effects as long-term use.
- *Glucose:* If hypoglycemia is present, glucose at 0.25 g/kg IV bolus can be given, followed by infusions of 2.5- 10% glucose solutions as needed to maintain normal blood glucose levels.
- *Bicarbonate:* Although very controversial, bicarbonate can be given if severe metabolic acidosis is present. The amount of bicarbonate to give can be calculated (i.e., base deficit x (0.3 x BW in kg)) or estimated (mild, moderate, or severe acidosis is treated with 1, 3, or 5 mEq bicarbonate/kg IV, respectively). Bicarbonate should be given slowly through IV (i.e., over 20 minutes or more).
- *Neutrophil-rich transfusions:* These transfusions have not been associated with beneficial responses in controlled trials. In addition, transfusion reactions and allosensitization to specific antigens of the granulocytes may occur, and increased prevalence of severe pulmonary reactions may also be noted.
- *Hematopoietic growth factors:* Canine recombinant granulocyte colony-stimulating factor (rcG-CSF, 5 µg/kg/day SQ) and canine recombinant granulocyte-

macrophage colony-stimulating factor (rcGM-CSF, 10 µg/kg/day SQ) have been associated with an increased rate of myeloid recovery in dogs and cats with neutropenia. These hematopoietic growth factors increase cell numbers and enhance neutrophil function, but are not yet widely available commercially. Human recombinant G-CSF and GM-CSF are commercially available; however, long-term use may induce antibody formation to the protein. Of the two human recombinant proteins, rhG-CSF induces the most profound increase in neutrophil numbers before development of antibodies is noted.

- Transfusions of fresh, whole blood.
- *Other options:* Tumor necrosis factor antiserum, antibody to tumor necrosis factor, interleukin and interferon therapy, pooled immunoglobulin preparations, activated protein C, antithrombin 3 and monoclonal antibodies to neutralize endotoxin may be future treatments of choice.

References

1. Dhaliwal RS: Tumor and tumor related complications. In: Henry CJ, Higginbotham ML (eds): *Cancer Mangement in Small Animal Practice*. St. Louis, Missori, Saunders Elsevier, 2010, pp 122-135.
2. Silverstein DC, Hopper K: *Small Animal Critical Care Medicine*. St. Louis, Missori, Saunders Elsevier, 2008, pp 18-20.
3. Ogilvie GK. Anemia, thrombocytopenia, and hypoproteinemia. In Wingfield WE. *Veterinary Emergency Medicine Secrets*. Hanley and Belfus, Philadelpha. pp 265-268, 2001.
4. Thamm DH, Vail DM: Aftershocks of cancer chemotherapy: managing adverse effects. *J Am Anim Hosp Assoc*. 43(1): 1-7, 2007.
5. Madewell BR, Feldman BF: Characterization of anemias associated with neoplasia in small Dogs. *JAVMA* 176: 419–425, 1980.
6. Comer KM: Anemia as a feature of primary gastrointestinal neoplasia. *Compend Contin Educ Pract Vet* 12(1): 13–22, 1990.
7. Yamauchi A, Ohta T, Okada T, et al: Secondary erythrocytosis associated with schwannoma in a dog. *J Vet Med Sci* 66(12): 1605-1608, 2004.
8. Bertazzolo W, Zuliani D, Pogliani E, et al: Diffuse bronchiolo-alveolar carcinoma in a dog. *J Small Anim Pract* 43(6): 265-268, 2002.
9. Sato K, Hikasa Y, Morita T, et al: Secondary erythrocytosis associated with high plasma erythropoietin concentrations in a dog with cecal leiomyosarcoma. *J Am Vet Med Assoc* 220(4):486-490, 2002
10. Helfand SC, Couto CG, Madewell BR: Immune-mediated thrombocytopenia associated with solid tumors in dogs. *JAAHA* 21: 787–794, 1985.
11. Hargis AM, Feldman BE: Evaluation of hemostatic defects secondary to vascular tumors in dogs: 11 cases (1983–1988). *JAVMA* 198: 891–894, 1991.
12. Chinn DR, Myers RK, Matthews HA: Neutrophilic leukocytosis associated with metastatic fibrosarcoma in the dog. *JAVMA* 186:806–809, 1985.
13. Couto CG: Tumor-associated eosinophilia in the dog. *JAVMA* 184:837– 838, 1984.
14. Ogilvie GK. Neutropenia, sepsis and thrombocytopenia. In Wingfield WE. *Veterinary Emergency Medicine Secrets*. Hanley and Belfus, Philadelphia. pp 235-241, 2001.
15. Haskins SC: Shock, in Kirk RW (ed): *Current Veterinary Therapy VIII*. Philadelphia, WB Saunders, 1983, pp 2–27.
16. Kirk RW, Bistner SI: *Shock, in Handbook of Veterinary Procedures Emergency Treatment*, ed 4. Philadelphia, WB Saunders, 1985, pp 59–68.
17. Parker MM, Parrillo JE: Septic shock, hemodynamics and pathogenesis. *JAMA* 250:2324–2230, 1983.
18. Hardie EM, Rawlings CA: Septic shock. *Compend Contin Educ Pract Vet* 5:369–373, 1983.
19. Wolfsheimer KJ: Fluid therapy in the critically ill patient. *Vet Clin North Am Small Anim Pract* 19:361–378, 1989.
20. Lazarus HM, Creger RJ, Gerson SL: Infectious emergencies in oncology patients. *Semin Oncol* 6: 543–560, 1989.
21. Couto CG: Management of complications of cancer chemotherapy. *Vet Clin North Am Small Anim Pract* 4:1037– 1053, 1990.
22. Woodlock TJ: Oncologic emergencies, in Rosenthal S, Carignan JR, Smith BD (eds): *Medical Care of the Cancer Patient*, ed 2. Philadelphia, WB Saunders, 1993, pp 236–246.
23. Hughes WT: Infectious Diseases Society of America: Guidelines for the use of antimicrobial agents in neutropenic patients with unexplained fever. *J Infect Dis* 161: 381–390, 1990.
24. Quadri TL, Brown AE: Infectious complications in the critically ill patient with cancer. *Sem in Oncology* 27: 335-346, 2000.

Table 8-5. Approach to the septic, neutropenic dog or cat[28,30]

Approach	Action
Identify the site of infection	Perform complete physical examination
	Acquire complete blood and platelet count, biochemical profile, urinalysis (FeLV and FIV tests)
	Acquire 4 blood cultures, cystocentesis for culture and sensitivity, thoracic radiographs, and transtracheal wash for culture and sensitivity
	If indicated, culture and sensitivity testing of CSF, catheters, joint fluid, and feces
Initiate supportive care	Establish indwelling intravenous catheter aseptically and initiate fluid therapy; for shock: 90 ml/kg (cats: 60 mls/kg) for the first hour divided into quarter aliquots administered every 15 minutes, followed by 10–12 ml/kg/hr with very close monitoring to adjust fluid rate every 15 minutes, then as needed
	Withhold any additional chemotherapeutic agents
Initiate intravenous antibiotic	Four quadrant (gram-positive, gram-negative, aerobic and anaerobic bacteria therapy) antimicrobial therapy after cultures are obtained:
	cefoxitin (22 mg/kg TID IV) or ampicillin (22 mg/kg TID IV) and Enrofloxacin (5-10 mg/kg IV slowly daily with caution in cats due to risk of blindness) If aminoglycosides are considered, they should be given with extreme caution due to risk for dehydration, renal disease, low renal blood flow. Monitor for nephrotoxicity (urinalysis, evaluate sediment for casts, monitor BUN/Creatinine) if aminoglycosides, particularly gentamicin, administered consider IV maintenance fluids.
	Granulocyte colony stimulating factor, if available (5 µg/kg/day SQ)
Redefine antibiotic therapy based on culture and sensitivity results	Monitor fever and neutrophil count
Discharge for home care	Appropriate antibiotic therapy (e.g., trimethoprim-sulfa 15 mg/kg BID PO)

Table 8-6. Antibiotics used to treat dogs with septic cancer[28]

Antibiotic	Potential toxicoses
Gram-negative bacteria	
Gentamicin (2.2 - 4.4 mg/kg, TID, IV	Caution: Nephrotoxicity, especially when pre-existing renal damage, dehydration, hypotension is present; ototoxicity; ensure adequate hydration and check frequently for renal damage during use
Cefazolin (22 mg/kg (10 mg/lb), q 8 hr, IV)	Phlebitis, muscle pain after IV or IM administration; rare prevalence of nephrotoxicity
Cefoxitin (22 mg/kg IV TID)	Phlebitis; discomfort with rapid IV injection; rare prevalence of nephrotoxicity
Gram-positive bacteria	
Na or K penicillin (22,000 units/kg IV QID)	Allergy to penicillin can cause anaphylaxis, hives, fever, and pain; neurologic signs may occur with rapid infusion
Cefoxitin (22 mg/kg IV TID)	See above
Enrofloxacin (10 mg/kg IV BID)	Hives, fever, and pain
Anaerobic bacteria	
Metronidazole (15 mg/kg IV or IM TID)	Anorexia, vomiting, and neurologic signs
Cefoxitin (22 mg/kg IV TID)	See above

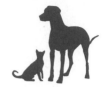

Chapter 9

Emergencies associated with hypergammaglobulinemia

HYPERGAMMAGLOBULINEMIA

> **Key point**
>
> Hypergammaglobulinemia, also known as M-component disorder or hyperviscosity syndrome, is common in dogs and cats with a variety of malignancies, particularly multiple myeloma.

Hypergammaglobulinemia, also known as M-component disorder or hyperviscosity syndrome, is common in dogs with a variety of malignancies, particularly multiple myeloma.[1-8] These diseases result from excessive secretion of immunoglobulin by a monoclonal line of immunoglobulin-producing cells (figure 9-1). These globulins include IgG, IgA, IgM, and light-chain protein classes. Light chains, also known as Bence-Jones proteins, may be present in the urine. Tumors of plasma cells, termed plasmacytoma or multiple myeloma, exhibit M-component disorders about 75% of the time. Disorders associated with the production of large quantities of immunoglobulins include:[1,2,5-9]

- Acute inflammation.
- Malignancy.
- Trauma.
- Necrosis.
- Infarction.
- Burns.
- Chemical injury.

Monoclonal gammopathies are associated with a clonal or occasionally a biclonal process that is malignant or potentially malignant, including: [1,2,5-9]

- Multiple myeloma.
- Waldenstrom's macroglobulinemia.
- Solitary plasmacytoma.
- Monoclonal gammopathy of undetermined significance.

- Plasma cell leukemia.
- Heavy chain disease.
- Amyloidosis.
- Rickettsial disease.

The quantity of M protein, the results of bone marrow biopsy, and other characteristics can help differentiate multiple myeloma from the other causes of monoclonal gammopathy. Paraneoplastic syndromes occur only in tumors that increase globulin concentration as an indirect, distant effect of the malignancy. In contrast, polyclonal gammopathies may be caused by any reactive or inflammatory process.

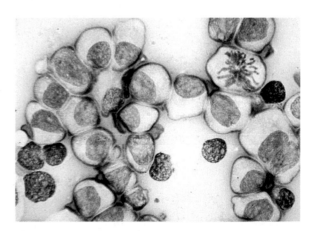

Figure 9-1: Hypergammaglobulinemia, also known as M-component disorder or hyperviscosity syndrome, is common in dogs with a variety of malignancies, particularly multiple myeloma. These diseases result from excessive secretion of immunoglobulin by a monoclonal line of immunoglobulin-producing cells as depicted here. Note these cells from the bone marrow of a dog with multiple myeloma and a monoclonal gammopathy generally have distinct cytoplasmic boarders, eccentric nuclei and a clear region near the nucleus in several of the cells.

Clinical presentation

Clinical signs associated with M-component disorders arise from increased viscosity associated with elevated globulins and from the tumor's direct effect on surrounding structures. Excessive bleeding from any site results from elevated proteins that interfere with normal platelet function.[1,2,5-9] Hyperviscosity syndrome, which decreases blood fluidity, causes:[1,2,5-9]

- Polydipsia.
- CNS signs including confusion and seizures.
- Retinopathies including retinal hemorrhage.
- Visual disturbances.
- Secondary renal problems.
- Congestive heart failure.
- Hemarthrosis.
- Epistaxis.
- Hemothorax.
- Hemoabdomen.

> **Key point**
>
> Renal decompensation often succeeds renal amyloidosis or monoclonal gammopathy induced proteinuria; increased serum viscosity decreases renal perfusion, and concentrating ability is impaired.

Renal decompensation often succeeds renal amyloidosis or Bence-Jones proteinuria; increased serum viscosity decreases renal perfusion, and concentrating ability is impaired. Neurologic signs arise when altered blood flow and diminished delivery of oxygen to neural tissue produce hypoxia in the CNS. Increased blood volume and viscosity place greater demands on the heart. This can produce decompensation of stable pre-existing cardiac conditions or development of a hypertrophic cardiomyopathy-like state.

Diagnosis

Each case of hypergammaglobulinemia must be assessed to determine the underlying cause by performing the following baseline tests [1-9]

- CBC, biochemical profile, and urinalysis.
- Immunoelectrophoresis of serum and urine (± Bence-Jones protein test of urine).
- Bone marrow aspiration and cytology.
- Thoracic and abdominal radiographs.
- Survey skeletal radiographs (± nuclear scintigraphy of skeletal system).
- Retinal examination.
- Coagulogram (APTT, OSPT, ACT, platelet count, fibrin degradation products (FDPs), and antithrombin III).
- Rickettsial titers including for Ehrlichia, Borreliosis.

> **Key point**
>
> In the presence of a monoclonal gammopathy, initial screening tests are performed primarily to detect evidence of bone marrow involvement by tumor or Ehrlichia, monoclonal gammopathy, renal failure secondary to hyperglobulinemia, coagulopathy distinct from increased globulins, lytic bone lesions suggestive of multiple myeloma, myelophthisis, or hypertension and bleeding.

Initial screening tests are performed primarily to detect evidence of bone marrow involvement by tumor or Ehrlichia, monoclonal gammopathy, renal failure secondary to hyperglobulinemia, coagulopathy distinct from increased globulins, lytic bone lesions suggestive of multiple myeloma, myelophthisis, or hypertension and bleeding. Since it determines not only whether monoclonal gammopathy is present but, also, which class of immunoglobulins is involved, immunoelectrophoresis generally is preferred to serum protein electrophoresis. Multiple myeloma, which does not engender paraneoplastic syndrome, is diagnosed by the prescence of monoclonal gammopathy, Bence-Jones proteinuria or monoclonal gammopathy-induced proteinuria, "punched out" bone lesions that may appear with a nuclear bone scan, and by more than 20% to 30% plasma cells in bone marrow. Resolution of clinical signs occurs when malignancy is controlled. If increased globulin concentrations are in response to *Ehrlichia* infection, titers should disclose the organism.

Treatment [1,2,8]

If an emergency condition exists causing a life threatening loss of blood, cognitive dysfunction, blindness, renal failure, etc., then the patient should be treated aggressively with fluid therapy (10 ml/kg/hr). Plasmapheresis rapidly reduces protein levels and is useful in cases where hyperviscosity requires symptomatic treatment.[1,2,8] In locations where that is not feasible, blood is removed using large bore catheters or needles as if to obtain blood for blood banking (ACD bags for the dog, heparin spiked syringe for the cat) with the intent to spin down the cellular component of the blood with subsequent resuspension of these cells with saline after discarding the globulin rich plasma. The goal is to harvest off and process half the blood volume (45 ml/kg in the dog and 30 ml/kg in the cat), while ensuring renal output is at least 2 ml/kg/hr. Once the fluids are administered to support the circulatory volume, the blood is harvested off and processed for immediate administration back to the pet. Patients generally respond quite dramatically, even if the reduction in the globulins is limited.

Key point

As an alternative to plasmapheresis, blood can be harvested from dogs and cats with clinically significant hypergammaglobulinemia; the plasma can then be removed and the RBCs resuspended in an equal volume of 0.9% NaCl for immediate reintroduction into the patient.

The long-term treatment of choice for multiple myeloma is melphalan (0.1 mg/kg daily for 10 days, then 0.5-1 mg/kg every other day PO) and prednisone (0.5-1 mg/kg daily for 21 days, then every other day thereafter PO).

In one study involving dogs,[8] multiple myeloma was confirmed in each case by observation of greater than 5% plasma cells on examination of a bone marrow aspirate and detection of monoclonal gammopathy of immunoglobulin. Treatment with melphalan, cyclophosphamide, and prednisone was associated with long-term survival (median, 540 days). Negative prognostic factors included hypercalcemia and Ig light chain proteinuria. Similar results are seen in the cat.

Other supportive care involves fluid therapy for dehydration. Because myeloma cells are believed to secrete a substance that suppresses macrophage and lymphocyte function, administration of prophylactic, broad-spectrum antibiotics should be considered, particularly in the early phases of therapy.

References

1. Ogilvie GK: Paraneoplastic syndromes, in Withrow SJ, MacEwen EG (eds): *Clinical Veterinary Oncology*. Philadelphia, JB Lippincott, 1989, pp 29–40.
2. Ogilvie GK: Paraneoplastic syndromes, in Ettinger SJ, Feldman EC (eds): *Textbook of Veterinary Internal Medicine*, ed 5. Philadelphia, WB Saunders, 2000, pp 498–506.
3. Griffin TW, Rosenthal PE, Costanza ME: Paraneoplastic and endocrine syndromes, in Cady B (ed): *Cancer Manual*, ed 7. Boston, American Cancer Society, 1986, pp 373–390.
4. Ogilvie GK: Metabolic emergencies and the cancer patient, in Wingfield WE (ed): *Veterinary Emergency Medicine Secrets*. Philadelphia, Hanley and Belfus, 2001, pp 247–251.
5. O'Connell TX, Horita TJ, Kasravi B: Understanding and interpreting serum protein electrophoresis. *Am Fam Physician* 71(1):105-112, 2005.
6. Ramaiah SK, Seguin MA, Carwile HF: Biclonal gammopathy associated with immunoglobulin A in a dog with multiple myeloma. *Vet Clin Pathol* 31(2):83-89, 2002.
7. Lautzenhiser SJ, Walker M C, Goring RL: Unusual IgM-secreting multiple myeloma in a dog. *J Am Vet Med Assoc* 223(5):611-648, 2003.
8. Matus RE, Leifer CE, MacEwen EG, et al: Prognostic factors for multiple myeloma in the dog. *J Am Vet Med Assoc* 188(11):1288-1292, 1986
9. Lane IF, Roberts SM, Lappin MR: Ocular manifestations of vascular disease: Hypertension, hyperviscosity, and hyperlipidemia. *JAAHA* 29:28–36, 1993.

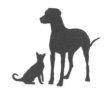

Chapter 10

Emergencies associated with extravasation of chemotherapeutic agents

Many chemotherapeutic agents are known to induce significant tissue injury after extravasation. Some of these agents are severe irreversible vesicants; others induce irritation to tissue. The agents commonly used in canine and feline medicine are listed in box 10-1. Each and every member of the veterinary health care team must be completely aware of this issue and must do everything possible to prevent drug extravasations.

The best key to prevention is awareness and training for each member of the veterinary health care team. Atraumatic placement of "first-stick" catheters, appropriate use of butterfly catheters, and adequate patient restraint, coupled with careful monitoring during administration, will prevent extravasations and the devastating consequences. Management of extravasations in human, canine and feline medicine is anecdotal and extremely controversial. Despite this controversy, guidelines (table 10-1) have been established for clinical use.

Key point

Atraumatic placement of "first-stick" catheters, appropriate use of butterfly catheters, and adequate patient restraint, coupled with careful monitoring during administration, will prevent extravasations and the devastating consequences.

PREDISPOSING FACTORS

As expected, accurate and secure "first stick" catheter placement is absolutely essential when administering drugs that can cause tissue damage if extravasated perivascularly. Generally, only small-gauge (22- to 23-ga) indwelling intravenous catheters should be used when treatment volumes exceed 1 ml; 23- to 25-ga butterfly needles can be used for administering small volumes of drugs, such as vincristine. Everyone involved in patient care should note when and where blood samples are taken by venipuncture and where catheters have been placed previously. This prevents administration of chemotherapeutic agents through veins that may leak because of previous procedures. Drawing blood samples from peripheral veins should be avoided if at all possible to preserve these veins for catheter access. Preferably all blood samples should be taken from the jugular veins to reduce damage to the peripheral veins. Only catheters that have been very recently placed (within 4 hours) should be used for administration of chemotherapeutic agents. Extreme care should be taken when administering drugs to all dogs and cats; however, there are patients that have even greater fragility of their veins. These would include extremely debilitated patients, diabetics, some aged dogs and cats, and patients that have been receiving weekly or biweekly therapy for a significant

Box 10-1. Selected drugs used in canine and feline medicine that may be vesicants or irritants when administered extravascularly [1-4]

Actinomycin D	Etoposide	Vinblastine
Daunorubicin	Mechlorethamine	Vincristine
Doxorubicin	Mithramycin	Vinorelbine
Epirubicin	Mitoxantrone	

General principle	Specific details
Table 10-1. General outline for immediate treatment of extravasation of drugs commonly used in veterinary medicine	
Minimize amount of drug at site	Do not remove the catheter or needle
	With a syringe, immediately withdraw as much drug as possible from the tissue, tubing, and catheter
	Administer antidote (see below) or sterile saline to neutralize or dilute the drug
Extravasated agent	**Antidote**
Doxorubicin, daunorubicin, epirubicin, idarubicin, and actinomycin D	Apply topical cooling with ice or cold compresses and DMSO for 6–10 hours to inhibit vesicant cytotoxicity; *do not apply heat.*
	Controversial:
	Infiltrate area with 1 mg/kg hydrocortisone
	Surgical debridement, plastic surgery, or limb amputation may be indicated in rare cases
Vincristine, vinblastine, and etoposide	Infiltrate area with 1 ml of hyaluronidase (150 units/ml) for every ml extravasated to enhance absorption and to disperse the drug
	Apply warm compresses to the site for several hours to enhance systemic absorption
	Controversial:
	• Topical DMSO
	• Infiltrate area with 1 mg/kg hydrocortisone
Mecloretamine	Locally injected sodium thiosulfate (sodium hyposulfite)

period of time. The catheter should be checked for patency with a very large injection of saline (e.g., 12–15 ml) prior to and after administration of the drug. In addition, it is mandatory that the catheter is visually monitored closely and checked for patency throughout drug infusion.

> **Key point**
>
> The catheter should be checked for patency with a very large injection of saline (e.g., 12–15 ml) prior to and after administration of the drug. The catheter must be visually monitored closely and checked for patency throughout drug infusion.

DIAGNOSIS

Usually, there is no doubt whether an extravasation has occurred. Some agents are very caustic if given perivascularly; dogs and cats may vocalize or physically react to pain at the injection site. Note that with small volumes there may be no reaction from the patient, so lack of these signs does not rule out extravasation. Treatment for extravasation must begin immediately. Evidence of tissue necrosis generally does not appear for 1 to 10 days after injection and may progress for 3 to 4 weeks. The lesions occur early with vinca alkaloids and late with anthracycline antibiotics, such as doxorubicin. Lesions may begin as mild erythema and progress to

open, draining wounds. These wounds will not heal without extensive debridement and plastic surgery weeks to months after the perivascular slough begins, when all damage is evident.

> **Key point**
>
> The perivascular administration of doxorubicin should be immediately treated, in part, with the application of cold compresses.

> **Key point**
>
> The perivascular administration of vinca alkaloids should be treated immediately, in part, with warm compresses.

TREATMENT[1-4]

Extensive training and awareness is the first step to prevention. Everyone involved with the administration of chemotherapeutic agents should be aware of procedures for treatment of extravasation (table 10-1). The procedures should be posted in a common area, and all materials needed to treat extravasations should be readily available and accessible. Because of their extensive use in canine and feline practice, doxorubicin and the vinca alkaloids are the most common causes of perivascular sloughs. Many agree that applying cold packs to a doxorubicin and warm packs to a vinca alkaloid perivascular injection may be helpful. Some believe that dexrazoxane may be of value for doxorubicin-induced perivascular injections. Regardless, no method effectively eliminates tissue necrosis. Sodium bicarbonate, corticosteroids, α-tocopherol, N-acetylcysteine, glutathione, lidocaine, diphenhydramine, cimetidine, propranolol, and isoproterenol are not known to be effective for the treatment of doxorubicin extravasations.[4]

Once tissue damage is identified, analgesics, an Elizabethan collar and bandages with nonstick pads are essential to allow the area to heal without self-trauma. Bandages should be changed daily as long as the area is draining or has the potential for infection. If a bacterial infection is noted,

culture and sensitivity testing, and appropriate administration of antimicrobials are essential. Frequent cleansing and debridement may be necessary. In some cases, reconstructive surgical repair techniques are necessary. In the event of doxorubicin extravasations, it may become necessary to amputate the limb.

References

1. Ogilvie GK: Extravasation of chemotherapeutic agents, in Wingfield WE (ed): *Veterinary Emergency Medicine Secrets*. Philadelphia, Hanley and Belfus, 2001, pp 259-260.
2. Jordan K, Grothe W, Schmoll HJ: Extravasation of chemotherapeutic agents: prevention and therapy. *Dtsch Med Wochenschr* 130(1-2):33-37, 2005.
3. Hubbard SM, Jenkins JF: Chemotherapy administration: Practical guidelines, in Chabner BA, Collins JM (eds): *Cancer Chemotherapy: Principals and Practice*. Philadelphia, JB Lippincott, 1990, pp 449–464.
4. Bertelli G. Prevention and management of extravasation of cytotoxic drugs. *Drug Saf. Apr*,12(4):211-255, 1995.

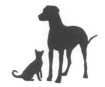

Chapter 11

Emergencies associated with chemotherapy-induced anaphylaxis and hypersensitivity

Although anaphylaxis or an anaphylaxis-like reaction can occur with any drug, these potentially life-threatening reactions usually happen soon after the administration of L-asparaginase. Hypersensitivity reactions can occur with any drug but most commonly occur with doxorubicin,[1] Taxol,[2] and etoposide.[3]

> **Key point**
>
> Although anaphylaxis or an anaphylaxis-like reaction can occur with any drug, these potentially life-threatening reactions usually happen soon after the administration of drugs such as L-asparaginase. Hypersensitivity reactions can occur with any drug but most commonly occur with doxorubicin,[1] Taxol,[2] and etoposide.[3]

L-asparaginase is well known for inducing anaphylaxis hemorrhagic pancreatitis, diabetes mellitus, and coagulopathies in humans. Anaphylaxis associated with the administration of L-asparaginase in the cat is rare. Forty-eight percent of dogs given L-asparaginase intraperitoneally developed adverse effects[4], thirty percent of these dogs exhibited signs of anaphylaxis. These findings are similar to those in children that were given L-asparaginase intravenously.[5] The same study showed that administration of the drug intramuscularly completely eliminated signs associated with anaphylaxis but did not reduce remission rates. Note that while hemorrhagic pancreatitis, diabetes mellitus, and coagulopathies may be seen in people with this drug, they were not reported by this study, nor in any others, where L-asparaginase was administered to a large number of dogs.

L-asparaginase-induced anaphylaxis and hypersensitivity are common because of enzyme immunogenicity. Anaphylaxis usually is caused by IgE-mediated mast cell degranulation; however, certain substances (e.g., bacterial and fungal cell walls) can trigger anaphylaxis by activating the alternate complement pathway. During the activation of this alternate pathway, C3a and C5a are formed. These are known potent anaphylatoxins capable of degranulating mast cells and basophils.[6] Although the exact mechanism of L-asparaginase-induced anaphylaxis in dogs and cats is largely unexplored, induction of anaphylaxis in children with acute lymphoblastic leukemia is believed to result, in part, from complement activation induced by formation of immune complexes of L-asparaginase and specific antibodies.[7] Anaphylaxis usually occurs within seconds to minutes after administration of L-asparaginase, however, some dogs and cats may have a delayed response that results in the same clinical signs hours after the drug is given.

The hypersensitivity reaction secondary to doxorubicin therapy is believed to be related, in part, to mast cell degranulation. Cremophor EL and polysorbate, the carriers used in formulations of Taxol and etoposide, respectively, are responsible for the hypersensitivity reaction induced by these drugs. It should be noted that these two carriers are sometimes found in other medications marketed for use in human patients; therefore, off label use of drugs should be used with caution for this and other reasons.

PREDISPOSING FACTORS

One predisposing factor related to anaphylaxis secondary to L-asparaginase or other drug therapy is a history of prior exposure to the drug. Because

L-asparaginase is a ubiquitous bacterial product in mammalian systems, anaphylaxis may occur after the first administration. In addition, anaphylactic and hypersensitivity reactions are worse in animals that have a prior condition such as atopy, which results in a buildup of mast cells and eosinophils prior to the drug treatment. As mentioned earlier, the route of administration of the drug may be a contributing factor to development of an anaphylactic or hypersensitivity reaction.

DIAGNOSIS

The most common clinical signs associated with drug-induced anaphylaxis are acute collapse and cardiovascular failure, which lead to shock and death. The event usually occurs within minutes after a parenteral injection of the offending drug, although some anaphylactic reactions that occur hours to days after drug therapy have been reported. The patient generally is pale and weak and usually exhibits a bradycardia or tachycardia as well as a rapid, thready pulse. Mucous membranes generally are pale to cyanotic. Peripheral extremities are often cool to the touch, and blood pressure is low.

> **Key point**
>
> The most common clinical signs associated with drug-induced anaphylaxis are acute collapse and cardiovascular failure, which lead to shock and death.

Hypersensitivity reactions may result in profound pruritus during or after administration of the drug. Pruritus may result in head shaking, and there may be swelling of the ears, lips, paws, or near the vein or area being treated. The erythematous reaction usually lasts for the duration of treatment. Occasionally, the edematous and erythematous reaction may last for hours after the treatment is finished. Alanine aminotransferase elevations may be severe necessitating supportive medication for liver disease including Denamarin and intravenous fluid therapy. Given that ALT has a half life of 60 hours in the dog and 24 hours in the cat, elevations in this parameter may lag behind evidence of clinical recovery.

THERAPY [6,8,9]

Prevention

Eighty-one dogs with histologically confirmed, measurable malignant tumors were used in a prospective study[8] to determine whether the prevalence of anaphylaxis is associated with intramuscular administration of 232 doses of L-asparaginase ($10,000 \text{ U/m}^2$). None of the dogs exhibited clinical signs associated with anaphylaxis.

Therefore, to reduce the probability of anaphylaxis, L-asparaginase should be given IM rather than IV or intraperitoneally. In addition, because L-asparaginase is a potent inducer of anaphylaxis, administration of a test dose is advised.

> **Key point**
>
> The risk of L-asparaginase-induced anaphylaxis can be reduced substantially by giving the drug intramuscularly rather than intravenously or intraperitoneally.

Hypersensitivity reactions secondary to the administration of doxorubicin can be almost completely eliminated by slow infusion the drug. One method includes diluting the drug into 150 to 500 ml of 0.9% NaCl and administering the anthracycline over 20 to 40 minutes. The author has administered literally thousands of dosages of doxorubicin, and less than 3% of patients showed any signs of hypersensitivity reactions. Some advocate pretreatment with diphenhydramine and glucocorticoids prior to doxorubicin therapy to reduce the prevalence of hypersensitivity reactions. Since these drugs have their own adverse effects and cost, the benefits of premedication may be limited.

The reactions secondary to the carriers in Taxol and etoposide can be reduced by slowing the rate of infusion and by pretreating with dexamethasone (1–2 mg/kg IV), diphenhydramine (2–4 mg/kg IM), and cimetidine (2–4 mg/kg IV slowly) one hour before infusion of the chemotherapeutic agent. If a reaction is noted, the infusion can be discontinued temporarily until the animal is more comfortable.

Treatment

Anaphylaxis is a potentially fatal condition and should be treated immediately with supportive care, fluids, glucocorticoids, H1 receptor antagonists, and epinephrine. The treatment outline is detailed in box 11-1.

Hypersensitivity reactions can be treated by terminating drug therapy. Reactions usually subside within minutes. The patient can then be treated with H1 receptor antagonists (see box 11-1) prior to re-initiating drug treatment at a much slower rate.

References

1. Ogilvie GK, Curtis C, Richardson RC, et al: Acute short term toxicity associated with the administration of doxorubicin to dogs with malignant tumors. *JAVMA* 195:1584–1587, 1989.
2. Ogilvie GK, Walters LM, Powers BE, et al: Organ toxicity of NBT taxol in the rat and dog: A preclinical study. *Proc 13th Ann Vet Canc Soc Conf*:90–91, 1993.
3. Ogilvie GK, Cockburn CA, Tranquilli WJ, Reschke RW: Hypotension and cutaneous reactions associated with etoposide administration in the dog. *Am J Vet Res* 49:1367–1370, 1988.
4. Teske E, Rutteman GR, Heerde P van, Misdorp W: Polyethylene

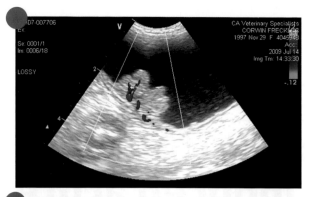

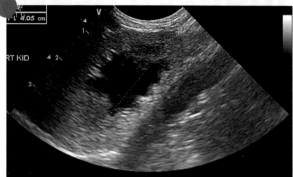

Figure 12-1: Renal failure sometimes occurs due the presence of a wide variety of malignant conditions such as transitional cell carcinoma or prostatic carcinoma or when these malignancies exist and potential nephrotoxins are administered such as NSAIDS. In this patient, a transitional cell carcinoma of the bladder (A) resulted in renal failure secondary to obstruction of the ureters and a secondary hydronephrosis (B).

Key point

Existing disease of the urinary tract and the concurrent use of nephrotoxic agents enhances the risk of developing renal disease due to the administration of chemotherapeutic agents.

As mentioned previously, cisplatin is not the only drug to cause some degree of nephrotoxicity. Doxorubicin, documented to cause chronic renal failure cats[9], has rarely been noted to cause renal failure in dogs. Another unrelated drug, methotrexate, is eliminated primarily by the kidneys and has been associated with the development of nephrotoxicity. Streptozocin, used to treat insulinomas, is a known nephrotoxin in the dog, however an appropriate 0.9% saline diuresis as is used for cisplatin is effective to mitigate this toxicity. It is not recommended in the cat.

Dogs with transitional cell carcinoma of the bladder, urethra, or prostate commonly have urethral obstruction that may lead to hydroureter, hydronephrosis, and renal dysfunction. The concurrent septic cystitis seen in most patients with bladder tumors may induce secondary pyelonephritis. This can result in acute and chronic renal failure. The drug that is commonly used to treat transitional cell carcinoma, piroxicam, can also enhance the progression of renal disease, especially when it is used in combination with the nephrotoxic chemotherapeutic agent, cisplatin.[13]

PREDISPOSING FACTORS

In veterinary medicine, the most common predisposing factors associated with the development of acute renal failure are cancer and nephrotoxic drugs, including chemotherapeutic agents. Therefore, when chemotherapeutic agents are used in veterinary patients, other nephrotoxic drugs, such as aminoglycosides, should be avoided. Other risk factors associated with the development of acute and chronic renal failure in dogs and cats are decreased cardiac output, urinary tract infection, sepsis, pre-existing renal disease, advanced age, dehydration, fever, liver disease, hypokalemia, and hypercalcemia. Several studies have shown that pre-existing renal disease may be one of the most important predisposing factors for the development of cisplatin-induced acute renal failure.

DIAGNOSIS

Acute and chronic renal failure is a result of decreased glomerular filtration rate, with or without tubular damage. Therefore, to diagnose these syndromes, the parameters used are related to damage of these structures. There may be significant renal disease for variable periods before clinical, hematologic, and biochemical abnormalities were identified, because at least two thirds of the kidney function must be abnormal before overt evidence of renal disease occurs.

Acute renal failure may occur with non-oliguria, oliguria, or anuria. Regardless of the amount of urine, it is usually isosthenuric or minimally concentrated with a high sodium content (>40 mEq/L). Glucose, protein, and renal epithelial cells may be noted in the urine. There is an acute rise in serum urea nitrogen, creatinine, and phosphorus concentrations. In oliguric or anuric renal failure, body weight, heart rate, and central venous pressure may increase if fluids are administered before urine flow is re-established.

THERAPY

The best treatment for acute or chronic renal failure is prevention. Substantial data exist to show that cisplatin nephrotoxicity can be reduced and almost eliminated with adequate hydration. The incidence of chemotherapy-induced renal failure can be reduced by not treating dogs and cats with pre-existing renal disease and by increasing the duration of time the drug is administered. Because cisplatin is a profound nephrotoxin, a brief discussion on hydration schemes used to reduce kidney damage is followed by a review of acute renal failure treatment.

Prevention

Prevention of chemotherapy-induced nephrotoxicity is best done by identifying and treating patients with underlying renal disease before chemotherapy is initiated. Performing a creatinine clearance may be helpful in predicting if pre-existing renal disease exists. In human medicine, the creatinine clearance is used to guide the reduction of the dosage of drugs as noted in table 12-1. Few guidelines exist in veterinary medicine however the general concept is logical. In the event that chemotherapy must be given, concurrent administration of fluids is essential. Cisplatin nephrotoxicity may be reduced with the administration of amifostine (WR-2721).

Many diuresis protocols exist to prevent or delay the onset of nephrotoxicity in the patient.[1,2] Because the six and four-hour protocols are most commonly used today, a brief discussion of each ensues:

Six-hour diuresis protocol: A study completed using normal dogs suggested that one dose of cisplatin could be administered safely at 70 mg/m^2 of body surface using a 6-hour diuresis protocol.[7] In that study, cisplatin was administered intravenously to six healthy dogs over a 20-minute period after 0.9% NaCl solution was administered intravenously for 4 hours at a rate of 18.3 ml/kg/hr. After the cisplatin injection, saline diuresis was continued at the same rate for 2 hours. All dogs vomited within 8 hours after the drug was administered. Clinical status, weight gain, and food consumption remained normal throughout the 27 days after the drug was administered. Nadirs in the daily neutrophil count were observed on days 6 and 15. There were no significant gross or histologic abnormalities referable to cisplatin administration when the dogs were necropsied at the conclusion of the study.

To ensure that the 6-hour diuresis protocol was safe and effective in older, tumor-bearing dogs, cisplatin (70 mg/m^2 body surface area IV every 21 days) was given to 61 dogs with malignant neoplasia for a total of 185 doses in one (n = 9 dogs), two (n = 26 dogs), three (n = 4 dogs), four (n = 9 dogs), five (n = 2 dogs), and six (n = 11 dogs) treatments. The cisplatin was given over a 20-minute period, after 0.9% NaCl solution (saline) was administered intravenously for 4 hours at a rate of 18.3 ml/kg/hr. After the cisplatin infusion, saline diuresis was continued at the same rate for 2 hours. Before each treatment with cisplatin, dogs were evaluated with at least a physical examination, CBC, serum urea nitrogen, and, in most cases, determination of serum creatinine and urine specific gravity. Four of the 61 dogs (6.6%) developed clinically evident renal disease after two (one dog), three (two dogs), and four (one dog) doses of cisplatin were administered. Three of the four dogs had pre-existing disease of the urinary tract prior to the beginning of therapy. Survival time in dogs that developed renal disease (median 145 days; range 15 to 150 days) was similar to all of the dogs in this study (median 154 days; range 30 to 500 days); 13 dogs were still alive at the conclusion of the study. Three of the four dogs that developed renal disease were euthanatized because of tumor-related causes and chronic renal failure; the fourth dog died as a direct result of the nephrotoxicity. Therefore, the 6-hour saline diuresis protocol used to administer cisplatin in this study seems to be effective in preventing nephrotoxicity in tumor-bearing dogs that did not have pre-existing urinary tract disease.

Four-hour diuresis protocol: After the 6-hour diuresis protocol was determined to be safe and effective for administering cisplatin, a 4-hour diuresis protocol was designed.10 In this study, cisplatin (70 mg/m^2 of body surface, IV, every 21 days) was given to 64 dogs that had malignant neoplasia for a total of 179 doses in one to four treatments. The cisplatin was given over a 20-minute period after 0.9% NaCl solution was administered intravenously for 3 hours at a rate of 25 mg/kg/hr. After the cisplatin infusion, saline solution diuresis was continued at the same rate for one hour. Before each treatment with cisplatin, dogs were evaluated with at least a physical examination, CBC, and determination of serum phosphorus concentration and urine specific gravity. Exogenous creatinine clearance was evaluated in eight dogs. Five of the 64 dogs developed clinically evident renal disease after two and three doses of cisplatin were administered. Two of the five dogs had pre-existing disease of the urinary tract prior to the beginning of treatment. Median survival time in dogs that developed renal disease was 114 days; the range was from 5 to 586 days. Thirty dogs were still alive at the conclusion of the study. Three of the five dogs that developed renal disease were alive at the conclusion of the study, one died of the cancer, and the fifth dog died as a result of renal damage. The neutrophil counts decreased and the creatinine concentrations increased prior to the third and fourth treatments compared to pretreatment values. It was concluded from this study that up to four doses of cisplatin can be safely administered using the 4-hour diuresis protocol with minimal nephrotoxicity. Because the 4-hour diuresis protocol was relatively safe, an additional study was initiated to see if a 1-hour diuresis protocol was safe.

Treatment for acute renal failure [12,13]

The initial goals for treating drug- and tumor-related acute renal failure in dogs and cats are to discontinue all drugs that may be nephrotoxic, document prerenal or postrenal abnormalities, and initiate fluid therapy (table 12-2). The primary objectives for fluid therapy are to:

- Correct deficits (such as dehydration) and excesses (such as volume overload) seen in oliguric renal failure.
- Supply maintenance needs.
- Supplement ongoing losses that occur with vomiting and diarrhea.

Key point

Maintenance requirements differ for each individual, however a quick formula that can be used to approximate the fluid needs is 66 ml/kg/day in dogs and 44 ml/kg/day in cats, plus an amount of fluid equal to external fluid losses, such as vomiting and diarrhea. Patients with renal failure require 1.5 to 3 times this amount to achieve a diuresis.

Table 12-2. Example of fluid therapy needs for a 10-kg dog that is 5% dehydrated and has diarrhea	
Fluids needed	**Calculation**
To correct dehydration	5% (0.05) × 10 kg body weight = 0.5 kg of water needed to correct dehydration
	1000 ml/kg of water × 0.5 kg = 500 ml of water needed to correct dehydration
	75% (0.75) × 500 ml = 375 ml of fluid should be administered to replace 75% dehydration
To meet daily needs	66 ml/kg (daily requirements) × 10 kg body weight = 660 ml needed on a daily basis
	Increase this amount from 1.5–3 times to induce a mild to moderate diuresis in renal failure patients, ensuring urine output exceeds 2 ml/kg/hr
To replace ongoing losses	Estimated losses through diarrhea = 200 ml
Total (first 24 hrs)	375 ml + 660 ml + 200 ml = 1235 ml; increase fluid therapy judiciously to increase urine output, sustaining a mild to moderate diuresis

Each patient must be assessed carefully, and a treatment plan must be tailored based on the hydration status, cardiovascular performance, and biochemical data. A general approach to patients in renal failure is shown in table 12-3. Maintenance requirements vary from 44 to 110 ml/kg body weight; smaller animals generally require the larger amount as their metabolic rate per kilogram is higher than larger animals. Maintenance requirements differ for each individual, however a quick formula that can be used to approximate the fluid needs is 66 ml/kg/day plus an amount of fluid equal to external fluid losses, such as vomiting and diarrhea. This is the amount of fluid that is needed daily for maintenance. In patients with renal failure, 1.5 to 3 times this amount of fluid is administered daily to achieve a diuresis. Care should be directed to ensure that excessive amounts of fluids are not being administered by monitoring body weight, blood pressures and central venous pressures. The success of this diuresis can be monitored by documenting adequate urine output (>2 ml/kg/hr). Fluid therapy should meet daily needs, replace excessive losses, and correct dehydration. The percentage of dehydration should be determined; approximately 75% of the fluid needed to correct the dehydration should be administered during the first 24 hours. Fluid therapy should be altered to correct electrolyte and acid–base abnormalities. For animals in acute renal failure, potassium-containing fluids generally are not good choices, because systemic hyperkalemia often occurs in these patients. Until more is known about the systemic effects of sepsis, lactate-containing fluids should be avoided because sepsis and cancer are associated with hyperlactatemia, which worsens with the administration of lactate-containing fluids.

If oliguric renal failure is present, a diligent and aggressive approach should be made to increase urine output. This can be done by first increasing glomerular filtration rate and renal blood flow. Additionally, an osmotic diuresis can be used with caution to increase urine flow. If urine output is less than 0.5 to 2.0 ml/kg/hr despite aggressive fluid therapy, furosemide should be administered every 1 to 3 hours. Furosemide will increase glomerular filtration rate and enhance diuresis in many patients. If furosemide is not effective, mannitol or 50% dextrose can be used as an osmotic diuretic to enhance urine production. The advantage of dextrose over mannitol is that dextrose can be detected on a urine glucose test strip. If the furosemide and osmotic diuretics are not effective, dopamine can be administered as a constant rate infusion. Dopamine enhances renal blood flow and increases urine output secondarily.

Key point

If oliguric renal failure is present, a diligent and aggressive approach should be made to increase urine output.

Treatment for acute renal failure should be continued until the patient improves substantially and until abnormal biochemical parameters have been corrected or are at least stabilized. The therapy should then be tapered off over several days, and a home treatment plan should be developed that includes avoiding nephrotoxic drugs; feeding a high-quality, low-quantity protein diet; maintaining a low-stress environment; and providing fresh, clean water ad libitum.

References

1. Page R, Matus RE, Leifer CE, et al: Cisplatin, a new antineoplastic drug in veterinary medicine. *J Am Vet Med Assoc* 186:288–290, 1985.
2. Mehlhaff CJ, Leifer CE, Patnaik AK, et al: Surgical treatment of pulmonary neoplasia in 15 dogs. *J Am Vet Med Assoc* 20:799–803, 1984.
3. Himsel CA, Richardson RC, Craig JA: Cisplatin chemotherapy for metastatic squamous cell carcinoma in two dogs. *JAVMA* 89:1575–1578, 1986.
4. Shapiro W, Fossum TW, Kitchell BE, et al: Use of cisplatin for treatment of appendicular osteosarcoma in dogs. *J Am Vet Med Assoc* 192:507–511, 1988.
5. LaRue SM, Withrow SJ, Powers BE, et al: Limb-sparing treatment for osteosarcoma in dogs. *JAVMA* 195: 1734–1744, 1989.
6. Cvitkovic E, Spaulding J, Bethune V, et al: Improvement of cis-dichlorodiammineplatinum (NSC 119875): Therapeutic index in an animal model. *Cancer* 39:1357–1361, 1977.
7. Ogilvie GK, Krawiec DR, Gelberg HB, et al: Evaluation of a short-term

General principle	Specific details
Stop nephrotoxins	E.G.: discontinue cisplatin, methotrexate, doxorubicin, and aminoglycosides; avoid anesthesia

Assess patient	CBC, urinalysis, and biochemical profile
	Urine culture and sensitivity
	Specifically, determine:
	    Percentage of dehydration
	    Amount of ongoing losses (e.g., vomiting, diarrhea, blood loss, etc.)
	    Maintenance fluid requirements
	    Electrolyte and biochemical abnormalities
	    Cardiovascular performance
	    Urine output

Administer fluids	Tailor therapy to needs of each patient:
	    Isotonic polyionic fluid initially
	    Correct dehydration first over 6 to 8 hours to prevent further renal ischemia while watching carefully for pathologic oliguria and subsequent volume overload
	    Meet maintenance requirements (approximately 66 ml/kg/day)
	    Meet ongoing losses (e.g., vomiting and diarrhea)
	    Induce a mild to moderate diuresis (>2 mls/kg/hr)

Monitor urine output	Metabolism cage or indwelling catheter
	For inadequate output (<0.5–2.0 ml/kg/hr):
	    Mannitol or dextrose 0.5–1.0 g/kg in a slow IV bolus
	    Furosemide 2–4 mg/kg IV q 1–3 hours PRN
	    Dopamine 1–3 µg/kg/min IV (50 mg dopamine in 500 ml of 5% dextrose = 100 µg/ml solution)

Correct acid–base and electrolytes	Rule out hypercalcemia of malignancy; treat specifically for that, if identified
Induce diuresis	Urine output: 2–5 ml/kg/hr; monitor body weight, heart and respiratory rate, and central venous pressure for signs of overhydration
Consider peritoneal dialysis if not responsive	Temporary or chronic ambulatory peritoneal dialysis with specific dialysate solution may be helpful
Initiate long-term plans	Continue diuresis until BUN and creatinine normalize or until these values stop improving despite aggressive therapy and a clinically stable patient, then gradually taper fluids Control hyperphosphatemia, if indicated (e.g., aluminum hydroxide, 500 mg at each feeding) Treat gastric hyperacidity, if indicated (cimetidine, 4 mg/kg every 6 hrs, IV or PO)

Table 12-3. Support for patient in renal failure

saline diuresis protocol for the administration of cisplatin. *Am J Vet Res* 49:1076–1078, 1988.

8. Rassnick KM, Frimberger AE, Wood CA, et al: Evaluation of ifosfamide for treatment of various canine neoplasms. *J Vet Intern Med* 14(3):271-276, 2000.

9. Cotter SM, Kanki PJ, Simon M: Renal disease in five tumor-bearing cats treated with Adriamycin. *J Am Anim Hosp Assoc* 21:405–412, 1985.

10. Ogilvie GK, Straw RC, Jameson VJ, et al: Prevalence of nephrotoxicosis associated with a four hour saline solution diuresis protocol for the administration of cisplatin to dogs with sarcomas: 64 cases (1989–1991). *JAVMA* 202:1845–1848, 1993.

11. Ogilvie GK, Fettman MJ, Jameson VJ, et al: Evaluation of a one hour saline diuresis protocol for the administration of cisplatin to dogs. *Am J Vet Res* 53: 1666–1669, 1992.

12. Couto CG: Management of complications of cancer chemotherapy. *Vet Clin North Am Small Anim Pract* 21:1037–1053, 1990.

13. Mohammed SI, Craig BA, Mutsaers AJ, et al: Effects of the cyclooxygenase inhibitor, piroxicam, in combination with chemotherapy on tumor response, apoptosis, and angiogenesis in a canine model of human invasive urinary bladder cancer. *Mol Cancer Ther* 2(2):183-188, 2003.

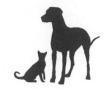

Chapter 13

Emergencies associated with acute tumor lysis syndrome

Acute tumor lysis syndrome (ATLS) is an under-reported, rare condition of acute collapse that may lead to death soon after administration of a chemotherapeutic agent or radiation therapy for a chemotherapy or radiation sensitive tumor.[1-3] ATLS most often occurs shortly after the treatment of lymphoma and lymphoid leukemia, or may occur after effective chemotherapy in dogs and cats with rapidly growing, bulky, chemosensitive tumors.[4,5] Affected dogs and cats present to the veterinary health care team with a history of acute decompensation over a short period, sometimes to the point of imminent death. Rapid diagnosis and therapy are essential to reduce mortality.

> **Key point**
> Rapid tumor lysis causes an acute release of intracellular phosphate and potassium resulting in clinical signs associated with hypocalcemia, hyperkalemia, and hyperphosphatemia.

PREDISPOSING FACTORS

The actual pathophysiology of ATLS in dogs and cats is unstudied and therefore unknown. In humans, and probably in dogs and cats, rapid tumor lysis may cause an acute release of intracellular phosphate and potassium.[1-5] This release of electrolytes causes hypocalcemia, hyperkalemia, and hyperphosphatemia. In human patients who undergo ATLS, hyperuricemia is also seen.[1-3] As noted earlier, ATLS is most common in lymphoma or leukemia patients, partly because the intracellular concentration of phosphorus in human lymphoma and leukemic cells is 4 to 6 times higher than in normal cells.[1] Unpublished clinical experience suggests that acute tumor lysis syndrome is most common in dogs and cats with some degree of volume contraction and a large tumor mass that responds rapidly to cytolytic therapy. In addition, septic dogs and cats, or pets with extensive neoplastic disease that

infiltrates the parenchyma of organs, are predisposed to ATLS. Canine and feline patients at highest risk are volume-contracted dogs with stage IV or V lymphoma that are treated with chemotherapy or radiation therapy and that undergo very rapid remission; therefore, this condition may be identified within 48 hours after the first treatment.

> **Key point**
> The metabolic disturbances associated with tumor lysis syndrome can lead to life-threatening complications including arrhythmias and acute renal failure.

DIAGNOSIS

Dogs and cats with suspected cases of ATLS are presented with clinical signs similar to those seen with neutropenic, septic dogs and cats and are often diagnosed after acute collapse and decompensation hours to days after the administration of chemotherapy.[4,5] To reduce morbidity and mortality, rapid diagnosis and therapy for ATLS is essential. Patients with ATLS may show cardiovascular collapse, vomiting, diarrhea, and ensuing shock. The hyperkalemia may rarely result in bradycardia with diminished P-wave amplitude and spiked T-waves on an electrocardiogram. Biochemical analysis of blood may confirm the presence of hypocalcemia, hyperkalemia, and hyperphosphatemia. However, if several hours have passed after decompensation, hyperkalemia and hyperphosphatemia may have corrected. Hyperuricemia (seen in humans with ATLS) has not been identified in dogs and cats. In the presence of elevated serum phosphate levels, hypocalcemia develops as a result of calcium and phosphate precipitation. Without effective treatment, cardiovascular collapse, shock or renal failure may occur in this syndrome; therefore, the blood urea nitrogen (BUN) and creatinine concentrations should be monitored closely.

General principle		Specific details
Treat decompensation (hours to days after therapy for a chemoresponsive tumor)	Evaluate the patient	Determine whether tumor has responded rapidly and dramatically
		Perform complete physical examination to evaluate for systemic disease, hydration status, cardiac output, etc.
		Rule in or out neutropenia, sepsis, coagulopathies, and organ failure with complete blood count, biochemical profile, urinalysis, blood cultures, etc.
Initiate specific support	Treat for shock.	Consider non-lactate-containing fluids
	Provide daily fluid needs, correct dehydration, correct electrolyte abnormalities, and compensate for external fluid losses	In ATLS, 0.9% NaCl may be ideal until hyperkalemia and hyperphosphatemia are corrected
		Fluids can be administered during acute shock or shock-like states at a rate of 40–60 ml/kg/hr for the first hour, followed by 10-12 ml/kg/hr with very close monitoring to adjust fluid rate as needed
		If hypocalcemia secondary to hyperphosphatemia causes clinically significant clinical signs (rare), exogenous parenteral calcium supplementation may be indicated
Monitor	Monitor hydration, electrolytes, and renal and cardiovascular function	Rate of fluid administration must be "fine-tuned" based on ongoing re-evaluation of hydration, cardiovascular, renal, and electrolyte status

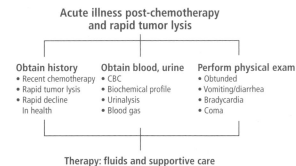

Acute illness post-chemotherapy and rapid tumor lysis

- **Obtain history**
  - Recent chemotherapy
  - Rapid tumor lysis
  - Rapid decline In health
- **Obtain blood, urine**
  - CBC
  - Biochemical profile
  - Urinalysis
  - Blood gas
- **Perform physical exam**
  - Obtunded
  - Vomiting/diarrhea
  - Bradycardia
  - Coma

Therapy: fluids and supportive care

Figure 13-1: Clinical approach to acute tumor lysis syndrome (ATLS).

Key point

Dogs and cats with acute tumor lysis syndrome often present with a history of acute decompensation, sometimes to the point of imminent death (within hours of presentation).[1-3]

Treatment

The best treatment is prevention. Because the kidneys are the main source of electrolyte excretion, metabolic abnormalities may be exacerbated in dogs and cats with renal dysfunction. Identification and correction of any volume depletion or azotemia prior to initiation of therapy may reduce the risk of ATLS; chemotherapy should be delayed until metabolic disturbances, such as azotemia, are corrected.

If ATLS is identified, the condition should be treated with aggressive crystalloid fluid therapy (table 13-1) and careful monitoring of electrolytes and renal parameters. The following general steps are taken:[1-5]

- Establish central venous access.
- Obtain blood and urine samples, pretreatment.
- Assess ECG continually.
- Start fluid therapy. Consider non-lactate containing fluids. Consider isotonic or hypotonic saline.
- Perform serial laboratory evaluations to assess changes in electrolytes (serial lactate, Na+, K+, creatinine, BUN, phosphorus, Ca+).
- Monitor urine output.
- Initiate hemodialysis if recovery is not rapid. Further chemotherapy should be withheld until the patient is clinically normal and all biochemical parameters have stabilized.

References

1. Marcus SL, Einzig AI: Acute tumor lysis syndrome: Prevention and management, in Dutcher JP, Wiernik PH (eds): *Handbook of Hematologic and Oncologic Emergencies.* New York, Plenum Press, 1987, pp 9–15.
2. Woodlock TJ: Oncologic emergencies, in Rosenthal S, Carignan JR, Smith BD (eds): *Medical Care of the Cancer Patient*, ed 2. Philadelphia, WB Saunders, 1993, pp 236–246.
3. Couto CG: Management of complications of cancer chemotherapy. *Vet Clin North Am Small Anim Pract* 4:1037–1053, 1990.
4. Page RL : Acute tumor lysis syndrome: *Semin Vet Med Surg* (Small Anim) 1(1):58-60, 1986.
5. Piek CJ, Teske E: [Tumor lysis syndrome in a dog] *Tijdschr Diergeneeskd* 121(3):64-66, 1996.

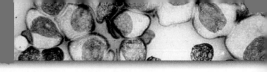

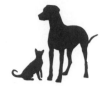

Chapter 14

Emergencies associated with disseminated intravascular coagulation

Disorders of hemostasis are an under-reported and under-recognized cause of morbidity and mortality in veterinary and human cancer patients.[1-10] This phenomenon is commonly recognized in veterinary medicine and can be almost diagnostic for certain types of malignancies. In one study,[3] the incidence of one type of coagulopathy, disseminated intravascular coagulopathy, was 9.6% in the 208 dogs explored with a malignant tumor. In that same study, the incidence of DIC was 12.2% of 164 dogs with malignant solid tumors. The incidence of DIC in dogs with hemangiosarcoma, mammary gland carcinoma, and adenocarcinoma of the lung was significantly higher than in dogs with other malignant tumors. Mast cell tumors can not only induce coagulopathies systemically, but also a localized, compartmentalized coagulopathy recognized clinically as significant bruising, or surgically as uncontrolled hemorrhage. These results suggested that special care in looking for DIC should be taken in dogs with a malignant solid tumor.

The etiology of this condition is not as clearly defined in cats as in dogs and people. Until more is known, some find it helpful to characterize this condition in the following categories:[1-4]

1. Disseminated intravascular coagulopathy.
2. Malignancy-associated fibrinolysis.
3. Platelet abnormalities.
4. Clinical syndrome of the hypercoagulable state of malignancy.
5. Chemotherapy-associated (e.g., L-asparaginase) thromboembolism.

Disseminated intravascular coagulation is a consumptive coagulopathy that often results in a life-threatening condition. Disseminated intravascular coagulopathy has been associated with the above parameters 2 through 5 and occurs with many malignancies. The malignancy sometimes induces DIC when clotting factors are activated by tumor-induced procoagulants or when the tumor directly or indirectly stimulates platelet aggregation. The resultant formation of clots in the circulation consumes clotting factors and platelets, which leads to widespread bleeding. In addition, deposition of fibrin throughout the body may result in concurrent microangiopathic hemolytic anemia. To reduce morbidity and mortality, DIC must be prevented or identified and treated early.

PREDISPOSING FACTORS

Disseminated intravascular coagulopathy occurs with a wide variety of malignant conditions including hemangiosarcoma, lymphoma, mast cell tumors, lung tumors, and mammary adenocarcinoma. Treatment with chemotherapeutic agents, surgery, or concurrent infection may induce or exacerbate DIC. Renal failure and loss of low molecular weight coagulation factors through glomeruli may increase the risk of coagulation abnormalities. Thrombosis with or without DIC has been identified in dogs with hyperadrenocorticism and in dogs that have been treated with high doses of glucocorticoids. The syndrome is more common in dogs than in cats. Other predisposing factors include:[1-4]

- Extrinsic vascular compression and/or tumor invasion.
- Tissue necrosis.
- Production of procoagulants by the cancer.
- Activation of platelets and increased accumulation of platelets around the cancer.
- Inflammation induction of factor VIII, fibrinogen, and von Willebrand factor.
- Deficiencies in endogenous anticoagulants.
- Presence of intravenous catheters.
- Damage to endothelial cells by chemotherapeutic agents.
- Doxorubicin-induced heart failure.
- Immobility due to lethargy, anorexia and anemia.

DIAGNOSIS

Clinical signs supportive of a diagnosis of DIC include, but are not limited to, oozing from venipuncture sites, nosebleeds, oral bleeding, melena, ecchymoses and petechial hemorrhages anywhere on the body, and hematuria.[1-4,5-7] Widespread thrombosis can cause multi-organ failure that may result in a variety of clinical signs, such as acute renal failure and acute onset of respiratory distress. Laboratory abnormalities associated with DIC vary depending on the organs involved and whether the DIC is acute or chronic (see table 5-1); the chronic form of DIC is rarely associated with clinical signs. In addition, alterations in red blood cell morphology, such as fragmentation, may result from microangiopathic events that occur in this syndrome. There are many causes for the decreased platelet count and coagulation factor deficiencies seen with DIC. Diagnosis is based on clinical findings and laboratory parameters (table 14-1), including: [1-4,5-7]

- Decreased PCV (<37%) that may be evident within a few hours.
- Hypoproteinemia (<5.5 g/dl) with external blood loss.
- Prolonged buccal mucosal bleeding time (>4 minutes) seen in thrombopathies and von Willebrand disease.
- Reduced von Willebrand factor (<65%) as seen in von Willebrand disease.
- Increased prothrombin time (PT) >16 seconds as seen with extrinsic and common coagulopathies.
- Increased activated partial thromboplastin time (APTT), >16 seconds as seen with intrinsic and common coagulopathies.
- Thrombocytopenia (<8-15 per high power field or <150,000/ul).
- Prolonged activated coagulation time (ACT), >110 seconds as seen with intrinsic and common coagulopathies.
- Decreased antithrombin III (AT-III) concentrations <90% seen with thrombosis.
- Hypofibrinoginemia < 100 mg/dl.
- Increased fibrin degradation products (FDPs) >1:5 seen with fibrin degradation.
- D-dimers >250 ug/dl seen with fibrin degradation.

> **Key point**
> Clinical signs supportive of a diagnosis of DIC include, but are not limited to, oozing from venipuncture sites, nosebleeds, oral bleeding, melena, ecchymoses and petechial hemorrhages anywhere on the body, and hematuria.

There are many causes for DIC-associated abnormalities.[1-4,5-7] Decreased platelet count can be caused by bone marrow failure, increased platelet consumption, or splenic pooling of platelets.

Prolonged PT may result from lack of one or more of the following clotting factors: VII, X, V, II (prothrombin), and I (fibrinogen). Increased APTT time may be cause by a deficiency in one or more of the following clotting factors: XII, XI, IX, VIII, X, V, II, and I. Heparin and oral anticoagulant therapy prolongs the APTT. Low fibrinogen levels are associated with decreased production or increased consumption of this protein.

One of the consequences of DIC is deep venous thrombosis. Diagnosis of these thromboses often relies on one or more of the following: [1-4,5-7]

- Contrast venography.
- [^{125}I]-fibrinogen scan.
- [^{99m}Technetium]-apcitide scintigraphy.
- Contrast ultrasonography.
- Lung scintigraphy.
- Duplex ultrasound.
- Magnetic resonance venography.
- Helical computerized tomography.
- D-dimer levels, although these are less sensitive for cancer.

TREATMENT [1-4]

The clinical signs associated with DIC are often not exhibited until quite late in the course of the disease in dogs and cats. Therefore treatment must begin as soon as possible. Specific treatment for DIC is controversial, but certain procedures are uniformly accepted despite the fact that few data document their efficacy. Treatment revolves around the following:

- Eliminate the underlying cause: The most important therapy for DIC is treatment of the underlying cause.
- Fluids: Fluid therapy is essential to correct volume contraction and to reduce the possibility of ensuing renal failure and acid-base abnormalities. Fluid administration, body weight and urine output must be carefully monitored in all dogs and cats. Increases in body weight, heart and respiratory rates, and central venous pressure may suggest volume overload. Volume overload is especially threatening in dogs and cats that are anuric secondary to acute renal shutdown.
- Transfusion support: In dogs and cats with severe bleeding diatheses, fresh blood or plasma with clotting factors and platelets may be useful for replacing components of the blood that are consumed.
- Heparin therapy: If thrombosis appears to be the most clinically evident problem, heparin therapy may reduce the formation of thrombi. The amount of heparin to be used is controversial. Methods include administration of heparin by intermittent subcutaneous or intravenous dosages, or by constant-rate infusion, to prolong the APTT by 1.5-2 times. Minidose heparin therapy may be helpful in some cases. The following treatment protocols are used, however data on efficacy is limited:

Tests/Observations	Acute DIC	Chronic DIC
Clinical signs	Clinically evident coagulopathies	Few clinical signs
Onset and duration	Rapid onset and quick progression	Insidious and prolonged
PT, APTT, and ACT	Prolonged	Normal to decreased
Platelets	Decreased	Often normal
FDPs/D-Dimers	Very high	High
Fibrinogen	Decreased to normal	Normal
Antithrombin III	Reduced	Normal
Prognosis	Grave	Good

- Mini dose: 5 to 10 IU/kg SQ q8h
- Low dose: 50 to 100 IU/kg SQ q8h
- Intermediate dose: 300 to 500 IU/kg SQ or IV q8h
- High dose: 750 to 1000 IU/kg SQ or IV q8h
- Discontinuation of therapy: Chemotherapeutic agents, including prednisone, should be withheld until all evidence of DIC is eliminated and the patient has recovered completely. It is known that dogs and humans that receive glucocorticoid therapy are at major risk for thromboembolic events that can initiate or perpetuate DIC; this is likely true for cats as well.

Key point

The clinical signs associated with DIC are often not exhibited until quite late in the course of the disease, therefore treatment must begin as soon as possible.

Dogs and cats with acute DIC have a poor prognosis; therefore, identification of patients at high risk and initiation of prophylactic treatment are of great value. Routine monitoring of ACTs and platelet counts can identify dogs and cats in the early phases of DIC.

Key point

Dogs and cats with acute DIC have a poor prognosis; therefore, identification of patients at high risk and initiation of prophylactic treatment are of great value.

References

1. Ogilvie GK. Acute tumor lysis syndrome. In Wingfield WE. *Veterinary Emergency Medicine Secrets.* Hanley and Belfus, Philadelphia. P 28-243, 2001.
2. Smith MR: Disorders of hemostasis and transfusion therapy, in Skeel RT (ed): *Handbook of Cancer Chemotherapy*, ed 3. Boston, Little, Brown & Co, 1991, pp 449–459.
3. Maruyama H, Miura T, Sakai M, et al: The incidence of disseminated intravascular coagulation in dogs with malignant tumor: *J Vet Med Sci* 66(5):573-575, 2004.
4. Woodlock TJ: Oncologic emergencies, in Rosenthal S, Carignan JR, Smith BD (eds): *Medical Care of the Cancer Patient*, ed 2. Philadelphia, WB Saunders, 1993, pp 236–246.
5. Hackner SG: Approach to the diagnosis of bleeding disorders. *Compend Contin Educ Pract Vet* 17:331-349, 1995.
6. Bateman SW, Mathews KA, Abrams-Ogg AC et al: Diagnosis of disseminated intravascular coagulation in dogs admitted to an intensive care unit. *J Am Vet Med Assoc* 215(6):798-804, 1999.
7. Nelson OL, Andreasen C: The utility of plasma D-dimer to identify thromboembolic disease in dogs. *J Vet Intern Med* 17(6):830-834, 2003.
8. Golden DL, Langston VC: Use of vincristine and vinblastine in dogs. JAVMA 193:1114-1117, 1988.
9. Slappendel RJ: *Disseminated* intravascular coagulation. *Vet Clin North Am Small Anim Pract* 18:169-84, 1988.
10. Couto CG: Disseminated intravascular coagulation in dogs. *Vet Med* 94:513-554, 1999.

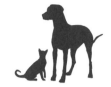

Chapter 15

Emergencies of cancer related disorders of the central nervous system

Cancer or cancer therapy-related disorders of the brain, spinal cord, and peripheral nerves are being recognized more and more often in veterinary medicine. Many of the causes of these disorders impact the central and peripheral nervous systems simultaneously, however some of the more important conditions will be discussed below under neurologic disorders of the brain, spinal cord and peripheral nerves. The ultimate therapeutic goal is to eliminate the underlying cause and to mitigate the clinical signs that can range from very subtle weakness to overt seizures or paralysis.

DISORDERS OF THE BRAIN

The most common disorders of the brain include subtle neurologic clinical signs secondary to a paraneoplastic syndrome to serious, life-threatening emergencies due to meningitis, a brain tumor, bleeding secondary to drug-induced thrombocytopenia, or chemotherapy-induced neurotoxicity.[1-5] The paraneoplastic syndromes most commonly recognized in veterinary medicine as having an impact on the central nervous system include hypercalcemia of malignancy (e.g.: secondary to anal sac adenocarcinoma or lymphoma), hypoglycemia (e.g.: secondary to insulinoma or carcinoma of the liver), hyperviscosity syndrome caused by hyperglobulinemia (e.g.: secondary to multiple myeloma), or erythrocytosis (e.g.: polycythemia). Other, less defined paraneoplastic syndromes that cause disorders of the central nervous system are also suspected in the dog and cat and are reviewed below. Radiation can cause late effects within the brain, especially when larger dosages are given over a short period of time resulting in mental dullness, depression and, on occasion, seizures and death. Chemotherapy-induced seizures in dogs are reported with 5-fluorouracil (contraindicated in cats). Additional drugs that have been shown to

cause this clinical sign in human beings include:
- L-asaparaginase, which may cause seizures by inducing cerebrovascular events.
- Cisplatin, which may cause a cortical blindness, reversible encephalopathy syndrome and ototoxicity (fatal in cats).
- Cytosine arabinoside, which may cause a leukoencepalopathy.
- Ifosfamide, which may cause an encephalopathy.
- Methotrexate, which is associated in rare situations with a leukoencephalopathy.
- Thalidomide causes a profound somnolence that can last for hours or days after each dosage.

Because brain herniation and seizures are relatively common life-threatening emergencies, they are reviewed in more detail below.

Brain herniation
Predisposing factors

Brain herniation can be caused by a wide variety of primary or secondary malignancies of the brain or by intracerebral hemorrhage and intradural hematoma, brain abscess, and acute hydrocephalus. Primary lung tumors, hemangiosarcoma, and malignant melanoma are examples of tumors that metastasize to the brain. Regardless of the cause, diagnosis must be made swiftly and therapy initiated without hesitation to prevent irreparable neurologic damage or death.

Clinical signs

Brain herniation is characterized by any CNS abnormality, including progressive drowsiness, small reactive pupils, periodic respirations (Cheyne-Stokes), and, in the most severe cases, bilateral extensor rigidity.[2,4] As the herniation evolves, hyperventilation, disconjugate eye movements, pupillary fixation, and abnormal motor postures can be noted. The "brain–heart syndrome" may be evident if the brain stem is compressed. This syndrome is associated with potentially fatal arrhythmias due to the presence of a central nervous system disturbance.

> **Key point**
>
> In the "brain–heart syndrome," the clinician may be distracted by the occurrence of bizarre arrhythmias that are actually caused by compression of the cardiac control center and centers of the brain that regulate autonomic control of the heart.

Diagnosis

The diagnosis and decision to treat are based primarily on the presence of relatively rapidly developing abnormal neurologic signs. Because the decision to withhold therapy may result in death or severe neurologic abnormalities that persist for the remainder of a pet's life, treatment should be initiated immediately or concurrently with diagnostic methods, such as computerized tomography (CT), magnetic resonance imaging (MRI), nuclear scans, and, if available, an electroencephalogram. A CSF tap at the cisterna magna may actually cause or exacerbate brain herniation; therefore, this procedure should not be used if increased intracranial pressure is suspected.

Treatment

The goals are to prevent further herniation and to treat existing herniation and the underlying cause.[2,4] Intubation and control of respiration may be required when hyperventilation produces cerebral vasoconstriction, decreased blood volume, and decreased intracranial pressure. Mannitol (1–2 g/kg QID IV slowly) can reduce brain water content, reduce brain volume, and decrease intracranial pressure rapidly. Steroids (e.g., dexamethasone NaPO$_4$ [2 mg/kg IV once, followed by 0.25 mg/kg QID IV]) can be administered acutely but may take hours to have full effect. Hydrocortisone (10–50 mg/kg IV) given at the time of brain trauma may be beneficial.[2,4] In rare cases, surgical decompression may be beneficial. Once treatment is underway, plain and contrast CT or other imaging techniques may help identify the cause of decompensation in the neurologic patient.

Seizures

Predisposing factors

A variety of metastatic and nonmetastatic conditions can cause seizures in veterinary cancer patients. Vascular disorders, such as intracerebral hemorrhage, subdural hematomas, and thrombosis of the CNS vessels, may be associated with seizures. Hypoglycemia secondary to insulinoma or hepatic tumor may induce CNS abnormalities.[1,2,4,5] Several chemotherapeutic agents (e.g., 5-fluorouracil, cisplatin, mitoxantrone, and vincristine), radiation therapy, and radiosensitizers are reported to cause seizures.[3,4]

Clinical presentation

Seizures may appear clinically as one of the following: partial (focal or local), simple partial (symmetric and rarely associated with loss of consciousness), complex partial (alterations in consciousness plus complex behavior), generalized seizures (involuntary, uncontrolled motor activity), and generalized nonconvulsive seizures (loss of consciousness with lack of spontaneous motor activity and transient collapse).[1,2] There is generally an aura or period of behavioral change before each type of seizure, followed by ictus or the actual clinical seizure, and finally a postictal period that lasts for approximately 30 minutes, during which the animal exhibits abnormal behavior that may include weakness and blindness. If malignancy is associated with the condition, the seizures generally get progressively worse over time because of the enlarging intracranial mass or because of progressive worsening of hypoglycemia in insulin-producing tumors.

Diagnosis

The diagnosis generally is evident from the historical or physical findings. In an emergency situation (often associated with a dog or cat in status epilepticus), a definitive diagnosis is made after the patient is stabilized. A diagnosis is generally made with imaging techniques that include skull radiographs, CT, nuclear imaging, or MRI of the brain. If a neoplasm is suspected, a complete staging scheme must be initiated as soon as the animal is stable. This should include a complete history, complete physical and neurologic examinations, CBC, biochemical profile, urinalysis, thoracic and abdominal radiographs, fasting (>24 hours) blood glucose and insulin levels, a CSF tap if the animal is not at risk for brain herniation, and an electroencephalogram, if available.

Treatment

Caution should be used when handling the seizuring patient. The general schema for a seizuring patient is noted in table 15-1; table 15-2 lists anticonvulsants used in acute situations to treat seizuring dogs and cats. If a seizure is in progress, diazepam should be administered intravenously. Respiration should be monitored and, when necessary, intubation and ventilation should be considered. In these patients, phenobarbital can be given via a loading dose, which is followed by a maintenance dose. Phenobarbital therapy also may be valuable when a single seizure is expected to continue or if clusters of seizures occur within a short period.

Table 15-1. Emergency procedures for status epilepticus

General principle	Specific details
Evaluate the patient	Brief history and physical examination
Place indwelling catheter	Acquire blood samples; determine glucose and calcium levels while therapy is initiated
Stop the seizures	Administer diazepam IV (2.5–15.0 mg)
	For hypoglycemia, administer 0.5 g dextrose as a 25% solution given IV over 5 minutes; for hypocalcemia, administer 1.0–1.5 ml/kg of 10% calcium gluconate solution ; if necessary, repeat diazepam bolus every 10 minutes for 3 dosages
	If diazepam is inadequate for seizure control, administer phenobarbital intravenously (see table 15-2)
	Acid–base status, ability to ventilate, body temperature, electrolyte balance, and hydration status are monitored and treated appropriately
Monitor during recovery	Phenobarbital may be administered (0.5 mg/kg TID IV) to reduce seizures; monitor blood levels. When seizures are controlled and the patient is able to swallow, oral phenobarbital therapy should be continued
Initiate definitive diagnostics	CBC, biochemical profile and fasting blood glucose and insulin measurement, CSF tap, CT or MRI of the brain (if indicated), and electroencephalogram (if available)

Table 15-2. Anticonvulsants used in an acute situation to treat seizures

Anticonvulsant	Recommended dosages	General indications, and precautions
Phenobarbital	5–16 mg/kg/day divided BID–TID	Drug of choice for long-term seizure control; half-life: 40 hours
		(Grand mal seizures and partial seizures; this drug is most effective in delaying progressive activity known as kindling; monitor for sedation, ataxia, polydipsia, and polyuria; these adverse effects usually abate with time)
Bromide	Loading dosage dogs, 400-600 mg/kg divided; maintenance 35-45 mg/kg q24 hrs	Caution when using with cats: 30 mg/kg
Benzodiazepines	Diazpepam: 0.5-1 mg/kg IV bolus, 1-2 mg/kg rectum, 0.5-2 mg/kg/hr CRI	Half-life: 2–4 hours
	Midazolam: 0.25-2 mg/kg IV bolus, 0.25-2 mg/kg/hr CRI	(Grand mal seizures and status epilepticus; monitor for sedation)
Felbamate	Dogs: 15-60 mg/kg PO q8 hours	
Levetiracetam	Dogs: 20 mg/kg PO, IV, IM q8 hrs; cats: 20 mg/kg PO q8 hrs	
Zonisamide	Dogs 5-20 mg/kg PO q12 hrs, cats: 5-10 mg/kg/day	
Gabapentin	Dogs: 10-20 mg/kg PO q6-8 hrs; cats: 10 mg/kg q8 hrs	

DISORDERS OF THE SPINAL CORD

Like the brain, disorders of the spinal cord may range from almost undetectable to serious, life threatening emergencies. Causes range from meningitis, tumor of the spinal cord, radiation- or chemotherapy induced neurotoxicity and drug induced thrombocytopenia.[1-5] Paraneoplastic syndromes can and do impact the spinal cord, however they are more commonly recognized as having an effect on the brain. Examples of these paraneoplastic syndromes include hypercalcemia of malignancy (e.g.: secondary to anal sac adenocarcinoma or lymphoma), hypoglycemia (e.g.: secondary to insulinoma or carcinoma of the liver) or hyperviscosity syndrome secondary to hyperglobulinemia (e.g.: secondary to multiple myeloma). Radiation can and does cause late effects within the spinal cord, especially when larger dosages are given over a short period of time resulting in paresis or occasionally paralysis. Because spinal cord compression is an important, relatively common, life threatening emergency, it is reviewed in more detail below.

Spinal cord compression

Predisposing factors

Many malignancy-induced spinal cord compressions in veterinary cancer patients are extradural.[3,6] With the increased use of CT and MRI, the antemortem diagnosis of intradural and extradural lesions are increasing.

Diagnosis

Clinical signs include back pain, a root signature, paresis, or paralysis.[6] Significant spinal cord compression may occur before clinical signs are evident because of slow progression of the tumor and compensation of the nervous tissue. In some cases, such as with neurofibrosarcomas, lower motor neuron signs (e.g., muscle atrophy, weakness, and lack of spinal reflexes) may precede clinical signs that are referable to the spinal cord.

The importance of early diagnosis cannot be overemphasized. When spinal cord compression is identified, immediate action must be taken to ensure that the underlying cause is specifically diagnosed and treated. Diagnosis is based on clinical findings, which include back pain, spinal tenderness, a root signature, abnormal findings on MRI, CT or contrast myelogram, and bone scans via scintigraphy. In many animals with spinal cord compression, a diagnosis can be made by performing a surgical spinal cord decompression and biopsy.

Treatment [3,4,6]

The optimal treatment for epidural spinal cord compression caused by metastatic disease is debated in human medicine. Corticosteroids (i.e., prednisone, 2 mg/kg BID initially) and radiotherapy are the mainstays of therapy for most patients that have solid tumors of the spinal cord. Steroids reduce spinal cord edema and may be beneficial when administered before and during radiation treatment. Surgical intervention is indicated if tissue diagnosis is required, if the cause of the spinal cord compression is uncertain, if relapse occurs in the area of prior irradiation, if spinal instability is present, or if radiation therapy and steroid treatment fail.

DISORDERS OF THE PERIPHERAL NERVES

Like the brain and spinal cord, cancer and cancer therapy may disrupt the function of the peripheral nerves. The results range from subtle neurologic clinical signs secondary to a paraneoplastic syndrome to serious, life threatening emergencies. As with the brain and the spinal cord, causes may be due to chemotherapy-induced neurotoxicity, tumor related disruption in neurotransmission, and disruptions of the entire peripheral nervous system due to paraneoplastic syndromes.[1-5] Examples of these paraneoplastic syndromes include hypercalcemia of malignancy (e.g.: secondary to anal sac adenocarcinoma or lymphoma), hypoglycemia (e.g.: secondary to insulinoma or carcinoma of the liver), thymoma induced myasthenia gravis, or hyperviscosity syndrome secondary to hyperglobulinemia (e.g.: secondary to multiple myeloma). Radiation can and does cause late effects within the peripheral nervous system, especially when larger dosages are given over a short period of time resulting in paresis or occasionally paralysis. Cisplatin, vincristine, cytosine arabinoside, paclitaxel, procainamide, and thalidomide can rarely cause a peripheral neuropathy. Because paraneoplastic syndromes are important and relatively common, it is reviewed in more detail below with emphasis on effects to the peripheral nervous system.

Neurologic syndromes

In both human and veterinary patients, the remote effects of cancer on the nervous system induce a wide variety of clinical signs[1-9] of unknown causes. Cancer-induced neuropathies in dogs include cases of peripheral neuropathy, trigeminal nerve paralysis, and Horner's syndrome.[6-11] Dogs and cats also exhibit neurologic signs secondary to endocrine, fluid, and electrolyte disturbances attributable to neoplasia. Examples of these include hypercalcemia, hyperviscosity syndrome, and hepatoencephalopathy. The neurologic syndromes of myasthenia gravis (e.g., megaesophagus and acetyl cholinesterase-responsive neuropathy) secondary to thymoma are well described in the literature.[6-11]

Site Involved	Syndrome
Brain	Optic neuritis
	Progressive multifocal leukoencephalopathy
	Cerebellar degeneration
Spinal cord	Subacute motor neuropathy
	Subacute necrotic myelopathy
Peripheral nerves	Peripheral neuropathy
	Autonomic GI neuropathy
	Sensory neuropathy
Muscle and neuromuscular junction	Dermatomyositis and polymyositis
	Myasthenic syndrome (Eaton-Lambert syndrome)
	Myasthenia gravis

Key point

In both human and veterinary patients, the remote effects of cancer on the nervous system induce a wide variety of clinical signs including peripheral neuropathy, trigeminal nerve paralysis, Horner's syndrome, hypercalcemic nephropathy, hyperviscosity syndrome, hepatoencephalopathy and myasthenia gravis.

Clinical signs

Manifestations of neurologic paraneoplastic syndrome comprise virtually any change in normal nervous system function. These abnormalities include behavioral changes; peripheral and spinal cord neuropathies; and alterations in the function of the cerebrum, cerebellum, medulla, and neuromuscular junction in both humans and dogs. Some of these aberrations are noted in table 15-3.

Diagnosis

The diagnosis of this paraneoplastic syndrome includes eliminating nonneoplastic causes using CBC, biochemical profile, urinalysis, tests of the thyroid and adrenal axes, brain or spinal cord imaging (CT, MRI, and contrast radiography), biopsy of the affected nerves, CSF tap, and (if indicated) electrodiagnostics.

Treatment

Elimination of the neoplastic condition may result in resolution of neurologic syndromes. Immune-mediated conditions of the CNS or peripheral nervous system may require the use of immunosuppressive therapy, including glucocorticoids.

References

1. Fenner WR: Seizures, narcolepsy and cataplexy, in Birchard SJ, Sherding RG (eds): *Saunders Manual of Small Animal Practice*. Philadelphia, WB Saunders, 1993, pp 1147–1156.
2. Fenner WR: Diseases of the brain, in Birchard SJ, Sherding RG (eds): *Saunders Manual of Small Animal Practice*. Philadelphia, WB Saunders, 1993, pp 1126–1146.
3. Couto CG: Management of complications of cancer chemotherapy. *Vet Clin North Am Small Anim Pract* 4:1037–1053, 1990.
4. Woodlock TJ: Oncologic emergencies, in Rosenthal S, Carignan JR, Smith BD (eds): *Medical Care of the Cancer Patient*, ed 2. Philadelphia, WB Saunders, 1993, pp 236–246.
5. Bunch SE: Anticonvulsant drug therapy in companion animals, in Kirk RW (ed): *Current Veterinary Therapy IX, Small Animal Practice*. Philadelphia, WB Saunders, 1986, pp 836–844.
6. Luttgen PJ: Spinal cord disorders, in Birchard SJ, Sherding RG (eds): *Saunders Manual of Small Animal Practice*. Philadelphia, WB Saunders, 1993, pp 1157–11644.
7. Shahar R, Rosseau C, Steiss J: Peripheral polyneuropathy in a dog with functional islet B-cell tumor and widespread metastases. *J Am Vet Med Assoc* 187:175, 1985.
8. Bergman PJ, Bruyette DS, Coyne BE, et al: Canine clinical peripheral neuropathy associated with pancreatic cell carcinoma. *Prog Vet Neurol* 5:57–62, 1994.
9. Duncan ID: Peripheral neuropathy in the dog and cat. *Prog Vet Neurol* 2:111–121, 1990.
10. Braund KG, McGuire JA, Henderson RA: Peripheral neuropathy associated with malignant neoplasms in dogs. *Vet Pathol* 24:16–24, 1987.
11. Braund KG: Remote effects of cancer on the nervous system. *Semin Vet Med Surg [Small Anim]* 5:262–273, 1990.

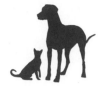

Chapter 16

Emergencies associated with chemotherapy or radiation-induced congestive heart failure

Primary cardiac disease is a cause of morbidity and mortality in the cancer patient. In addition, heart disease secondary to anthracycline or anthracycline-like drugs is an uncommon problem that can become life-threatening in the dog, but not the cat. Other drugs and treatments have the potential to induce cardiac damage (table 16-1). Doxorubicin is the anthracycline most commonly associated with the development of such cardiac diseases as arrhythmias or dilatative cardiomyopathy. Other anthracyclines that have been shown to cause heart disease in human patients include daunorubicin, epirubicin, and idarubicin.[1,2] Cardiomyopathy may occur in response to the administration of any number of dosages of doxorubicin, but the risk of developing this cardiac condition increases significantly in dogs that receive a total cumulative dosage exceeding 240 mg/m^2.[1,2]

Radiation can induce cardiomyopathy if the heart is in the radiation therapy field and if sufficiently high dosages are used.[3] Histologic and clinically significant pericardial effusion can develop approximately 3 months after a 3-week radiation treatment schedule is completed. Radiation can induce a thinning of the myocardium and development of significant amounts of fibrosis 1 year after treatment.

> **Key point**
> Radiation can induce cardiomyopathy if the heart is in the radiation therapy field and if sufficiently high dosages are used.

Radiation therapy and doxorubicin may be synergistic in causing cardiotoxic effects.

PREDISPOSING FACTORS

Doxorubicin-induced cardiac disease may occur more frequently in breeds with a predisposition to develop cardiomyopathy (e.g.: Boxers, Dobermans, Newfoundlands), those that have had pre-existing cardiac disease such as a viral myocarditis or endocarditis, and in those that cannot metabolize or eliminate the drug adequately after administration. Similarly, rapid infusion of the drug, which establishes very high serum

Cancer therapy	Potential cardiovascular complication	Reported?
Anthracyclines	Cardiomyopathy, CHF, dysrhthmias	Yes (not cats)
Mitoxantrone	Cardiomyopathy, CHF	No
Cyclophosphamide	CHF, hemorrhagic myocarditis, pericardial effusion	No
Ifosfamide	CHF	No
5-Fluorouracil	CHF (contraindicated cats)	No
Paclitaxel (Taxol)	Dysrhythmias, ECG changes	Yes?
Thalidomide	Embolic events	No
Radiation	CHF, pericarditis, pericardial effusion	Yes

Table 16-1. Cancer therapies and reported impact to the cardiovascular system in humans or dogs

CHF, congestive heart failure; ECG, electrocardiogram.

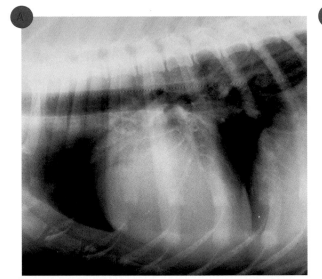

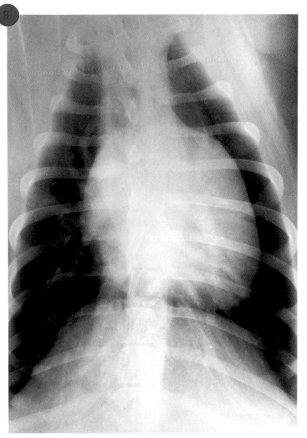

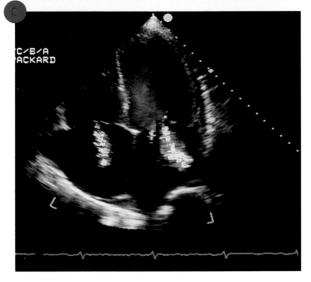

Figure 16-1: Two chest radiographs and one image of an echocardiogram from a dog who presented with biventricular dilated cardiomyopathy with mild concentric atrial valve leaks secondary to annular dilation of the tricuspid and mitral valves secondary to doxorubicin cardiomyopathy.

concentrations, may increase the prevalence of cardiac disease. Therefore, increased duration of infusion of a dosage of doxorubicin may reduce the prevalence of acute and chronic cardiac disease.

Ideally, breeds at risk should be carefully screened for pre-existing heart disease before treating with therapies that are known to be cardiotoxic. Screening patients for heart disease with a physical exam, thoracic radiographs and an echocardiogram is ideal.

DIAGNOSIS

The diagnosis of heart disease is best performed first with a physical examination to monitor for arrhythmias, murmurs, weak pulses, poor capillary refill, jugular pulses, hepatomegaly, splenomegaly, etc. Thoracic radiograph, electrocardiogram, or radionuclide scan may also be helpful. Monitoring should intensify in those dogs with compatible clinical signs and if they have received around 180 mg/m² total cumulative dose of doxorubicin. Endomyocardial biopsies are still the

gold standard, however few centers routinely perform this test. Measuring serum levels of troponin C, T or I is being evaluated as a non-invasive test to monitor for myocardial damage. [6]

> **Key point**
>
> The diagnosis of heart disease is best performed first with a physical examination to monitor for arrhythmias, murmurs, weak pulses, poor capillary refill, jugular pulses, hepatomegaly, splenomegaly, etc.

In one study,[4] 32 of 175 dogs treated with doxorubicin developed clinically evident cardiac disease at cumulative doses of doxorubicin of >1580 mg/m²). Thirty-one dogs had electrocardiographic abnormalities, including arrhythmias (i.e., atrial premature complexes, atrial fibrillation, paroxysmal atrial and sinus tachycardia, ventricular arrhythmias, bundle branch blocks, and atrioventricular dissociation) and nonspecific alterations in R wave, ST segment, or QRS duration. Seven dogs had overt congestive heart failure that resulted in death within 90 days, despite supportive therapy. In contrast a recent study found that of 303 dogs with osteosarcoma receiving 5 doses of doxorubicin (cumulative dose 150mg/m^2), 23 developed cardiomyopathy (7.6%). Dobermans, Great Danes, Newfoundlands and Great Pyrenees accounted for 11 of these dogs. Careful screening and limiting the cumulative dose may reduce the incidence of cardiac disease in dogs receiving doxorubicin. (Moore and Ogilvie, unpublished data) Arrhythmias may occur at the time of treatment or within a variable period after treatment is complete. In humans with doxorubicin-induced cardiac diseases, significant dysrhythmias often occur in the absence of other physical or historical abnormalities.[5]

In dogs with cardiomyopathy and fulminant congestive heart failure, clinical signs vary from anorexia, lethargy, and weakness to more common signs associated specifically with decreased cardiac output and ensuing congestive heart failure. Owners may complain that their pet has exercise intolerance; coughing spells late at night, which may develop into a persistent cough at all times of the day; abdominal distention; increased respiratory effort and rate; and generalized malaise.

The physical examination can reveal much useful information and may include identification of a jugular pulse; rapid heart and respiratory rates; ascites; cool extremities; blue mucous membranes; delayed capillary refill time; pitting edema of lower extremities; enlarged liver and spleen; and rapid, weak pulses. The lung fields may sound dull because of pleural effusion, or pulmonary edema may cause crackling lung sounds. Heart murmurs or an abnormal rhythm are frequently auscultated; heart sounds from dogs with atrial fibrillation may sound like "jungle drums" (i.e., irregularly irregular) on auscultation. Electrocardiography may suggest heart chamber enlargement or may be diagnostic for arrhythmias, which may be supraventricular or ventricular in origin.

Thoracic and abdominal radiographs are very valuable in identifying evidence of cardiac disease, including pericardial or pleural effusion, enlargement of the heart, liver, spleen, and pulmonary veins, and pulmonary edema, which usually is first noted around the hilar region. Echocardiography is extremely valuable for confirming pericardial effusion and for documenting chamber size, myocardial wall thickness, and dynamic parameters (e.g., ejection fraction, cardiac output, and contractility). Blood pressure measurements may assist in documentation of hypertension or hypotension. An elevated central venous pressure aids in making a diagnosis of cardiac insufficiency. Finally, there are more specific tests that can further clarify a diagnosis of drug- or radiation therapy-induced cardiac disease.

These include fluid analysis of thoracic or abdominal effusion (usually a modified transudate with reactive mesothelial cells and macrophages) and contrast radiography. Unfortunately, no evaluation method can be performed routinely in veterinary practice to predict whether cardiotoxicity will occur in dogs that receive anthracycline agents or radiation therapy. This precludes withdrawal of therapy before overt signs of cardiac insufficiency occur. In humans, nuclear medicine imaging techniques may be able to predict the development of doxorubicin cardiomyopathy before it becomes clinically evident.

THERAPY

Prevention

The hallmark of doxorubicin-induced heart disease is development of dilated cardiomyopathy. Many methods to prevent the development of this condition have been explored. Vitamin E, thyroxine, coenzyme Q10, IP-6 and selenium treatments are ineffective for prevention of cardiomyopathy. In humans, weekly low-dose doxorubicin therapy or the administration of the dosage over 24-72 hours reduces the prevalence of cardiomyopathy.[6] The compound ICRF-187 (dexrazoxane) is more effective. This compound substantially reduces the occurrence of cardiomyopathy in dogs treated concurrently with doxorubicin. ICRF-187 is administered intravenously just prior to the administration of doxorubicin at a dosage of 30 mg of ICRF-187 for every 1 mg of doxorubicin to be administered.

- Identify patients at risk.
  - Boxers, Dobermans, other predisposed breeds should be screened, or perhaps not treated at all.
- Minimize the cumulative dose.
  - Cumulative dosing is the most important factor in doxorubicin cardiomyopathy. Limit to 180-240mg/m^2.
- Use different dosing schedule.
  - Risk of cardiac toxicity is related to peak plasma level rather than the area under the curve of the drug. There is evidence that continuous infusion causes less risk of cardiomyopathy than does slow bolus infusion. In human patients the rate was 21% with bolus, and only 6% with a 6-hour infusion.
- Liposomal encapsulation.
  - Taken up by the reticuloendothelial system, but clinical trials in people do not support the reduction in toxicity.
- Minimize cardiac irradiation if concurrent doxorubicin to be used.

Treatment

The development of cardiomyopathy may be associated with a profound decrease in contractility without substantial alterations in quality of life. Indeed, some indoor pets live a normal life despite significant reductions in contractility and ejection fraction. Other patients exhibit signs of heart failure. Once these alterations in cardiovascular performance are documented, doxorubicin administration should be discontinued indefinitely. The important lesson to be learned from these data is that the presence or absence of clinical signs should dictate whether cardiac drugs should be initiated, rather than basing the decision on results of diagnostic tests.

Treatment of cardiomyopathy begins with the indefinite discontinuation of the inciting cause (e.g., radiation therapy or doxorubicin). Diuretics, a low-salt diet, rest, oxygen therapy, positive inotropes, and vasodilators should be used as dictated by the clinical status of the patient. For example, furosemide may be used two to three times a day in a compensated animal, whereas the drug may be used every few hours, if necessary, in patients in respiratory distress from severe, fulminant pulmonary edema. Digoxin, a positive inotrope, can be given orally or parenterally in combination with a preload or afterload reducer. It is falling out of favor due to the current widespread use of pimobendan. When given orally, therapeutic levels of digoxin generally are not achieved for a few days, which may be adequate for animals that are

relatively stable. Factors such as dehydration and electrolyte disturbances may promote development of digoxin toxicoses. Because digoxin toxicity is a serious problem that occurs frequently, intravenous loading dosages should not be used unless absolutely necessary. Regardless of the method of digitalization, periodic determination of serum digoxin concentration is essential for adjustment of drug dosage to maintain therapeutic levels.

Pimobendan is a positive ionotrope with vasodilatory effects that is rapidly absorbable when given orally. It is quite effective for treating myocardial failure and is often combined with furosemide.

In an acutely decompensated dying dog with cardiomyopathy, a constant rate infusion of dobutamine or oral pimobendan combined with intravenous furosemide. If digoxin is used, then an intravenous (e.g., nitroprusside) or transdermal application (e.g., 2% nitroglycerin) of a preload or afterload reducer may be more logical than oral treatment. Dobutamine may increase cardiac output within minutes to hours, whereas improvement of cardiac output with oral pimobendan therapy may take days. Oxygen is indicated for all patients as needed. A more detailed treatment regimen for cardiomyopathy is outlined in table 16-2.

Table 16-2. Potential therapeutic approach for dogs with drug- or radiation-induced dilative cardiomyopathy	
General principle	**Specific details, drug dosages, and toxicities**
Discontinue cardiotoxic	All cardiotoxic drugs should be discontinued indefinitely; additional radiation therapy to the heart should be avoided agents
Enforce complete rest	Avoidance of any stressful environment is essential; consider cage rest
Oxygenate	Acquire and maintain a patent airway
	Provide supplemental oxygen if needed; fifty percent oxygen should not be used for more than 24 hours to avoid pulmonary toxicity
	Perform thoracocentesis to reduce pleural effusion
	Initiate diuretic therapy for pulmonary edema (see below)
Reduce pulmonary edema	Furosemide (drug of choice; monitor for dehydration, hypokalemia, etc.) 2-4 mg/kg IV or IM every 2-12 hours depending on the severity of edema; decrease to 1-4 mg/kg SID-TID PO for maintenance therapy
	Hydrochlorothiazide/spironolactone combination (use with furosemide or as maintenance therapy; monitor for dehydration and electrolyte abnormalities) 2-4 mg/kg BID PO
Increase contractility	Perform pericardiocentesis if pericardial effusion is present in significant amounts to reduce contractility
	Digoxin (monitor blood levels to acquire and maintain therapeutic blood levels [1-2 ng/ml]; watch for anorexia, vomiting, diarrhea, and ECG abnormalities suggestive of digoxin toxicity) Extreme caution in cats due to unique sensitivity
	Pimabendan (0.25 mg/kg PO BID) has been used with success in dogs with CHF secondary to dilated cardiomyopathy and mitral valve insufficiency. Pimobendan is a phosphodiesterase-III inhibitor that sensitizes the myocardium to calcium, and improves inotropic activity in addition to causing arteriolar and venous dilation. In addition to its use as a long-term inodilator in the treatment of dogs with CHF, Pimobendan is also recommended for use in emergency therapy of CHF, as it can have an onset of effects within one hour

Table 16-3. Drugs used to treat supraventricular and ventricular tachyarrhythmias induced by anthracycline antibiotics or radiation therapy

Drug	Trade name	Drug dosages
Procainamide	Procan SR® Procainamide HCL	20 mg/kg PO q 8 hrs 6-8 mg/kg IV bolus, 20-40 µg/kg/min CRI
Quinidine	Sustained release	5-20 mg/kg PO q 8 hrs
Lidocaine	Lidocaine HCL	2-4 mg/kg IV bolus, 6-80 µg/kg/min CRI
Mexiletine	Mexitil®	4-10 mg/kg PO q 8 hrs
Atenolol	Tenormin®	0.25-1 mg/kg PO q 12-24 hrs
Propranolol	Indural®	0.04-0.06 mg/kg IV slowly or 0.2-1.0 mg/kg BID-TID PO, often in combination with digoxin for supraventricular arrhythmias
Sotalol	Betapace®	
Diltiazem	Cardizem®	0.5-2 mg/kg PO q 12 hrs
Digoxin		0.5-1.5 mg/kg PO q 8 hrs 0.003-0.005 mg/kg PO q 12 hrs

Key point

In an acutely decompensated dying dog with cardiomyopathy, a constant rate infusion of dobutamine and/or oral pimobendan combined with intravenous furosemide is often quite helpful.

Arrhythmias may occur during infusion of a chemotherapeutic agent (see table 16-1). If arrhythmias persist, interfere with an animal's quality of life, or serve as a serious threat to the animal's survival, therapy should be instituted and the underlying cause identified and eliminated. In each case, the potential adverse effects of the antiarrhythmic agents must be evaluated and considered before therapy is initiated. Treatments and their indications are as below:

- Digoxin: supraventricular premature complexes, supraventricular tachycardia, and atrial fibrillation.
- Lidocaine: premature ventricular contractions and ventricular tachycardia.
- Procainamide: premature ventricular contractions and ventricular tachycardia.
- Atenolol, sotalol, propranolol: supraventricular premature complexes and tachyarrhythmias, atrial fibrillation, and ventricular premature complexes.
- Diltiazem: supraventricular premature complexes and tachyarrhythmias and atrial fibrillation.

References

1. Keefe DL. Anthracycline-induced cardiomyopathy. *Semin Oncol* 28(4 Suppl 12):2-7, 2001.
2. Speyer JL, Ewer MS, Freedberg RS: Cardiac effects of cancer therapy in, Abeloff MD, Armitage JO, Niederhuber JE et al: *Clinical oncology*, 3rd edition, Philadelphia, Elsevier, 2004, pp 1251-1268
3. McChesney SL, Gillette EL, Powers BE: Radiation-induced cardiomyopathy in the dog. *Radiation Res* 113:120–132, 1988.
4. Mauldin GE, Fox PR, Patnaik AK, et al: Doxorubicin-induced cardiotoxicosis: Clinical features of 32 dogs. *J Vet Intern Med* 6:82–88, 1992.
5. Jakacki RI, Larsen RL, Barber G, et al: Comparison of cardiac function tests after anthracycline therapy in childhood. *Cancer* 72:2739–2745, 1993.
6. DeFrancesco TC, Atkins CE, Keene BW, et al: Prospective clinical evaluation of serum cardiac troponin T in dogs admitted to a veterinary teaching hospital. *J Vet Intern Med* 16(5):553-557, 2002.

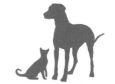

Chapter 17

Care beyond a cure: the power of being a healer

Most veterinarians enter the profession with a passion to heal animals through knowledge, compassion and caring. Relief of pain and suffering is first and foremost on the minds of the most compassionate veterinarians. Most veterinarians have come to the realization that the greatest responsibility is to bring health and wellness to animals, as well as the people and surrounding society in a "one medicine" approach. The importance of healing via this approach is especially vital when dealing with cancer, a frightening disease that requires the very best care from the heart and science possible regardless of the species that is afflicted. Thus, recognizing the power, responsibility and impact of being a healer who cares beyond the benefits of natural or pharmaceutical medicines, surgery, radiation or manipulative arts is key to reaching one's full potential.

DEFINING "HEALER"

In Western cultures, the word "healer" has many dictionary definitions including someone who has spiritual gifts to bring health and balance. However, for our purposes, the term healer is defined by the American Heritage Dictionary as "someone who makes healthy, whole, or sound, to restore to health, free from ailment." This includes cancer. Veterinarians, like physicians, are regarded by society as healers; many consider the single most important attribute of an extraordinary veterinarian or veterinary nurse is the ability to heal with compassionate care independent of potions, medicines, bandages, surgery, etc. This unique brand of healing or caring is defined as meeting not only the medical needs of the animal, but also the non-medical needs of the people who care for the pet. There is no doubt that the medicines, potions, manipulative therapies, radiation, acupuncture and surgery bring healing; our goal is to ask, "What evidence exists that veterinarians bring healing by their very presence and actions?" Caring for companion animals has direct benefit on these pets but the health of animals has many well-documented health gains for people and society, as

well. These include, but are not limited to, enhanced mental wellness, lower blood pressure, decreased depression, enhanced immunity, and impacts on society such as decreased violence among children and criminals, as well as decreased costs associated with decreased hospitalization and enhanced quality and quantity of survival among the elderly.

Key point

Many consider the single most important attribute of an extraordinary veterinarian or veterinary nurse is the ability to heal with compassionate care independent of potions, medicines, bandages, surgery, etc.

HEALING: A DISSIPATING GIFT AND RESPONSIBILITY?

In veterinary and human medical education, it has been suggested that students, interns and residents are growing more cynical and less compassionate over the course of their education.[1-3] This is unfortunate in that some agree that the most desirable characteristics of extraordinary veterinarians and physicians are disappearing.[4,5] These traits include positive patient/client directed attitudes such as compassion, caring, and respect. In order to foster these critical skills, medical educators for pre and post DVM/MD educational opportunities must teach not only facts or moral reasoning processes, but also the motivational network of values, attitudes, and feelings that underlie moral behavior and compassionate care.[5-7] In short, veterinarians and veterinary students need to be reunited with the passion to care from the heart as much as from the science while recasting animal doctors as members of a profession whose responsibilities extend far beyond the patient/veterinary relationship. This is especially true in cancer care where clients are frightened and need support. Similarly, the challenges of treating cancer are many and thus require a dedicated, focused, compassionate veterinary health care team.

Key point

The most desirable characteristics of extraordinary veterinarians and physicians are disappearing including positive patient/client directed attitudes such as compassion, caring and respect.

HEALING BY RELIEVING ANXIETY

The first gift of any compassionate healer is the alleviation of anxiety which has profound healing effects.[8-13] There is no greater way to witness the power healing through the alleviation of anxiety than in a veterinary cancer center or in a general practice that cares for community animals and their families, including those with cancer. It is there that people listen to veterinary oncologists and practitioners who not only provide bad news about the disease but also frightening treatment options such as chemotherapy, radiation and surgery. During these discussions, anxiety levels are very high and this emotional state is very likely to interfere with the ability to hear the information they need in order to make rational decisions. There is evidence that the clinician's behavior during the diagnostic consultation can and does influence the client's psychological adjustment and their willingness to embrace the plan to care for their pet. That experience may, at worse, confound, or, at best, resolve prior misconceptions, fears and anxieties about cancer, death, dying, and recovery from a serious disease that is unrelated to the pet's problems. Thus, it appears that reducing the client's anxiety during those initial evaluation periods may lead to better client understanding, a stronger veterinary-client relationship and enhanced patient well being.

Key point

There is evidence that the clinician's behavior during the diagnostic consultation can and does influence the client's psychological adjustment and their willingness to embrace the plan to care for their pet.

The question arises: how can a veterinarian or other member of the veterinary health care team extend care to reduce anxiety and therefore enhance the patient's quality of life? Substantial information exists to support the practice of dispelling the myths and empowering the client with information about the cancer and its treatment.[8-14] Few studies have been done in veterinary medicine to illustrate, however a growing knowledge base is developing in human medicine. The following three studies illustrate the value of providing compassionate care to reduce anxiety. In the first publication, the authors assessed 34 intervention studies designed to increase breast cancer patients' psychosocial and informational preparedness.[13] Spending time with patients to empower them with information to enhance their understanding of the disease, as well as treatment, reduced their pain and subsequent use of analgesics, and decreased their hospital stay by two days in 85% of the studies. In another study,[14] the study's authors assessed 30 human breast cancer patients who were given information about the risks and benefits of radiation therapy. These patients scored significantly higher on a knowledge questionnaire at the beginning of treatment and had lower anxiety scores during the last week of treatment, compared with the control group. Educating clients about treatments and their benefit and risks may also decrease morbidity. In one study, cancer patients who were given training on active participation in the doctor-patient interaction and were given their medical charts before the physician consultation had fewer symptoms during their treatment with chemotherapy.[15]

CULTIVATING EMPATHY AND COMPASSION

Few would disagree that a critical aspect of being an effective healer is being a respected, authoritative, compassionate source of information. The very act of empowering others with information about the disease or disorder and the treatments increases a client's perception of the healer's compassion, caring and ability to be empathetic. Indeed, empathy and compassion are considered the foundation of an ethical veterinary practice. The question arises therefore, how does one acquire these skills of compassion and enhanced client and patient outcomes? In one study, Hall et al[16] found three dimensions of communication in effective healers. These three dimensions include informative-ness, interpersonal sensitivity and partnership building. Others have defined compassionate caring as an affiliated style defined as friendliness, interest and empathy in the client's psychosocial issues, social orientation, courtesy and competence.[16-19] Additionally, one study involving breast cancer patients[20] found favorable impressions when the physician was noted to understand their fears, appeared warm and caring, and was informative. This resulted in significantly better psychologic adjustment six months after breast cancer surgery suggesting that compassion brings about positive patient (client) outcomes. Since veterinarians care not only for the pet but also the family and other people involved in the relationship, these factors should be taken into consideration.

Key point

The very act of empowering others with information about the disease or disorder and the treatments increases a client's perception of the healer's compassion, caring and ability to be empathetic.

HEALING WITH ROUTINE AND RITUAL

Many members of the veterinary health care team often recognize that creating an environment and a ritual with clients and their animals can be healing all in itself. At California Veterinary Specialists' Angel Care Cancer Center in Southern California, the staff does everything possible to meet with each client in a comfortable environment that was designed to include warm colors and windows with views of nature. The first meeting includes a chat with a veterinary nurse who begins to introduce the concepts of cancer and cancer care. Subsequent to that, the same members of the team care for the patient and client in the familiar setting that the client was initially introduced to. In essence, the team tries to create a ritual of comfort. The healing value to the client is obvious, but it is also therapeutic for the animal patient (most agree that when the client is at ease and is less anxious, the patient is likely to be less stressed and anxious as well). Most recognize that animals and people come to enjoy and even express satisfaction and contentment when being petted, touched, or spoken to in unique ways, especially when in a comforting environment. Establishing healing rituals such as American Indian dances and healing drumming can create receptive patients and clients who are susceptible to the influences of authoritative, culturally sanctioned "powers" that are separate, but just as important as traditional medical, surgical, radiological, acupuncture, herbal and other treatments.[21] Experimental research into placebo effects demonstrates that routine biomedical pharmacological and procedural interventions contain significant dimensions in rituals. This research also suggests that ritual healing not only represents changes in effect, self-awareness and self-appraisal of behavioral capacities, but involves modulations of symptoms through neurobiological mechanisms.

Key point

This research also suggests that ritual healing not only represents changes in effect, self-awareness and self-appraisal of behavioral capacities, but involves modulations of symptoms through neurobiological mechanisms.

THE MIND BODY CONNECTION: POWER OF PLACEBO

As suggested above, the placebo effect must be accounted for when understanding the effect of a healer on the client and therefore, directly or indirectly, on the patient. This effect occurs in part because of the beliefs of the clients and care providers. Montgomery and Kirsch[22] demonstrated the benefit of the placebo effect on human patients by telling people that a placebo that they called trivaricane appeared to be a powerful analgesic when applied to the finger. The placebo material was applied and a painful stimulus was initiated on the treated finger and another without the placebo. The subjects rated the intensity of the pain and the unpleasantness of the experience. As you might expect, the subjects firmly believed the placebo treated finger experienced less irritation than the untreated finger. It is unknown if animal patients can experience the same thing, however, since they are powerfully influenced by the attitude and actions of people around them, it is likely that an indirect placebo effect would be beneficial. In addition, in his work Pavlov confirmed that certain rituals and actions can condition animals to act, believe, and respond in a favorable fashion. In addition, many clients will affirm their conviction that their pets can "sense" when they are being helped and trust in this action. Thus, the placebo effect, or mind-body connection must be recognized as an important aspect of healing. Rather than diminishing the value of a healer, the mind-body connection should be considered a powerful tool that should be acknowledged as a method as effective as a medication or even surgery. In fact, when patients with knee problems were treated with an actual therapeutic surgical procedure or a sham operation (an incision but no further surgery before the incisions were sutured closed in all patients), there was no difference in recovery between the two groups of patients: The sham treated patients willed themselves to health because they believed in the healing power of their healer, the surgeon.[23]

SPIRITUAL HEALING

Finally, a discussion on healing cannot proceed without a brief mention of the healing power of spirituality.[25-29] While few data exist on the importance of faith and healing in veterinary medicine, data does exist in human medicine. This includes one study indicating that almost 80 percent of people polled felt that spiritual faith was effective for the treatment of disease including cancer.[25] Sixty three percent of these same people felt that their physicians should talk to patients about spiritual faith[26] and 48 percent of patients wanted their physicians to pray for them.[27] Given the importance of spirituality and healing in the minds of so many people, more medical and veterinary schools are addressing the importance of both spiritual and medical care. These schools are including courses on religion, spirituality, prayer, and health[1] and this subject is being addressed more openly in educational forums for graduates. The trend seems prudent due to the fact that 90 percent of 296 physicians surveyed during a recent American Academy of Family Physicians meeting were convinced that religious beliefs can heal and three quarters believed that prayer could enhance a patient's recovery.[25] A recent study reported that in a National Health Interview Survey of 22,306 adults in the United States confirmed that 49 percent of people had prayed about their health, an increase of 14 percent over a similar survey done in 2002.[29] This study, published in the May 2011 issue of Psychology of Religion and Spirituality, the increase in prayer occurred in adults of all ages. It is hypothesized by us that the same trend is likely occurring as people pray for the health of their pets. Thus, for those inclined in the veterinary health care team, including a discussion on faith and healing among receptive clients may be something to consider. The merit thereof is rooted in many religions including Christianity. For example, the apostle Paul wrote in 1 Corinthians 12 (7-10):

"A spiritual gift is given to each of us so we can help each other. To one person the Spirit gives the ability to give wise advice; to another the same Spirit gives a message of special knowledge. The same Spirit gives great faith to another, and to someone else the one Spirit gives the gift of healing. He gives one person the power to perform miracles, and another the ability to prophesy."

Key point

Given the importance of spirituality and healing in the minds of so many people, more medical and veterinary schools are addressing the importance of both spiritual and medical care.

The gift and power of being a healer cannot be understated and nor explained in the few short paragraphs above. Regardless, it is important enough to introduce in this venue and to serve as a stepping-stone for further exploration.

References

1. Peabody FW: The care of the patient. *JAMA* 88:877–82, 1927.
2. Subcommittee on Evaluation of Humanistic Qualities in the Internist: American Board of Internal Medicine Evaluation of humanistic qualities in the internist. *Ann Intern Med* 99:720–4, 1983.
3. Self DJ, Schrader DE, Baldwin DC, Jr, Wolinsky FD: The moral development of medical students: a pilot study of the possible influence of medical education. *Med Educ.*27:26–34, 1993.
4. Feudtner C, Christakis DA, Christakis NA: Do clinical clerks suffer ethical erosion? Students' perceptions of their ethical environment and personal development. *Acad Med* 69:670–9, 1994.
5. Lipkin M: Integrity, compassion, respect. *J Gen Intern Med* 1:65–7, 1986.
6. Pellegrino ED: Teaching medical ethics: some persistent questions and some responses. *Acad Med.*64:701–3, 1989.
7. Sulmasy DP, Geller G, Levine DM, Faden R: Medical house officers' knowledge, attitudes, and confidence regarding medical ethics. *Arch Intern Med.*150:2509–13, 1990.
8. Dermatis H, Lesko LM: Psychosocial correlates of physician-patient communication at time of informed consent for bone marrow transplantation. *Cancer Invest* 9:621-628, 1991.
9. Fallowfield LJ, Hall A, Maguire GP, et al: Psychological outcomes of different treatment policies in women with early breast cancer outside a clinical trial. *BMJ* 301:575-580, 1990.
10. Jepson C, Chaiken S: Chronic issue-specific fear inhibits systematic processing of persuasive communications. *J Soc Behav Pers* 5:61-84, 1990.
11. Eagly AH, Chaiken S: *The Psychology of Attitudes.* Orlando, FL, Harcourt Brace Jovanovich, 1993.
12. Roberts CS, Cox CE, Reintgen DS, et al: Influence of physician communication on newly diagnosed breast cancer patients' psychological adjustment and decision-making. *Cancer* 74:336-341, 1994.
13. Mumford E, Schlesinger HJ, Glass GV: The effects of psychological intervention on recovery from surgery and heart attacks: An analysis of the literature. *Am J Public Health* 72:141-151, 1982.
14. Rainey LC: Effects of preparatory patient education for radiation oncology patients. *Cancer* 56:1056-1061, 1985.
15. Kaplan SH, Greenfield S, Ware JE Jr: Assessing the effects of physician-patient interactions on the outcomes of chronic disease. *Med Care* 27:S110-S127, 1989.
16. Hall JA, Roter DL, Katz NR: Meta-analysis of correlates of provider behavior in medical encounters. *Med Care* 26:657-675, 1988.
17. Buller MK, Buller DB: Physicians' communication style and patient satisfaction. *J Health Soc Behav* 28:375-388, 1985.
18. Bertakis KD, Roter D, Putnam SM: The relationship of physician medical interview style to patient satisfaction. *J Fam Pract* 32:175-181, 1991.
19. Willson P, McNamara JR: How perceptions of a simulated physician-patient interaction influence intended satisfaction and compliance. *Soc Sci Med* 16:1699-1704, 1982.
20. Blanchard CG, Labrecque MS, Ruckdescel JC, et al: Information and decision-making preferences of hospitalized adult cancer patients. *Soc Sci Med* 27:1139-1145, 1988.
21. Kaptchuk TJ. Placebo studies and ritual theory: a comparative analysis of Navajo, acupuncture and biomedical healing. *Philos Trans R Soc Lond B Biol Sci.* 366(1572):1849-1858, Jun 27, 2011.
22. Montgomery G, Kirsch: Mechanisms of placebo pain reduction: An empirical investigation. *Psychological Science* 7(3):174-176, 1996.
23. Mosley J, Bruce K, O'Malley N et al: A controlled trial of arthroscopic surgery for osteoarthritis of the knee. *New England Journal of Medicine* 220;347(2):81-88.
24. Levin JS, Larson DN, Puchalski CM: Religion and spirituality in medicine: research and education. *JAMA* 278: 792–93, 1997.
25. Eisenberg DM, Kessler RC, Foster C, Norlock FE, Calkins DR, Delbanco TL: Unconventional medicine in the United States: prevalence, costs, and patterns of use. *N Engl J Med* 328:246–52, 1993.
26. King DE, Bushwick B: Beliefs and attitudes of hospital inpatients about faith healing and prayer. *J Family Practice* 39: 349–52, 1994.
27. Marwick C: Should physicians prescribe prayer for health? Spiritual aspects of well-being considered. *JAMA* 273: 1561–62, 1995.
28. Matthews DA, McCullough ME, Larson DB, Koenig HG, Swyers JP, Milano MG: Religious commitment and health status. *Arch Family Medicine* 7: 118–24, 1998.
29. Wachholtz, A, Sambamoorthi U: National trends in prayer use as a coping mechanism for health concerns: Changes from 2002 to 2007. *Psychology of Religion and Spirituality* (2); 67-77, 2011.

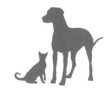

Chapter 18

Safe handling of chemotherapeutic agents

The health and well being of the veterinary health care team, including the client, is paramount regardless of whether one is dealing with anesthetic agents, antibiotics, or chemotherapeutic agents. Like all drugs, chemotherapeutic agents have potential risks if they are handled inappropriately. Fortunately, new, practical systems are available, such as the PhaSeal® injectable drug mixing and administration system (Carmel Pharma, Mölndal, Sweden) that can reduce the risk associated with the handling of these agents. As the benefits of anticancer drugs become more apparent, their use is rapidly expanding, which in turn puts the veterinary health care team at increased risk of exposure during drug preparation and administration. All chemotherapeutic agents must be considered potentially toxic, most are mutagenic or teratogenic, and at least some are carcinogenic. Reliable information regarding the amount of drug exposure needed for any of these effects is difficult to obtain; however, some toxicities have been seen in caregivers who prepare and administer chemotherapy for human patients without appropriate protection and precautions, including:[1, 2]

- Chromosome damage. Some authors have found increases whereas others have found decreases in chromosomal aberrations including sister chromatid exchanges, structural aberrations (e.g., gaps, breaks, translocations), and micronuclei in peripheral blood lymphocytes.[2-6] The biological effects of these findings are unknown.
- Reproductive effects. Hemminki et al[7] found no difference in exposure between nurses who had spontaneous abortions and those who had normal pregnancies with regard to exposure to cytotoxic drugs, whereas Selevan et al[8] and others[9] found a relationship between cytotoxic drug exposure and adverse reproductive outcomes.
- Hepatocellular toxicity. Liver damage has been reported in nurses working in human oncology wards.[10]

Key point

All chemotherapeutic agents must be considered potentially toxic, most are mutagenic or teratogenic, and at least some are carcinogenic.

Whenever possible, the practitioner should minimize exposure to all work place hazards including chemotherapeutic agents. All institutional, city, regional, state, and national regulations and law must be reviewed and followed to the letter. Whenever possible, the team should contract the duties of preparing the chemotherapeutic agents to institutional, city, or regional pharmacies who prepare chemotherapeutic agents routinely. All regulations and procedures for handling, mixing, and administering chemotherapeutic agents and other hazards should be readily available and used during routine training periods for the entire team. Exposure to cytotoxic agents can occur in four ways: [1, 11–13]

- Inhalation due to aerosolization during mixing and/or administration of the drug.
- Absorption of the drug through the skin.
- Ingestion through contact with contaminated food or cigarettes.
- Accidental inoculation.

Common clinical examples of situations in which exposure may occur include:
- Withdrawal of a needle from a pressurized drug vial (the "pssst" as the needle is removed).
- Transfer of drugs between containers.
- Opening of glass ampules.
- Expulsion of air bubbles from drug-filled syringes.
- Failure or improper set up of equipment.
- Exposure to excreta from patients treated with certain cytotoxic drugs.
- Crushing or breaking of tablets.

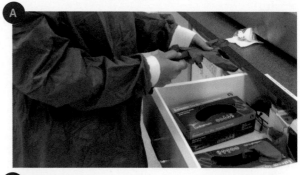

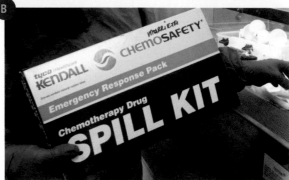

Key point

Whenever possible, the team should contract the duties of preparing the chemotherapeutic agents to institutional, city, or regional pharmacies who prepare chemotherapeutic agents routinely.

Safe drug handling is possible in veterinary practice, especially when employing a biological safety cabinet (figure 18-1 A and B) with the PhaSeal® system. Because of the relatively small doses of chemotherapy delivered by most practitioners, the risk of exposure is relatively low if the drugs are handled appropriately. Everyone who prepares or administers antineoplastic drugs should be appropriately trained, equipped, and have routine health examinations. Women of childbearing age should exercise extreme caution when handling cytotoxic agents, and pregnant women should not handle antineoplastic drugs at all. Procedures for handling chemotherapeutic agents must meet or exceed the guidelines outlined by OSHA, NIOSH and any state or local regulations. OSHA regulations should be followed and clients, as well as all personnel contacting chemotherapy agents, should be protected to the best of the veterinarian's abilities. A chemotherapy logbook, which includes identification of patients treated and personnel involved in treatments, should be maintained in order to track exposures. The risk of exposure can be greatly reduced by understanding the hazardous properties found in the Material Safety Data Sheets (MSDS) for each drug and by using appropriate protective equipment. The information contained in each MSDS includes the specific health hazards including carcinogenicity, primary routes of exposure, protective equipment, treatment of personnel acutely exposed, chemical activators, solubility, stability, volatility, and specific procedures to be undertaken in case of a spill. The MSDS should be requested with the initial shipment of any chemotherapy agent and should be kept on file in an easily accessible location.

Key point

Safe drug handling is possible in canine and feline practice especially when employing a biological safety cabinet with the PhaSeal® system.

A hazardous drug safety and health plan should be developed for each hospital and clinic that handles chemotherapeutic agents. This plan should include at least: [1, 11–13]

- A standard operating procedure for the mixing, handling, and exposure of or to hazardous drugs.
- Control measures the employer will use to determine and implement control measures to reduce employee exposure to hazardous drugs.
- A ventilation system and other protective

Figure 18-1: A biologic safety cabinet should be used when possible (A). Gloves designed for chemotherapy and a nonpermeable gown should be worn when preparing chemotherapeutic agents. Eye protection must be worn in addition to appropriate gloves and a non-permeable gown whenever spills or chemotherapeutic agents are handled with a spill kit (B) outside the hood.

equipment necessary to mix, administer, and clean up chemotherapeutic agents.
- Provisions for information and training.
- Provisions for medical examinations of exposed personnel.
- Assignment of people in leadership position to ensure that personnel apply and adhere to all safety measures.
- Establishment of a designated area to mix, handle, and administer chemotherapeutic agents.
- Procedures to safely remove contaminated waste.
- Decontamination procedures.

Antineoplastic agents should be stored according to the manufacturers' directions. Drugs that require refrigeration should be kept in a separate refrigerator away from other medications and foodstuffs. If a reconstituted drug is stored, the vial should be placed in a sealable plastic bag labeled with the date of reconstitution.

The following information is provided for people involved in the day-to-day technical aspects of chemotherapy preparation and administration (see box 18-1). The reader is advised to review this section and all OSHA guidelines for information that can reduce the risks inherent in handling these drugs.

Box 18-1. Guidelines for handling chemotherapeutic agents

Minimizing exposure to chemotherapy drugs requires the use of appropriate equipment. The following are considered the essentials of personal protective equipment: [1, 11–13]

- Nonpowdered appropriate-thickness gloves for chemotherapy. Change them at least every hour.
- Protective disposable gown made of lint-free, low-permeability fabric with a closed front, long sleeves, and elastic or knit closed cuffs.
- When a biological safety cabinet is NOT available, an approved respirator with a high-efficiency filter is essential.
- In absence of biological safety cabinet, eye and face protection must be provided with an appropriate plastic face or splash goggles shield whenever splashes, sprays, or aerosols may be present.

PREPARING CHEMOTHERAPEUTIC AGENTS

Mixing chemotherapeutic agents must be done with care and respect because these drugs can be dangerous if they are not handled appropriately. The following are some high points of handling chemotherapeutic agents followed by a narrative on their use: [1, 11–13]

- Wear a disposable, closed, moisture-barrier gown with elastic or knit cuffs, appropriate thickness gloves designed for chemotherapy, and safety glasses or face shield.
- Use a class II, type A vertical laminar air flow cabinet exhausted outside the facility, even that meets or exceeds the current National Sanitation Foundation Standard and the PhaSeal® system. Alternatively have the drugs mixed up at a distant facility or pharmacy that has the appropriate equipment.
- Mix agents in a quiet area.
- Use absorbent plastic-backed liners to collect spills.
- Use Luer-Lock syringes.
- Hands should be washed before donning and after removing gloves. Gowns or gloves that become contaminated should be changed immediately. Employees should be trained in proper methods to remove contaminated gloves and gowns. After use, gloves and gowns should be disposed of in accordance with standard recommendations.
- Infusion sets and pumps, which should have Luer-Lock fittings, should be observed for leakage during use. A plastic-backed absorbent pad should be placed under the tubing during administration to catch any leakage.
- Priming IV sets or expelling air from syringes should be carried out in a biological safety cabinet and use the PhaSeal® system. If done at the administration site, lines should be primed with nondrug-containing solution or a back-flow closed system should be used. IV containers with venting tubes should not be used.
- Syringes, IV bottles and bags, and pumps should be wiped clean of any drug contamination with sterile gauze. Needles and syringes should not be crushed or clipped. They should be placed in a puncture-resistant container, then into the chemotherapy disposal bag with all other contaminated materials.

Key point

Mixing chemotherapeutic agents must be done with care and respect because these drugs can be dangerous if they are not handled appropriately.

The PhaSeal® system

The PhaSeal® system was designed to allow medical specialists to mix and administer chemotherapy without contaminating either the facility, patient or staff involved in the process. The system is available worldwide and can be adapted with ease. PhaSeal® (Carmel Pharma, Mölndal, Sweden), a closed, double-membrane system for ensuring leak-free transfers of drugs, has been shown to reduce environmental and personnel exposure compared with existing processes for the preparation and administration of antineoplastic agents. PhaSeal® uses a dry connections system to ensure a leak-free transfer of drugs. Each element is sealed-off with a membrane cover. Transfer of the injectable drug is made via a specially cut injection cannula. When the components of the PhaSeal® system are separated after transfer, the membranes act as tight seals preventing leakage. In this way, the cytotoxic drugs have no contact with the atmosphere and thus, workers and all connections are kept dry. At present, the system cannot be deployed for use with ampules.

This system is ideal for use in veterinary medicine. In a study at Ängelholm Hospital, Sweden, PhaSeal® was tested for one year. The results were reported on the PhaSeal® web site. No safety cabinet was used during preparation of the drugs. After one year, contamination levels were determined. No cytotoxic drugs were found in the environment. This study suggests that the use of PhaSeal® alone is sufficient to prevent environmental contamination. In another study performed in veterinary medicine, the PhaSeal® system resulted in dramatic reduction of contamination in a veterinary hospital. The manufacturers of the PhaSeal® system suggest that their system may preclude the need for a cabinet however this is not recommended by the author. The biologic safety cabinet or hood is the preferred site for mixing or preparing all chemotherapeutic agents and is essential for practices that handle large volumes of these drugs. Many pharmacies will prepare chemotherapeutic agents for a fee. Practitioners should take advantage of this option when possible. However, because most practices handle small volumes of these drugs, this section is designed for those situations. Even when a biologic safety cabinet is being used, the safety principles involved in drug handling and reconstitution are the same.

Key point

The biologic safety cabinet or hood is the preferred site for mixing or preparing all chemotherapeutic agents.

When chemotherapeutic agents are mixed with PhaSeal®, all needed materials should always be available in the biological safety cabinet that is located in a quiet, low-traffic drug preparation area (figure 18-2 A and B). Eating, drinking, and smoking should not take place in the drug preparation area. The components should include the following PhaSeal® components:

- An infusion adapter with an inline spike to connect the bag to the external intravenous set. The adapter and set have a built-in connector to allow for sealed transfer of the medication to the bag.
- A Luer-Lock connector, to ensure a sealed connection between the injector and the intravenous administration set.
- An Luer-Lock injector, an encapsulated, specially cut cannula that is permanently attached to a syringe and allows for sealed transfer of the medication by means of a double membrane.
- A protector unit, a pressure-equalizing device that permanently attaches to the medication vial. The expansion chamber makes sure that neither overpressure nor vacuum occurs during drug preparation. This effectively prevents vapor leakage. The drugs have no contact with the atmosphere, and hence, no spreading of aerosols or vapor.

The other materials that should be available in the cabinet or within easy reach include:

- A plastic-backed absorbent liner to absorb any leaks and spills (the liner should be changed if it becomes contaminated with any drug and when the area is cleaned).
- Heavy-duty gloves specifically designed for handling and mixing chemotherapy.
- An infusion pump and IV lines prefilled with NaCl (if appropriate).
- A stack of gauze squares.
- A large, sealable plastic bag or container should be available for chemotherapy waste.
- A puncture-proof container for all contaminated sharps.

When preparing cytotoxic agents, a gown with long sleeves, closed cuffs, and a closed front should be worn.

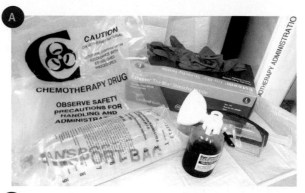

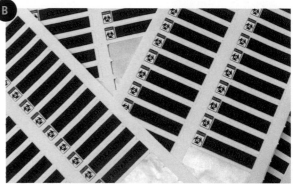

Figure 18-2: All materials that should be on hand for preparing or handling chemotherapeutic agents include appropriate gloves, all Phaseal pieces to prevent contamination of the bottle or exposure to the handler, Luer-Lock syringes and prefilled IV drip sets (A). Everything must be clearly labeled (B).

The gown should be made of a disposable fabric with low permeability. Gloves designed for chemotherapy should be pulled over the cuffs of the gown to protect the skin from drug exposure. Vinyl gloves should not be used— they are more permeable and thus more likely to allow skin contamination. Goggles or protective eyewear are necessary. The use of a dust-and-mist respirator or a mask with a filter to prevent inhalation of aerosolized drugs is recommended if a biological safety cabinet is not used with the PhaSeal® system. A conventional surgery mask does not provide adequate protection.

To prepare the chemotherapeutic drug, the plastic lid is first removed from the vial. The top of the vial is wiped with an alcohol swab. The vial is kept upright, and placed upright into the PhaSeal® clamping device provided. The plastic protector unit is then placed into the clamping device (figure 18-3 A-C). The clamping device is closed to seal the device permanently to the protector unit to ensure pressure changes are contained within the system. The vial and protector are removed from the clamping device for reconstituting or to withdraw the contents.

When reconstituting a drug, the syringe is prefilled with air or diluent to be added, and the air is attached to the injector that has the needle guarded (figure 18-4 A-F). The injector/syringe combination is then

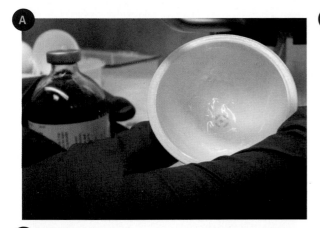

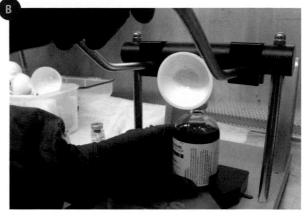

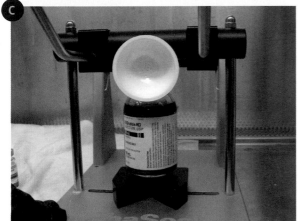

Figure 18-3: To prepare the chemotherapeutic drug, the plastic lid over the injection port of the chemotherapy vial is first removed and the top of the vial is wiped with an alcohol swab (A). The vial is kept upright, and placed upright into the Phaseal clamping device provided. The plastic protector unit is then placed into the clamping device (B). The clamping device is closed to seal the device permanently to the protector unit to ensure pressure changes are contained within the system (C). The vial and protector are removed from the clamping device for reconstituting or to withdraw the contents.

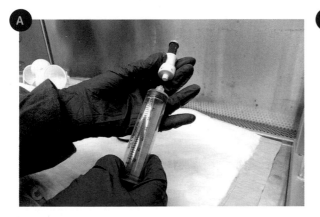

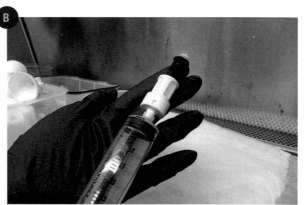

Figure 18-4: When reconstituting a drug, the syringe is attached to the injector by twisting it onto the Leur-lok (A, B).

connected to the protector device that is attached to the drug in question. The injector/syringe combination is then rotated to the "locked" position in the protector device. The safety latch of the injector is released and the needle is advanced into the vial to subsequently inject air or diluent. The injector/syringe is then withdrawn from the vial so that the needle is no longer within the vial. The injector/syringe is then disconnected. Note that the double membrane system prevents drug from ever being in contact from the operator.

When the diluent is slowly pushed into the vial, and the bottle is gently rolled or shaken. A Luer-Lock syringe can remain attached while mixing. After the drug is completely dissolved the vial is turned upside down, and the drug is aspirated into the syringe slowly to avoid excess air bubbles (figure 18-5 A-D). When the correct amount has been retrieved, any air or excess drug should be pushed back into the vial.

If the syringe contents are to be administered into a Luer-Lock connector is placed between the IV bag and

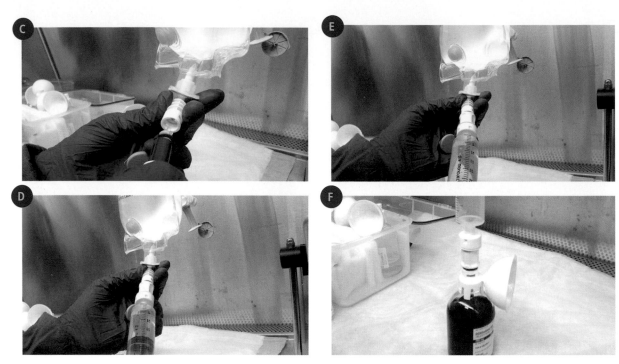

Figure 18-4 (*cont*): A connector is pushed into place into one of the ports on the bag of diluents. This connector has a special adaptor to receive the injector/syringe complex. The syringe and injector with the needle guarded is then attached to the connector and rotated into the "locked" position. The needle is advanced into the diluents and the desired amount of diluents is withdrawn and the needle is then withdrawn and disconnected (C-E). The injector/syringe/diluent combination is then connected to the protector device that is attached to the drug in question (F) and then rotated to the "locked" position in the protector device. The needle is advanced into the vial to subsequently add the diluents to the vial of drug.

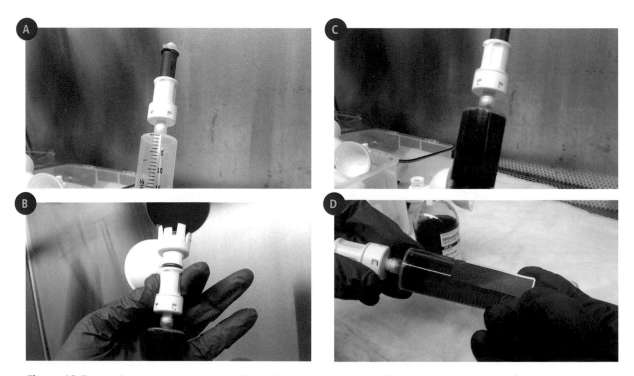

Figure 18-5: In order to remove a quantity of drug from a vial, a volume of air equal to the amount of drug to be drawn up (A) is added to the vial via the connector after ensuring that the drug is completely dissolved in the vial. The syringe/needle/vial combination is turned upside down, and the drug is aspirated into the syringe slowly to avoid excess air bubbles (B, C). When the correct amount has been retrieved, any air or excess drug should be pushed back into the vial. The syringe is then labled (D).

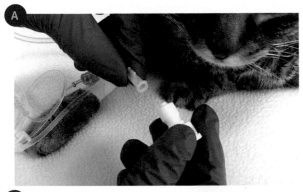

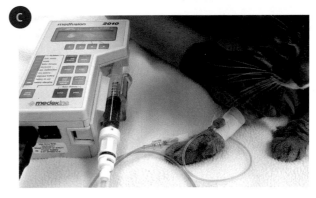

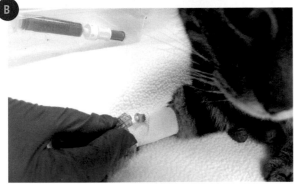

Figure 18-6: If the drug is to be administered directly into the patient's IV line (A), a separate connector is attached to the IV catheter or associated tubing (B). The injector and its associated syringe containing the drug is then attached to the IV connector and injected (C) and then removed as before.

the IV tubing to ensure a sealed connection between the injector and the intravenous administration set. The IV tubing leading to the connector is then clamped off. This connector has a special adaptor to receive the injector/syringe complex. The injector/syringe combination is advanced into the adaptor and then rotated to fix it into place. The safety latch of the injector is released and the needle is advanced into the connector to subsequently inject the drug into the bag. The needle is withdrawn from the injection port of the IV bag connector and the injector is withdrawn.

If the drug is to be administered directly into the patient's IV line, a separate connector is attached to the IV catheter or associated tubing (figure 18-6 A-C). The injector and its associated syringe containing the drug is then attached to the IV connector and injected and then removed as before.

Alternate approach

The alternate approach should only be used when all efforts to use a biological safety cabinet and PhaSeal® have failed. In this approach, chemo-pins are used prevent aerosolization of the drug and pressure from building in the vials when reconstituting drugs and are thus recommended when preparing injectable drugs. Luer-Lock syringes (figure 18-8) are required because they prevent the syringe from separating from the chemo-pin or needle. To prepare injectable drugs, the first step is removing the plastic lid from the vial and aseptically wiping the top of the vial with an alcohol swab. A chemo-pin is then inserted into

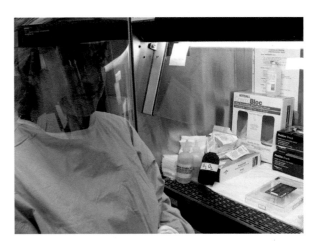

Figure 18-7: Chemotherapeutic agents should be mixed and administered in a biological safety cabinet however if not available, these drugs can be safely mixed if the handler wears a gown, a face shield, and gloves specifically designed for use with chemotherapy.

the vial. The vial is kept upright while the syringe is attached to the chemo-pin and twisted tight. When reconstituting a drug, diluent is slowly pushed into the vial, and the bottle is gently rolled or shaken. A Luer-Lock syringe can remain attached while mixing. After the drug is completely dissolved the vial is turned upside down, and the drug is aspirated into the syringe slowly to avoid excess air bubbles. When the correct amount has been retrieved, any air or excess drug should be pushed back into the vial. The

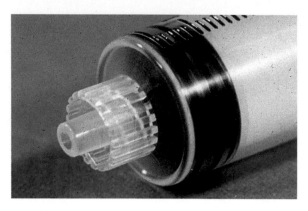

Figure 18-8: Luer-Lock syringes should be used whenever possible because their screw-on end allows a secure connection with the needle.

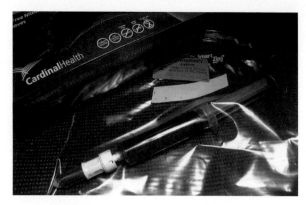

Figure 18-9: Drugs and syringes should be placed in plastic bags to contain any inadvertent spills during transportation in the hospital.

vial should then be turned upright and put down. An alcohol-moistened gauze square is wrapped around the top of the pin and syringe and the syringe is gently removed from the pin. The gauze will trap any drug that leaks or aerosolizes. A covered needle should be placed on the syringe and the chemo-pin capped after clearing the filter with an air-filled syringe. The labeled syringe should then be put into a sealable plastic bag (figure 18-9). If the remaining drug is to be stored, the chemo-pin is left inserted into the vial to allow access for multiple doses.

Key point
The alternate approach should only be used when all efforts to use a biological safety cabinet and PhaSeal® have failed.

If chemo-pins are not available, the diluent must be slowly added to the drug directly through the needle and the displaced air allowed to escape back into the syringe to avoid excess pressure in the vial. Once the drug has been reconstituted and the correct dose retrieved, an alcohol-moistened gauze square should be wrapped around the top of the vial and the needle. Then the needle should be slowly pulled out of the vial. Any air bubbles that are present should be injected into an alcohol-soaked cotton ball and discarded in the appropriate waste container. The cap should be carefully placed on the needle and the syringe put into a sealable plastic bag and labeled. As a general rule, needles should not be recapped, although sometimes this is not possible.

Regardless whether one uses the PhaSeal® system or the standard administration technique, it is extremely important to label all chemotherapeutic drugs. All syringes, fluid bags, pill bottles, and so forth must have a chemotherapy label listing the drug name, milligrams of drug, patient's name, and

dose. The drug vial should be put into a sealable plastic bag to be stored in a refrigerator or discarded according to storage instructions. Every drug has a package insert that states the expiration date and storage conditions.

All nonsharp materials used in drug preparation should be placed into a large sealable plastic bag, and all sharps must be placed in a puncture-proof container labeled as chemotherapy waste (figure 18-10). Once everything is discarded and all vials and syringes are inside sealable plastic bags, gloves should be removed by rolling them off the hands; they can then be placed in the plastic bag with the rest of the items. Care must be taken to avoid touching the outside of the gloves.

Key point
All nonsharp materials used in drug preparation should be placed into a large sealable plastic bag, and all sharps must be placed in a puncture-proof container labeled as chemotherapy waste.

Bags containing the drugs should be sealed before protective gear is removed. If protective garments are contaminated during drug preparation, they should be discarded and replaced immediately. Thorough hand washing after drug preparation is strongly recommended to remove any potential drug residues. A large, clearly labeled barrel or chemotherapy waste container should be kept in the drug preparation area for full waste bags (containing contaminated gauze squares, cotton balls, and the like) and all contaminated safety gear (e.g., gowns, gloves, masks).

When preparing a drug to be delivered by IV drip infusion, it is a good idea to prime the administration set by filling the fluid lines with diluent from the bag before the chemotherapeutic agent is added. This reduces the risk of exposure when connecting the drip set to the patient. Once reconstituted, the drug

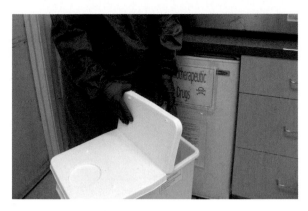

Figure 18-10: Chemotherapeutic agents and all material that may be contaminated with chemotherapy must be disposed of appropriately.

> **Key point**
>
> Although the risks are low, due to metabolism of chemotherapeutics, l gloves designed for handling chemotherapy should be worn when handling bodily fluids or stool (including disposal of litter) from patients that have received chemotherapeutic agents.

should be slowly injected into the bag. A gauze square wrapped around the injection port as the needle is withdrawn helps prevent aerosolization of drug. The fluid that contains the drug should be stored in a labeled, sealable bag until it is administered. Again, materials should be discarded appropriately. An infusion pump will allow the rate of administration of any infusion to be constant, and is preferred when the drug is diluted in a fluid bag.

Some chemotherapy agents are prepared for oral administration. When preparing or administering pills, nonporous gloves designed for chemotherapy are strongly recommended. Cytotoxic powder has been found as far as 12 inches away from where tablets are crushed or split; therefore drugs are best dispensed in whole tablets only. When small quantities of some orally administered drugs are needed, they may be prepared from the injectable formulation for use as an elixir (rather than splitting tablets). When crushing or splitting of pills cannot be avoided—and especially if a safety hood is not available—gown, goggles, and respirator mask are mandatory, and the preparation surface must be well cleaned afterwards. Oral medications should be placed in clearly labeled containers with a warning label for dispensing to owners. Owners should wear gloves designed for chemotherapy when administering oral agents to their pets and should return empty vials to the veterinarian for proper disposal. Detailed information about how owners should administer and dispose of these medications should accompany each prescription. Although the risks are low, due to metabolism of chemotherapeutics, l gloves designed for handling chemotherapy should be worn when handling bodily fluids or stool (including disposal of litter) from patients that have received chemotherapeutic agents. Caution should be employed to reduce aerosolization of bodily waste, for example high pressure hosing.

Intralesional injections consisting of a cytotoxic agent mixed with a vehicle (e.g., bovine collagen matrix, sterile sesame oil, or some other biodegradable polymer or material that acts to slowly release drug into the tumor) have been recommended by some for select localized cancers. The mixture is injected into a tumor, providing a very high drug concentration to the tumor cells but minimal systemic drug levels, thereby avoiding the risk of systemic toxicity. These mixtures are prepared in the biologic safety cabinet, but two Luer-Lock syringes, one containing the cytotoxic agent and one containing the vehicle, should be prepared. Each agent should be placed into a syringe with sufficient capacity to contain both liquids when combined (i.e., 5 ml of drug and 5 ml of vehicle each in a 10-ml syringe). The syringes are attached to a three-way stopcock, and the two liquids can then be rapidly mixed between the syringes to create an oily emulsion. The syringe that now contains all of the mixture should be detached after covering the attachment with an alcohol-moistened gauze swab to prevent aerosolization, and a needle is attached. The remaining syringe and stopcock should be discarded as contaminated waste.

It is preferable to mix multiple small volumes of drug in this way rather than a single large volume, because separation of drug from vehicle may occur rapidly, thereby reducing the efficacy of the treatment. Likewise, the drug-vehicle mixture should be administered soon after preparation. If a delay is encountered, the drug can be remixed with its vehicle using a new syringe and three-way stopcock; gloves, mask, goggles, and a gown must be worn. It may be wise to mix inside a sealable plastic bag. The needles on used syringes should not be recapped. All materials should be disposed of as contaminated waste. Note that some of the drugs reported for intralesional chemotherapy rely on reconstitution of the lyophilized drug to a higher concentration than would normally be administered systemically. Some of those drugs (e.g., cisplatin, carboplatin) are available as reconstituted drug, which is too dilute for intralesional use.

ADMINSTERING CHEMOTHERAPY

When administering chemotherapeutic agents, the same principles and caution are utilized as maintained for the mixing and handling of chemotherapeutic agents. Specifically, it is important to:[1, 11–13]

- Wear personal protective equipment including a disposable, closed, moisture-barrier gown with elastic or knit cuffs, appropriate thickness gloves designed for chemotherapy, safety glasses or face shield.
- Wear disposable non-powdered gloves designed for mixing and administering chemotherapeutic agents.
- Use absorbent plastic-backed liners to catch spills.

First 48 hours after chemotherapy

When chemotherapeutic agents are spilled or if there is elimination of any bodily excreta within 48 hours after the drug is administered, the contaminated area should be closed and traffic rerouted. Personal protective equipment must be used appropriately by all individuals involved. Commercially available "spill kits" should be used when possible. The following recommendations should be followed: [1, 11–13]

- Wear two pairs of doubled nonpowdered gloves designed for mixing and administering chemotherapeutic agents.
- Wash skin with soap and water upon contact with drug.
- Clean minor spills with 70% isopropyl alcohol.
- Decontaminate large spills with neutralizing agent or high pH soap.
- Protective clothing should be worn when cleaning up fecal matter and urine for approximately 48 hours after the administration of chemotherapeutic agents.

Disposal

Chemotherapy is considered a biological hazard and therefore must be disposed of appropriately using the following guidelines: [1, 11–13]

- Properly dispose of contaminated needles and syringes in appropriate container.
- During use, containers for contaminated sharps should be replaced routinely and not be allowed to overfill.
- During use, containers for contaminated sharps should be easily accessible to personnel and located as close as feasible to the immediate area where sharps are used or can be reasonably anticipated to be found.
- Contaminated sharps and contaminated materials must be appropriately discarded as soon as feasible in containers that are puncture-resistant, closable, leak-proof, and labeled.
- Hazardous drug-related waste should be handled separately from other hospital trash and disposed of in accordance with applicable Environmental Protection Agency (EPA), state, local, NIOSH and OSHA regulations for hazardous waste.

The health care team

Cancer chemotherapy requires a team approach; team members include the veterinarian, who listens, diagnoses, and prescribes therapy, the animal health technicians or nurses, who provide care, information, and technical expertise, and the receptionist, who informs, coordinates, and enables the caregiver and the health care team. The team approach also involves extended team members, such as the attending or consulting oncologist or internist, pharmacist, and radiologist; these members are a vital link in the advanced care of the cancer patient, especially when it comes to chemotherapy.

Key point

When the caregiver is recognized, enabled, and empowered with information and the ability to extend care to his or her best friend, compassionate care can truly be delivered.

The most important members of the team are the caregivers/clients. When the caregiver is recognized, enabled, and empowered with information and the ability to extend care to his or her best friend, compassionate care can truly be delivered. This empowering process involves giving detailed oral and written information about the cancer and chemotherapy, providing ongoing intellectual and emotional support via the entire team, and assuring that the caregiver understands and is able to provide continual and seamless care at home.

The following information summarizes the technical procedures associated with the administration of chemotherapy, however the most important aspects of providing this type of care are dependent on the ability of the health care team to extend compassionate care to the patient and the caregiver.

ADMINISTERING CHEMOTHERAPEUTIC AGENTS

Chemotherapeutic agents can be administered via several routes: intravenous, intramuscular, intracavitary, subcutaneous, intralesional (with a vehicle to slow absorption), and oral (box 18-2). Intrathecal and intraarterial administration are used less commonly in canine medicine. Regardless of the route of administration or who is administering the drugs, personal protection apparel including gloves designed for chemotherapy, gown, eyewear and facemask should be worn when handling cytotoxic agents.

Dosing

The dosing of chemotherapy also requires a team approach. Because many of the drugs used to treat

---

Box 18-2. Methods of chemotherapy administration

- Intracavitary (e.g., carboplatin, mitoxantrone).

- Intralesional (e.g., carboplatin, cisplatin, 5-fluorouracil [fatal in cats], bleomycin).

- Intramuscular (e.g., L-asparaginase).

- Intravenous: over-the-needle or indwelling catheter (e.g., vincristine, doxorubicin, mitoxantrone, cisplatin).

- Oral (e.g., cyclophosphamide, chlorambucil, melphalan).

- Subcutaneous (e.g., bleomycin).

---

cancer can have serious, potentially life-threatening side effects and the margin of safety is not as great as with other medications, team members must constantly check and recheck dosages, labels, and administration procedures. The safety of the patient, caregiver, and the veterinary health care team must be paramount.

Key point

Drugs used to treat cancer can have serious, potentially life-threatening side effects, thus the margin of safety is not as great as with other medications. Team members must constantly check and recheck dosages, labels, and administration procedures.

There has recently been discussion in the literature about the validity of dosing chemotherapeutic agents using body surface area (BSA) in square meters.[1, 11–13] These studies have shown that this dosing method may not be ideal for all veterinary patients, especially smaller animals, in which increased toxicity may be

observed.[6] The best known example is doxorubicin: the standard dose of 30 mg/m^2 may be too high for very small dogs and cats, and a dose of 1 to 1.1 mg/kg (or 20 to 25 mg/m^2) is more routinely used. Until a better dosing scheme is developed, many chemotherapeutic agents will continue to be dosed on a square meter basis.

General concepts in calculating and administering doses

- Convert weight in pounds to kilograms by dividing by 2.2. A 22-lb dog or cat weighs 10 kg (22 ÷ 2.2 = 10).
- Weight in kilograms can then be found on a weight to BSA conversion table (table 18-1).
- Determine the dose of a drug (in this example, vincristine) by multiplying the dosage (0.5 to 0.7 mg/m^2) by the patient's BSA (m^2). The patient's metabolic status should be evaluated by assessing the biochemical profile to help select the type of drug to be used (table 18-2). The severity of chemotherapy-induced myelosuppression should also be considered (box 18-3).

Table 18-1. Conversion of body weight (kg) to body surface area (m^2)*											
Dogs								**Cats**			
kg	m^2	kg	m^2	kg	m^2	kg	m^2	kg	m^2	kg	m^2
0.5	0.06	13	0.55	26	0.88	39	1.15	2	0.159	8.5	0.416
1	0.10	14	0.58	27	0.90	40	1.17	2.5	0.184	9	0.432
2	0.15	15	0.60	28	0.92	41	1.19	3	0.208	9.5	0.449
3	0.20	16	0.63	29	0.94	42	1.21	3.5	0.231	10	0.464
4	0.25	17	0.66	30	0.96	43	1.23	4	0.252		
5	0.29	18	0.69	31	0.99	44	1.25	4.5	0.273		
6	0.33	19	0.71	32	1.01	45	1.26	5	0.292		
7	0.36	20	0.74	33	1.03	46	1.28	5.5	0.311		
8	0.40	21	0.76	34	1.05	47	1.30	6	0.330		
9	0.43	22	0.78	35	1.07	48	1.32	6.5	0.348		
10	0.46	23	0.81	36	1.09	49	1.34	7	0.366		
11	0.49	24	0.83	37	1.11	50	1.36	7.5	0.383		
12	0.52	25	0.85	38	1.13	51	1.38	8	0.400		

*Most chemotherapeutic agents are dosed on a body surface area basis.

Table 18-2. Possible effect of organ dysfunction on dosing of select chemotherapeutic agents

Drug	Critical organ	Dose modifications
Doxorubicin	Liver	Initial dose reductions of as much as 50% when bilirubin is >1.5
Vincristine	Liver	Dose reduction is directly proportional to liver dysfunction
Vinblastine	Liver	Dose reduction is directly proportional to liver dysfunction
Carboplatin	Kidney	Dose reduction is directly proportional to creatinine clearance
Bleomycin	Kidney	Decrease initial dose by as much as 50%–75% if creatinine clearance is <25 ml/min/m^2
Cyclophosphamide	Kidney, liver	Decrease initial dose by as much as 50%–75% if creatinine clearance is <25 ml/min/m^2; because the liver is necessary to activate the drug, liver disease may warrant dose modification
Cisplatin	Kidney	Do not use with clinically evident renal failure; use caution in animals with any renal problems. NEVER use in cats
Methotrexate	Kidney	Dose reduction is directly proportional to creatinine clearance

---

Box 18-3. Myelosuppressive potential of some commonly used chemotherapeutic agents in veterinary medicine*

Highly myelosuppressive

Doxorubicin

Vinblastine

Cyclophosphamide

Actinomycin D

Moderately myelosuppressive

Melphalan

Chlorambucil

5-fluorouracil (fatal if used in cats)

Methotrexate

Mildly myelosuppressive

L-asparaginase*

Vincristine*

Bleomycin

Corticosteroids

*Myelosuppression can occur if these two drugs are administered concurrently.

- Before the quantity of drug is drawn up or obtained, the concentration (mg/ml or mg/pill or capsule) of the chemotherapeutic agent is checked. For example, doxorubicin (and some other drugs) has a concentration of 2 mg/ml, so it is necessary to divide the milligrams by 2 to determine how many milliliters to administer. If the drug is a pill or capsule, the amount to be administered is rounded down to the next whole tablet. Chemotherapy pills or capsules must never be split, crushed, reformulated, or repackaged to prevent inadvertent exposure of the handler to cytotoxic drugs and/or overdose of the patient.

- Before the drug is administered, the dose and results of the CBC are double-checked. If the neutrophil count is below 3000/µl, administration of myelosuppressive drugs (e.g., doxorubicin, cyclophosphamide) should be postponed and the CBC rechecked in 3 to 7 days.

- A CBC is sometimes obtained 7 days after administering the first dose of any potentially myelosuppressive drug (7 days is the neutrophil nadir for most drugs; refer to drug tables in the following section for individual variation). If the neutrophil count is below 1,500/µl 7 days after treatment, the drug dose may be reduced by 25 percent, especially if the dog or cat demonstrates clinical signs relating to neutropenia. The new dose can be administered subsequently, assuming the patient does well with the reduced dose. Doses can then be increased by increments of 10 percent until the originally calculated "full" dose is reached provided the patient continues to tolerate the lower doses.

- Anorexia is a common side effect of many chemotherapeutic agents in dogs and cats. If severe or accompanied by more than 10 percent loss of body weight, a dose reduction should be considered. A good rule of thumb is 25 percent, although the dose may subsequently be increased by increments of 10 percent if no further anorexia is observed.

- For some drugs, the results of a serum chemistry profile should be reviewed before the drug is administered. For example lomustine (CCNU) can result in liver failure if not discontinued when serum ALT activity rises; carboplatin may be poorly excreted when renal dysfunction is present, resulting in more severe myelosuppression than would be predicted.

Intravenous administration

Many chemotherapeutic agents are administered IV. Because some of these agents are vesicants or irritants, every attempt must be made to ensure that the veins are cared for and that catheters are placed as cleanly and atraumatically as possible. As a general rule, peripheral veins should never be used for venipuncture to collect blood samples to ensure that the veins are preserved for catheter placement only. Chemotherapeutic agents are usually administered by butterfly catheter, over-the-needle catheter, a through-the-needle intracatheter (such as used for central venous access), or a vascular access port. Vascular access ports can be placed subcutaneously and the catheter placed in a free-flowing vein such as the jugular.

Peripheral vessels are preferred for IV drug administration because of the ease of monitoring for drug extravasation. Regardless of the type of catheter used, certain preparatory steps should be taken. The leg to be used should be clipped at the site of injection and prepared using aseptic technique. When a drug is known to be a vesicant, an indwelling catheter or a vascular access device should be placed, particularly if the drug is not being administered as a bolus.

Drugs should never be administered when venipuncture is less than perfect (i.e., when the vein is entered more than once); another leg should be used instead. If another leg is unavailable, the first venipuncture site should be allowed to clot before another attempt is made proximal to that site. A second venipuncture should never be attempted distal to the site of a failed attempt. It is a good idea to alternate and record the veins being used to allow them to recover between administrations.

Key point

Drugs should never be administered when venipuncture is less than perfect.

The catheter should be flushed with nonheparinized 0.9% NaCl (minimum, 10 ml) before and after each drug administration to determine patency. When multiple drugs are being given, the catheter should be flushed between agents. Nonheparinized 0.9% NaCl is recommended because heparin causes precipitates to form when mixed with some drugs (e.g., doxorubicin).

The catheter and leg should be monitored constantly during drug administration to detect any extravasation. If the catheter is to be secured, use only one piece of tape and ensure that visualization of the injection site, the area surrounding the site, and the leg proximal to the site is not obscured.

It is important to check whether there is a specific rate at which a drug should be administered to minimize toxicity. For example, undiluted doxorubicin should be given at a maximum rate of 1 ml/minute whereas vincristine can be given as a bolus. Alternatively, doxorubicin can be placed in 35 ml of 0.9% NaCl and administered over 10 to 15 minutes. The drug should be injected slowly and evenly to prevent excessive pressure to the vein and leakage of drug around the needle or catheter.

After the drug has been administered and the catheter flushed, a piece of gauze or an alcohol-soaked cotton ball should be placed (with a gloved hand) over the needle as it is withdrawn from the injection port or over the catheter as it is removed from the vein; this minimizes drug aerosolization. All of the drug should be flushed through the catheter without re-aspirating the catheter, as re-aspirating at this time allows diluted drug to remain in the catheter. A cotton ball can be taped over the insertion site after the catheter is removed and pressure applied for several minutes.

All materials should be discarded into appropriate chemotherapy waste containers. Syringes and needles should be placed in a puncture- and leak-proof container that is clearly marked as containing hazardous or chemotherapeutic waste. Even though gloves designed for chemotherapy are always worn, it is important to wash hands thoroughly after every drug administration.

Intravenous over-the-needle catheter

Generally, drugs that are to be given as a bolus (but over a period of minutes) are given through IV over-the-needle catheters. Over-the-needle catheters should be used for doxorubicin administration, for which a slow rate of delivery is important to prevent an allergic reaction. It is preferable to place the catheter while wearing gloves designed for chemotherapy, but it may be placed before drugs are prepared as long as patency is reconfirmed before drug administration.

For over-the-needle catheter administration, long, clear, male-adapter injection ports allow for better viewing of the flush back of blood and the drug being administered. In addition, these plugs allow the person administering the drug to determine when all of the drug has been flushed out of the catheter at the end of the procedure.

Once the catheter has been placed, a 4 by 4-inch gauze square should be folded in half and slipped under the injection cap to absorb any drug that may leak out of the injection cap during administration. Needles should be inserted as far as possible into the injection port to allow for easier flushing of residual drug after injection.

Continuous intravenous infusion

An indwelling catheter should be used when drugs (e.g., cytosine arabinoside, ifosfamide) are to be administered over a long period (6 to 48 hours).[1, 11–13] or for saline diuresis that accompanies nephrotoxic drugs such as cisplatin or streptozotocin. In these administrations, an infusion pump is recommended. Free-flowing fluid administration, even when monitored continuously, may not ensure continued diuresis, or could result in uneven delivery of the drug dose. Both could affect the risk of toxicity. A calibrated infusion pump will allow predictable administration of the chemotherapy dose.

The catheter site and all connections in the IV line should be monitored frequently for patency and leakage. The patient must be prevented from chewing or disconnecting the IV line.

During long periods of drug administration, disposal of contaminated waste, particularly urine, becomes important. When the patient or any waste is handled, gloves designed for chemotherapeutic agents, a gown, goggles, and a mask should be worn to reduce the risk of exposure to excreted active metabolites. Cages, runs, or excreta should not be hosed, because this aerosolizes the drug and distributes it more widely. All waste, including litter material, should be discarded as contaminated material.

Key point

When the patient or any waste is handled, gloves designed for chemotherapeutic agents, a gown, goggles, and a mask should be worn to reduce the risk of exposure to excreted active metabolites.

Subcutaneous infusion ports

Many veterinary patients are small, and their vascular integrity may be compromised by multiple anesthesias (surgery, radiation therapy) prior to receiving chemotherapy. With the risk of extravasation reactions being high in these patients, an indwelling, subcutaneously located implantable vascular access port may assure timely drug delivery and also reduce patient stress during restraint for catheter placement and administration of chemotherapy. Such a port may be maintained for the duration of the chemotherapy protocol and then removed. The implantable vascular access port must be placed surgically, in a similar manner to a tunneled catheter, with a subcutaneous pocket for positioning of the port. Ports for veterinary patients are available from Norfolk Vet Products, Skokie, Illinois.

Intramuscular or intralesional administration

IM injections are administered in the normal fashion, but gloves designed for chemotherapy should be worn. Because L-asparaginase can cause an anaphylactic reaction when given IV, the syringe must be checked for blood to ensure that a vessel has not been inadvertently entered before injecting the drug IM. Preferred sites of injection include well-muscled areas such as the caudal thigh region or lumbar musculature.

Intralesional chemotherapy is always administered as a suspension in oil or other vehicle, not as pure drug. Gloves designed for chemotherapy, goggles, and a protective gown should be worn when administering intralesional chemotherapy, and it is important to watch the area carefully for any leakage of chemotherapeutic agent. If leakage occurs, the area should be swabbed and cleaned with soap and water and the cleaning materials disposed of as hazardous waste. When repositioning the needle during intralesional therapy, there is often pressure on the syringe contents that will cause the mixture to leak out when the needle is withdrawn from the tumor. Negative pressure on the syringe when withdrawing will help reduce leakage.

Oral administration

Wearing specially designed gloves for mixing and administering chemotherapy is necessary when administering pills. The patient is given the pills in the normal fashion. It is important to assure oneself that the patient has indeed swallowed the pill; it may be helpful to follow pill administration with water given via syringe. If owners are to administer oral chemotherapy, they must be instructed to wear disposable protective chemotherapy gloves and wash their hands immediately after administration.

Intracavitary administration

Some chemotherapeutic agents (e.g., cisplatin (dogs only), carboplatin, mitoxantrone) can be administered into body cavities (thorax, abdomen, pericardial sac, urinary bladder).[1, 4] Both the person administrating the drug and the one restraining the animal should wear gloves. As with IV administration, the IV line needs to be primed *before* the drug is added to the bag. The diluent should be warmed to body temperature or slightly above before drug is added and the solution administered.

For both thoracic and abdominal administration, and particularly for pericardial administration, ultrasonographic guidance may be very helpful in avoiding needle puncture of organs or structures.

For thoracic administration, the patient is placed in lateral recumbency and the injection site is aseptically prepared. The right side is preferred, and the area of the cardiac notch provides the least risk of lung puncture. The area is infiltrated with lidocaine, and an 18-gauge rigid plastic IV cannula is inserted between the ribs and flushed with a minimum of 12 ml of warm saline to ensure a patent pathway. If there is resistance to the flush or if the dog or cat appears uncomfortable or coughs, the cannula should be removed and a new one inserted.

For abdominal administration, the patient is placed in dorsal recumbency and a midline site caudal to the umbilicus is used. The site chosen should be caudal enough to avoid the spleen. Allowing the patient to urinate before administration reduces the risk of bladder puncture. The site is aseptically prepared, and the catheter should be placed as described for thoracic administration.

Once the patency is determined, the fluid line is attached and the drug is administered. A maximum volume of 250 ml/m² should be infused into the thoracic cavity and 1000 ml/m² into the abdominal cavity to ensure adequate exposure of all surfaces with minimal discomfort to the patient. The fluid should flow fairly easily into the cavity. If the fluid drip slows or is intermittent, the cannula can be adjusted slightly. The area should be monitored constantly to make sure the fluid is not being administered SC. Once the bag is empty, the IV line should be turned off; a piece of gauze should be wrapped around the cannula and the cannula slowly removed. At this point, the person restraining the animal should hold an alcohol-moistened gauze square over the site and apply pressure to stop any bleeding and/or leakage

that may occur. Finally, the patient should be allowed to move around for a few minutes to allow the drug to distribute through the entire cavity. All materials must be discarded as contaminated waste.

References

1. OSHA Work Practice Guidelines for Personnel: Dealing with Cytotoxic Drugs. *OSHA Instructional Publication* 8-1.1, Washington DC, Office of Occupational Medicine, 1986.
2. Nikula E, Kiviniitty K, Leisti J, Taskinen P: Chromosome aberrations in lymphocytes of nurses handling cytostatic agents. *Scand J Work Environ Health* 10:71-74, 1984.
3. Norppa H, Sorsa M, Vainio H, et al: Increased sister chromatid exchange frequencies in lymphocytes of nurses handling cytostatic drugs. *Scand J Work Environ Health* 6:299-301, 1980.
4. Pohlova H, Cerna M, Rossner P: Chromosomal aberrations, SCE and urine mutagenicity in workers occupationally exposed to cytostatic drugs. *Mutat Res* 174:213-217, 1986.
5. Stiller A, Obe G, Bool I, Pribilla W: No elevation of the frequencies of chromosomal aberrations as a consequence of handling cytostatic drugs. *Mutat Res* 121:253-259, 1983.
6. Stucker I, Hirsch A, Doloy T, et al: Urine mutagenicity, chromosomal abnormalities and sister chromatid exchanges in lymphocytes of nurses handling cytostatic drugs. *Int. Arch Occup Environ Health* 57:195-205, 1986.
7. Hemminki, K, Kyyronen P, Lindbohm ML: Spontaneous abortions and malformations in the offspring of nurses exposed to anaesthetic gases, cytostatic drugs, and other potential hazards in hospitals, based on registered information of outcome. *J Epidem Comm Health* 39:141-147, 1985.
8. Selevan SG, Lindbolm ML, Hornung RW, Hemminki K: A study of occupational exposure to antineoplastic drugs and fetal loss in nurses. *New Engl J Med* 313:1173-1178, 1985.
9. Stucker I, Caillard JF, Collin R, et al: Risk of spontaneous abortion among nurses handling antineoplastic drugs. *Scand J Work Environ Health* 16:102-107, 1990.
10. Rosner F: Acute leukemia as a delayed consequence of cancer chemotherapy. *Cancer* 37:1033-1036, 1976.
11. Kandel-Tschiederer B, Kessler M, Schwietzer A, Michel A: Papers Reduction of workplace contamination with platinum-containing cytostatic drugs in a veterinary hospital by introduction of a closed system. *Veterinary Record 166*, 822-825, 2010.
12. Takada S: Principles of chemotherapy safety procedures. *Clin Tech Small Anim Pract* 18(2):73-74, 2003.
13. Kandel-Tschiederer B, Kessler M, Schwietzer A, Michel A: Reduction of workplace contamination with platinum-containing cytostatic drugs in a veterinary hospital by introduction of a closed system. *Vet Record 166*, 822-825, 2010.

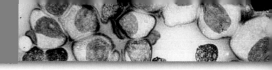

Chapter 19

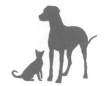

Healing with chemotherapy

Most veterinarians, veterinary nurses and the general public have one thing in common: They are all frightened by the concept of chemotherapy. This innate fear is a learned bias that begins very early in life. In order to dispel the myths and misperceptions associated with chemotherapy, the entire veterinary health care team must become very aware of the facts associated with the properties, benefits, and risks associated with anticancer agents. This must occur before clients and patients are cared for. Everyone must be committed to the goals that chemotherapy must only be employed if it will likely improve quality of life. Once the team has taken these steps, then they are then able to discuss the fears, myths and misperceptions that many clients have about chemotherapy. From that point, every effort must be taken to prevent toxicities before they occur and aggressively treat them if they do occur. The purpose of this section is to review select, clinically relevant information about cancer therapies.

GENERAL PRINCIPLES OF CANCER THERAPY

Before a therapeutic strategy can be defined and instituted, the patient should be fully evaluated and stabilized and the tumor identified histologically and staged to determine the extent of disease. In addition, the client, veterinarian, and the rest of the veterinary health care team need to be aware of the:

- Potential benefits and toxicoses associated with the administration of chemotherapeutic agents—both parties should be committed to preventing toxicosis from developing and promptly resolving it if it does occur.
- Need to follow the treatment protocol, including timing, dosages, and treatment intervals whenever possible.
- Expenses associated with chemotherapy (fortunately, many chemotherapeutic agents are becoming available as generic products at a fraction of the cost of the patented parent drug).
- Time, equipment and expertise required to safely and effectively provide optimal treatment.

When a practice decides to treat patients with chemotherapy, the following management decisions must be made:

- Chemotherapy must be readily available for routine use. Treatment delays can abolish any efficacy that the drugs provide.
- Ideally, localized, solid malignancies should be removed surgically to the greatest extent possible before therapy. Alternatively, radiation therapy, either palliative or definitive, can be used to provide local control of the malignancy prior to chemotherapy; these drugs can be used to enhance the effect of radiation as well as to delay or prevent spread or regrowth of the cancer.
- Adjuvant chemotherapy should begin as soon after surgery as possible while maintaining quality of life.
- Therapy should be given at appropriate dosages for limited periods of time.
- Procedures should be set up to manage urgent care situations, 24 hours a day.
- Clients should be given oral and written information about the chemotherapeutic agents and protocol being used as well as medication that can prevent nausea, vomiting, diarrhea, and anorexia (e.g., metoclopramide).

Key point

Clients should be given oral and written information about the chemotherapeutic agents and protocol being used as well as medication that can prevent nausea, vomiting, diarrhea, and anorexia (e.g., maropitant, metronidazole).

Box 19-1. Stages of a combination treatment protocol [5-9]

Induction is the often intensely scheduled initial treatments during which time a patient has a relatively higher risk of toxicity but usually also greatest chance of response; (e.g., the first 12 weeks of VELCAP [vincristine, asparaginase, cyclophosphamide, doxorubicin, prednisone]).

Consolidation is sometimes used at the end of induction using unrelated, effective drugs to further reduce the proportion of surviving cancer cells (e.g., MOPP [mechlorethamine, vincristine, procarbazine, and prednisone] and lomustine in VELCAP).

Maintenance is a less intense (usually decreased frequency of administration) phase using drugs already used during induction. Maintenance therapy probably has little influence on whether an animal is cured but may prolong survival in animals by slowing the time to relapse.

Rescue is a term used for therapy given when the previously used drugs are no longer effective. Unrelated drugs, often alkylating agents are used as they are less likely to show cross resistance.

Chemotherapeutic agents are used to induce remission and for intensification, consolidation, and maintenance therapy. The following definitions are important when discussing classical clinical chemotherapy:

Remission: The standard definitions in the past for remission are as follows: *complete remission* exists when all clinical evidence of a tumor has disappeared; in contrast, the term *partial remission* is often used when the sum of the products of the two longest diameters of the tumor in question is reduced in size by at least 50% and there is no additional evidence of new tumors anywhere. Progressive disease occurs when the tumor increases in size by at least 50% of the sum of the products of two largest diameters. More recently, an adaptation of the human Response Evaluation Criteria for Solid Tumors (RECIST) has been used to assess responses in veterinary patients, including those with lymphoma. This criteria assesses the change in tumor size in target and non-target lesions. *Target* lesions are those tumors that can be repeatedly measured clinically without imaging techniques. These target lesions should be measurable with a longest diameter (LD) ≥ 20 mm at baseline measurement. A minimum of one and a maximum of five involved tumors are identified as target lesions and measured and recorded at pretreatment baseline and at stipulated intervals during treatment and follow-up. All remaining measurable and non-measurable lesions are also be categorized as *non-target* lesions. The mean of the sums of the longest diameters of all target lesions is determined and that is defined as the Mean Sum LD.

In the RECIST system, the following definitions are included:

- Complete response (CR): A complete response of target lesion such that there is a disappearance of all evidence of disease. Any pathologic non-target lesions must be considered to have returned to normal size and no new sites of disease should be observed.

- Partial response (PR): At least a 30% decrease in the mean sum LD of target lesions.
- Progressive disease (PD): At least a 20% increase in the mean sum LD of target lesions.
- Stable disease (SD): Neither sufficient change in size to qualify for PR or PD.

Adjuvant treatment: After surgery or radiation therapy, adjuvant chemotherapy may be given to slow the progress of metastatic disease or to potentially provide a cure. The optimum time to administer primary chemotherapy is when the patient has microscopic disease rather than when there are gross metastases. An example of successful adjuvant veterinary chemotherapy is the use of platinum compounds and doxorubicin after surgery for canine osteosarcoma.

Intensification, which is introduced after remission has been obtained, involves the administration of chemotherapeutic agents with different mechanisms of action in an attempt to kill any resistant tumor cells. This is often discussed, but rarely employed in veterinary chemotherapy protocols.

Consolidation, which also takes place after a patient is in remission, is the phase of treatment in which different drugs are administered to improve clinical response by reducing the microscopic tumor burden.

Maintenance therapy refers to the drugs used to keep the patient in remission. Consolidation and maintenance therapies were classically used in the treatment of hematopoietic tumors (e.g., lymphoma) than solid tumors (e.g., carcinomas and sarcomas), however most chemotherapy protocols used now are shorter and more intense with similar results to those with maintenance periods.

Metronomic chemotherapy is the use of tiny dosages of chemotherapeutic agents, most notably cyclophosphamide, CCNU and chlorambucil to delay or prevent progression of cancer via an antiangiogenic mechanism rather than through a direct cytotoxicity.

Neoadjuvant therapy is used to decrease the bulk of primary tumors with chemotherapy before surgery or radiation.

Molecular therapeutics is the use of drugs or agents that delay or prevent the progression or spread of cancer by changing the way a cell functions or divides by precisely impacting one or more molecular mechanisms. A perfect example includes the tyrosine kinase inhibitors. Tyrosine kinase inhibitors are an innovative class of drug that has recently become available to veterinary medicine. This targeted therapy inhibits enzymes involved in cellular signaling pathways that regulate key cell functions and cell survival. Over the last decade, tyrosine kinase inhibitors have revolutionized the management of certain human cancers and are now making inroads into veterinary medicine, with canine mast cell tumor being their first major success story. Tyrosine kinase inhibitors used in the veterinary setting, either having been borrowed from human medicine or developed especially to address unmet veterinary needs, include imatinib, masitinib, and toceranib. Of these, the latter two have been approved for use in many parts of the world for the treatment of canine mast cell tumor.

Cancer prevention by delay is defined as the use of treatments to enhance the disease-free interval, survival, and quality of life after surgery, chemotherapy, or radiation.[1] While the ultimate goal for the treatment of high-grade malignancies is to eliminate all evidence of cancer, resulting in a cure, this is often not accomplished unless additional therapies can be initiated. Cancer prevention by delay is currently of great interest, in part because the medical definition of success of cancer therapy is being re-defined. Cancer has traditionally been defined as a chronic disease. With many of the molecular cancer therapies available today, the goal is not to eliminate the cancer but to arrest its growth to prevent it from becoming a clinically evident problem. The importance of this approach is underscored with the fact that, despite decades of intense effort and billions of dollars of expenditure, the cure rate in human and veterinary patients by these approaches has remained elusive. This concept is based on the use of treatments designed to enhance disease-free interval, survival, and quality of life after surgery by reducing the rate of cancer development or incidence. Cancer prevention by delay is an important mechanism behind the successes of several therapeutic agents, including:[1]

- Tamoxifen has been shown to significantly diminish the risk of breast cancer in people, but this has not been documented in dogs and cats.
- Retinoids and interferon-α to reduce the risk of head and neck cancer in some human and rodent tumors. Tretinoin has been shown to be of benefit in treating mycosis fungoides in dogs and cats.
- NSAIDs have been shown to delay or reduce the development of soft tissue sarcomas, hemangiosarcoma in dogs and colorectal cancer in people.
- Polyunsaturated fatty acids of the n-3 series have been shown to decrease the risk of breast cancer recurrence in women and lymphoma and hemangiosarcoma in dogs.
- Anti-angiogenesis agents have been shown to reduce the risk of cancer recurrence.

The delay of cancer growth and development, also known as clinical cancer chemoprevention, is a valuable clinical tool until permanent or absolute cancer prevention can be achieved. Piroxicam may have the same effect against transitional cell carcinoma and head and neck squamous cell carcinoma in dogs and cats.

The beneficial effects of chemotherapy are inversely proportional to tumor size; therefore, whenever anticancer drugs are being used as adjuvants, the tumor should be reduced to its smallest volume and number of cells, such as with surgery or radiation therapy, before chemotherapy is initiated. To use chemotherapeutic agents to their fullest advantage, clinicians should be knowledgeable about a drug's indications for use, doses, and timing of administration, resistance, and toxicity. Chemotherapy should be considered for patients with such malignancies as leukemia, lymphoma, multiple myeloma, and other hematopoietic tumors or with highly malignant tumors that metastasize rapidly.

Key point

The beneficial effects of chemotherapy are inversely proportional to tumor size; therefore, whenever anticancer drugs are being used as adjuvants, the tumor should be reduced to its smallest volume and number of cells, such as with surgery or radiation therapy, before chemotherapy is initiated.

DRUGS

Chemotherapy-induced cures for lymphoproliferative malignancies may be possible with combination chemotherapy protocols and almost never with single-agent protocols. Other, non hematopoietic malignancies are often benefited with chemotherapy by delaying or preventing progression or metastases, but the probability of cures is very rare. Importantly, each drug in a combination protocol *must* be effective for the treatment of the cancer in question. Compared with multiple-drug regimens, single-drug regimens are less toxic, less expensive, and require less time for clients and the veterinary health care team. However, multiple-drug protocols are believed to be more effective—especially for lymphoid malignancies—because a combination of drugs is used and resistance develops more slowly. Currently in veterinary medicine, however, few multiple-drug protocols have been shown to be more effective than single-agent protocols for the treatment of nonlymphoid malignancies. This is probably because the doses used to treat dogs and cats with cancer are an order of magnitude lower than those used in human cancer patients.

Doses

With few exceptions, the most effective dose of chemotherapeutic agents is often very close to the toxic dose. In addition, a given dose of a drug kills a constant fraction of cells regardless of the number of cells present at the start of therapy. Doses of chemotherapeutic agents are often given on the basis of metabolic rate, described as body surface area (BSA) in square meters. Most antineoplastic agents seem to be metabolized or excreted in a complex fashion and thus should be dosed on a square meter basis. A chart for converting weight in kilograms to BSA is recommended. Be extremely cautious *not* to use the weight in pounds when reading the kilogram chart. This can result in serious toxicity.

Dosing and toxicity can depend on many factors, including an animal's ability to metabolize and eliminate chemotherapeutic agents. The selection of drug dosage can also be influenced by organ dysfunction. While there are no established guidelines, it may be safest to reduce the dosage of hepatically metabolized drugs by 50% if the serum bilirubin is greater than 1.5 mg/dL, and by 75% if serum bilirubin is greater than 3.0 mg/dL. Dosages can then be slowly increased following each cycle that occurs without toxicity.

Because carboplatin is renally excreted, carboplatin dosage should ideally be based on glomerular filtration rate (GFR). If GFR cannot be estimated, an arbitrary dose reduction of 50% to 75% should be performed for animals with renal azotemia, after which dosages can be increased after each cycle with no toxicity.

Timing

The timing of administration of antitumor drugs is critical. Delays in therapy can ultimately result in a regrowth of tumor cells that are developing resistance to the drugs being used. Unlike some tumor cells, normal cells have repair mechanisms that are able to correct cellular damage. Therefore, cytotoxic drugs must be given at proper intervals to allow the tumor cells to die while normal cells recover. An improper administration schedule results in either excess toxicity or a lack of antitumor activity.

Resistance

As mentioned earlier, in contrast to normal cells, most tumor cells develop resistance to antitumor medicine. Resistance is one of the limiting factors in tumor chemotherapy. This resistance results from an acquired or induced phenomenon known as *multiple drug resistance* (MDR), which is caused by a cell membrane protein that literally pumps out cellular toxins, such as chemotherapeutic agents. Because chemotherapeutics diffuse into cells passively, the pump mechanism is able to prevent intracellular accumulation of these drugs. Certain anticancer drugs (e.g., doxorubicin, paclitaxel) are eliminated from the cell by this mechanism even though they have different molecular structures. Fortuitously, there seems to be little cross-resistance among alkylating agents (e.g., cyclophosphamide, chlorambucil, melphalan). Resistance to other drugs, such as the enzyme L-asparaginase, is induced when antibodies are formed against the drug, thereby causing a rapid destruction of the substance after administration. The introduction of the tyrosine kinase inhibitors has enhanced the ability to control cancer in dogs and cats, however resistance develops to this class of drugs.

Toxicity

Select chemotherapeutic agents and their toxicities are noted elsewhere in this section (table 19-1). Most of these agents kill or damage rapidly dividing cells. The most clinically important toxicoses include bone marrow suppression, alopecia, and gastrointestinal toxicity (BAG). Methods of identifying and treating some of the more common side effects are discussed below.

Bone marrow toxicity

Many antitumor drugs cause a decrease in the number of blood cells present days to weeks after administration. Neutropenia and thrombocytopenia are the early signs of bone marrow suppression. Clinical signs may include those related to sepsis, petechial and ecchymotic hemorrhages, pallor, and weakness. Many animals are physically normal despite low leukocyte and platelet counts, so only patients exhibiting clinical signs should be treated. The treatment of clinically significant bone marrow toxicity includes using aseptic techniques when placing indwelling devices (e.g., catheters), minimizing trauma, and controlling any bleeding with prolonged application of direct pressure or cold packs.

Table 19-1. Properties associated with some anticancer drugs

Common drugs	Potential toxicoses*	Reported indications
Alkylating agents		
CCNU (lomustine)	BA, cumulative thrombocytopenia, hepatic and renal toxicity	Lymphoma, mycosis fungoides, mast cell tumor, brain tumor
Chlorambucil	BAG, cerebellar toxicity	Chronic lymphocytic leukemia, lymphoma
Cyclophosphamide	BAG, sterile hemorrhagic cystitis	Lymphoma, sarcoma, mammary adenocarcinoma
Hydroxyurea	BAG, anemia	Myelogenous leukemia, primary erythrocytosis
Ifosfamide	BAG, sterile hemorrhagic cystitis	Soft tissue sarcoma, lymphoma, hemangiosarcoma
Melphalan	BAG	Multiple myeloma
Mechlorethamine (Mustargen)	BAG, perivascular slough	Lymphoma
Dacarbazine	BAG	Lymphoma, sarcoma
Procarbazine	BAG	Lymphoma
Thiotepa	BAG	Transitional cell carcinoma
Antimetabolites		
Cytarabine	BAG	Lymphoma, leukemia
Fluorouracil	Neurotoxicity, BAG, Fatal in cats	Sarcomas, carcinomas
Gemcitabine	BAG, neurotoxicity	Hepatic and pancreatic carcinomas, lymphoma, bladder tumors
Methotrexate	BAG	Lymphoma
Antibiotics		
Bleomycin	Pulmonary fibrosis, BAG	Squamous cell carcinoma, lymphoma
Dactinomycin	BAG, perivascular slough	Lymphoma
Doxorubicin	BAG, perivascular slough, allergic reaction during administration, anorexia and weight loss, renal failure (rare), cardiomyopathy	Lymphoma, sarcoma (including hemangiosarcoma), thyroid carcinoma, mammary adenocarcinoma
Idarubicin	BAG	Lymphoma
Mitoxantrone	BAG	Lymphoma, mammary adenocarcinoma, squamous cell carcinoma
Plicamycin (Mithramycin)	BAG, vesicant	Hypercalcemia of malignancy
Enzymes		
L-asparaginase/ pegaspargase	Anaphylaxis, disseminated intravascular coagulopathy, pancreatitis, pain on injection	Lymphoma
Vinca alkaloids		
Vinblastine	BAG, peripheral neuropathy, perivascular slough	Lymphoma, mast cell tumor
Vincristine	BAG, peripheral neuropathy, perivascular slough	Lymphoma, sarcoma, mast cell tumor, thrombocytopenia
Hormones		
Prednisone/prednisolone	iatrogenic Cushing's syndrome	Lymphoma, mast cell tumor

(Continued)

Table 19-1. Properties associated with some anticancer drugs *(cont.)*

Common drugs	Potential toxicoses*	Reported indications
Miscellaneous agents		
Amifostine	Hypotension, nausea	To reduce cisplatin and/or radiation toxicity in the dog
Carboplatin	BAG, nephrotoxicity (rare), emesis (rare)	Osteosarcoma (dogs), squamous cell carcinoma, germinal cell tumor, transitional cell carcinoma
Cisplatin	BAG, nephrotoxicity, ototoxicity. Fatal if used in cats	Osteosarcoma, squamous cell carcinoma, transitional cell carcinoma
Dexrazoxane		To reduce doxorubicin-induced cardiotoxicity in the dog only
Epoetin alfa	Hypertension, fever, lethargy	Cancer-related anemia
Gallium nitrate	Nephrotoxicity, nausea, vomiting, diarrhea	Hypercalcemia of malignancy
Isotretinoin	Keratoconjunctivitis sicca, hypertriglyceridemia, hepatotoxicity	Cutaneous neoplasms such as sebaceous adenoma, mycosis fungoides
Mesna		To prevent cystitis secondary to ifosfamide toxicity
Mitotane	Signs associated with hypoadrenocorticism	Adrenocortical carcinoma
Streptozocin/ streptozotocin	Nephrotoxicity, emesis, occasional hypoglycemic-induced weakness postinfusion, alanine transaminase elevation	Insulinoma in the dog only
Pamidronate disodium	Nephrotoxicity, emesis	Bone metastasis, osteosarcoma
Paclitaxel	BAG, diluent Cremophor EL and alcohol cause an acute allergic reaction, hypotension, and collapse on administration	Mammary adenocarcinoma, osteosarcoma, malignant histiocytosis (preliminary data) in the dog only
Piroxicam	GI ulceration and nephrotoxicity	Transitional cell carcinoma, squamous cell carcinoma, pain relief

* **Bone marrow suppression is dose-dependent.**
BA = bone marrow suppression and alopecia; BAG = bone marrow suppression, alopecia, and gastrointestinal toxicity (anorexia and weight loss are sometimes the only observable clinical signs in BAG)

If an animal develops a fever or becomes septic, urine, blood, and, if indicated, material obtained via a transtracheal aspirate should be analyzed and cultured immediately prior to the initiation of therapy unless the delay is likely to be life threatening. The affected animal should be treated with broad-spectrum bactericidal antibiotics (e.g., cephalosporins, sulfamethoxazole-trimethoprim [SMZ-TMP]) until results of culture and sensitivity testing are available. Do not delay antibiotic treatment while awaiting culture results. In addition, the patient should be supported with fluids, warmth, and nutritional therapy and given transfusions of fresh whole blood (collected in plastic containers) or specific cell lines as needed.

The availability of recombinant human granulocyte colony-stimulating factor now makes it possible to treat bone marrow toxicity by boosting endogenous production of neutrophils. The drug(s) that induced the bone marrow suppression should be discontinued until blood counts have recovered; subsequent doses of that myelosuppressive drug should be reduced (e.g., decrease cyclophosphamide doses by 25%).

The use and misuse of antibiotics is an important issue facing the entire biomedical community. In general, antibiotics are not use prophylactically when administering chemotherapy. Having said that, there appears to be a benefit when dogs with lymphoma are being given doxorubicin for the first treatment to induce remission. Indeed, the administration of SMZ-TMP to dogs with lymphoma for 14 days from the day of treatment with doxorubicin markedly reduces the likelihood for gastrointestinal (GI) toxicity (vomiting or diarrhea), hospitalization, and lower quality of life (modified Karnofsky) score.[3] The effect may be due to reduced bacterial translocation in damaged intestinal epithelial layers.

Anemia may develop later in response to the administration of chemotherapeutic agents but, unlike neutropenia, is rarely acute or severe because red blood cells have a longer life span. It is not uncommon for dogs and cats to present with a mild anemia prior to chemotherapy due to anemia of chronic disease.

Recombinant human erythropoietin may be useful in treating dogs and cats with nonregenerative anemia secondary to chemotherapy or the underlying malignancy. Human cancer patients treated with erythropoietin for anemia report that they have greater energy and a better quality of life while on chemotherapy. No similar data exist for dogs and cats. Caution is advised when using recombinant human products because antibodies to these foreign proteins can develop in approximately 3 to 6 weeks and occasionally may react with the patient's own hematopoietic growth factors.

Alopecia

Alopecia is an uncommon complication of chemotherapy but often a major concern for caregivers. Dogs and cats can lose their whiskers, but the development of generalized alopecia is relatively uncommon except in dogs with constantly growing hair coats, such as poodles, schnauzers, Old English sheep dogs, cats, and terriers (figure 19-1). Coat color and texture changes, however, are common during prolonged courses of chemotherapy. Finally, light skin may turn dark and dark skin may turn light.

Gastrointestinal toxicity

The clinical signs of this relatively common side effect include vomiting, anorexia, and diarrhea (figure 19-2). Diagnostics should proceed to eliminate chemotherapy and non–chemotherapy-induced causes, such as internal parasites, *Giardia*, and clostridial colitis. The treatment varies depending on the cause but may include antiemetics (e.g., metoclopramide, maropitant, dolasetron, ondansetron), protectants and absorbents (e.g., bismuth-containing compounds), antidiarrheals (metronidazole and tylosin) and broad-spectrum antibiotics, if indicated. In addition, support with fluids, warmth, and nutritional therapy should be provided. As a preventive measure, some clinicians dispense maropitant and metoclopramide to the client to initiate therapy at home when a medication with the potential to cause nausea is administered.

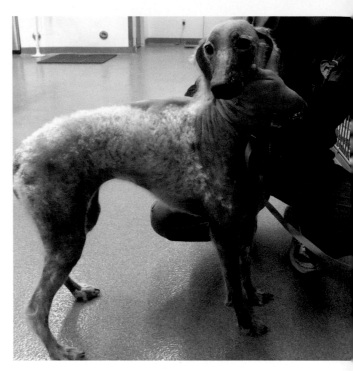

Figure 19-1: Cats almost never develop significant alopecia, but dogs with a constantly growing hair coat can develop some degree of alopecia such as this poodle. Dogs and cats do lose whiskers in response to chemotherapy. This poodle, unlike most, developed generalized alopecia that completely resolved after chemotherapy.

Clients may be instructed to give maropitant and metoclopramide, even if nausea and vomiting are not noted, both as a preventive measure and because nausea may be difficult for caregivers to assess accurately. Maropitant and metoclopramide are preferred because of their overall efficacy and lack of systemic side effects; chlorpromazine may induce the clinically worrisome side effect of sedation. Serotonin antagonists, such as dolasetron and ondansetron, may be superior to metoclopramide, but the cost of these drugs is greater.

Small and large bowel diarrhea can occasionally be seen in response to the administration of chemotherapeutic agents and antibiotics. Metronidazole and tylosin are helpful in mitigating these adverse effects. Doxorubicin is periodically associated with the development of colitis that can cause blood and mucus in the stool (figure 19-2). Metronidazole and tylosin can be helpful for this condition as well.

Anorexia in dogs and cats can often be resolved with antiemetics, adequate hydration, pain relief, and administration of the appetite-stimulating drugs mirtazapine, cyproheptadine and megestrol acetate. Subsequent doses of the specific chemotherapy agent that caused the anorexia should be reduced by 25%.

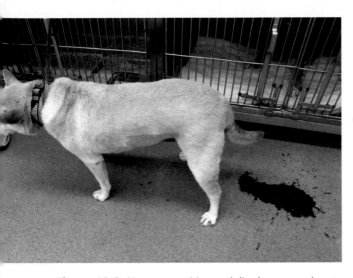

Figure 19-2: Nausea, vomiting and diarrhea secondary to chemotherapy can be prevented in most cases with the use of prophylactic antiemetics (maropitant, metoclopramide) and antidiarrheals (metronidazole, tylosin). Doxorubicin is unique in that it can induce colitis with blood and mucus in the stool as depicted here. Metronidazole and/or tylosin can be very helpful in treating colitis.

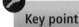

Key point

Anorexia in dogs and cats can often be resolved with antiemetics, adequate hydration, pain relief, and administration of the appetite-stimulating drugs mirtazapine, cyproheptadine and megestrol acetate.

Allergic reactions

Signs of L-asparaginase hypersensitivity include urticaria, vomiting, diarrhea, hypotension, and loss of consciousness soon after administration. These signs can essentially be eliminated by administering the medication intramuscularly. Doxorubicin- or paclitaxel-induced allergic reactions include cutaneous hyperemia, intense pruritus, head shaking, and vomiting during administration. These reactions are due to histamine release from mast cells and can be reduced substantially by slowing the infusion rate (e.g., give the entire dose over approximately 20 to 30 minutes). Other drugs that can induce allergic reactions include bleomycin, cytosine, and procarbazine. Both etoposide and paclitaxel induce dramatic cutaneous reactions and hypotension during administration, not because of the medication itself but rather the vehicle that keeps each drug in solution.

Treatment for allergic reactions includes immediately discontinuing drug administration and giving epinephrine, diphenhydramine, and glucocorticoids for acute allergic reactions. Premedication with diphenhydramine, cimetidine, and glucocorticoids may prevent or reduce allergic reactions to doxorubicin, paclitaxel, or etoposide; for doxorubicin, simply slowing the infusion rate is often sufficient to prevent allergic reactions during administration.

Key point

Anaphylaxis caused by administration of L-asparaginase can be substantially reduced if the drug is given by IM route, instead of IV or intraperitoneal route.

Cardiac toxicity

Doxorubicin has been shown to induce dose-dependent dilated (congestive) cardiomyopathy and transient dysrhythmias during administration in dogs, but almost never in cats. This occurs in those predisposed to cardiac disease or with underlying acquired myocardial disease. Until more is known, most oncologists limit the cumulative dose of doxorubicin to 180 to 240 mg/m^2 (six to eight treatments) during a dog's lifetime. Breeds or individual lines of dogs known to have a high prevalence of clinically important cardiac disease such as cardiomyopathy (e.g., Doberman pinschers, great Danes, Newfoundlands, boxers) should be screened for cardiac disease prior to treatment with doxorubicin, or a less cardiotoxic alternative should be considered. Routine cardiac auscultation to assess for unexplained tachyarrhythmias should be performed before any pet is treated with doxorubicin. Echocardiograms and electrocardiograms should be performed on dogs and cats given more than 180 mg/m^2 of doxorubicin.

Key point

Doxorubicin has been shown to induce dose-dependent dilated (congestive) cardiomyopathy and transient dysrhythmias during administration in dogs, but almost never in cats.

Cystitis

Cyclophosphamide and ifosfamide have been reported to induce sterile chemical cystitis in dogs and much less commonly in cats. Cyclophosphamide and ifosfamide are hepatically metabolized to their active forms as well as to compounds that can cause urothelial damage (acrolein). Prolonged contact time between the bladder wall and acrolein results in hemorrhagic cystitis. Clinical signs include stranguria, hematuria, and dysuria. Furosemide given as a single dose (2 mg/kg) at the time of cyclophosphamide administration almost completely abrogates this toxicity and is recommended even in dogs receiving concurrent prednisone. Allowing ample opportunity for the dog and cat to void urine is equally important, and cyclophosphamide is preferably administered in the morning rather than late in the day. Mesna is a thiol drug that is active only in urine, binding to acrolein and avoiding the toxicity of urothelial damage. The cost of mesna is high, which usually limits its use to dogs and cats receiving ifosfamide that have a much higher risk of urothelial damage.

Treatment includes replacing cyclophosphamide with another alkylating agent (e.g., chlorambucil) or discontinuing the ifosfamide to prevent exacerbation of the condition. Secondary infections are common, so urine should be collected for culture and sensitivity any time cystitis is suspected. Appropriate antibiotics must be administered if cystitis becomes septic. If renal function is normal, piroxicam (0.3 mg/kg PO q24-48h in the dog, 0.1 mg/kg q48h in the cat) may be helpful in reducing adverse effects, and for prolonged cases intravesicular dimethyl sulfoxide (DMSO) may accelerate recovery. Most cases resolve with time, but it may take several weeks to subside; this is a toxicity best prevented. The risk of developing cystitis can be decreased by administering cyclophosphamide in the morning (thereby allowing the animal maximum opportunity to urinate during the day), encouraging fluid intake and, if a combination protocol that includes prednisone is being used, giving cyclophosphamide at the same time as the glucocorticoid (steroids tend to induce polydipsia and secondary polyuria).

Nephrotoxicity

Cisplatin and streptozocin, have been occasionally linked with the development of nephrotoxicity in dogs, especially those with preexisting renal disease. Dogs and cats may develop nephrotoxicity in response to the following drugs: lomustine, doxorubicin, methotrexate, and carboplatin. Identifying animals with evidence of kidney disease, ensuring adequate hydration, and eliminating the concurrent administration of nephrotoxic agents are essential steps to limit this problem.

Neurotoxicity

Vincristine, vinblastine, lomustine, and fluorouracil are examples of drugs that are linked directly or indirectly to neurotoxicity in dogs and cats. Cisplatin is an example for the dog only, as it is lethal when administered to cats. Peripheral neuropathy is associated with vincristine and vinblastine in humans but is rare in dogs and cats; fluorouracil has been shown to cause severe seizures and disorientation in dogs and cats. Cisplatin can cause ototoxicity. Finally, chlorambucil, when used at high dosages for prolonged periods, may be linked to central neurotoxicity. Lomustine and many other drugs may

cause hepatotoxicity and subsequent disorders of the central nervous system.

Key point

Vincristine, vinblastine, lomustine, and fluorouracil are examples of drugs that are linked directly or indirectly to neurotoxicity in dogs and cats.

Local dermatologic toxicity

Doxorubicin, actinomycin D, mechlorethamine, vincristine, and vinblastine have been known to cause severe localized cellulitis if they are extravasated. Many other drugs are classified as irritants if administered perivascularly. These reactions and their prevention are discussed in detail in the Oncologic Emergencies section. Treatment includes stopping the injection, aspirating the drug and 5 ml of blood back into the syringe, and then withdrawing the syringe. For perivascular injections of vincristine and vinblastine, infiltrating the area with 4 to 6 ml of saline and approximately 8 mg of dexamethasone and then applying warm compresses may be helpful. In contrast, cold packs should be applied to areas of doxorubicin extravasation and hot packs to areas of vincristine and vinblastine administration; the area is *not* infused with saline as this will enlarge the affected area. Aggressive surgical debridement and skin grafts may be necessary for deep, ulcerative lesions.

Key point

Cold packs should be applied to areas of doxorubicin extravasation and hot packs to areas of vincristine and vinblastine extravasation.

Pulmonary toxicity

Bleomycin has rarely been associated with the development of severe pulmonary fibrosis.

APPLIED CHEMOTHERAPY

The word chemotherapy is taking a broader definition with the use of single agent and combination chemotherapy, metronomic chemotherapy, molecular chemotherapeutics such as tyrosine kinase inhibitors, and cancer vaccines. The purpose of this brief section is to introduce each general category by giving some common applications of each starting with:

- Canine and feline lymphoma and transitional cell carcinoma where single and multiagent chemotherapy is common.
- Soft tissue sarcomas where metronomic chemotherapy has been shown to be quite helpful.

- Oral malignant melanoma, where a DNA xenogeneic melanoma vaccine has been shown to be helpful.

As noted previously, there are many benefits to multiple-drug treatment protocols. Tumor resistance generally develops more slowly than with single-drug regimens, and multiple-drug protocols are more effective, especially with lymphoid tumors. Disadvantages associated with the use of multiple antineoplastic agents include increased cost and the potential for toxicity. Cures attributable to chemotherapy were not seen in human medicine until effective combinations were employed. Whenever drugs are used in combination, several important points must be kept in mind:[5-9]

- Each drug must be effective when used alone to treat a specific malignancy.
- Combinations of drugs with overlapping toxicities should be avoided unless they are arranged in a protocol to prevent superimposition of toxicoses.
- Drugs should be used with an intermittent treatment schedule for maximum efficacy.
- Combined chemotherapeutics are most effective when they have different mechanisms of action and act at different stages of the cell cycle.

Canine lymphoma

Lymphoma accounts for approximately 90% of canine hematopoietic tumors and is the hematopoietic malignancy most responsive to chemotherapy in dogs (figure 19-3 A and B). Simplistically, response to therapy is related to the extent of disease, regardless if this is a B-cell or T-cell tumor, and the treatment that is chosen. In order to determine the extent of disease, standard staging schemes include, but not necessarily limited to, a biopsy and/or cytology, chest radiographs, abdominal ultrasound, bone marrow aspirate, complete blood cell count, biochemical profile and either flow cytometry or immunohistochemistry to define if the lymphoma is of T or B-cell lineage.

Each client should be given all the options and the best option be used first. As a general rule, combination chemotherapy is superior to single-agent therapy. While methotrexate has been used in combination chemotherapy protocols for the treatment of canine lymphoma, the general consensus is that it has minimal efficacy and is therefore not recommended. Some of the more effective protocols in dogs and cats include:

- Prednisone.
- Doxorubicin (marginally effective in the cat).
- CCNU.
- COP protocol: Cyclophosphamide, Oncovin (vincristine) and prednisone.
- COPA protocol: Cyclophosphamide Oncovin (vincristine), prednisone and Adriamycin (doxorubicin).

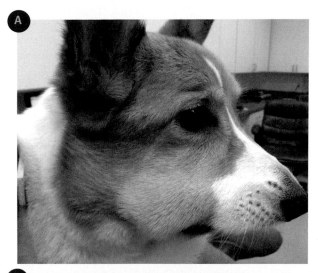

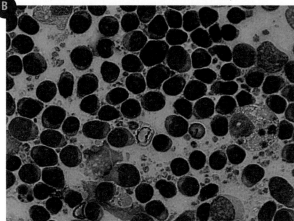

Figure 19-3: Lymphoma is is the most responsive cancer in dogs and cats to chemotherapy. Dogs commonly present with generalized lymphadenopathy that can occasionally be associated with significant facial swelling as depicted here. This lymphadenopathy responds quickly to chemotherapy, with combination chemotherapy protocols being the most effective for inducing and maintaining a durable remission. Cats with lymphoma do not commonly develop lymphadenopthy (A). Large and intermediate cell lymphoma is very common in the dog. This type of lymphoma is very responsive to therapy. Flow cytometry or immunohistochemistry can be used to determine if the malignancy is T-cell or B-cell lymphoma. This may influence therapy and prognosis. Note the large round lymphoma cells depicted her with very discrete cytoplasmic borders, characteristic for this disease (B).

- CHOP protocol: Cyclophosphamide Oncovin (vincristine), prednisone, Adriamycin (doxorubicin), and L-asparaginase

Each time an effective drug is added to the COP protocol, the remission duration increases; however, so does the cost and the potential for toxicity. It is also important that clients realize that a second or third remission is possible with appropriate therapy but that these subsequent remissions are more difficult to attain and that their duration is generally half the duration of the previous remission.

Single agent chemotherapy

For clients who cannot afford or will not accept a combination chemotherapy protocol due to the risks of toxicity, a protocol using prednisone alone (40 mg/m^2 PO daily for 7 days then every other day) or in combination with chlorambucil (6 to 8 mg/m^2 PO every other day) may provide palliation with few risks of side effects.

Prednisone: Approximately 50% of dogs treated with prednisone have a PR or CR;[92,101,102]; this response usually lasts between 14 and 240 days (average: 53 days).[11-13]

CCNU: CCNU (lomustine) has been used to treat lymphoma. Some believe that it has special benefit for the treatment of T cell lymphoma, such as mycosis fungoides. Indeed, it was used to treat 36 dogs with epitheliotropic lymphoma. Twenty-eight of 36 (78%) dogs had a measurable response to CCNU for a median duration of 106 days. Six dogs (17%) had a complete response, twenty-two dogs (61%) had a partial response.[15]

Doxorubicin: Doxorubicin is considered the most active single agent in the treatment of canine lymphoma, and protocols that contain doxorubicin are considered superior to those that do not. Doxorubicin was reported to be successful as a rescue agent.[110] Overall, doxorubicin causes CR in about 70% of dogs treated, for a median ranging from 4-7 months.[15]

Combination protocols with maintenance therapy

The most effective chemotherapy protocols use a five-drug combination of L-asparaginase, vincristine, cyclophosphamide, doxorubicin, and prednisone (CHOP or VELCAP protocols). However, the cyclophosphamide, Oncovin (vincristine) and prednisone protocol (COP) is simpler and less expensive. Similar remission rates and survival times have been obtained for the five drug protocols. Although these protocols require more intense client–veterinarian communication and monitoring for toxicity, the overall level of satisfaction for owners, pets, and veterinarians is high. Most oncologists recommend discontinuous protocols such as VELCAP-S or the Wisconsin protocol.

COP protocol: COP is a well-tolerated protocol and is relatively inexpensive (table 19-2). Its efficacy has been evaluated in seven published reports with minor variations in dosage and schedule. Overall, COP chemotherapy causes complete remission in about 70% of dogs with lymphoma for a median of 4-5 months.

CHOP protocols: vincristine, cyclophosphamide, prednisone, doxorubicin, and L-asparaginase: Currently, short-term protocols are generally recommended over the longer-term variants. In one such study, 82 dogs with lymphoma received a single 15-week course of chemotherapy and then no treatment until relapse.[16,17] At relapse, reinduction followed by maintenance chemotherapy (VELCAP-L) is used. In the study, 56 dogs (68%) achieved CR for a median first remission duration of 5 months. Of 48 dogs that relapsed, 30 repeated the induction cycle.

Table 19-2. COP protocol for canine lymphoma

Vincristine is administered at 0.75 mg/m^2 IV. Cyclophosphamide* is given at 250 mg/m^2 PO or 200 mg/m^2 IV. The dose for prednisone is 1 mg/kg daily for 7 days, then PO every other day.

Week	Vincristine	Cyclophosphamide*	Prednisone
1	•	•	↓
2	•		
3	•		
4	•	•	
5			
6			
7	•	•	
10	•	•	
	↓	↓	
	every 3 weeks		

*If hemorrhagic cystitis occurs, chlorambucil is substituted on the same schedule at 15 mg/m^2 PO daily for 4 consecutive days (or 6 to 8 mg/m^2 PO daily continuously).

The second remission rate for all 30 dogs was 87% (26 dogs). Overall disease control for the 38 dogs that remained on protocol lasted 11 months. A shorter protocol called the VELCAP-S protocol was found to be of similar efficacy (table 19-3)

A similar study that used a 25-week induction (Wisconsin protocol) had a high remission rate.[18] In that study, fifty-three dogs with multicentric lymphoma were treated with a 6-month modified version of the University of Wisconsin (UW)-Madison chemotherapy protocol (UW-25). Remission rate was 94.2% (complete remission = 92.3%, partial remission = 1.9%). The median disease free interval and survival was 282 and 397 days (table 19-4).

Feline lymphoma

Feline lymphoma is very common in cats and is best treated with chemotherapy, although radiation therapy has been shown to be quite effective for the treatment of extranodal lymphoma such as lymphoma of the nasal cavity. Most cats with lymphoma respond well to therapy, however unique subtypes such as large granular cell lymphoma appears to be more refractory to the beneficial effects of chemotherapy than many other forms. Response to therapy is dependent on the extent of disease, the lymphocyte subtype involved, and the treatment that is chosen. Standard staging scheme includes a hemogram, biochemical profile, thyroid evaluation, determination of FeLV and FIV positivity, abdominal ultrasound, chest radiographs, bone marrow aspirate as well as histopathology and/or cytology of involved tissue.

Chemotherapy is the principal modality used to treat feline lymphoma. Small cell lymphoma is effectively treated with chlorambucil and prednisolone, whereas intermediate or large cell lymphoma is largely unaffected by this approach but is effectively treated with CCNU and prednisolone. Other single agents such as mitoxantrone, idarubicin, L-asparaginase and cyclophosphamide may have short-term benefits for the treatment of lymphoma in cats. While doxorubicin is the best single agent for the treatment of lymphoma in dogs, it is of limited benefit in cats unless combined with other drugs. The most commonly used single agent chemotherapy protocols for the treatment of cats with lymphoma include prednisone or prednisolone, and CCNU. Prednisolone is inexpensive but of limited benefit for the treatment of lymphoma as a single agent with approximately a third of the treated cats achieving a complete remission. The median duration of remission is approximately one month. CCNU (60 mg/m^2 body surface area PO q3-4 weeks) has been shown to have some efficacy for the treatment of lymphoma in cats, especially high-grade lymphoma of the gastrointestinal tract.

Combination chemotherapy is almost always superior in efficacy to single agent chemotherapy, however knowledge of the latter provides a basis for providing shorter-term control for select patients or for constructing combination chemotherapy protocols. While methotrexate has been used in combination chemotherapy protocols for the treatment of feline lymphoma, the general consensus is that it has minimal efficacy and is therefore not recommended. Some of the more effective protocols in the cat include:

Table 19-3. VELCAP-S protocol for canine lymphoma[11]

Vincristine is administered at 0.75 mg/m^2 IV. Cyclophosphamide* is given at 250 mg/m^2 PO. The dose for L-asparaginase is 10,000 IU/m^2 IM (maximum treatment dose = 10,000 IU). Doxorubicin is administered at 25 mg/m^2 IV. Prednisone is given at 40 mg/m^2 PO sid for 7 days, then every other day.

Week	Vincristine	Cyclophosphamide*	L-asparaginase	Doxorubicin
1	•			
2	•			•
3	•			•
4				•
5				
6				
7	•	•	•	
8			•	
9			•	
12		•	•	

*If hemorrhagic cystitis occurs, chlorambucil is substituted on the same schedule at 15 mg/m^2 PO daily for 4 consecutive days (or 6 to 8 mg/m^2 PO daily continuously).

Table 19-4. Modified CHOP lymphoma protocol treatment for the dog[18]	
Week 1	Vincristine, 0.7 mg/m² IV Asparaginase, 400 IU/kg or 10,000 IU/m² IM Prednisone, 2 mg/kg PO q24hrs
Week 2	Cyclophosphamide, 250 mg/m² IV Asparaginase, 400 IU/kg or 10,000 IU/m² IM Prednisone, 1.5 mg/kg PO q24hrs
Week 3	Vincristine, 0.7 mg/m² IV Prednisone, 1.0 mg/kg POq24hrs
Week 4	Doxorubicin, 30 mg/m² IV Prednisone, 0.5 mg/kgq24 hrs
Week 6	Vincristine, 0.7 mg/m² IV
Week 7	Cyclophosphamide, 250 mg/m² IV
Week 8	Vincristine, 0.7 mg/m² IV
Week 9	Doxorubicin, 30 mg/m² IV
Week 11	Vincristine, 0.7 mg/m² IV
Week 13	Cyclophosphamide, 250 mg/m² IV
Week 15	Vincristine, 0.7 mg/m² IV
Week 17	Doxorubicin, 30 mg/m² IV
Week 19	Vincristine, 0.7 mg/m² IV
Week 21	Cyclophosphamide, 250 mg/m² IV
Week 23	Vincristine, 0.7 mg/m² IV
Week 25	Doxorubicin, 30 mg/m² IV

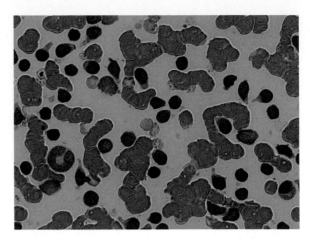

Figure 19-4: Small lymphocytes as depicted here are noted in small cell lymphoma infiltrated organs. Small cell lymphoma responds very well to chlorambucil and prednisolone therapy. Many cats respond for months or years with an excellent quality of life.

- CCNU and prednisolone.
- COP protocol: cyclophosphamide, Oncovin (vincristine) and prednisolone.
- COPA protocol: cyclophosphamide Oncovin (vincristine), prednisolone and Adriamycin (doxorubicin).
- CHOP protocol: cyclophosphamide Oncovin (vincristine), prednisolone, adriamycin (doxorubicin), and L-asparaginase.

Chlorambucil and prednisolone for small cell lymphoma

Small cell lymphoma is perhaps the most common form of lymphoma in the cat (figure 19-4). Unlike large or intermediate cell lymphoma, small cell lymphoma responds very well to just chlorambucil and prednisolone. In one series of twenty-nine cats with well-differentiated lymphoma that were treated with prednisone and chlorambucil alone; twenty cats (69%) achieved a CR for up to 49 months (median, 16 months).[19] The median survival for all twenty-nine cats regardless of response was 17 months, while those achieving CR lived a median of 23 months. In contrast, eleven cats with lymphoblastic lymphoma in the same study received multiple-agent chemotherapy but

only 2 (11%) had a CR.[20] In a second, separate study, twenty-eight cats were diagnosed with small-cell GI lymphoma and also treated with a combination of chlorambucil and glucocorticoids. The overall clinical response rate was 96%, with median clinical remission duration of 786 days.

COP protocol (cyclophosphamide, vincristine, and prednisone)

The COP protocol used most often involves a 4-week induction period (table 19-4) followed by maintenance therapy every 3 weeks until 1 year, at which time all treatment is stopped. In one study,[21] thirty-eight cats were treated with COP and maintenance therapy for various anatomic forms of lymphoma. The CR rate varied from 100% for multicentric lymphoma to 50% for extranodal lymphoma. Similarly, the median duration of remission ranged from 4.5 months for alimentary lymphoma to 28 months for cats with peripheral nodal lymphoma. All groups contained individuals that lived longer than a year. The overall CR rate was 30 of 38 cats (74%), with six cats having a partial response and two having no response. The duration of CR ranged from 2 to 42 months.[21]

In another study, sixty-one cats with malignant lymphoma were more recently treated with the COP chemotherapy protocol (table 19-5).[22] Most cats were FeLV negative. Complete remission (CR) was achieved in 46 of the 61 cats (75.4%). The estimated 1- and 2-year disease-free periods in the 46 cats with CR were 51.4 and 37.8%, respectively. The median duration of remission was 251 days. The overall estimated 1-year survival rate in all cats was 48.7%, and the 2-year survival rate was 39.9%, with a median survival of 266 days. The median survival time and

Table 19-5. COP protocol for treatment of feline lymphoma [22]

Agent	Week						
	1	2	3	6	9	12	15[a]
Vincristine (0.75 mg/m² IV)	•	•	•	•	•	•	• →
Cyclophosphamide (250 mg/m² PO [to nearest 25 mg])	•			•	•	•	•
Prednisone (10 mg PO daily throughout the protocol)	• ——————————————————————————→						

[a]After week 15, administer protocol every 3 weeks to 1 year, then stop therapy.

the 1-year survival rate for mediastinal lymphoma that is not commonly seen in the United States were 262 days and 49.4%, respectively.

CHOP protocol: cyclophosphamide Oncovin (vincristine), prednisolone, Adriamycin (doxorubicin), and L-asparaginase

The addition of doxorubicin to the COP protocol improved response to therapy. In one study where thirty-eight cats with lymphoma were treated with the modified CHOP protocol, also known as the Wisconsin protocol (table 19-6).[23] The overall median survival time was 210 days, and overall duration of first remission was 156 days. Eighteen of the thirty-eight (47%) cats had complete remission, 14 (37%) had partial remission, and six (16%) had no response. Median survival time for cats with complete remission (654 days) was significantly longer than median survival time for cats with partial remission (122 days) and for cats with no response (11 days).

Transitional cell carcinoma

Transitional cell carcinoma is a common tumor in dogs. Unlike in people, this disease is almost always invasive through the bladder wall and is most commonly observed at or around the trigone of the bladder. The most common clinical signs include hematuria, pollakiuria and stranguria

The same disease occurs in cats, however it is much less commonly diagnosed and it appears to be more aggressive than in the dog. TCC is the most common bladder tumor in cats and appears to involve the trigonal region of the bladder. The clinical signs of bladder cancer are indistinguishable from those seen with feline urologic syndrome or urinary tract infection. Hematuria, pollakiuria and stranguria

Table 19-6. Modified CHOP lymphoma protocol treatment for the cat[23]

Week 1	Vincristine, 0.5 mg/m² IV Asparaginase, 400 IU/kg or 10,000 IU/m² IM Prednisone, 2 mg/kg PO q24hrs.
Week 2	Cyclophosphamide, 250 mg/m² IV Asparaginase, 400 IU/kg or 10,000 IU/m² IM Prednisone, 1.5 mg/kg PO q24hrs
Week 3	Vincristine, 0.5 mg/m² IV Prednisone, 1.0 mg/kg POq24hrs
Week 4	Doxorubicin, 1 mg/kg IV Prednisone, 0.5 mg/kgq24 hrs
Week 6	Vincristine, 0.5 mg/m²
Week 7	Cyclophosphamide, 250 mg/m² IV
Week 8	Vincristine, 0.5 mg/m²
Week 9	Doxorubicin, 1mg/kg IV
Week 11	Vincristine, 0.5 mg/m²
Week 13	Cyclophosphamide, 250 mg/m² IV
Week 15	Vincristine, 0.5 mg/m²
Week 17	Doxorubicin, 1 mg/kg IV
Week 19	Vincristine, 0.5 mg/m²
Week 21	Cyclophosphamide, 250 mg/m² IV
Week 23	Vincristine, 0.5 mg/m²
Week 25	Doxorubicin, 1mg/kg IV

are commonly seen. Other less specific signs such as straining and anorexia may occur, and some cats may have a palpable caudal abdominal mass. Tenesmus and rectal prolapse are periodically seen.

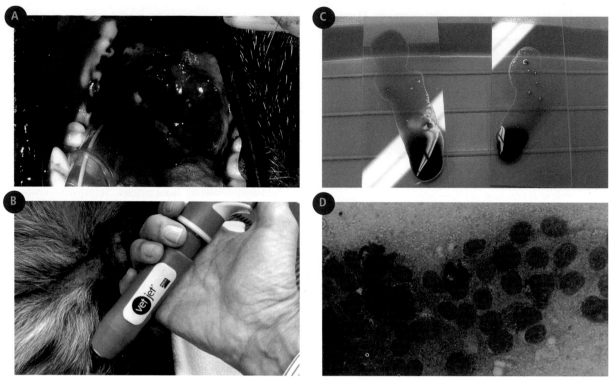

Figure 19-6: Oral melanoma of the oral cavity (A), including of the hard palate as depicted here is associated with a very poor prognosis unless the primary disease is treated with surgery and radiation therapy and the metastatic disease is delayed or prevented with chemotherapy or the DNA xenogeneic melanoma vaccine (B). Oral melanoma can and often does metastasize to the regional lymph node. Metastases may be present even though the lymph node is normal in size. The lymph node aspirate with metastatic disease may be associated with a black liquid (C). The cytology of malignant melanoma is often associated with fine granular "dust-like" material in and around the malignant cells (D).

achieved were entered into a study to evaluate the efficacy of a DNA xenogeneic melanoma vaccine. Four vaccines were given every two weeks followed by booster vaccines every six months by a needle-free IM vaccination device. Kaplan-Meier analysis of survival time until death attributable to malignant melanoma was determined to be significantly improved for dogs that received the huTyr vaccine, compared with that of historical controls. Median survival time could not be determined for vaccinates because less than 50% died of malignant melanoma before the study was completed.

References

1. Lippman SM, Hong WK: Cancer prevention by delay. [Commentary: JA O'Shaughnessy, et al: Treatment and prevention of intraepithelial neoplasia: An important target for accelerated new agent development. *Clin Cancer Res* 8:314–346, 2002.] *Clin Cancer Res* 8(2):305–313, 2002.
2. Chretin JD, Shaw NA, Hahn KA, Ogilvie GK, Rassnick KM, Moore AS: Prophylactic trimethoprim Sulfadiazine during chemotherapeutic induction: A double blind, placebo controlled study. Proc 20th *Annu Conf Vet Cancer Soc*. 2000;47.
3. Kirpensteijn J, Teske E, Kik M, et al: Lobaplatin as an adjuvant chemotherapy to surgery in canine and feline appendicular osteosarcoma: A phase II evaluation. *Anticancer Res* 22(5):2765–2770, 2002.
4. Poirier VJ, Hershey AE, Burgess KE, et al: Efficacy and toxicity of paclitaxel (Taxol) for the treatment of canine and feline malignant tumors. *J Vet Intern Med* 18(2):219–222, 2004.
5. Simon D, Schoenrock D, Ueberschaer S, Nolte I: Adjuvant chemotherapy with docetaxel and doxorubicin in canine and feline invasive mammary gland tumors: First results. Proc 19th *Annu Conf Vet Cancer Soc* 74, 1999.
6. Perry MC, Anderson CM, Donehower RC: Chemotherapy In: Abeloff MD, Armitage JO, Niedenhuber JE, et al (eds): *Clinical Oncology* ed 3. Philadelphia, Elsevier Churchill Livingston. 2004, pp 483–535.
7. Chabner BA: Principles of cancer therapy, in Wyngaarden JB, Smith LH (eds): *Cecil Textbook of Medicine*. Philadelphia, WB Saunders, 1982, p 1032-1045.
8. Ogilvie GK: Principles of oncology, in Morgan RV (ed): *Handbook of Small Animal Internal Medicine*. Philadelphia, Churchill Livingston, 1992, pp 799–812.
9. Moore AS, Kitchell BE: New chemotherapy agents in veterinary medicine. *Vet Clin North Am Small Anim Pract* 33[3]:629–649, 2003.
10. Brick JO, Roenigk WJ, Wilson GP: Chemotherapy of malignant lymphoma in dogs and cats. *JAVMA* 153:47–52, 1968.
11. Moldovenu G, Friedman M, Miller DG: Experience with the management of malignant lymphoma in dogs. *Sangre (Barc)* 17:253–262, 1964.
12. Bell R, Cotter S, Lillquist A, et al: Characterization of glucocorticoid receptors in animal lymphoblastic disease: correlation with response to single-agent glucocorticoid treatment. *Blood* 63:380–383, 1984.
13. Squire RA, Bush M, Melby EC, et al: Clinical and pathologic study of canine lymphoma: Clinical staging, cell classification, and therapy. *J Natl Cancer Inst* 51:565–574, 1973.
14. Postorino NC, Susaneck SJ, Withrow SJ, et al: Single agent therapy with adriamycin for canine lymphosarcoma. *J Am Anim Hosp Assoc* 25:221–225, 1989.
15. Williams LE, Rassnick KM, Power HT, Lana SE, Morrison-Collister KE, Hansen K, Johnson JL: CCNU in the treatment of canine epitheliotropic lymphoma. *J Vet Intern Med*. 2006;20(1):136-143.
16. Moore AS, Cotter SM, Rand WM, et al: Evaluation of a discontinuous treatment protocol VELCAP-S) for canine lymphoma. *J Vet Intern Med* 15:348–354, 2001.
17. Baskin CR, Couto CG, Wittum TE: Factors influencing first remission and survival in 145 dogs with lymphoma: a retrospective study. J Am Anim Hosp Assoc 36:404–409, 2000.

18. Garrett LD, Thamm DH, Chun R, Dudley R, Vail DM: Evaluation of a 6-month chemotherapy protocol with no maintenance therapy for dogs with lymphoma. *J Vet Intern Med.* 16(6):704-709, 2002.

19. Fondacaro JV, Richter KP, Carpenter JL, et al: Feline gastrointestinal well differentiated lymphocytic lymphoma: 39 cases. Abstract 123. *J Vet Intern Med* 13:257, 1999.

20. Stein TJ, Pellin M, Steinberg H, Chun R: Treatment of feline gastrointestinal small-cell lymphoma with chlorambucil and glucocorticoids. *J Am Anim Hosp Assoc.* 46(6):413-417, 2010.

21. Cotter SM: Treatment of lymphoma and leukemia with cyclophosphamide, vincristine, and prednisone: II. Treatment of cats. *JAAHA* 19:166–172, 1983.

22. Teske E, van Straten G, van Noort R, Rutteman GR: Chemotherapy with cyclophosphamide, vincristine, and prednisolone (COP) in cats with malignant lymphoma: new results with an old protocol. *J Vet Intern Med.* 16(2):179-186, 2002.

23. Milner RJ, Peyton J, Cooke K, Fox LE, Gallagher A, Gordon P, Hester J: Response rates and survival times for cats with lymphoma treated with the University of Wisconsin-Madison chemotherapy protocol: 38 cases (1996-2003). *J Am Vet Med Assoc.* 227(7):1118-22, 2005.

24. Knapp DW, Glickman NW, Widmer WR, et al: Cisplatin versus cisplatin combined with piroxicam in a canine model of human invasive urinary bladder cancer. *Cancer Chemother Pharmacol* 46:221-226, 2000.

25. Boria PA, Mutsaers AJ, DiBernardi L, et al: Carboplatin and piroxicam therapy in 31 dogs with transitional cell carcinoma. *Proc 22nd Ann Conf Vet Cancer Soc.*25, 2002.

26. Henry CJ, McCaw DL, Turnquist SE, et al: Clinical evaluation of mitoxantrone and piroxicam in a canine model of human invasive urinary bladder carcinoma. *Clinical Cancer Research* 9:906-911, 2003.

27. Arnold EJ, Childress MO, Fourez LM, Tan KM, Stewart JC, Bonney PL, Knapp DW. Clinical trial of vinblastine in dogs with transitional cell carcinoma of the urinary bladder. *J Vet Intern Med.* 2011 ;25(6):1385-1390.

28. Rassnick KM, Bailey DB, Flory AB, Balkman CE, Kiselow MA, Intile JL, Autio K. Efficacy of vinblastine for treatment of canine mast cell tumors. *J Vet Intern Med.* 2008 ;22(6):1390-1396.

29. Hosoya K, Kisseberth WC, Alvarez FJ, Lara-Garcia A, Beamer G, Stromberg PC, Couto CG. Adjuvant CCNU (lomustine) and prednisone chemotherapy for dogs with incompletely excised grade 2 mast cell tumors. *J Am Anim Hosp Assoc.* 2009 ;45(1):14-18.

30. Rassnick KM, Bailey DB, Russell DS, Flory AB, Kiselow MA, Intile JL, Malone EK, Balkman CE, Barnard SM. A phase II study to evaluate the toxicity and efficacy of alternating CCNU and high-dose vinblastine and prednisone (CVP) for treatment of dogs with high-grade, metastatic or nonresectable mast cell tumours. *Vet Comp Oncol.* 2010 Jun;8(2):138-152.

31. Hahn KA, Legendre AM, Shaw NG, Phillips B, Ogilvie GK, Prescott DM, Atwater SW, Carreras JK, Lana SE, Ladue T, Rusk A, Kinet JP, Dubreuil P, Moussy A,Hermine O. Evaluation of 12- and 24-month survival rates after treatment with masitinib in dogs with nonresectable mast cell tumors. *Am J Vet Res.* 2010 ;71(11):1354-1361.

32. Carlsten KS, London CA, Haney S, Burnett R, Avery AC, Thamm DH. Multicenter prospective trial of hypofractionated radiation treatment, toceranib, and prednisone for measurable canine mast cell tumors. *J Vet Intern Med.* 2012 Jan-Feb;26(1):135-141.

33. Elmslie RE, Glawe P, Dow SW. Metronomic therapy with cyclophosphamide and piroxicam effectively delays tumor recurrence indogs with incompletely resected soft tissue sarcomas. *J Vet Intern Med.* 2008;22(6):1373-1379.

34. Grosenbaugh DA, Leard AT, Bergman PJ, Klein MK, Meleo K, Susaneck S, Hess PR, Jankowski MK, Jones PD, Leibman NF, Johnson MH, Kurzman ID,Wolchok JD. Safety and efficacy of a xenogeneic DNA vaccine encoding for human tyrosinase as adjunctive treatment for oral malignant melanoma in dogs following surgical excision of the primary tumor. *Am J Vet Res.* 2011 ;72(12):1631-1638.

count is required and doses may need to be adjusted. This drug can cause anemia in cats and dogs.

Note: Hydroxyurea has been used to treat chronic myelogenous leukemia and polycythemia (primary erythrocytosis).

Lomustine (CCNU)

Dose supplied: 10, 40, and 100 mg capsules.
Feline dosage: 50–60 mg/m^2 every 6 weeks.
Canine dosage: 60–90 mg/m^2 q4-6wk.
Route of administration: PO.
Storage: Store at room temperature.
Mechanism of action: Alkylating agent.
Metabolism: Rapidly absorbed from the GI tract and metabolized by the liver.
Toxicity: Myelosuppression (neutropenia) can be rapid and marked (nadir, approximately 1 week but often 2 to 5 weeks). This drug can cause a cumulative thrombocytopenia in dogs and may also do so in cats. Hepatic and renal toxicities are rare in dogs but may occur in cats.
Note: CCNU has shown efficacy in the treatment of lymphoma and mast cell tumors in cats and dogs. Because it is lipophilic, it has been effective in treating brain tumors in dogs, and the same may be true for cats.

Mechlorethamine (Mustargen)

Dose supplied: 10 mg vials.
Canine/Feline dosage: 3 mg/m^2 as per protocol (usually MOPP protocol).
Route of administration: Slow IV push (Note: this is a strong vesicant when administered extravascularly). Reconstitute vial with 10 ml 0.9% NaCl to concentration of 1 mg/ml.
Storage: Store unopened vials at room temperature; discard unused reconstituted material.
Mechanism of action: Nitrosourea alkylating agent.
Metabolism: Rapidly metabolized through spontaneous hydrolysis.
Toxicity: Myelosuppression (neutropenia) can be rapid and marked (nadir, 1 week). Nausea and vomiting may occur 30 minutes to 2 hours after administration and last for up to 8 hours. This drug is a strong vesicant and can cause tissue necrosis and sloughing if extravasated.
Note: Mechlorethamine has shown efficacy against lymphoma in cats and dogs when used in combination protocols (e.g., MOPP).

Procarbazine

Dose supplied: 50 mg capsules (10 mg capsules can be reformulated by a compounding pharmacy).
Canine dosage: 50 mg/m^2 daily for 14 days.
Feline dosage: 10 mg/cat daily for 14 days.
Route of administration: PO.
Storage: Store at room temperature.
Mechanism of action: Nonclassic alkylating agent.

Metabolism: Rapidly absorbed from the GI tract and metabolized by the liver.
Toxicity: Myelosuppression (neutropenia) is seen in other species, but whether this occurs in dogs and cats is uncertain, as the drug is usually given concurrently with mechlorethamine. Nausea and vomiting occur commonly and can be dose limiting; diarrhea and anorexia also occur frequently. If these side effects are noted, cease drug administration and reinstitute when resolved with antinausea medications and/or at an every-other-day schedule; use prophylactic antinausea medications for future administration.
Note: Procarbazine has shown efficacy against lymphoma in dogs and cats when used in combination protocols (e.g., MOPP).

Ifosfamide

Dose supplied: 1 and 3 g vials (mesna is included in the package).
Feline dosage: 900 mg/m^2 every 3 weeks (investigational).
500 mg/m^2 every 3 weeks (investigational).
1 g vial: Reconstitute with 20 ml 0.9% NaCl = 50 mg/ml.
3 g vial: Reconstitute with 30 ml 0.9% NaCl = 100 mg/ml.
Canine dosage: 350 (dogs <10 kg) to 375 mg/m^2 q3wk.
1-g vial: Reconstitute with 20 ml 0.9% NaCl = 50 mg/ml.
3-g vial: Reconstitute with 30 ml 0.9% NaCl = 100 mg/ml.
Route of administration: IV as continuous infusion diluted in 0.9% NaCl and given over 30 minutes. Must be preceded (for 30 minutes) and followed (for 5 hours) by fluid diuresis (with 0.9% NaCl) at a rate of 18.3 ml/kg/hr. To help prevent hemorrhagic cystitis, mesna should be administered in three doses, each equal to 20% of the ifosfamide dose. Mesna is given as an IV bolus at the start of pretreatment diuresis and 2 and 5 hours after ifosfamide infusion.
Storage: Store unopened vials at room temperature. Reconstituted solution is chemically stable for 7 days at room temperature and 6 weeks refrigerated.
Mechanism of action: Alkylating agent.
Metabolism: Hepatic metabolism to active form (as for cyclophosphamide).
Toxicity: Myelosuppression (neutropenia; nadir, 1 week). Monitor serum creatinine and urinalysis before each treatment, as hemorrhagic cystitis may occur; renal toxicity has been seen in humans.
Note: Ifosfamide has shown efficacy against soft tissue sarcoma and lymphoma in dogs and cats.

Dacarbazine (DTIC)

Dose supplied: 100 and 200 mg vials.
Canine dosage: 800 mg/m^2 q3-4 wk; or 200 mg/m^2/d for 5 consecutive days every 3 weeks.

Route of administration: IV infusion over 5 hours.
Storage: Store refrigcrated.
Mechanism of action: Nonclassic alkylating agent.
Metabolism: Metabolized by the liver; some excreted unchanged in urine.
Toxicity: Nausea and vomiting at administration controlled by single dose of dolasetron before drug is administered; diarrhea may occur. Myelosuppression (neutropenia) is seen.
Note: Dacarbazine has shown efficacy against lymphoma in dogs, particularly when administered with doxorubicin.

Streptozocin/streptozoticin

Dose supplied: 1 g vials.
Canine dosage: 500 mg/m^2 IV q2-3wk. IV saline at 18.3 ml/kg/hr for 7 hours. The dose of streptozocin is included in the infusion during hours 3 and 4. Butorphanol tartrate 0.4 mg/kg IM may be given at the end of the streptozocin portion of the infusion as an antiemetic, although ondansetron or dolasetron may be more effective.
Storage: Room temperature.
Mechanism of action: Nitrosourea alkylating agent. Selective toxicity for beta cells.
Metabolism: Liver.
Toxicity: Nephrotoxicity, emesis, occasional hypoglycemic-induced weakness post-infusion, alanine transaminase elevation (usually resolves on discontinuing drug), diabetes.
Note: Used to treat insulinomas.

ANTIMETABOLITES

Antimetabolites interfere with biosynthesis of nucleic acids by substituting them for normal metabolites and inhibiting normal enzymatic reactions. The dosing of each drug varies by protocol.

Capecitabine

Dose supplied: 150 and 500 mg capsules.
Canine dosage: Investigational; advise checking for updated recommendations from oncologists.
Route of administration: Oral.
Storage: Store at room temperature.
Mechanism of action: Antimetabolite.
Metabolism: Metabolized in vivo to fluorouracil in the liver and then in the peripheral and tumor tissues to thymidine phosphorylase.
Toxicity: Neurotoxicity is theoretically possible. Myelosuppression and the canine equivalent to palmar plantar syndrome seen in people.
Note: May have efficacy in lymphoma.

Methotrexate

Dose supplied: 2.5 mg tablets; 5, 20, 50, 100, 200, and 250 mg and 1 g vials for injection.
Canine/Feline dosage: 2.5 mg/m^2 daily.

Route of administration: PO, IV, IM, SQ.
Storage: Store at room temperature. The drug must be protected from light. Vials may be frozen.
Mechanism of action: Antimetabolite; inhibits the conversion of folic acid to tetrahydrofolic acid by binding to the enzyme dihydrofolate reductase, which inhibits synthesis of thymidine and purines essential for DNA synthesis.
Metabolism: A large percentage of the drug is excreted unchanged in the urine. The drug is bound to serum albumin, so simultaneous administration of drugs that displace the methotrexate from the plasma protein (e.g., sulfa drugs, aspirin, metoclopramide, chloramphenicol, phenytoin, tetracycline) should be avoided to prevent excessive toxicity. Daily dose should be reduced if serum creatinine level is elevated.
Toxicity: Anorexia and vomiting occur frequently but may be prevented by premedication with antiemetics. The nadir of myelosuppression is 6 to 9 days in some species, but has not been documented in dogs or cats. Alopecia (whisker loss) may also be seen.
Note: Methotrexate has been used in combination with other drugs to treat lymphoma. It is a folic acid-inhibitor and can be given at a very high dose and then reversed ("rescued") with leucovorin calcium to prevent potentially fatal toxicities. Its actual efficacy as a single agent is in question.

Mercaptopurine

Dose supplied: 50 mg tablets.
Canine/Feline dosage: 50 mg/m^2 daily (Note: Because of the tablet size, may need to be re-compounded or dosed at 50 mg q48-72h).
Route of administration: PO.
Storage: Store at room temperature.
Mechanism of action: Purine antimetabolite; inhibits nucleotide synthesis required for RNA and DNA synthesis.
Metabolism: Metabolized by the liver and degraded by the enzyme xanthine oxidase. Xanthine oxidase is inhibited by allopurinol, so concurrent use of other drugs that use this enzyme necessitates a 75% dosage reduction.
Toxicity: Myelosuppression.
Note: Mercaptopurine has been suggested as a treatment for leukemia and lymphoma; results are varied.

Fluorouracil (5-FU)

Dose supplied: 500 mg, 5 g ampules or vials; 1% or 2% topical ointment or solution.
Canine dosage: 5–10 mg/kg weekly IV.
Feline dosage: CONTRAINDICATED IN CATS.
Route of administration: IV push; topical.
Storage: Store at room temperature; protect from light.
Mechanism of action: Pyrimidine antimetabolite;

blocks methylation reaction of deoxyuridylic acid to thymidylic acid, interfering with synthesis of DNA and, to a lesser extent, RNA.

Metabolism: The drug is metabolized by the liver and partially excreted by the kidneys.

Toxicity: This drug is neurotoxic. Myelosuppression (neutropenia and thrombocytopenia) reaches a nadir in 9 to 14 days. Vomiting, nausea, alopecia, and GI toxicity are possible.

Note: This drug has had limited use in veterinary medicine because of its neurotoxicity. It reportedly is effective for the treatment of tumors of the GI tract. 5-FU is available as a topical cream and has been used to treat superficial malignancies, including cutaneous lymphoma and squamous cell carcinoma, with varying results.

Cytarabine

Dose supplied: 100 and 500 mg and 1 and 2 g vials.

Canine/Feline Dosage: 100 mg/m²/d IV continuous infusion for 4 days; if no toxicity, increase to 150 mg/m²/d for 4 days or 10 mg/m² SQ once or twice daily. Can be administered intrathecally.

Canine dosage: Low dose: 10 mg/m² SQ or IM q12-24hr; High Dose: 60 mg/m² SQ, IM, or IV q24hr for 4 days q3wk. For granulomatous meningoencephalitis: 200 mg/m² as a constant rate infusion over 48 hours or 50 mg/m² SQ bid for 2 consecutive days – repeat dosage schedule every 3 weeks.

Feline dosage: 60-100 mg/m² IV constant rate infusion daily for 2-4 days; if no toxicity, increase to 150 mg/m² daily for 4 days OR 10 mg/m² SQ q12-24hr.

Route of administration: IV, SQ. If administered IV, infuse via a Buretrol over 10 to 20 minutes or as continuous infusion.

Storage: Store at room temperature. Reconstituted solution is stable at room temperature for 48 hours. Discard solution if a slight haze develops.

Mechanism of action: Antimetabolite; pyrimidine analogue; inhibits DNA synthesis.

Metabolism: The drug is activated and inactivated by liver enzymes.

Toxicity: Myelosuppression is the major toxicity. Leukopenia and thrombocytopenia (nadir, 7 to 14 days in dogs) frequently occur and apparently are related to the dose and frequency of administration. Fever and thrombophlebitis are rarely seen. Alopecia may be seen.

Note: This drug has been used alone or in combination with other agents to treat lymphoreticular neoplasms and myeloproliferative disorders. It has been administered intrathecally to dogs and cats to treat CNS lymphoma. The actual efficacy of this drug as a single agent is not clear.

Cytarabine, liposomal

Dose supplied: 50 mg vials.

Canine dosage: Investigational, advise checking for updated recommendations from oncologists.

Route of administration: Intrathecal administration results in prolonged effect with minimal systemic effects.

Storage: Refrigerated.

Mechanism of action: Antimetabolite; pyrimidine analogue; inhibits DNA synthesis.

Metabolism: The drug is activated and inactivated by liver enzymes, however liposomes prolong half-life dramatically.

Toxicity: Myelosuppression is the major toxicity. Leukopenia and thrombocytopenia may theoretically occur and may be related to the dose and frequency of administration; however, intrathecal therapy should minimize systemic effects.

Note: Applications are primarily for CNS lymphoma.

Gemcitabine

Dose supplied: 200 mg and 1 g vials.

Canine dosage: 250–300 mg/m² IV weekly for 4 weeks with a 1-week rest. Toxicity and probably efficacy depend on the rate the drug is infused. Preliminary studies suggest that the drug should be infused over a 30–90 minute period.

Route of administration: IV, SQ. If administered IV, infuse via a Buretrol over 10 to 20 minutes or as continuous infusion. Note that longer infusions will increase the effective dose proportionally.

Storage: This drug has a very short half-life. Discard unused solution.

Mechanism of action: Antimetabolite; cell phase specificity, primarily killing cells undergoing DNA synthesis (S-phase) and also blocking the progression of cells through the G1/S-phase boundary.

Metabolism: The drug is metabolized by the liver and kidneys.

Toxicity: Myelosuppression is the major toxicity. Leukopenia and thrombocytopenia (nadir, 3–5 days in dogs) frequently occur and apparently are related to the dose and frequency of administration. Alopecia may be seen. Pulmonary toxicity is reported in people.

Note: This drug has been used to treat a wide variety of tumors; however, a consensus on what tumors are best treated with this agent has yet to be reached. In people, pancreatic, bladder, and breast cancers are successfully treated with this drug.

ANTIBIOTICS

Antibiotics form stable complexes (intercalate) with DNA and therefore inhibit DNA or RNA synthesis.

Doxorubicin

Dose supplied: 10, 20, 50, 150, and 200 mg vials.

Canine dosage: 30 mg/m² or 1 mg/kg or 25 mg/m² for small (<10 kg) dogs IV q3wk; total cumulative dose of up to 180 mg/m² to 240 mg/m².

Feline dosage: 20–25 mg/m² or 1–1.1 mg/kg IV every 3 weeks; total cumulative dose of up to 180 to 240 mg/m².

Route of administration: Dilute with 30 ml of 0.9% NaCl and administer IV over 15 to 30 minutes, or give undiluted drug IV at a rate of 1 ml/min. (Do not heparinize, as this will cause precipitation. Doxorubicin hydrochloride is reportedly physically incompatible with aminophylline, cephalothin sodium, dexamethasone sodium phosphate, diazepam, fluorouracil [as an IV additive only], furosemide, heparin sodium, and hydrocortisone sodium succinate.)

Storage: Store at room temperature. Reconstituted solution is stable for months if refrigerated. Avoid storing with aluminum-hub needles.

Mechanism of action: Antitumor antibiotic; inhibits DNA and RNA synthesis.

Metabolism: Metabolized predominantly by the liver. Approximately 50% of the drug is excreted in bile. In animals with bilirubin levels above 2 mg/dl, the dose should be decreased by 50% to reduce toxicity. The drug is also excreted in urine and causes a red color in urine for up to 2 days after administration.

Toxicity: Leukopenia and thrombocytopenia (nadir, 7 to 10 days). GI toxicity, anorexia, vomiting, and hemorrhagic colitis are possible (2 to 5 days after administration). GI toxicity and quality of life improved when administered concurrently with sulfamethoxazole-trimethoprim (*Journal of Veterinary Internal Medicine, Vol. 21, Issue 1, pgs. 141-148*). The cumulative dose likely to cause cardiotoxicity in dogs and cats has not been clearly elucidated, but most oncologists limit this agent to 180 to 240 mg/m^2. Extravasation causes severe tissue necrosis. Immediately apply ice or cold compresses to the area of extravasation for 6 to 10 hours. The drug has been reported to cause renal toxicity in dogs and cats. Allergic reactions occur occasionally but may be eliminated by slowing the infusion or by pretreating with antihistamines. Alopecia may be seen in some dogs and cats.

Note: Doxorubicin is used to treat lymphoma, thyroid carcinoma, sarcoma, and mammary carcinoma. This antineoplastic agent seems to have a broad spectrum of activity against a variety of tumors.

Doxorubicin, liposomal

Dose supplied: 20 and 50 mg vials.

Canine dosage: 1 mg/kg IV q3wk.

Route of administration: Administer IV over 15 to 30 minutes or give undiluted drug IV at a rate of 1 ml/min. (Do not heparinize as this will cause precipitation. Doxorubicin hydrochloride is reportedly physically incompatible with aminophylline, cephalothin sodium, dexamethasone sodium phosphate, diazepam, 5-fluorouracil (as an IV additive only), furosemide, heparin sodium, and hydrocortisone sodium succinate).

Storage: Store at room temperature. Avoid storing with aluminum-hub needles.

Mechanism of action: Antitumor antibiotic; inhibits DNA and RNA synthesis. The liposomal

preparation can decrease toxicity and may, in some cases, enhance efficacy.

Metabolism: Metabolized predominantly by the liver. Approximately 50% of the drug is excreted in bile. In animals with bilirubin levels above 2 mg/dl, the dose should be decreased by 50% to reduce toxicity. The drug is also excreted in urine and causes a red color in urine for up to 2 days after administration.

Toxicity: Leukopenia and thrombocytopenia. Less cardiotoxicity than with native doxorubicin. Extravasation causes severe tissue necrosis. Immediately apply ice or cold compresses to the area of extravasation for 6 to 10 hours. The drug may cause renal toxicity in dogs. Allergic reactions occur occasionally but may be eliminated by slowing the infusion or by pretreating with antihistamines. Alopecia may be seen in some dogs. More importantly, palmar–plantar erythrodysesthesia syndrome is possible and may be reduced by administering concurrent pyridoxine.

Note: Doxorubicin is used to treat lymphoma, thyroid carcinoma, sarcoma, and mammary carcinoma. This antineoplastic agent seems to have a broad spectrum of activity against a variety of tumors but may not be more efficacious than native doxorubicin in many patients.

Mitoxantrone

Dose supplied: 20, 25, and 30 mg multidose vials.

Canine dosage: 5.5 mg/m^2 IV (administered over at least 3 minutes) q3wk.

Feline dosage: 6.5 mg/m^2 IV (administered over at least 3 minutes) q3wk.

Route of administration: IV.

Storage: Store at room temperature. The drug is incompatible with heparin. Do not freeze.

Mechanism of action: Intercalates DNA; inhibits DNA and RNA synthesis.

Metabolism: Liver.

Toxicity: Unlike doxorubicin, this drug does not readily cause allergic reactions, cardiomyopathy, cardiac arrhythmias, or severe tissue damage at the site of extravasation. It is more myelosuppressive than doxorubicin and can cause alopecia and GI disturbances.

Note: Mitoxantrone is moderately effective for the treatment of lymphoma, squamous cell carcinoma, transitional cell carcinoma, mammary gland tumors, and a number of other neoplastic conditions.

Idarubicin

Dose supplied: 2 mg capsules; 5 and 10 mg vials.

Canine dosage: Investigational; advise checking for updated recommendations from oncologists.

Feline dosage: 2 mg/cat for 3 days every three weeks vs. every 3 weeks.

Route of administration: PO, IV (limited availability worldwide).

Storage: Store at room temperature. Injectable form is stable for 7 days if refrigerated. Incompatible with heparin.

Mechanism of action: Antitumor antibiotic; inhibits DNA and RNA synthesis.

Metabolism: Metabolized predominantly by the liver.

Toxicity: Bone marrow suppression, GI disturbances, and alopecia.

Note: Orally administered idarubicin has shown to be effective for the treatment of lymphoma in cats.

Bleomycin

Dose supplied: 15 unit vials (1 unit = 1 mg).

Canine/Feline dosage: 0.3 to 0.5 U/kg/wk IM or SQ to total cumulative dose of 125–200 U/m². IV push over at least 10 minutes.

Route of administration: IM, SQ; may be used intralesionally. May cause pain at injection site. IV administration should be slow (1 U/min).

Storage: Can be stored for 24 hours at room temperature, 1 to 2 months if refrigerated, and 2 years if frozen. It should not be used with heparin.

Mechanism of action: Antitumor antibiotic; inhibits DNA synthesis and, to a lesser extent, RNA and protein synthesis.

Metabolism: Rapidly excreted by the kidney. Dose should be decreased if serum creatinine level is elevated because of renal disease.

Toxicity: Pulmonary fibrosis has been reported in some species and seems to be dose-related. A maximum cumulative dose of 200 mg/m² is recommended. In addition, allergic reactions (fever) have been reported.

Note: Bleomycin has been suggested as a treatment for squamous cell carcinoma and, intralesionally, for acanthomatous epulis.

Plicamycin (mithramycin)

Dose supplied: Lyophilized powder in vials containing 2.5 mg of drug.

Canine dosage: 0.1 mg/kg/wk for 2 weeks for the treatment of hypercalcemia of malignancy.

Route of administration: Slow IV (over a minimum of 20 minutes).

Storage: Room temperature.

Mechanism of action: Antitumor antibiotic.

Metabolism: Metabolized by the liver.

Toxicity: Bone marrow suppression, GI toxicity, alopecia, and extravasation reactions can occur with this drug.

Note: Mithramycin has been suggested as a treatment of hypercalcemia of malignancy and it may have anticancer properties.

Dactinomycin

Dose supplied: 0.5 mg vials.

Canine/Feline dosage: 0.5 to 0.9 mg/m² slow IV infusion every 1 to 3 weeks.

Route of administration: Slow IV (over a minimum of 20 minutes); may cause pain at injection site.

Storage: Use within 24 hours of reconstitution because of the absence of preservatives.

Mechanism of action: Antitumor antibiotic that inhibits DNA synthesis and, to a lesser extent, RNA and protein synthesis.

Metabolism: Excreted by the liver.

Toxicity: Bone marrow suppression, GI toxicity, alopecia, and extravasation reactions can occur with this drug.

Note: This drug has been used to treat lymphoma.

TOPOISOMERASE-1 INHIBITORS

Interferes with the action of topoisomerase enzymes, which are enzymes that control the changes in DNA structure by catalyzing the breaking and rejoining of the phosphodiester backbone of DNA strands during the normal cell cycle.

9-Aminocamptothecin (9-AC)

Dose supplied: Investigational vials.

Canine dosage: 3.35 to 3.69 mg/m² IV.

Route of administration: As a continuous 72-hour IV infusion q3wk.

Storage: Use within 24 hours of reconstitution because of the absence of preservatives.

Mechanism of action: Inhibition of topoisomerase-1 interferes with DNA synthesis.

Metabolism: Metabolized by the liver.

Toxicity: Bone marrow suppression, mild GI.

Note: This drug has been used to treat lymphoma in investigational trials.

ENZYMES

Any of numerous proteins or conjugated proteins produced by living organisms and functioning as biochemical catalysts. The most commonly used enzyme in veterinary and human medicine is L-asparaginase.

L-asparaginase

Dose supplied: 10,000 U vials.

Canine dosage: 10,000 to 20,000 U/m² or 400 U/kg weekly or less frequently.

Feline dosage: 10,000 U/m² or 400 U/kg q7-21d.

Route of administration: IM.

Storage: Refrigerate. Reconstituted drug may be active for up to 7 days. Do not use if cloudy.

Mechanism of action: Enzyme; inhibits protein synthesis by depriving tumor cells of the amino acid asparagine.

Metabolism: Not completely understood.

Toxicity: Allergic and anaphylactic reactions are seen, especially after several doses have been given. The incidence of anaphylaxis is minimal when administered IM. If administered IV, the potential for inducing an acute anaphylactic reaction is high. Pretreatment with antihistamines and steroids may reduce risk of reactions. If anaphylaxis occurs, L-asparaginase should be discontinued indefinitely. Other toxicities include fever and vomiting shortly after administration. The drug has been associated with acute pancreatitis in dogs and humans. Myelosuppression may occur if this drug is administered concurrently with vincristine.

Note: The drug is used to treat lymphoma and lymphoblastic leukemia and may be combined with other antineoplastic agents. L-asparaginase does not induce a sustained remission when used alone in the treatment of lymphoma.

Pegaspargase

Dose supplied: 750 U/ml in a 5 ml vial. No reconstitution or dilution necessary.

Canine dosage: 10,000 to 20,000 U/m² or 400 U/kg weekly or less frequently.

Route of administration: IM.

Storage: Refrigerate. Reconstituted drug may be active for up to 7 days. Do not use if cloudy.

Mechanism of action: Enzyme; inhibits protein synthesis by depriving tumor cells of the amino acid asparagine.

Metabolism: Polyethylene glycol added to naturally occurring enzyme to prolong half-life.

Toxicity: The drug is less immunogenic than native L-asparaginase. Toxicity similar to L-asparaginase, although specific toxicity in the dog is not clearly described in the literature. Coagulopathies, hypercholesterolemia, fever, chills, anorexia, lethargy, confusion, and tachycardia all theoretically possible.

Note: Pegaspargase can be effective for the treatment of lymphoma when L-asparaginase cannot be used and yet when this enzyme may be effective.

VINCA ALKALOIDS

Vinca alkaloids bind to the microtubules to prevent the normal formation and function of the mitotic spindle, thus arresting the cell division in metaphase.

Vincristine

Dose supplied: 1, 2, and 5 mg vials; Hyporets (1 and 2 mg/ml disposable syringes).

Canine/Feline dosage: 0.5 to 0.75 mg/m² weekly.

Route of administration: Administer through a patent IV catheter; follow with adequate saline flush (10 ml).

Storage: Refrigerate. Protect from light until immediately before injection.

Mechanism of action: Plant alkaloid. Causes metaphase arrest by binding to microtubular protein used in formation of mitotic spindle.

Metabolism: Rapidly cleared from plasma and excreted in bile. Decrease dose by 50% in animals with bilirubin levels above 2 mg/dL.

Toxicity: Can cause neurotoxicity and resultant paresthesia, constipation, and paralytic ileus.

Anorexia in treated dogs and cats may be due to ileus. This drug is a potent irritant that can cause severe tissue irritation and necrosis if extravasated; if extravasation occurs, apply warm compresses immediately and infiltrate with saline and 8 mg dexamethasone. Myelosuppression is dose-related and uncommon unless drug is given in combination with L-asparaginase. Vincristine causes a marked increase in peripheral platelet count in animals with adequate megakaryocytes.

Note: Vincristine is most commonly used to treat lymphoma, sarcomas, immune-mediated thrombocytopenia, and mast cell tumors.

Vinblastine

Dose supplied: 10 mg vial.

Canine dosage: 2.5 mg/m² weekly.

Feline dosage: 1.5-2 mg/m² q2-3wk.

Route of administration: Potent irritant, avoid extravasation. Administer through a patent IV catheter; follow with adequate saline flush (10 ml).

Storage: Refrigerated reconstituted drug is stable for 30 days. Protect from light.

Mechanism of action: Plant alkaloid. Causes metaphase arrest by binding to microtubular protein used in the formation of mitotic spindle.

Metabolism: Rapidly cleared from plasma; excreted in bile. A 50% decrease in dose is recommended in animals with bilirubin levels above 2 mg/dL.

Toxicity: Unlike vincristine, vinblastine may cause severe bone marrow suppression (neutrophil nadir, 4 to 7 days after administration). Neurotoxicity and mild peripheral neuropathies occur but are less severe than with vincristine. Extravasation can cause severe tissue irritation and necrosis. If extravasation occurs, immediately pack with warm compresses and infiltrate the area with saline and dexamethasone.

Note: Vinblastine is used to treat lymphoma and mast cell tumors.

Vinorelbine

Dose supplied: 10 mg vial.

Canine dosage: 15–18 mg/m² weekly to every 2 weeks.

Route of administration: Potent irritant, avoid extravasation. Administer through a patent IV catheter; follow with adequate saline flush (10 ml).

Storage: Refrigerated reconstituted drug is stable for 30 days. Protect from light.

Mechanism of action: Plant alkaloid. Causes metaphase arrest by binding to microtubular protein used in the formation of mitotic spindle.

Metabolism: Rapidly cleared from plasma; excreted in bile. A 50% decrease in dose is recommended in animals with bilirubin levels above 2 mg/dL.

Toxicity: May cause severe bone marrow suppression, neurotoxicity and mild peripheral neuropathies. Extravasation can cause severe tissue irritation and necrosis. If extravasation occurs, immediately pack with warm compresses and infiltrate the area with saline and dexamethasone.

Note: Vinorelbine has been suggested as an effective treatment for primary lung tumors.

PLANT ALKALOIDS

Plant alkaloids are chemotherapy treatments derived made from certain types of plants.

Etoposide (VP-16)

Dose supplied: 50 mg capsules (erratic absorption in the dog), 100 mg multidose vials.

Canine dosage: 40 mg/m^2 reported to result in profound hypotension during administration due to carrier.

Route of administration: IV slow infusion or orally (poor and erratic bioavailability). Due to acute and potentially fatal degranulation of mast cells upon administration of VP-16, diphenhydramine, cimetidine, and dexamethasone must be administered 20 minutes prior to slow infusion with VP-16.

Storage: Vials of unreconstituted drug can be stored at room temperature.

Mechanism of action: Topoisomerase II inhibitor.

Metabolism: Metabolized by the liver and excreted in the urine.

Toxicity: Hypotension and death is possible during IV administration due to carrier polysorbate 80. Bone marrow suppression, alopecia, and nausea and vomiting. Has not been studied in cats, but the diluent causes an allergic reaction in dogs when administered IV. Not currently recommended for use in cats.

HORMONES

Hormones are believed to interfere with the cellular receptors that stimulate growth. The most common examples of hormones used to treat cancer are the corticosteroids used to treat lymphoma and mast cell tumors.

Prednisone

Dose supplied: 5, 10, 20, and 50 mg tablets; 1 mg/ml syrup; injectable solution.

Canine/Feline dosage: 30 to 40 mg/m^2 daily or every other day or 1 mg/kg/d for 4 weeks; 1 mg/kg every other day thereafter as long as the tumor is in remission and the patient is doing well.

Route of administration: PO, IV.

Storage: Store at room temperature.

Mechanism of action: Binds to cytoplasmic receptor sites, which then interact with DNA and prevent cell division.

Metabolism: Metabolized by the liver and excreted in the urine. Prednisone is activated by the liver to its active form, prednisolone; severe liver disease, however, does not significantly affect activation.

Toxicity: Polydipsia and polyuria are the major side effects. Long-term use may be associated with development of alopecia and other signs of iatrogenic Cushing's syndrome.

Note: Active in treatment of lymphoma and mast cell tumors. Prednisone does not induce a sustained remission when used alone in the treatment of lymphoma.

CYTOKINES, HEMATOPOIETIC GROWTH FACTORS

Cytokines are small cell-signaling protein molecules that are secreted by numerous cells and are a category of signaling molecules used extensively in intercellular communication. Cytokines can be classified as proteins, peptides, or glycoproteins; the term "cytokine" encompasses a large and diverse family of regulators produced throughout the body by cells of diverse embryological origin.

Hematopoietic growth factors are one of a group of proteins, including erythropoietin, interleukins, and colony-stimulating factors, that promote the proliferation of blood cells.

Epoetin alfa (erythropoietin)

Dose supplied: Vials of 2,000, 4,000, and 10,000 units as a human or canine recombinant protein.

Canine/Feline dosage: 100 units/kg three times weekly as needed for anemia.

Route of administration: IV, IM, or SQ route results in measurable levels for 24 hours.

Storage: Vials should be kept refrigerated.

Mechanism of action: Acts as a hematopoietic growth factor specifically to increase the production of red blood cells.

Metabolism: Proteolysis within the serum is common. If the recombinant human product is used, antibodies are possible resulting in destruction by the reticuloendothelial system.

Toxicity: Hypertension and flu-like syndrome seen in people. If antibodies are directed against the protein, this may cross-react against the native erythropoietin resulting in severe nonregenerative anemia that may be permanent.

Note: Erythropoietin can be used to resolve anemia.

Filgrastim (granulocyte colony-stimulating factor)

Dose supplied: Single-dose vials of 300 and 480 mg in solution as a human or canine (not commercially available) recombinant protein.

Canine dosage: 5 mg/kg/d until neutropenia has resolved.

Route of administration: SQ.

Storage: Vials should be kept refrigerated.

Mechanism of action: Acts as a hematopoietic growth factor specifically to increase the production of neutrophils.

Metabolism: Proteolysis within the serum is common. If the recombinant human product is used, antibodies are possible, resulting in destruction by the granulocytes.

Toxicity: Hypertension and flu-like syndrome seen in people. If antibodies are directed against the protein, this may cross-react against the native granulocytes, resulting in serious neutropenia.

Interferon alfa

Dose supplied: 3 to 50 million units per vial.

Canine dosage: Investigational; advise checking for updated recommendations from oncologists. 3 million units/three times per week.

Route of administration: IV, IM, or SQ.

Storage: Vials should be kept refrigerated.

Mechanism of action: Biological-response modifier, immunostimulant.

Metabolism: Proteolysis throughout the body.

Toxicity: Fatigue, fever, chills, anorexia, lethargy, diarrhea, and weight loss.

Interleukin-2

Dose supplied: 18 million units per vial.

Canine dosage: Investigational; advise checking for updated recommendations from oncologists.

Route of administration: IV, SQ.

Storage: Vials should be kept refrigerated.

Mechanism of action: Biological-response modifier, immunostimulant.

Metabolism: Proteolysis.

Toxicity: Fatigue, fever, chills, anorexia, lethargy, diarrhea, weight loss, capillary leak syndrome, and hypotension. CNS and hepatic toxicity possible.

Note: Intralesional or systemic therapy may have efficacy for solid tumors.

MISCELLANEOUS

Amifostine (WR-2721)

Dose supplied: 500 mg vial.

Canine dosage: Investigational; advise checking for updated recommendations from oncologists.

Route of administration: Poorly absorbed orally. IV administration is preferable.

Storage: Vials of unreconstituted drug can be stored at room temperature.

Mechanism of action: Cytoprotectant and free-radical scavenger. Documented as agent to reduce bone marrow, kidney, and nerve toxicity during concurrent administration of radiation and cisplatin.

Metabolism: Metabolized to active metabolites that are excreted in the urine.

Toxicity: Hypotension when administered intravenously. Nausea, vomiting, somnolence, and hypocalcemia occasionally seen.

Note: Amifostine may protect against radiation and cisplatin-induced toxicity to the bone marrow and kidney.

Cisplatin (*cis*-diamminedichloroplatinum II)

Dose supplied: 10, 50, and 100 mg vials.

Canine dosage: 50–70 mg/m^2 with a fluid diuresis at 18.3 ml/kg/hr 3 hours before and 1 hour after the administration of cisplatin. Because aluminum causes precipitation, do not use aluminum needles.

Feline dosage: IV USE CONTRAINDICATED IN CATS due to fatal pulmonary edema. Intralesional administration ONLY as a suspension in oil or collagen matrix at 1.5 mg/cm^3 of tumor and surrounding normal tissue. Because aluminum causes precipitation, do not use aluminum needles.

Canine route of administration: IV or intracavitary; intralesional administration as a suspension in oil or collagen matrix only.

Storage: Dry powder is stable at room temperature for 2 years. Reconstituted solution is stable at room temperature for 20 hours. The reconstituted solution should not be refrigerated because a precipitate will form.

Mechanism of action: Similar to alkylating agents and other heavy metals. Binds to DNA and causes cross-linkage.

Metabolism: When given IV to dogs, cisplatin is rapidly distributed to liver, intestine, and kidneys; less than 10% is in plasma after 1 hour, and 50% of the administered dose is excreted in urine in 24 to 48 hours.

Toxicity: Myelosuppression with a nadir at days 5 and 16, alopecia, vomiting, nephrotoxicity, and neurotoxicity, including ototoxicity. IV use in the cat is associated with fatal pleural effusions and pulmonary edema. Intralesional administration as a suspension in oil or collagen matrix is rarely associated with significant systemic absorption. Local reactions include necrosis, swelling, and inflammation.

Note: Cisplatin is effective for the intralesional treatment of squamous cell carcinoma and soft tissue sarcomas.

Carboplatin

Dose supplied: 50, 150, and 450 mg vials.

Canine dosage: 300 mg/m^2 q3wk (depending on size of patient).

Feline dosage: 220 mg/m^2 q4wk.

Route of administration: IV; must be diluted with 5% dextrose in water. Intralesional administration as a suspension in oil or collagen matrix. Intracavitary.

Storage: Dry powder is stable at room temperature

for 2 years. Reconstituted solution is stable at room temperature for 8 hours.

Mechanism of action: Similar to alkylating agents and other heavy metals. Binds to DNA and causes cross-linkage.

Metabolism: Metabolized by the liver and kidney. Dose should be reduced if serum creatinine level is increased because of renal disease.

Toxicity: Myelosuppression is the most significant toxicity (neutrophil nadir, 17 to 21 days and may be prolonged). Carboplatin should not be administered without the current neutrophil count being known. Unlike with cisplatin, nephrotoxicity and emesis are rare.

Note: Carboplatin is used in treatment of squamous cell carcinoma and possibly other carcinomas and sarcomas.

Oxaliplatin

Dose supplied: 50 and 100 mg vials of lyophilized powder.

Canine dosage: 35 mg/m^2 q3wk (investigational).

Route of administration: IV.

Storage: Dry powder is stable at room temperature for 2 years. Reconstituted solution is stable at room temperature for 8 hours.

Mechanism of action: Similar to alkylating agents and other heavy metals. Binds to DNA and causes cross-linkage.

Metabolism: Unchanged in circulation until excreted by the kidney. Dose should be reduced if serum creatinine level is increased because of renal disease.

Toxicity: Myelosuppression is the most significant toxicity (thrombocytopenia, neutropenia nadir; 7 to 10 days). Vomiting and depression rare. Unlike with cisplatin, nephrotoxicity is rare.

Note: Lobaplatin, an investigational drug similar to oxaliplatin, has been reported for treatment of osteosarcoma.

Dexrazoxane

Dose supplied: 500 mg vial with diluent.

Canine dosage: 30 mg for every 1 mg of doxorubicin

Route of administration: 15 to 30 minute IV infusion in 30 minutes prior to the administration of doxorubicin.

Storage: Vials of unreconstituted drug can be stored at room temperature.

Mechanism of action: Free-radical scavenger and chelating agent.

Metabolism: Metabolized by the liver and excreted in the urine.

Toxicity: Slight potentiation of doxorubicin toxicity reported in other species. Mild nausea, vomiting, diarrhea, and anorexia.

Note: Can be used to reduce the risk of doxorubicin cardiotoxicity.

Gallium nitrate

Dose supplied: 500 mg vials.

Canine dosage: Investigational, advise checking for updated recommendations from oncologists.

Route of administration: Continuous IV infusion.

Storage: Vials should be kept refrigerated.

Mechanism of action: Heavy metal that antagonizes iron metabolism in cancer cells. Causes hypocalcemia by similar mechanism.

Metabolism: Not metabolized.

Toxicity: Nephrotoxicity, nausea, vomiting, diarrhea, and mild bone marrow suppression.

Note: Used to treat hypercalcemia of malignancy.

Paclitaxel

Dose supplied: 50 mg/5 ml vials.

Canine dosage: 132 mg/m^2 q3wk.

Feline dosage: 5 mg/kg every 3 weeks (investigational).

Route of administration: IV. Must dilute with 0.9% NaCl to a concentration of 0.6 to 0.7 mg/ml. Prepare in a glass container; administer through a 0.22 μm inline filter using non-PVC tubing. Pretreat with corticosteroids, diphenhydramine, and H2-receptor antagonists.

Storage: Refrigerate vials before use. Reconstituted solution is stable at room temperature for 24 hours.

Mechanism of action: Inhibits microtubule disassembly.

Metabolism: Metabolized by the liver and kidney.

Toxicity: Myelosuppression and anaphylactoid reactions (due to the diluent Cremophor EL) and somnolence (alcohol also in the diluent) are the most significant toxicities.

Note: Paclitaxel is a relatively new chemotherapeutic agent. Studies are underway to define its usefulness in veterinary medicine. (Preliminary results are available for mammary carcinoma, histiocytosis, and osteosarcoma).

Docetaxel

Dose supplied: 80 mg/2 ml vials with separate diluent.

Canine dosage: 30 mg/m^2 (investigational).

Route of administration: IV. Must dilute with 0.9% NaCl to a concentration of 0.6 to 0.7 mg/ml. Prepare in a glass container; administer through a 0.22 μm inline filter using non-PVC tubing. Pretreat with corticosteroids, diphenhydramine, and H2-receptor antagonists.

Storage: Refrigerate vials before use. Reconstituted solution is stable at room temperature for 24 hours.

Mechanism of action: Inhibits microtubule disassembly.

Metabolism: Metabolized by the liver and kidney.

Toxicity: Myelosuppression and anaphylactoid reactions (due to the diluent polysorbate 80) and somnolence due to the alcohol also in the diluent) are the most significant toxicities.

Note: Docetaxel is a relatively new chemotherapeutic agent. Studies are underway to define its usefulness in veterinary medicine (preliminary results are available for mammary carcinoma and lymphoma).

Isotretinoin

Dose supplied: 10, 20, and 40 mg capsules.
Canine dosage: 1–3 mg/kg/day.
Route of administration: PO.
Storage: Room temperature
Mechanism of action: Induces apoptosis. Derivative of vitamin A that binds to nuclear receptors and changes gene expression.
Metabolism: Metabolized by the liver and kidney
Toxicity: Keratoconjunctivitis sicca, hypertriglyceridemia, hepatotoxicity, pruritis, conjunctivitis, xerostomia.
Note: This drug has been shown to be effective for a variety of cutaneous neoplasms and dysplasias.

Megestrol acetate

Dose supplied: 5, 20, 40 mg tablets and 40 mg/ml solution.
Canine dosage: 0.05 mg/kg/day for 3–5 days then every 48–72 hours thereafter to enhance appetite.
Route of administration: PO.
Storage: Room temperature.
Mechanism of action: Appetite stimulant.
Metabolism: Metabolized by the liver and eliminated via the kidney.
Toxicity: Edema, weight gain, anxiety, sleep disturbances.
Note: This drug is used in people and dogs to enhance weight gain and to reduce toxicity associated with chemotherapy, surgery, and radiation therapy.

Mitotane

Dose supplied: 500 mg tablet.
Canine dosage: Initially 50–75 mg/kg PO in daily divided doses for 10–14 days. May supplement with predniso(lo)ne at 0.2 mg/kg/day. If basal or post-ACTH serum cortisol values are decreased, but still above the therapeutic end-point (<1 µg/dl), repeat therapy for an additional 7–14 days and repeat testing. If post-ACTH serum cortisol values remain greatly elevated or unchanged, increase mitotane to 100 mg/kg/d and repeat ACTH stimulation test at 7 to 14 day intervals. If continues to remain greatly elevated, increase dosage by 50 mg/kg/d every 7 to 14 days until response occurs or drug intolerance ensues. Once undetectable or low-normal post-ACTH cortisol levels are attained, continue mitotane at 100–200 mg/kg/wk in divided doses with glucocorticoid supplementation.
Route of administration: PO.
Storage: Room temperature.
Mechanism of action: Adrenal cortical cytotoxin.

Metabolism: Metabolized by the liver and eliminated via the kidney.
Toxicity: Hypoadrenocorticism and associated clinical signs in addition to nausea, vomiting, diarrhea, and alteration of metabolism and clearance of other drugs.
Note: Mitotane has been shown to be effective for the treatment of adrenocortical carcinomas.

Pamidronate

Dose supplied: 30 and 90 mg vials.
Canine dosage: 1 mg/kg IV over 2 hours 3 hours after and 1 hour before a saline diuresis at 18.3 ml/kg/hr.
Route of administration: IV.
Storage: Store at room temperature.
Mechanism of action: Bisphosphonate inhibitor of bone metastasis and hypercalcemia.
Metabolism: Excreted by the kidneys.
Toxicity: Nausea, fever, constipation, hypocalcemia.
Note: Used to treat metastatic bone lesions and hypercalcemia of malignancy.

Piroxicam

Dose supplied: 10 and 20 mg capsules.
Canine dosage: 0.3 mg/kg/d PO; may need to be reformulated by a compounding pharmacy.
Feline dosage: 0.3 mg/kg PO q48h; may need to be reformulated by a compounding pharmacy.
Route of administration: PO. Avoid other GI irritants and nephrotoxins.
Storage: Store at room temperature.
Mechanism of action: Unknown; possible biologic-response modifier.
Metabolism: Metabolized by the liver and kidney.
Toxicity: Nephrotoxicity and GI irritation. Do not administer with other nonsteroidal or corticosteroid drugs. Administration of piroxicam concurrently with other nephrotoxic drugs may lead to worsening of renal toxicity.
Note: This NSAID has been shown to cause measurable regression in transitional cell carcinoma of the urinary bladder and squamous cell carcinoma in dogs, and therefore may be of value in dogs and cats.

Thalidomide

Dose supplied: 50-mg tablets.
Canine dosage: Investigational, advise checking for updated recommendations from oncologists.
Route of administration: PO.
Storage: Store at room temperature.
Mechanism of action: Novel antiangiogenic and immunomodulatory agent.
Metabolism: Unknown.
Toxicity: Profound somnolence, fatigue, nausea, vomiting, diarrhea.
Note: Antiangiogenic agent with at least theoretical benefit for the treatment of hemangiosarcoma and other malignant diseases.

Mesna

Dose supplied: Solution of 100 mg/ml as uroprotectant for cyclophosphamide and ifosfamide to prevent hemorrhagic cystitis.

Canine dosage: 60% of the daily ifosfamide mg dosage.

Route of administration: IV bolus before, 2 and 5 hours after chemotherapy with ifosfamide, or as a constant-rate infusion.

Storage: Store at room temperature.

Mechanism of action: Inactivates highly reactive metabolite of cyclophosphamide and ifosfamide called acrolein.

Metabolism: Filtered by the kidneys.

Toxicity: Nausea, vomiting, diarrhea.

Note: Used to prevent cystitis due to ifosfamide and cyclophosphamide.

Zoledronic acid

Dose supplied: Vials of 4 mg of drug in powder form.

Canine dosage: Investigational, advise checking for updated recommendations from oncologists.

Route of administration: IV.

Storage: Store at room temperature.

Mechanism of action: Bisphosphonate inhibitor of bone metastasis and hypercalcemia.

Metabolism: Excreted by the kidneys.

Toxicity: Nausea, fever, constipation, hypocalcemia, and renal insufficiency.

Note: Used to treat bone metastases and hypercalcemia of malignancy.

TYROSINE KINASE INHIBITORS

A pharmaceutical drug that inhibits tyrosine kinases, enzymes responsible for the activation of signal transduction cascades (through phosphorylation of various proteins). TKIs are typically used as anti-cancer drugs.

Toceranib phosphate

Dose supplied: 10, 15, and 50 mg tablets.

Canine/Feline dosage: 2.25-2.70 mg/kg PO Monday, Wednesday and Friday.

Route of administration: PO.

Storage: Store at room temperature.

Mechanism of action: Toceranib phosphate is a small molecule that has both direct antitumor and antiangiogenic activity. In non-clinical pharmacology studies, toceranib selectively inhibited the tyrosine kinase activity of several members of the split kinase receptor tyrosine kinase (RTK) family, some of which are implicated in tumor growth, pathologic angiogenesis, and metastatic progression of cancer. Toceranib inhibited the activity of Flk-1/KDR tyrosine kinase (vascular endothelial growth factor receptor, VEGFR2), platelet-derived growth factor receptor (PDGFR), and stem cell factor receptor (Kit) in both biochemical and cellular assays.

Metabolism: Metabolized by the liver.

Toxicity: Gastrointestinal toxicity; diarrhea, bloody diarrhea, loss of appetite, vomiting and weight loss. Use non-steroidal anti-inflammatory drugs with caution in conjunction with Palladia due to an increased risk of gastrointestinal ulceration or perforation.

Note: Indicated for the treatment of Patnaik grade II or III, recurrent, cutaneous mast cell tumors with or without regional lymph node involvement in dogs.

Masitinib

Dose supplied: 50 and 150 mg tablets.

Canine/Feline dosage: 12.5 mg/kg/day.

Route of administration: PO.

Storage: Store at room temperature.

Mechanism of action: Masitinib is a protein-tyrosine kinase inhibitor. Protein tyrosine kinases are thought to be activated in cancer cells and to drive tumor progression. Tyrosine kinase inhibitor drugs act by interfering with these cell communications and may prevent tumor growth. *In vitro*, masitinib selectively inhibits the mutated form of the c-Kit receptor (a receptor tyrosine kinase) in the juxtamembrane region and the c-Kit wild-type receptor. It also inhibits the platelet-derived growth factor receptor and the fibroblast growth factor receptor 3.

Metabolism: Metabolized by the liver.

Toxicity: Renal toxicity and protein loss syndrome, nonregenerative anemia and hemolytic anemia, neutropenia, hepatic toxicity, vomiting, diarrhea, and lethargy.

Note: Indicated for the treatment of recurrent (post-surgery) or nonresectable Grade II or III cutaneous mast cell tumors in dogs that have not previously received radiotherapy and/or chemotherapy except corticosteroids.

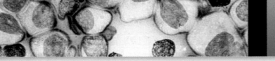

Chapter 21

Radiation therapy

Radiation therapy has been used for decades in veterinary and human oncology. The equipment is becoming more readily available around the world to large segments of the veterinary profession (primarily through referral centers or those who are willing to develop relationships with private or public radiation oncology businesses). Radiation therapy is effective for controlling many cancers as either a short to medium-term palliative care approach, or as a definitive approach. This treatment modality is used alone or in combination with other cancer therapies, including surgery and chemotherapy.

The readers of this section are almost certainly never going to do radiation therapy themselves. However, everyone interested in treating cancer should be aware of the different types of radiation therapy, the general indications, and potential benefits and risks of this modality. Radiation therapy is a local treatment; therefore, care should be taken to ensure that the animal is staged properly to delineate the extent of the neoplastic process. Dogs and cats with metastatic disease may not be good candidates for an intensive course of radiation therapy, but they may benefit from a palliative course of radiation. Consultation with an oncologist or a radiation oncologist is essential to determine whether a particular patient with a malignancy is likely to benefit from radiation therapy.

PROPERTIES AND USES OF RADIATION THERAPY

Ionizing radiation can be electromagnetic or particulate. Electromagnetic radiation is a wave and a packet of energy (a photon). There are two types of electromagnetic radiation; roentgen rays made by electrical machines (orthovoltage, linear accelerator), and gamma radiation produced intranuclearly most commonly by decay of radioactive isotopes such as cobalt (^{60}Co) or cesium (^{137}Cs). Linear accelerators are commonly used in veterinary medicine. Orthovoltage, cobalt, cesium source radiation therapy machines are becoming rare due to the dated nature of this technology. Radioactive isotopes administered orally or by injection such as ^{131}I are commonly used to treat thyroid tumors in dogs and cats.

The mechanism of radiation induced killing of cancer cells is complex. Ionizing radiation may kill cells directly, primarily through its effects on DNA and to a lesser extent through the effects on membranes. Alternatively, radiation may interact with water in the cells and intracellular matrix to form cytotoxic free radicals. Cells damaged by ionizing radiation may be killed directly through apoptosis, they may later attempt to divide and then die, or they may divide aberrantly. Some cells, however, remain functional but do not divide. These cells may be either terminally differentiated or sterile. In fact, if one biopsies a tumor that has been previously irradiated, tumor cells may be noted histologically but they are not able to divide, and therefore of no risk to the survival of the patient. Unfortunately, it can be very difficult to distinguish these radiation-induced "sterile" cancer cells from viable ones histopathologically. On the other hand, some tumor cells may only have minor damage that is repairable. It is these latter cells that are the source of tumor relapse. Radiation-resistant tumors may have increased capacity to repair potentially lethal damage.

Radiation-induced apoptosis occurs at low doses for lymphocytes, bone marrow, and germ cells as well as tumors derived from those tissues. Lymphoma is an example of a common malignancy of dogs and cats that is generally highly radiation sensitive. For tumors derived from other tissues, the proportion of cells undergoing apoptosis may be important in determining the response of that tumor to radiation therapy. Loss of apoptotic response may result in radiation resistance.

Cellular killing by radiation is executed by a constant proportion (rather than a constant number), hence tumor killing is exponential. Because some of the initial damage done by radiation is sublethal and repairable, there is a threshold dose that needs to be delivered before cell killing becomes exponential. Thus, it is important for clients to understand that the beneficial effects from radiation therapy may not be noted until late in the course of therapy or even weeks or months after the treatment is completed.

The cell cycle can be divided into four phases: G_1, S, G_2 and M. The distribution of tumor cells throughout the cell cycle may affect radiation response. As cells proceed through G_1, they become more resistant to radiation damage. Cells in late S phase (and those in resting phase G_0) are the most resistant. Cells that are in mitosis (M) and in G_2 are the most sensitive to radiation damage. Depending on the proportion of cells in each phase, there may be alterations of the threshold dose and exponential killing rate. Radiation therapy may cause some degree of cell cycle synchronization, but as a practical matter this is difficult to take advantage of before cells rapidly redistribute in the cell cycle.

Oxygen is critical to the clinical responsiveness of tumors to radiation therapy; greater doses of radiation are required under hypoxic conditions than in oxic conditions to provide equivalent cell killing. The enhanced cell killing occurs when oxygen is present because oxygen will react with DNA lesions, rendering them permanent. If there is less oxygen available, then there is an increased chance of repair before the damage is made permanent. Between well-oxygenated and necrotic zones in the tumor are hypoxic cells. Larger tumors are more likely to have abnormal blood supply and therefore more hypoxic cells; for this reason, radiation is most effective when treating small tumors or residual microscopic tumor tissue after surgery. Fractionation of the radiation dose (i.e.: giving small amounts of radiation repeatedly over time, such as Monday through Friday for 19 treatments) may allow hypoxic cells to become reoxygenated between fractions after oxygenated cells are killed. Drugs that act as hypoxic-cell sensitizers (oxymimetics such as nitroimidazoles) may improve the efficacy of radiation therapy by increasing susceptibility of the resistant hypoxic cells. Great interest has been focused on the potential value of using hyperbaric oxygen chambers to treat cancer patients immediately before or after therapy. Because veterinary patients often require anesthesia during radiation, it is possible that the inhaled oxygen rich air through the endotracheal tube during the anesthetic procedure may have a beneficial effect to radiation.

> **Key point**
>
> Fractionation of the radiation dose (i.e.: giving small amounts of radiation repeatedly over time, such as Monday through Friday for 19 treatments) may allow hypoxic cells to become reoxygenated between fractions after oxygenated cells are killed.

Interactions may occur between drugs and radiation therapy. For example, the antineoplastic drugs doxorubicin, cisplatin, and dactinomycin may enhance radiation damage to both tumor and normal cells, primarily by reducing the threshold for damage. Single strand DNA breaks are more reparable than double strand DNA breaks. Double strand breaks are more common when radiation sensitizers such as cisplatin are given concurrently with radiation resulting in greater efficacy. Doxorubicin that is administered even long after a course of radiation therapy may cause recurrence of acute effects of radiation (radiation recall). Hydroxyurea kills cells in S phase, when they are most resistant to radiation therapy. Radioprotective agents (sulfhydryl compounds) make cells more resistant by reducing the lifespan of oxygen-free radicals.

EXTERNAL BEAM, BRACHYTHERAPY, AND SYSTEMIC RADIATION THERAPY

External beam radiation therapy

The delivery of radiation therapy from a machine to the patient is called *teletherapy* or *external-beam radiation therapy*. In veterinary medicine, external-beam radiation therapy primarily is delivered by linear accelerators and less commonly by radioactive ^{60}Co, ^{137}Cs source units, or orthovoltage radiation therapy machines (figure 21-1). Because the source of radiation is external to the patient, teletherapy does not make the patient radioactive. Therefore, once the patient goes home, there is no radioactivity spread to people who care for the treated patient or their other pets. There is no period of isolation or quarantine required for patients treated with teletherapy.

Orthovoltage external beam radiation therapy

Orthovoltage radiation therapy is becoming less and less available, but it has been shown to be very effective for treating superficial tumors (e.g., mast cell tumors, soft tissue sarcomas) and tumors within air-filled cavities (e.g., nasal tumors). The radiation deposits most of its energy superficially because radiation produced by orthovoltage machines undergoes mainly photoelectric absorption. During photoelectric absorption, a photon interacts with tissue in the radiation field causing ejection of an orbital electron. During this interaction, most of the energy is lost. Photoelectric absorption also varies with the atomic number of the tissue. This means that the distance through tissue that radiation produced by an orthovoltage machine can travel is limited and, further, that when dense materials such as bone are within the treatment field the radiation travels an even shorter distance. In practical terms, penetration of orthovoltage radiation is limited to superficial tissues and the maximum dose is delivered to the skin. It also means that deep-seated tumors will not receive an adequate dose when orthovoltage is used. In addition, tumors that are surrounding or surrounded by bone may have areas of the tumor "protected" due to absorption of radiation dose.

Acute side effects are seen mostly in the superficial tissues where the highest dose is delivered. In addition, because bone absorbs higher radiation doses than surrounding tissues, late tissue effects are more common in bone when orthovoltage rather than megavoltage is the source of radiation.

Megavoltage external beam radiation therapy

Radiation produced by megavoltage machines (^{60}Co and linear accelerator) undergoes mostly Compton absorption. The clinical importance of this is that the energy is more deep penetrating than with orthovoltage machines. During Compton absorption, an incident photon dislodges an electron with low binding energy. Much of the energy is released as a secondary photon, which travels farther in the tissue. Because Compton absorption is not dependent on the atomic number of the tissue, penetration is not affected by tissue density and deeper structures can be irradiated than when using an orthovoltage source. Maximum dose in tissues is not achieved until a depth of approximately 0.5 cm below the surface; therefore, megavoltage radiation is "skin-sparing." Because megavoltage radiation is skin sparing, irradiation of superficial tumors is achieved by placing a layer of tissue-equivalent bolus material over the tumor that allows buildup of dose so the tumor is no longer "spared."

Intensity-modulated radiation therapy (IMRT) or conformal radiation is an advanced mode of high-precision radiation therapy used in some veterinary centers. This technique utilizes computer-controlled linear accelerators to deliver precise radiation doses to a cancer. The radiation dose is designed to conform to the three-dimensional shape of the tumor by modulating the intensity of the radiation beam to focus a higher radiation dose to the tumor while minimizing damage to the nearby surrounding tissue. Many beams are directed to the area in question from many different directions producing a sculpted radiation dose that maximizes tumor dose while also protecting adjacent normal tissues.

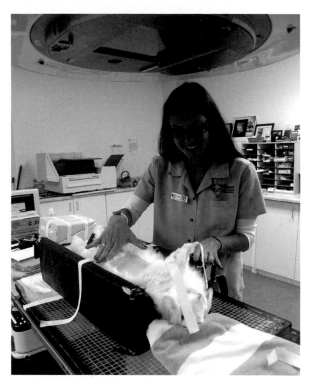

Figure 21-1: Megavoltage radiation is the preferred treatment for many neoplastic conditions. This linear accelerator, like all other megavoltage radiation therapy units, has excellent penetrating capability and is able to reach deep-seated tumors while minimizing injury to overlying tissues. The most advanced megavoltage machines can shape the beam of radiation to the size of the tumor and the nearby surrounding tumor to maximize tumor control and minimize adverse effects.

IMRT has been suggested to be so accurate that tissue more than 4 mm outside the beam has minimal radiation exposure. This is a great improvement over conventional radiation therapy but not as accurate as one-session intracranial radiosurgery where a precision of 0.33 to 1 mm can be obtained.

Electron-beam therapy

Electron-beam therapy may also be available with certain linear accelerators. With electrons, the maximum dose is delivered to the surface of the irradiated tissue without much deep penetration. Essentially, the dose is delivered to a much narrower volume of tissue. Because electrons can be given different energies, the distance they travel before energy reduces varies. With higher electron energies, penetration is greater and dose fall-off is not as steep. Lower-energy electrons are very useful for superficial tumors because deeper tissue is spared by a prompt fall in radiation dose; for example, this is useful with a mast cell tumor on the thoracic wall of a small dog or cat where underlying lung must be spared. One disadvantage of electron-beam therapy is the same as for orthovoltage: Bone may shield underlying tissues.

Thus, linear accelerators with photon and electron capability are very versatile because the oncologist can select which energy is needed to treat the disease.

Stereotactic radiosurgery

Stereotactic radiosurgery (SRS) and stereotactic body radiosurgery (SBRS) are collectively known as stereotactic radiation therapy. Stereotactic radiation therapy is a highly precise, intensified form of radiation therapy that is delivered in 1-5 treatments with a linear accelerator that is directed by a sophisticated computerized tumor targeting system. This form of therapy is becoming more and more readily available in veterinary medicine. SRS is a term that is most commonly used when discussing treatment of tumors of the brain or spinal cord whereas SBRS refers to the treatment of tumors elsewhere in the body. In either case, this targeting system accounts for the movement of the tumor due to respiration, heart beats and other movements. The term radiosurgery is misleading as the procedure does not involve removing the *tumor* with a surgical blade. Instead, a focused high-intensity beam of radiation is used to target a tumor. Standard radiation is normally administered daily for several weeks whereas SRS is delivered in 1-5 treatments. As a treatment method, radiosurgery has two important goals:

• Maximizing control of the growth of the malignancy.
• Minimizing exposure to the surrounding normal, healthy tissue.

Stereotactic radiosurgery (figure 21-2 A-C) may be delivered by several different types of machines including CyberKnife, Eclipse, Gamma knife, or a Proton Beam Unit. Each method requires highly detailed three dimensional imaging such as 64 slice computerized tomography, magnetic resonance imaging or positron emission tomography followed by sophisticated radiation planning. The end goal is better tumor control with fewer adverse effects.

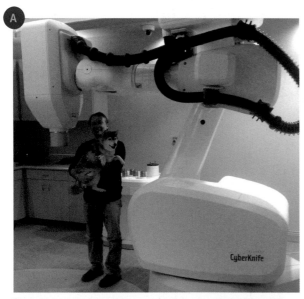

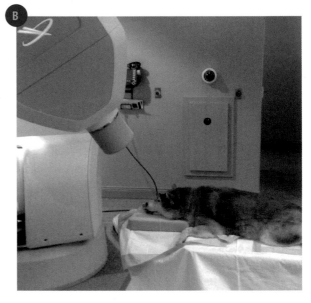

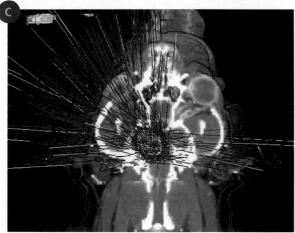

Figure 21-2: Stereotactic radiosurgery (SRS) is the use of highly sophisticated equipment that is designed to use computer directed beams of energy that are targeted to the tumor while compensating for patient and tumor movement via constant re-imaging. The equipment is CyberKnife that uses a robot to direct a miniaturized linear accelerator around the patient (A). The patient is monitored during therapy remotely so that a full dosage of radiation therapy can be delivered in 1-3 dosages rather than 12-25 dosages normally used in standard radiation treatment protocols (B). In stereotactic radiosurgery, tiny beams of radiation are directed to the tumor from as many as 200 directions. Where these beams intersect is within the tumor resulting in maximum tumor control with minimum normal tissue injury (C).

Brachytherapy

Radiation therapy is administered not only from external sources of energy but also from implanted radiation sources within or around the tumor (brachytherapy). Brachytherapy has a rapid drop-off in intensity with increasing distance from the source and is therefore very effective for delivering extremely high doses very specifically to a very localized site such as the prostate, with normal tissue damage usually being restricted to the immediate surrounding tissues. The amount of normal tissue injured is directly proportional to the energy of the radiation implanted as well as the time that the implant (radioactive source) is left in place.

Interstitial brachytherapy involves implanting "seeds" or "straws" of radioactive materials within the tumor. Interstitial brachytherapy seeds are often implanted in a removable package (e.g., Silastic tubing) and removed once the calculated dose has been delivered. Radiation therapy with a strontium-90 (^{90}Sr) hand-held source delivers a very high dose of beta-particle radiation that only penetrates 3 to 5 mm below the skin surface. Radioactive sources also can be administered into body cavities. Sources of radiation vary depending on the tissue to be implanted (e.g., cesium or radium for intracavitary placement, iridium for interstitial implants).

Because the source of radiation is implanted in the patient, interstitial brachytherapy makes the patient radioactive. Therefore, a period of isolation or quarantine is required for patients treated with interstitial brachytherapy.

Systemic therapy

Radiation can be targeted to a specific tissue by use of a radionuclide with special affinity for the tumor cells. Examples in veterinary medicine include iodine-131 (^{131}I) (figure 21-3 A and B) for treatment of thyroid carcinoma in dogs and cats and samarium-153 (^{153}Sm) (figure 21-4) targeted to bone for treatment of bone tumors in dogs.[1, 2] Radionuclides such as these emit beta particles that give up all their energy within a few millimeters of their source. It is therefore theoretically possible to deliver a very high dose to the tumor while restricting radiation of surrounding normal tissue.

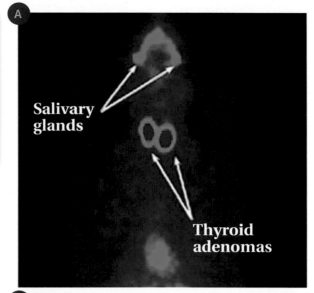

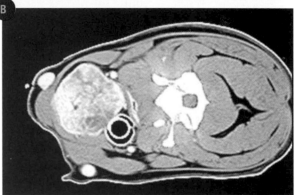

Figure 21-3: ^{131}I is effective for treating thyrotoxicosis in cats due to thyroid adenomas (A). Thyroid carcinomas that take up iodine can be successfully treated in the dog and cat. The image here depicts a CT scan of this contrast enhancing carcinoma of the peritracheal thyroid gland (B).

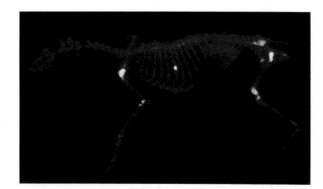

Figure 21-4: This is a bone scan outlining the skeletal system that has one bright spot defining at least a rib and pelvic tumor. These skeletal tumors can be treated with the systemically administered radioactive samarium-153 (^{153}Sm) targeted to bone for treatment of tumors of the bone in dogs.

Recently, radionuclides have been linked to monoclonal antibodies that "seek out" specific tumor tissues; this technique is also known as *radioimmunotherapy*.

Because the source of radiation is targeted to tissue within the patient, systemic radiotherapy makes the patient radioactive. Therefore, a period of isolation or quarantine is required for patients treated with systemic radiotherapy.

PALLIATIVE OR DEFINITIVE RADIATION THERAPY

One of the most important decisions is whether a patient should be treated with curative, coarse fractionated, or palliative intent. This decision influences not only the course of treatment but also the expectations of the caregiver for his or her pet.

Treatment with curative intent (definitive therapy) is often complicated, requiring frequent travel and multiple anesthesias if standard radiation therapy is employed. The total dose of radiation is usually higher than that required for palliation, and consequently the risks of unfavorable sequelae are greater. Such treatment is likely to be prolonged and expensive; however, for many patients the chance of long-term tumor-free survival (more than 3 years) is high. Typical definitive radiation schedules include the administration of daily (Monday through Friday) dosages for a total of 15 to 19 treatments.

Coarse fractionated radiation therapy is the administration of nearly a total dosage of definitive radiation in fewer treatments. This is being done more commonly now for cats due to their inherent tolerance of radiation and for dogs that are receiving radiation therapy for melanomas. Typical schemes include 6 to 9 treatments over 3 to 4 weeks.

Palliative radiation therapy is designed to relieve pain or symptoms of cancer while slowing the growth rate and occasionally the size of the tumor. If the palliative radiation is effective, it can be retreated. It is often performed when a specific site is causing a problem to the patient, but the rest of the cancer is unlikely to respond to any treatment (e.g., a painful digital metastasis from a pulmonary tumor that is not causing signs at any other site). For this reason, palliative therapy should minimize cost, inconvenience, discomfort, and risk of side effects, and it should be completed in the shortest reasonable time.

Key point

Palliative radiation therapy is designed to relieve pain or symptoms of cancer while slowing the growth rate and occasionally the size of the tumor. If the palliative radiation is effective, it can be retreated.

TREATMENT METHODS

A major component of successful radiation therapy is defining the extent of the disease and initiating treatment planning. The importance of planning is illustrated by a study in which all recurrences of soft tissue sarcomas were seen at the edge of, or beyond, the treatment field, implying that the field may have not been properly planned. Dogs that did not have local recurrence lived a median of 5 years after treatment, emphasizing the importance of these marginal failures.[6] Standard definitive or palliative treatments are best done by first doing a CT scan. Stereotactic radiosurgery, when done with CyberKnife or Trilogy based systems often requires high resolution 64-slice computerized tomography (CT) three-dimensional images fused with magnetic resonance imaging (MRI) or positron emission tomography (PET or PET/CT) images. Regardless, if standard radiation or stereotactic radiosurgery are used, the CT generated images are entered into a treatment planning computer that gives the radiation oncologist the best options for enhancing tumor control with the least chance for harming normal tissues and impacting quality of life (figure 21-5 A and B). Planning integrates beam distribution and homogeneity of dose within the target volume (tumor), while at the same time taking steps to minimize the dose to transit volume (normal tissue surrounding the tumor). This is achieved by port films, patient immobilization, marking techniques using tattoos and laser localization, and detailed computed tomography (CT)–based treatment planning. Gross tumor volume is the clinically evidenced tumor based on imaging. More relevant is the clinical tumor volume, which is the gross tumor volume plus the volume at risk for tumor extension. If only the clinical tumor volume is irradiated, margins that contain tumor cells may receive an insufficient dose due to patient movement during treatment and homogeneity of the beam at the edge of the field. The planning tumor volume is the final volume irradiated and consists of the clinical tumor volume plus a margin that allows for physiologic motion and beam variation (figure 21-6). CT-based radiation therapy planning also has the advantage of producing multiple images that can predict normal tissues that will be irradiated, allowing the radiation oncologist to block sensitive structures and to adjust the number and direction of the radiation fields.

The beam of radiation can be altered to make the dose conform to a specific target volume. Electrical machines deliver a beam that tends to have greater intensity in the center than on the sides. Wedges of a highly radiation absorptive material such as lead may allow a more uniform dose to be delivered to the patient. Lead may also be used to block sensitive structures within the radiation field, where blocking will not protect tumor tissue (e.g., eyes can be blocked when irradiating a brain tumor).

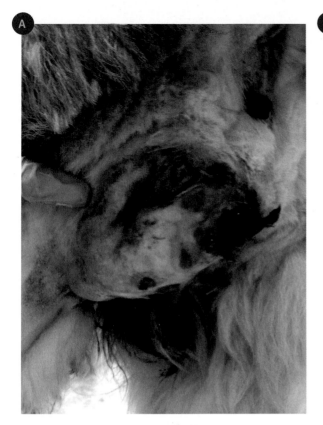

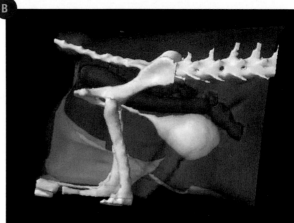

Figure 21-5: This dog with a metastatic anal gland, anal sac adenocarcinoma was imaged by CT (A). The CT images were imported into a computerized treatment program that reconstructed the body including the bladder (yellow), colon (pink) and tumor (orange) (B). This information was analyzed to create a treatment plan with the highest chance of delivering the full dosage of radiation to the tumor while sparing the sensitive normal colonic and bladder tissues.

After the treatment plan has been devised, a dosage is prescribed, and the least toxic method of administering the energy is determined. The dosage generally is limited by the tolerance of nearby normal tissues. The goal is to have less than 5% of the patients experiencing significant toxicity.

Port films are radiographs made by the therapy machine to define the anatomic structures exposed to radiation and to assess the accuracy of treatment delivery. They also help to determine if radiosensitive structures need to be blocked. One study used port films to assess the accuracy of planned treatment for animals treated with radiation.[7] Port films taken on day 1 identified a reason to move or change the size of the radiation field in 53% of cases.

Much of the accuracy problem in veterinary radiation is because skin marks are mobile and therefore difficult to use. Fields defined by palpable structures such as lymph nodes or bony landmarks give more consistency to radiation planning and treatment. Patient immobilization is best done using anesthesia. Short-acting injectable agents such as propofol are suitable prior to endotracheal intubation and isoflurane anesthesia, as radiation treatments are usually completed in minutes and there are no painful stimuli. Repeatable positioning is important to reduce variation in dosing. In a study of pets with head tumors, animals positioned using a head holder attached to the table and an inflatable pillow for the thorax and neck had the most repeatable positioning.[8] Similar immobilization strategies may be used for animals with tumors at other body sites.

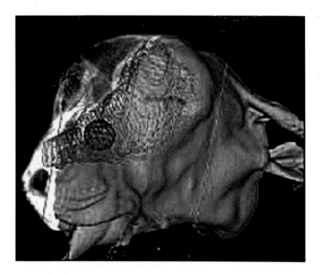

Figure 21-6: This is a reconstruction of the skull from CT images that allowed the identification of the tumor in red coloring. This is called the gross tumor volume that is the clinically evident tumor visualized on CT imaging. Clinical tumor volume is the gross tumor volume plus microscopic extension. The planning tumor volume is the final volume irradiated, and consists of the clinical tumor volume plus a margin that allows for physiologic movement that could result in a geographic "miss." The tissue that is very radiation sensitive is outlined in yellow which represents the eye. The treatment planning computer thus plans to treat the tumor and a surrounding region while sparing sensitive tissues.

TIMING OF RADIATION THERAPY

Radiation is most effective at the periphery of a tumor where there are small numbers of cells that are well vascularized. In contrast, surgery is limited by preservation of normal tissues adjacent to the tumor and therefore fails microscopically and peripherally due to residual tumor cells. Surgery and radiation therapy are therefore complementary.

Most radiation therapy in veterinary practice is delivered postoperatively to the residual microscopic tumor. Postoperative (adjuvant) radiation therapy has the advantage that it is possible to histologically identify patients with residual disease that would benefit most from radiation therapy. The major disadvantage is that surgery may reduce tumor vascular supply. Tumor cells along the surgical scar may survive radiation therapy because they are protected in a relatively hypoxic environment. In addition, a large surgical scar will increase the size of the radiation field and hence the risk of side effects.

One study evaluated the effect of starting radiation therapy the day after surgery, compared with delaying until 1 or 3 weeks after surgery. This study found that the strength of tissue healing was significantly less when radiation was started immediately after surgery, but healing was unaffected when the delay was 1 week or longer.[9]

Preoperative (neoadjuvant) radiation therapy has the advantage of sterilizing well-oxygenated cells at the periphery of a tumor before the vascular supply to these cells is compromised by surgery. Cells in the periphery that could be dislodged and seeded at the time of surgery are also irradiated. Preoperative radiation therapy may also reduce tumor volume in unresectable tumors, but this should not be used as a reason to reduce the size of the surgical field any more than is absolutely necessary to preserve normal structures. Disadvantages of preoperative radiation therapy include a delay of surgery while acute effects resolve; however, if peripheral cells are sterilized, this wait is not compromising the patient. A reduction in gross tumor size may lull the surgeon into attempting a less aggressive surgery. Another potential disadvantage is that fatally irradiated tumor cells may not die until they attempt mitosis, which can make histologic interpretation of surgical margins difficult.

Irradiation of a large volume of tissue leads to a poor outcome, regardless if the tumor is irradiated pre- or post-operatively. Some very large soft tissue sarcomas in cats are irradiated prior to surgical removal to reduce tumor recurrence (figure 21-7). When large areas are irradiated, planning is made more difficult and a larger volume of normal tissue is irradiated. This leads to a decreased chance of tumor control and an increased risk of complications. The earlier in the course of cancer that radiation is used, the more likely it is to result in a successful outcome and the less likely it is to result in severe toxicity.

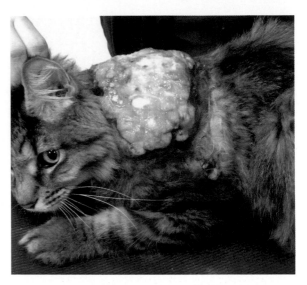

Figure 21-7: Large bulky tumors are best treated with either pre- or post-operative radiation therapy. This very large soft tissue sarcoma was treated with pre-operative radiation therapy to enhance the success of surgery that was performed 30-60 days post radiation therapy to reduce the probability of tumor recurrence. Another option for this type of patient is to treat with palliative radiation therapy which is designed to first provide comfort, second, to slow the rate of progression, and thirdly, to occasionally reduce the size of the tumor.

Key point

Irradiation of a large volume of tissue leads to a poor outcome, regardless if the tumor is irradiated pre- or post-operatively. Minimizing the treatment volume while concurrently maximizing tumor control is a critical balance.

Key point

Acute effects of radiation are common and should be expected when clinically relevant doses of radiation are administered. These effects occur toward the end of the treatment course and for days to weeks afterward.

ADVERSE EFFECTS AND PATIENT MANAGEMENT

The goal of radiation therapy is to increase tumor cell killing without increasing adverse effects of radiation. This therapeutic index should be as wide as possible. The dose (and therefore effectiveness) of radiation therapy is limited by the tolerance of normal tissues surrounding the tumor to the effects of radiation therapy. Differences in radiation response by normal tissues are determined not only by the actual cell type but more importantly by the proliferative requirements for tissue maintenance. If the proliferative requirement is high, these tissues are termed *radiosensitive*, whereas if the proliferative requirement is low, they are termed *radioresistant*. For example, liver and bone undergo little or no proliferation in steady state but there can be a problem if there is damage that requires cellular proliferation to reconstitute normal tissue, such as a bone fracture or liver damage. Tissues that are constantly renewing, such as skin, gastrointestinal mucosa, bone marrow, glands, and reproductive tissues, are considered to be radiosensitive, and these are the tissues in which the acute effects of radiation are most commonly seen (acutely responding). During radiation therapy, there may be differential recruitment of cells from un-irradiated adjacent areas in order to replace and repair acutely damaged tissue. This may be the major difference between tumor and normal tissues, as there is little opportunity for tumors to recruit new cells.

Most normal acutely responding tissues (except bone marrow stem cells) have a large threshold dose (see above), so dividing the total radiation dose into multiple smaller dose fractions may preserve these tissues by allowing repair between subthreshold fractions. Increasing the size of each fraction means that a biologically higher equivalent dose will be given to late-responding tissues rather than to acute-responding tissues and, therefore, the likelihood of late effects of radiation increases.

Acute effects

Acute effects of radiation are common and should be expected with clinically relevant doses of radiation toward the end of the treatment course and for days to weeks afterward. These effects arise in rapidly proliferating normal cells and may be exacerbated by release of catabolic products. Common acute side effects include mucositis, moist epidermal inflammation, and keratitis, depending on the tumor site and surrounding field irradiated. The occurrence of acute effects is felt to be acceptable, as healing is usually rapid and complete. Acute effects will be worsened when there is insufficient time between radiation fractions for recruitment of new normal tissue cells and for repair of sublethal damage. Shorter radiation courses with larger fractions of radiation will increase the severity of acute side effects compared with the same total dose given over a more protracted period in smaller dosages per fraction. For these reasons, excessive acute reactions can be ameliorated by a small decrease in fraction size or a short treatment break. This allows rapid resolution due to reconstitution of normal tissue. Small breaks, such as experienced over weekends, may ameliorate acute effects and allow re-oxygenation of tumor tissue. However, it is also possible that the same scheduling may protect rapidly proliferating tumors. Treatment of acute effects is usually symptomatic preceding repair or replacement of the damaged normal cells (see below).

Late effects

Late effects of radiation are less common than acute effects in veterinary medicine. Common limitations on all organ systems may be based on radiosensitivity of vascular connective tissue and endothelial cells. Those tissues whose functional activity does not require cell renewal such as muscle and nervous tissue are more resistant to the acute side effects of radiation. However, these tissues have vascular and connective tissue stromal cells, which may be required to divide and thereby show damage that translates into late effects of radiation. Radiation may also directly damage cell membranes and thus interrupt membrane transport leading to edema. This process may be important in the development of central nervous system damage.

Second malignancies are an uncommon late effect of radiation and are more likely at lower total doses since at higher doses the risk falls, presumably due to cell killing. The latent period for carcinogenesis is measured in years, so there may be an increased risk of second, radiation induced malignancy when patients are treated at a younger age for tumors that are potentially curable by radiation therapy.

Unlike acute effects, late effects of radiation occur months to years after a course of radiation therapy and are irreversible. Examples of late effects are necrosis, fibrosis, non-healing ulceration, central nervous system damage, and blindness. The occurrence of late effects is dependent on the size of each radiation fraction dose and somewhat on the total dose of radiation. The likelihood of late radiation effects is highest with large doses per treatment fraction. For example, late effects are higher with so-called hypofractionated or palliative treatment protocols, such as 8 Gy per fraction given weekly, than with small doses (3 Gy) given daily. Protraction of the total treatment course by taking breaks in treatment will probably not help to avoid late radiation effects. Late effects of radiation are considered to be dose limiting, and considerable emphasis is placed on their avoidance in the design of radiation protocols. In human patients, aggressive therapy results in a high cure rate. A long life expectancy, even in older patients, means that effects seen 5 years after therapy may still result in considerable morbidity. In veterinary medicine, patient lifespan is shorter, and particularly for older animals, survival times, even in cured patients, may be insufficient to see late radiation effects.

Other effects

Other effects of radiation are less common. Local radiation may cause a decreased immune response, presumably by irradiating circulating lymphocytes as they pass through irradiated volume and/or due to cytokine release. This rarely appears to be clinically significant. Mutagenesis is an uncommon problem.

Even if germ-line cells are affected, most radiation-induced mutations are recessive and so rarely lead to abnormal births.

Radiation therapy is a local treatment; therefore, side effects are confined to the area being treated. The only exception to this is when the entire body is irradiated, as with bone marrow transplantation, which is an uncommon procedure in veterinary medicine. It is important to educate clients about the ways in which different tissues will respond to radiation therapy and the timing of the appearance of adverse effects.

Acute effects of radiation are to be expected, but in nearly all cases such side effects resolve without limiting protocols. Protocols that use smaller doses per fraction (definitive or coarse) have a lower risk of late effects, thereby allowing higher total doses to be delivered, which leads to higher tumor control rates. In contrast, late effects of radiation are dose limiting and are more likely with higher doses per treatment fraction (hypofractionated or palliative). The higher risk of late effects is an excellent reason not to use a palliative protocol in a dog and cat that has a radiosensitive tumor and a high likelihood of long survival.

Skin

The skin is often injured in external-beam radiation therapy, particularly with orthovoltage and electron-beam sources. Acute reactions that generally appear toward the end of radiation therapy include erythema, dry desquamation with pruritus, and moist desquamation followed by a healing period where it is common to see alopecia as well as skin and hair color change (figure 24 A and B). The best treatment for these cutaneous injuries involves gently cleansing the area with mild soap and water, if symptomatic. This is often done under anesthesia or sedation. If self-mutilation is a problem, an Elizabethan collar or bandages over a Telfa pad should be employed. Non–petroleum-based vitamin E or Aloe vera based ointments have been used. Although controversial, some suggest that pets with severe pruritus or moist desquamation may benefit from cleansing the area with a 1:1 solution of hydrogen peroxide and normal saline and may require treatment with a topical or oral corticosteroid with tramadol or gabapentin. If a topical corticosteroid is used, a non–petroleum-based product is recommended. Combining cleansing with a wetting solution such as Cara-klenz with subsequent application of aloe vera gel extract (Carrington Dermal Wound Gel) has been recommended by some. Telfa pads should be used whenever the area needs to be covered. Occasionally, a patient may develop a pruritic rash that originates from the area of treatment and spreads to areas outside the treatment field. Systemic antihistamines, such as diphenhydramine, or topical corticosteroids may be indicated for these

patients. Late adverse effects include changes in pigmentation, telangiectasia, ulceration, and fibrosis, which, if extensive, can be quite painful. Debilitating late skin changes, which are extremely rare, can be repaired with reconstructive techniques using well-vascularized tissue.

Oral cavity and pharynx

Damage to the oral cavity and pharynx is very common in dogs and cats that receive radiation therapy for nasal and oral tumors. This area can be very frustrating to treat because radiation-induced oral mucositis may result in anorexia and secondary debilitation. Placing a gastrostomy or esophagostomy tube before initiating radiation therapy is recommended in any animal that does not have a good plane of nutrition and any time the oral cavity is to be included in the radiation field (e.g., oral melanoma in older or smaller dogs). Oral mucositis and anorexia are common in the acute phase of radiation therapy, and xerostomia (dry mouth) and dental caries may be seen in the chronic phase. Because oral damage can be so debilitating, care should be taken to ensure that all necessary dental work is completed prior to the start of radiation therapy. During treatment, owners may want to rinse their pet's mouth out with a solution of salt and water (1 teaspoon of salt in 1 quart of water). Some recommend Miracle Mouthwash (equal parts Benadryl, Maalox, and lidocaine with or without tetracycline a corticosteroid or the antifungal substance nystatin). Still others are advocates of mixing Maalox with saltwater solution to coat the mouth. Cool tea solutions can be used to lavage the mouth three to six times per day, which may reduce the discomfort of the oral cavity and freshen the breath. If the patient experiences pain when swallowing, 5 to 15 ml of 2% lidocaine (xylocaine viscous solution) may be squirted into the mouths of dogs several times a day. Because oral and nasal damage from radiation therapy may reduce smell and taste sensations, more palatable, warmed, aromatic foods should be prescribed. Increasing the amount of liquids given may help overcome xerostomia brought on by salivary gland radiation. Artificial saliva preparations, such as a mixture of sorbitol, sodium, carboxymethyl cellulose, and methylparaben (Salivart), may be beneficial in these patients. Some investigators have recommended oral glutamine supplementation to reduce the severity of oral mucositis. However, in one study, while changes in prostaglandin levels appeared less pronounced in supplemented dogs than in dogs not receiving glutamine, clinical mucositis did not differ.[10] Mucositis usually resolves within 3 weeks after radiation therapy is completed.

Late effects are rare; occasionally, bone necrosis of the mandible or maxilla may be seen years after irradiation of an oral tumor.

Colon and rectum

Occasionally, the colon and rectum are in the area of radiation. Irritation to the colon and rectum can be manifested by bleeding, tenesmus, and pain. A low-residue diet, a stool softener, metronidazole and/or tylosin may provide relief. Steroid enemas (e.g., Proctofoam) may be beneficial in select patients. Whenever the anus and perianal areas are injured by radiation therapy, the area should be kept clean by gently using soap and water and dried thoroughly. Sedation or anesthesia is often required to clean this region.

If radiation therapy is to be used for tumors of the caudal abdomen, small frequent fractions are more likely to avoid complications. In one study, dogs receiving more than 3.3 Gy per fraction to the pelvic area had an increased risk of developing severe colitis, and 60% of these dogs had intestinal perforation. In contrast, dogs treated with fractions of 2.7 Gy or less had only mild to moderate self-limiting complications.[11] Current treatment protocols taking this knowledge into account has nearly eliminated the more serious adverse effects.

Eye

The eye is often in the field of radiation therapy in dogs and cats with nasal tumors. The lens of the eye is considered sensitive to relatively low doses of radiation therapy, which can result in cataract formation months to years after radiation therapy is complete. In addition, retinal hemorrhages may result in blindness. The eye itself can be protected with creative radiation planning and by shielding the eye with a tungsten contact lens.

Conjunctivitis or keratoconjunctivitis sicca may occur acutely and it is important to monitor tear production in animals during and after therapy. For keratoconjunctivitis sicca, artificial tear preparations may be beneficial. It is important to confirm that no corneal ulcers are present before prescribing steroid-containing ophthalmic ointments.

Hematology

If a significant amount of the bone marrow is included in the radiation therapy field, such as with half body radiation therapy, or the inclusion of a large amount of marrow containing bone, bone marrow damage may occur. This may be a concern when large fields are irradiated and chemotherapy is also planned; myelosuppression may be enhanced in these patients. In addition, all lymphocytes that pass through the radiation field are lysed.

Bone

If bone is included in the radiation therapy field, a bone sequestrum due to necrosis may result. This late effect is much more likely to occur following orthovoltage radiation therapy than megavoltage radiation. Bone necrosis occurs many months to years after therapy. Removal of the sequestrum is indicated in such cases. Whenever brachytherapy is used to deliver radiotherapy to localized areas, radiation from these local sources can damage surrounding structures, including bone.

Lung

If lung is included in the radiation therapy field, radiation pneumonitis may be caused, even at relatively low radiation doses. Pneumonitis can cause decreased respiratory tidal volume if a large enough volume of lung is irradiated. Small volumes may not cause clinical problems, although pneumonitis still occurs. The use of electron-beam radiation therapy can reduce the risk of this toxicity, as electrons give up most of their energy in a narrow depth, so lung tissue underlying the irradiated tumor can be spared.

Miscellaneous sites

Other areas that can be damaged include the esophagus, stomach, small intestine, and liver.

The **endocrine system**, including the pituitary gland and thyroid, may be injured whenever radiation therapy to the head and neck is performed.

When the **heart** is included in the radiation therapy field, pericarditis and resultant pericardial effusion may be identified 4 to 6 months after radiation therapy is complete. A pericardectomy may be necessary to treat these animals.

Whenever the **urinary bladder** is in the radiation therapy field, high single doses of radiation, such as those used in intraoperative radiation therapy, can result in severe fibrosis and lack of elasticity. Fibrosis also may occur as a late effect of fractionated external-beam radiation therapy. This is rarely seen in well-designed and delivered radiation protocols.

Cranial radiation therapy occasionally results in headache, nausea, vomiting, and papilledema. Steroid therapy generally is indicated for these patients and should be considered during and after treatment. The most severe effect of radiation therapy to the brain includes brain necrosis, which can result in severe neurologic problems.

Fatty acids and radiation

Tumor sensitization to radiation by polyunsaturated fatty acids (PUFAs) has been investigated. One group studied the *in vitro* response of a chemically induced rat malignant astrocytoma cell line to radiation after the cell culture medium was supplemented with either gamma-linoleic acid or the long-chain n-3 PUFAs eicosapentaenoic acid or docosahexaenoic acid (DHA) and found that n-3 PUFAs enhanced radiation-induced cell cytotoxicity.[12, 13]

Another study documented enhanced radiosensitivity of rat autochthonous mammary tumors by dietary DHA.[14] Whether dietary n-3 PUFAs can lead to increased sensitivity of tumor tissue in the absence of a similar increase in the radiosensitivity of non-tumor tissue remains a critical issue. Several studies have suggested that PUFAs do not sensitize normal tissues to radiation. For example, since ionizing radiation generates reactive oxygen species, a study was initiated to determine whether dietary DHA might sensitize mammary tumors to irradiation using a model in which mammary tumors were induced by *N*-methylnitrosourea in Sprague-Dawley rats. In the study, it was shown that dietary DHA sensitized mammary tumors to radiation. The addition of vitamin E inhibited the beneficial effect of DHA, suggesting that this effect might be mediated by oxidative damage to the peroxidizable lipids.[14] Finally, in another study, the investigators hypothesized that menhaden fish oil would reduce inflammation from radiation damage and lower blood lactate levels in dogs with nasal carcinoma.[13] In a randomized, double-blind, placebo-controlled clinical study, 12 dogs with malignant carcinomas of the nasal cavity were given dietary menhaden oil [docosahexaenoic acid (DHA) and eicosapentaenoic acid (EPA)] or soybean oil (control) and then received radiation therapy. Megavoltage radiation was delivered in 18 fractions to a total dose of 56 Gy. They determined that dogs that are fed with menhaden oil had significantly higher plasma concentration of DHA by 500% and EPA by 200% and had significantly lower tissue inflammatory eicosanoids and decreased resting energy expenditure by 20% when compared with controls. Increased plasma DHA was significantly associated with decreased plasma lactic acid and matrix metaloproteinases. These data may suggest that dietary fish oil could reduce some detrimental inflammatory eicosanoids and metabolic consequences of radiation therapy. Thus, it appears that enhancing fatty acid levels to reduce adverse effects of radiation therapy seem prudent.

> **!** **Important point**
>
> Enhancing n-3 fatty acid levels to reduce adverse effects of radiation therapy seems prudent based on evidence based medicine.

CLINICAL USE OF RADIATION THERAPY

Radiation is becoming widely available to treat tumors in animals. Orthovoltage machines capable of delivering low-energy external-beam radiation are less versatile than linear accelerators and ^{60}Co machines that deliver megavoltage radiation. In addition, electron-beam capabilities that are available with some linear accelerators allow more targeted treatment in smaller patients. With the increased availability of computerized treatment planning and the delineation of the extent of the disease by CT and magnetic resonance imaging, the beneficial effects of radiation therapy are bound to increase substantially. The future of radiation therapy will be tied into the use of radiobiologic and tumor biology information to enhance the beneficial effects of radiation therapy. In addition, the combination of radiation therapy with surgery and chemotherapy may result in substantial improvement in the efficacy of this treatment modality.

Differences in control rates between studies of treatment of the same tumor type may depend on the total dose, the size of each fraction, and the protraction of the course of radiation. Veterinary radiation protocols can be broadly characterized as definitive, coarse, and hypofractionated (palliative):

- **Definitive fractionation**: Recent studies using higher total dosages (usually 2.7 to 3 Gy per fraction daily to a total dose of 51 to 60 Gy) and long-term follow-up have reported durable control for a variety of tumor types. Using these definitive fractionation protocols, cures are possible for dogs and cats with certain oral tumors, mast cell tumors, and brain tumors, and for dogs and cats with soft tissue sarcomas. Those who use stereotactic radiosurgery with CyberKnife or Trilogy machines may argue that the delivery of 1-5 dosages of radiation therapy to a full definitive total dosage due to the ability of this method to minimize normal tissue injury is appropriately categorized as definitive radiation therapy.
- **Coarse fractionation radiation therapy**: Many reports of radiation therapy in veterinary medicine have used relatively high doses per fraction (4 Gy or higher) delivered on an alternate-day schedule (Monday, Wednesday, and Friday) to a modest total dose (40 to 48 Gy). This relatively coarse fractionation would be expected to result in good tumor control for radiation-sensitive tumors and a modest prevalence of late effects. In Great Britain, radiation has been delivered weekly with very large dosages per fraction. It is considered state of the art to treat canine melanomas with coarse fractionated radiation therapy, such as twice weekly for six to eight treatments. Interestingly, the normal tissues in cats seem to be more radioresistant than that of dogs, therefore more and more protocols are taking advantage of this knowledge by the administration of larger dosages less frequently, such as the administration of radiation twice weekly (e.g.: Monday, Thursday) for six treatments to a total dosage that may be considered appropriate for what is usually administered in definitive radiation protocols.
- **Palliative radiation therapy**: The use of very large fractions (8 to 10 Gy fractions) to a moderate total dose (16 to 30 Gy) has been employed for palliation in pets that have a short life expectancy and, therefore, little risk of late radiation side effects.

Examples of clinical indications

In the section below, a few key examples of the efficacy of radiation are noted to illustrate the importance of this therapeutic modality. In some situations, palliative radiation therapy is mentioned. This is the use of a relatively small number of treatments to reduce pain and the growth rate of the cancer, and on occasion to reduce the size of the tumor. Coarse fractionated radiation therapy is also mentioned. If palliative radiation is quite effective, it can be repeated with close attention to ensure that normal tissues do not have a high chance of being irreparably injured. The difference between palliative radiation therapy and coarse fractionated radiation therapy can be difficult to define, however the latter is generally associated with more treatments over a larger segment of time, with the goal of obtaining a longer response to therapy than palliative radiation therapy. Definitive radiation therapy is an attempt to give a total dosage of radiation therapy that is generally higher than with palliative or coarse fractionated radiation therapy, with the goal of providing a longer response to therapy and even to enhance permanent tumor control in some cases. Definitive radiation is most commonly given in small dosages frequently (e.g.: 15-25 treatment sessions) over a relatively long period of time (e.g.: 3-4 weeks). The effect of the body's movement during these treatments can be taken into account through the use of newer equipment such as with intensity modulated radiation therapy (IMRT). Still more advanced is stereotactic radiosurgery, a sophisticated, technologically advanced way of delivering a full dosage of radiation therapy directly to the tumor with minimal effects to the surrounding normal tissues over 1-5 dosages while accounting for the location of the tumor within the body during respirations and unintentional movements during therapy via on-board imaging such as with Trilogy or CyberKnife-based technology.

> **! Important point**
>
> Palliative radiation therapy is the use of a relatively small number of treatments to improve comfort, reduce the growth rate of the cancer, and on occasion to reduce the size of the tumor.

Oral tumors

The most common oral tumors in dogs are malignant melanoma, squamous cell carcinoma (SCC), fibrosarcoma, and epulides. In the cat, oral squamous cell carcinoma is far more common than fibrosarcomas and lymphoma. Radiation therapy is effective for local control of many of these oral tumors.

Coarse fractionation: In one study, 105 dogs were treated for malignant oral tumors using megavoltage radiation therapy delivered by a linear accelerator to a total dose of 48 Gy.[15] Acute reactions in the final week of treatment were considered severe enough to result in discontinuation of therapy in 8% of dogs. Dogs with SCC and oral melanoma had high early local recurrence rates when compared with dogs with fibrosarcoma, but all tumors had a similar late recurrence rate.[15] Survival rates 3 years after treatment were 55% for SCC, 40% for fibrosarcoma, and 20% for oral melanoma. Large tumors of any histologic type were more likely to progress at an earlier time, and oral melanomas were more likely to metastasize.

The same protocol was used to treat 47 dogs with epulides.[16] These dogs were on average younger and had longer survival than dogs with malignant oral tumors due to successful long-term control by radiation. Survival rates 3 years after treatment were over 80%. In this study, 11% of dogs had late effects. Long-term survival in this group of dogs gives reliable information on late effects for this fractionation protocol.[16] It is possible that a lower dose per fraction may reduce the risk of late effects in dogs with oral tumors, but this has not yet been reported in the veterinary literature.

Hyperfractionation: The administration of multiple dosages of radiation therapy in a short period of time has some theoretical benefits. Very little has been done in this area in veterinary medicine, but one area hyperfractionated radiation seems to have a place is in oral squamous cell carcinoma (SCC).[16] Thirty-one cats with oral squamous cell carcinoma were treated with 14 fractions of 3.5 Gy of radiation therapy given within a 9-day period with the addition of carboplatin given at 90-100 mg/m² on day 1 and day 4.5. Median survival for all cats was 163 days. Cats with tumors of tonsillar origin or cheek responded best to therapy and were long-term survivors with a mean survival of 724 days, and the median had not been reached because of continued survival of 4 cats. Thus, hyperfractionated radiation therapy with carboplatin may be an effective alternative for cats with this aggressive disease.

Hypofractionation: Traditionally, melanomas have been considered to be radioresistant. Recent research suggests that melanomas may be one of the few tumors for which large-dose fractions are necessary to cause death of tumor cells. Therefore, high dose per fraction schedules may be warranted in patients with malignant melanomas. Oral melanomas have a high metastatic rate, especially when the tumor is large, restricting the beneficial results of radiation therapy for this tumor unless the tumor is concurrently treated with the DNA xenogeneic melanoma vaccine or other effective agents to reduce metastases and recurrence.

In one study, 36 dogs with oral melanoma received 36 Gy in four weekly fractions of 9 Gy each. Tumor size was reduced in all dogs, and 25 of them had complete remission. Median survival was 21 weeks, and acute radiation effects were predictably mild. Only 10 dogs survived for longer than 1 year, but late effects of bone necrosis or second malignancy were seen in five of these dogs.[17] Such hypofractionated protocols may not be ideal where long-term survival is possible, such as for dogs with small (early-stage) oral melanomas, as late effects of radiation should be of concern. Now that the DNA xenogeneic melanoma vaccine is available, distant metastatic disease is often delayed or prevented.

Squamous cell carcinoma of non-oral sites

Tonsillar SCCs typically have a poor response to therapy, primarily because of the high metastatic rate. In a study involving eight dogs with tonsillar SCC, median survival time was 4 months when radiotherapy was combined with surgical excision.[18] Another study used orthovoltage radiation therapy, cisplatin, and doxorubicin to treat tonsillar SCC in six dogs; the median disease-free interval was 8 months and median survival approximately 10 months.[19] SCC of th e nasal planum in dogs has been reported to be refractory to the beneficial effects of radiotherapy.[20] The reason for this difference in response rate for the same tumor type at different sites is unknown.

Ceruminous and salivary gland carcinoma

Coarse fractionation: Ceruminous gland carcinomas are frequently incompletely excised. Megavoltage radiation therapy (48 Gy in 12 fractions) was used to treat five dogs with ceruminous gland carcinoma.[21] Some dogs had been treated surgically with incomplete margins; therefore, radiation was administered as an adjuvant therapy. One dog with recurrence was treated with further radiation and survived another 20 months. Three dogs were alive and free of disease between 2 and 5 years after treatment.[21]

Nasal tumors

There is little doubt that radiation therapy is the treatment of choice for dogs and cats with nasal tumors (figure 21-8 A and B). There is much variation

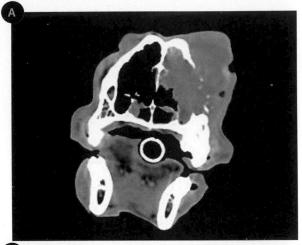

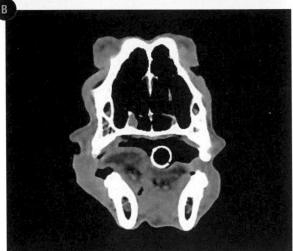

Figure 21-8: Nasal adenocarcinoma in the dog and the cat usually responds quite well to radiation therapy delivered palliatively or definitively. CT scans define the extent of the disease and the location of sensitive tissues and is taken into account via pre-treatment computer assisted radiation planning (A). Five doses of palliative radiation were delivered to the dog with the nasal adenocarcinoma imaged in figure 21-8 A. This CT image obtained one year after treatment confirms that there is nearly complete tumor control and remodeling of the tumor induced osteopenia of the skull. If and when the tumor recurs, it can be retreated with palliative radiation (B).

within the literature regarding response to therapy. The prognostic factors that may influence response to therapy include tumor histology, clinical stage, tumor size, type of radiation therapy, and the dose of energy delivered, as well as whether surgery was performed prior to radiation therapy.

Definitive and coarse fractionation: Nasal tumors in dogs and cats are conventionally treated with radiation therapy. In the past, if megavoltage was used, surgical debulking was not recommended because it was thought that the air-filled nasal cavity would result in inconsistent dosing due to the sparing of 0.5 cm of tissue as radiation absorption builds. This assumption has recently been questioned.[22] If orthovoltage is used, surgical debulking is necessary to enable dosing of residual tissue by the lower energy beam. Survival times for this tumor type are modest, ranging from 8 to 16 months depending on the study.[23–26] There is no difference between orthovoltage and megavoltage, and many dogs and cats have residual nasal signs. The poor response has led to studies that have attempted to improve control by dose and/or schedule manipulation.

Two studies investigated an *accelerated radiation* course for nasal tumors. Radiation was delivered in daily fractions over 11 to 13 days or twice a day over 21 days.[27, 28] Acute toxicities were common, including mucositis that was severe and protracted (up to 5 weeks); skin necrosis occurred in one dog. Few dogs lived longer than 6 months, and late effects were seen in nearly every dog. Unilateral or bilateral blindness occurred 6 months after treatment. Osteonecrosis was seen in three dogs and seizures in one. Five dogs died due to acute or late tissue reactions. Theoretically, these protocols should have resulted in equivalent or better tumor control and a reduced risk of late effects. However, there was no reduction in recurrence rate compared with standard protocols and survival times were actually worse.[29] In addition, the high incidence of late effects and the high rate of acute side effects made these approaches unacceptable.

Hypofractionated radiation consisting of four doses of 9 Gy given once a week was used to treat 56 dogs with nasal tumors. Clinical signs improved in most dogs by the end of the treatment schedule. Mild acute radiation side effects were observed in the majority of the dogs, but late radiation side effects were rare. The median survival time after the final dose of radiation was 7 months. The 1- and 2-year survival rates were 45% and 15%, respectively, which is little different than results with more conventional dosing schemes.[30] Some radiation oncologists now believe that hypofractionated protocols may offer a reasonable alternative for dogs and cats with a nasal carcinoma.

Soft tissue sarcomas

Soft tissue sarcomas are very common in the dog and in the cat (figure 21-9 A and B). These tumors can occur in response to injections in the cat and less commonly in the dog. These tumors frequently recur after incomplete surgical excision because they have many "fingers" that extend out into surrounding tissues and go beyond the margins of the excised tissues. Soft tissue sarcomas have been considered to be radiation resistant; however, higher total dosages provide long-term control of this tumor in the majority of dogs and cats. Radiation has been delivered in several prescribed courses including palliative, course fractionated, and definitive radiation therapy protocols.

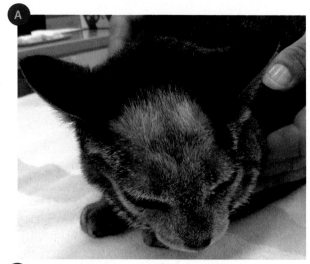

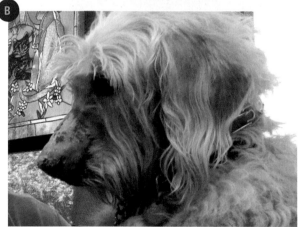

Figure 21-9: Note the hair color change in this cat that received definitive radiation for a nasal lymphoma. Cats are in general far more resistant to the adverse effects of radiation therapy compared to the dog. Nasal lymphoma usually responds well to radiation therapy and/or chemotherapy (A). This dog had a mast cell tumor that was cytoreduced with surgery followed by definitive radiation therapy and a tyrosine kinase inhibitor, masitinib. Note the alopecia and skin color change within the radiated field. Mast cell tumors generally respond quite well to radiation therapy. Tyrosine kinase inhibitors alone or in combination with radiation, surgery or chemotherapy are also commonly associated with long term control of mast cell tumors (B).

Coarse fractionation: Radiation therapy is frequently used postoperatively to treat incompletely excised sarcomas (figure 21-10). In addition, radiation therapy seems to be effective for treating gross evidence of malignant soft tissue sarcomas. For example, one study reported that 50% of dogs with soft tissue sarcomas have their disease controlled 1 year after receiving radiation therapy dosages ranging from 45 to 50 Gy delivered in10 fractions.[31] Predictably, smaller tumors respond

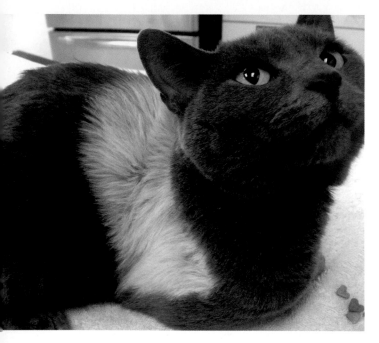

Figure 21-10: Injection site sarcomas in the cat commonly recur after surgical resection; therefore radiation delivered to a wide area after surgical extirpation of the tumor is ideal. Note the hair color change that occurred in the irradiated cat. Adjuvant carboplatin and/or doxorubicin have been reported to delay or prevent the development of metastatic disease associated with soft tissue sarcomas in the cat.

better to radiation therapy; 60% to 75% of such tumors were controlled at 1 year when treated with 52 Gy of radiation therapy.[32,33] When radiation therapy was used to treat soft tissue sarcomas after incomplete surgical excision, 41% of dogs were disease-free 2 years after treatment.[33]

Key point

Radiation therapy is commonly used postoperatively to treat incompletely excised sarcomas.

Definitive fractionation: Currently, if complete excision cannot be attained, debulking down to the level of microscopic disease followed by definitive radiation therapy is the recommended treatment for all soft tissue sarcomas in dogs and cats (figure 21-10). Smaller dose per fraction is an important factor in limiting late effects in dogs and cats. Treatment protocols utilizing 3-Gy fractions appear to have a lower risk of causing late effects and allow the delivery of higher total doses to provide longer term control of the cancer with fewer adverse effects. A protracted course of radiation to a total dose of 63 Gy in 3-Gy fractions on alternate days was given postoperatively to 48 dogs and cats with soft tissue sarcomas.[6] By 1

and 5 years after treatment, 87% and 76% of dogs were alive, respectively; most deaths were unrelated to the tumor. Acute effects were mild, and no treatment delays were reported. The only late effect reported was a dog that developed osteosarcoma in the treatment field 6 years after radiation.

Doxorubicin is believed to be a radiation sensitizer and may increase the effect of radiation on cancer cells when given at low dosages. In a recent study, doxorubicin (10 mg/m^2 IV) was given once weekly 1 hour prior to a 3-Gy fraction of orthovoltage radiation (total dose 51 Gy) to 39 dogs with incompletely excised soft tissue sarcomas.[34] Seven dogs (18%) developed local recurrences a median of 7 months after treatment, and this was more likely in dogs with grade 2 or 3 tumors. Six dogs (15%) developed distant metastases, two without local recurrence. The 1, 2, and 4-year survival rates were 85%, 79%, and 72%, respectively. Tumor control and patient survival were longer for dogs that had grade 1 tumors.[34] This control was similar to that seen with higher doses of radiation therapy.

Mast cell tumors

Mast cell tumors in dogs and cats (see figure 21-9) are very responsive to radiation therapy; however because these tumors degranulate when they die or are disrupted, significant adverse effects can be noted systemically or regionally. These adverse effects include bruising, bleeding, swelling, stomach ulcers, hypotension, and acute death. Therefore, whenever possible, mast cell tumors should be downsized with surgery, chemotherapy, or with tyrosine kinase inhibitors prior to radiation with either surgery or radiation therapy. The three most common types of radiation for mast cell tumors include course fractionated and definitive radiation therapy.

Key point

Mast cell tumors in dogs and cats are very responsive to radiation therapy; however because these tumors degranulate when they die or are disrupted, significant adverse effects can be noted systemically or regionally.

Hypofractionated: Hypofractionated radiation therapy (four weekly 8-Gy fractions) was used to treat 35 dogs with non-resectable mast cell tumors of all grades on the head or limbs; 17 dogs had cytologic evidence of lymph node metastasis.[39] All dogs received concurrent prednisolone (40 mg/m^2/d) for 10to 14 days prior to radiation therapy and at half that dose for 2 months after. A complete response was seen in 12 dogs and a partial response in 19. The median tumor control was 34 months, with 1- and 2-year control rates of 60% and 52%, respectively.

Definitive and coarse fractionation: Long-term control is likely for dogs and cats with incompletely excised grade 1 mast cell tumors after radiation therapy. Approximately 90% of dogs with this tumor treated to a total dose of 48 to 54 Gy in 3- or 4-Gy fractions given three times a week postoperatively were still alive and tumor-free 3 years after radiation.[35, 36] This treatment is clearly the best choice for this tumor regardless of the protocol. Acute effects are the same as those reported for similar protocols and schedules. Late effects were seen in only one dog.[35,36]

Some investigators have recommended prophylactic irradiation of the regional lymph node in dogs with grade 2 mast cell tumors that have mast cells observed on cytologic examination of a lymph node needle aspirate.[37] Because of the difficulties in determining whether mast cells seen on cytology are inflammatory or neoplastic, most radiation oncologists now include the regional lymph node adjacent to a mast cell tumor in the radiation field regardless of whether they have mast cells on cytology or not.

Radiation therapy (52.2 Gy in 2.9-Gy fractions given three times a week) was used to treat 31 dogs that had only residual microscopic disease after surgery for grade 3 mast cell tumor.[38] In all cases, the regional lymph node was irradiated as well. Local control of the mast cell tumor was excellent, with a median remission time of 28 months. More than half of the dogs (16 of 31) eventually developed lymph node metastases, underscoring the need for systemic therapy in this disease.[38]

Brain tumors

Radiation therapy either alone or when combined with surgery has been very effective when used to treat dogs and cats with brain tumors. Meningiomas and hypophyseal macroadenomas appear to be the most radioresponsive; however, responses have been seen in dogs and cats with other types of malignant disease.

Coarse fractionation: In a study of 20 dogs with meningiomas treated with megavoltage radiation to a total dose of 48 Gy in 4-Gy fractions on alternate days, the 2-year progression-free survival was 42% for dogs with rapidly proliferating tumors and 91% for those with slowly proliferating tumors. [40] Late effects were seen in 20% of long-term survivors: Of 14 dogs that lived longer than 12 months, two had presumed radiation-induced brain signs and one developed a radiation-induced glioma. In another study, the median survival for 65 dogs with brain tumors was 13.5 months.[41]

Definitive fractionation: Late effects were not seen in 29 dogs with brain tumors that received 48 Gy in 16 daily fractions of 3 Gy; however, the median survival was 8 months and therefore the population at risk may have been low.[42]

Hypofractionation/palliative: Recent studies have adapted hypofractionated protocols for treatment of tumors where long-term survival is possible, and where late effects of radiation should be of concern. In one study, 83 dogs with brain tumors were treated using a total of 38 Gy in five weekly fractions of 7.6 Gy.[43] Median survival was 11 months, although 12 dogs died due to late effects of treatment.[43]

Stereotactic radiosurgery: A linear accelerator mounted on a rotating gantry that is centered on the brain tumor allows a single large dose (10 to 15 Gy) of radiation to be delivered. In a preliminary report, control of tumors for more than 1 year was seen in three dogs, despite the relatively low total dose of radiation.[4] A preliminary report indicated that radiosurgery may be more effective in treating pituitary macroadenomas than other brain tumors.[5] Stereotactic radiosurgery has been used to treat osteosarcoma, nasal tumors, and spinal cord tumors among others.

> **Key point**
>
> Radiation therapy either alone or when combined with surgery has been very effective when used to treat dogs and cats with brain tumors. Meningiomas and hypophyseal macroadenomas appear to be the most radioresponsive; however, responses have been seen in dogs and cats with other types of malignant disease.

Thyroid tumors

Radioisotopes: Radiation therapy using ^{131}I has been used to treat thyroid tumors in dogs and cats even when they are not actively secreting hormone. This is the method of choice for treating thyrotoxicosis in the cat.

Coarse fractionation: Radiation to a dose of 48 Gy was reported for treatment of 25 dogs with unresectable thyroid carcinomas. [44] Of those, 72% were free of disease 3 years after treatment. Acute toxicities were common and resulted from mucositis in the larynx, trachea, and esophagus. Late effects were seen in 30% of 20 dogs that lived longer than a year, including chronic tracheitis, hypothyroidism, and hypoparathyroidism.[44]

Hypofractionated: Another study reported four once-weekly fractions of 9 Gy to treat 13 dogs with invasive thyroid carcinoma; most responses were partial, with only one complete remission seen. Four of the dogs died of progression of the primary disease and four from metastatic spread. The median survival time for all dogs was 22 months (range, 2 to 57 months).[45] Side effects were similar to those described above. Radiation therapy for this disease may be more effective when given in small fractions rather than in larger "coarse" fractions.

In a compilation of three studies, metastases occurred in 14 of 46 dogs (30%), indicating a need for adjunctive chemotherapy in addition to radiation therapy.

Thymoma

Coarse fractionation or definitive: Radiation therapy is important in the treatment of thymoma in humans. In dogs and cats, radiation may reduce tumor size to a point at which surgical excision is feasible or not even needed, but risks of radiation toxicity to lungs and myocardium are dose limiting (figure 21-11 A and B). In one report, 13 dogs were treated for thymoma with megavoltage radiation therapy. Radiation protocol varied but mostly consisted of 3- to 4-Gy fractions given daily or three times a week to 21 to 54 Gy (definitive) or weekly (hypofractionated) 5-Gy fractions to 15 Gy through parallel opposed portals. Three dogs had a complete and five had partial (more then 50%) reduction in tumor size for a median of 3 to 6 months.[46]

Transitional cell carcinoma of the urinary bladder

Coarse fractionation: A pilot study using ^{60}Co teletherapy (44 and 48 Gy) and preradiation cisplatin chemotherapy (50 mg/m^2 twice, divided into three doses before the first three and last three radiation treatments) found a minor shrinkage in tumor volume but few severe side effects. Survival times were 6 and 7 months**.**[47] Eight dogs in a group of 15 treated with mitoxantrone and piroxicam also received radiation therapy. The response rate was higher in the group receiving radiation therapy than in the group treated with chemotherapy alone, although survival times were not statistically significantly different.[48]

Hypofractionated: In another pilot study of 10 dogs, the addition of once-weekly coarse fraction radiation therapy (six fractions of 5.75 Gy weekly) to mitoxantrone and piroxicam did not improve on survival times seen with mitoxantrone and piroxicam chemotherapy alone.[49]

Mammary tumors

Radiation therapy has a role to play in preservation of breast tissue in women with mammary cancer, but its use in the treatment of canine and feline mammary cancer has not been reported. It is possible that radiation therapy may play a role in reducing the risk of local recurrence for aggressive tumors such as inflammatory carcinomas or in tumors that cannot be completely removed.

Other tumors

Rectal, colonic, and prostate tumors have been treated successfully with radiation therapy. In each case, the extent of the disease must be clearly defined and the animal appropriately staged with at least abdominal radiography, ultrasonography or CT, hemogram, biochemical profile, and urinalysis. When radiation therapy is delivered to these particular sites,

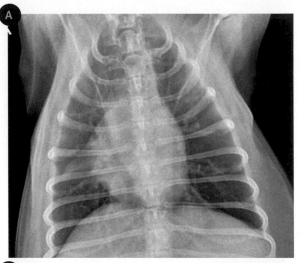

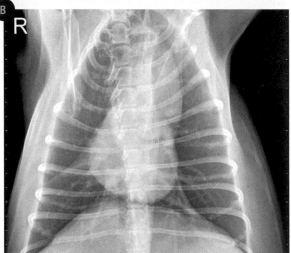

Figure 21-11: Thymomas in the dog and the cat have variable lymphocyte content and therefore a different response to chemotherapy and radiation therapy. Radiation is however quite effective and reducing the size of many thymomas as noted in this pre (A) and post (B) radiation treatment radiographs.

problems such as dysuria, colitis, and prostatitis must be expected. If radiation therapy is to be used for tumors of the caudal abdomen, small frequent fractions are more likely to avoid complications (see discussion of the effects on the colon and rectum above). Whenever possible, radiation therapy should be combined with other treatment modalities to enhance their beneficial effects.

Osteosarcoma

Palliative radiation therapy of osteosarcoma is a logical and often effective mode of improving quality of life for patients in which surgical removal or amputation is not an option.

Hypofractionation: Radiation delivered in weekly fractions of 8 to 10 Gy has been reported as a palliative treatment for dogs with pain from osteosarcoma or other clinical signs related to the tumor. Improved limb function was seen in approximately 75% of the dogs treated with either 10 Gy on days 0, 7, and 21 or 8 Gy on days 0 and 7. Improvement lasted for a median of 2 months regardless of the protocol, and toxicities were rare and acute.[50, 51]

Some radiation oncologists believe that a reasonable clinical approach may be to deliver a single large dose to the affected site and then to repeat a single dose as necessary to maintain pain control. Others administer two to five dosages 24 hours apart to the affected site until discomfort returns when the treatment may be repeated.

Radioisotope: Samarium-153-ethylenetetramethylenen phosphate (Sm-153-EDTMP) emits radioactive particles and accumulates in areas of increased bony activity, thereby providing high-dose localized radiation therapy. This compound was given to 28 dogs with osteosarcoma of the appendicular (*n* = 20) or axial (*n* = 8) skeleton.[1] Many dogs showed functional improvement; however, the average survival for the 20 dogs with appendicular osteosarcoma was 240 days. This treatment may palliate in a manner similar to external-beam radiation. Another study found that, with the exception of one dog that had a long-lasting complete response, pain relief was poor in a series of nine dogs with presumed osteosarcoma; survival was for a median of 4 months.[52] There are anecdotal reports of long-term survival after surgery and Sm-153-EDTMP.[2, 53]

Other techniques: Targeted stereotactic radiosurgery may offer some advantages in delivering a single high dose of 30 Gy to the tumor alone. Preliminary results are encouraging.[3]

OTHER RADIATION TECHNIQUES

Whole- or half body-body irradiation has been little used in the clinical setting in dogs and cats. In normal dogs, the highest tolerated whole-body irradiation dose was 2.6 Gy, but 50% of dogs were dead within 30 days.[54] More recently, clinical use of whole-body irradiation doses of 1.0 Gy to treat in dogs resulted in infrequent biochemical changes consistent with tumor lysis syndrome, transient partial responses, and unexpected long-term thrombocytopenia.[55] In cats, half body radiation when combined with chemotherapy has been shown to be helpful for the treatment of lymphoma of the abdominal cavity.

Another clinical technique using half-body irradiation has been reported; half the body receives 7 Gy of megavoltage radiation on day 1, and 28 days later the other half is irradiated. In one study, acute radiation sickness was seen in all eight normal dogs when they received caudal irradiation.[56] The second treatment, regardless of anatomy, was more likely to cause bone marrow toxicity and platelets were more affected. Pneumonitis was common, and there was permanent bone marrow atrophy (cellularity less than 20%) 1 year after radiation, implying that combining this technique with chemotherapy would be risky. Similar toxicities were seen when 14 dogs with failed lymphoma were treated; five dogs had a complete or partial response.[57] Again, acute radiation sickness was seen in 30% of dogs after cranial irradiation and in 80% of dogs after caudal irradiation. Deaths occurred in four dogs due to acute tumor lysis, thrombocytopenia, and gastrointestinal signs ascribed to parvovirus. Pneumonitis was seen in six dogs and was progressive until death in two. Clearly this technique has toxicities that are difficult to justify.

In contrast, when half-body radiation therapy was given to dogs with lymphoma in two consecutive daily 4-Gy fractions (instead of a single dose) toxicities were mainly mild and self-limiting. Dogs in remission from lymphoma after chemotherapy appeared to benefit from the addition of radiation as a consolidation phase.[58]

References

1. Lattimer JC, Corwin LA, Stapleton J, et al: Clinical and clinicopathologic response of canine bone tumor patients to treatment with samarium-153-EDTMP. *Nucl Med* 31:1316–1325, 1990.
2. Moe L, Boysen M, Aas M, et al: Maxillectomy and targeted radionuclide therapy with 153Sm-EDTMP in a recurrent canine osteosarcoma. *J Small Anim Pract* 37:241–246, 1996.
3. Farese JP, Milner R, Thompson M, et al: Stereotactic radiosurgery for the treatment of lower extremity canine appendicular osteosarcoma [abstract]. *Proc 23rd Annu Conf Vet Cancer Soc*: 69, 2003.
4. Lester NV, Hopkins AL, Bova FJ, et al: Radiosurgery using a stereotactic headframe system for irradiation of brain tumors in dogs. *JAVMA* 219:1562–1567, 2001.
5. Fidel J, Kippenes-Skogmo H, Gavin PR, et al: Radiosurgery for selected canine and feline brain tumors, a retrospective analysis [abstract]. *Proc 23rd Annu Conf Vet Cancer Soc*: 48, 2003.
6. McKnight JA, Mauldin GN, McEntee MC, et al: Radiation treatment for incompletely resected soft-tissue sarcomas in dogs. *JAVMA* 217:205–210, 2000.
7. McEntee MC, Thrall DE: Use of portal radiography to increase accuracy of dose delivery in radiation therapy. *Vet Radiol Ultrasound* 36:69–77, 1995.
8. Kippenes H, Gavin PR, Sande RD, et al: Comparison of the accuracy of positioning devices for radiation therapy of canine and feline head tumors. *Vet Radiol Ultrasound* 41:371–376, 2000.
9. Henry C, Stoll MR, Higginbotham ML, et al: Effect of timing of radiation initiation on post-surgical wound healing in dogs [abstract]. *Proc 23rd Annu Conf Vet Cancer Soc*: 52, 2003.
10. Lana SE, Hansen RA, Kloer L, et al: The effects of oral glutamine supplementation on plasma glutamine concentrations and PGE2 concentrations in dogs experiencing radiation-induced mucositis. *J Appl Res Vet Med* 1:259–265, 2003.
11. Anderson CR, McNiel EA, Gillette EL, et al: Late complications of pelvic irradiation in 16 dogs. *Vet Radiol Ultrasound* 43:187–192, 2002.
12. Vartak S, Robbins ME, Spector AA: Polyunsaturated fatty acids increase the sensitivity of 36B10 rat astrocytoma cells to radiation-induced cell kill. *Lipids* 32:283–292, 1997.
13. Hansen RA, Anderson C, Fettman MJ, Larue SM, Davenport DJ, Gross KL, Richardson KL, Ogilvie GK. Menhaden oil administration to dogs treated with radiation for nasal tumors demonstrates lower levels of tissue eicosanoids. Nutr Res. 2011 31(12):929-936, 2011.
14. Colas S, Paon L, Denis F, et al: Enhanced radiosensitivity of rat autochthonous mammary tumors by dietary docosahexaenoic acid. *Int J Cancer* 109:449–454, 2004.
15. Théon AP, Rodriguez C, Madewell BR: Analysis of prognostic factors and patterns of failure in dogs with malignant oral tumors treated with megavoltage irradiation. *JAVMA* 210:778–784, 1997.

16. Fidel J, Lyons J, Tripp C, Houston R, Wheeler B, Ruiz A. Treatment of oral squamous cell carcinoma with accelerated radiation therapy and concomitant carboplatin in cats. *J Vet Intern Med.* 25(3):504-510, 2011.

17. Blackwood L, Dobson JM: Radiotherapy of oral malignant melanomas in dogs. *JAVMA* 209:98–102, 1996.

18. MacMillan R, Withrow SJ, Gillette EL: Surgery and regional irradiation for treatment of canine tonsillar squamous cell carcinoma: retrospective review of eight cases. *J Am Anim Hosp Assoc* 18:311–314, 1982.

19. Brooks MB, Matus RE, Leifer CE, et al: Chemotherapy versus chemotherapy plus radiotherapy in the treatment of tonsillar squamous cell carcinoma in the dog. *J Vet Intern Med* 1988; 2:206–211, 1988.

20. Lascelles BDX, Parry AT, Stidworthy MF, et al: Squamous cell carcinoma of the nasal planum in 17 dogs. *Vet Rec* 147:473–476, 2000.

21. Theon AP, Barthez PY, Madewell BR, Griffey SM: Radiation therapy of ceruminous gland carcinomas in dogs and cats. *JAVMA* 205:566–569, 1994.

22. Cohen M, Brawner WR, Henderson R, et al: Use of a soft tissue equivalent material inside the canine nasal cavity to maximize megavoltage dose distribution to the floor [abstract]. *Proc 22nd Annu Conf Vet Cancer Soc:*18, 2002.

23. Northrup NC, Etue SM, Ruslander DM, et al: Retrospective study of orthovoltage radiation therapy for nasal tumors in 42 dogs. *J Vet Intern Med* 15:183–189, 2001.

24. Evans SM, Goldschmidt M, McKee LJ, Harvey CE: Prognostic factors and survival after radiotherapy for intranasal neoplasms in dogs: 70 cases (1974–1985). *JAVMA* 194:1460–1463, 1989.

25. Theon AP, Madewell BR, Harb MF, Dungworth DL: Megavoltage irradiation of neoplasms of the nasal and paranasal cavities in 77 dogs. *JAVMA* 202:1469–1475, 1993.

26. Henry CJ, Brewer WG Jr, Tyler JW, et al: Survival in dogs with nasal adenocarcinoma: 64 cases (1981–1995). *J Vet Intern Med* 12:436–439, 1998.

27. Adams WM, Miller PE, Vail DM, et al: An accelerated technique for irradiation for malignant canine nasal and paranasal sinus tumors. *Vet Radiol Ultrasound* 39:475–481, 1998.

28. Thrall DE, McEntee MC, Novotney C, et al: A boost technique for irradiation of malignant canine nasal tumors. *Vet Radiol Ultrasound* 34:295–300, 1993.

29. LaDue TA, Dodge R, Page RL et al: Factors influencing survival after radiotherapy of nasal tumors in 130 dogs. *Vet Radiol Ultrasound* 40:312–317, 1999.

30. Mellanby RJ, Stevenson RK, Herrtage M, et al: Long-term outcome of 56 dogs with nasal tumours treated with four doses of radiation at intervals of seven days. *Vet Rec* 151:253–257, 2002.

31. McChesney SL, Withrow SJ, Gillette EL, et al: Radiotherapy of soft tissue sarcomas in dogs. *JAVMA* 194:60-63, 1989.

32. McChesney SL, Gillette EL, Dewhirst MW, Withrow SJ: Influence of WR 2721 on radiation response of canine soft tissue sarcomas. *Int J Radiat Oncol Biol Phys* 12:1957–1963, 1986.

33. Evans SM: Canine hemangiopericytoma: A retrospective analysis of response to surgery and orthovoltage radiation. *Vet Radiol Ultrasound* 28:13–16, 1987.

34. Simon D, Ruslander DM, Rassnick KM, et al: Combination of orthovoltage radiation therapy and weekly low-dose doxorubicin for incompletely excised soft tissue sarcomas in 39 dogs. *Vet Record* 2005 (in press).

35. Frimberger AE, Moore AS, LaRue SM, et al: Radiotherapy of incompletely resected, moderately differentiated mast cell tumors in the dog: 37 cases (1989–1993). *J Am Anim Hosp Assoc* 33:320–324, 1997.

36. Al Sarraf R, Mauldin GN, Patnaik AK, Meleo KA: A prospective study of radiation therapy for the treatment of grade 2 mast cell tumors in 32 dogs. *J Vet Intern Med* 10:376–378, 1996.

37. Chaffin K, Thrall DE: Results of radiation therapy in 19 dogs with cutaneous mast cell tumor and regional lymph node metastasis. *Vet Radiol Ultrasound* 43:392–395, 2002.

38. Hahn KA, King GK, Carreras JK: Efficacy of radiation therapy for incompletely resected grade-III mast cell tumors in dogs: 31 cases (1987–1998). *JAVMA* 224:79–82, 2004.

39. Dobson J, Cohen S, Gould S: Treatment of canine mast cell tumours with prednisolone and radiotherapy. *Vet Comp Oncol* 2:132–141, 2004.

40. Thèon AP, LeCouteur RA, Carr EA, Griffey SM: Influence of tumor cell proliferation and sex-hormone receptors on effectiveness of radiation therapy for dogs with incompletely resected meningiomas. *JAVMA* 216:701–707, 2000.

41. LaRue SM, Gillette EL: Recent advances in radiation oncology. *Comp Contin Educ Pract Vet* 15:795–804, 1993.

42. Spugnini EP, Thrall DE, Price GS, et al: Primary irradiation of canine intracranial masses. *Vet Radiol Ultrasound* 41:377–380, 2000.

43. Brearley MJ, Jeffery ND, Phillips SM, Dennis R: Hypofractionated radiation therapy of brain masses in dogs: A retrospective analysis of survival of 83 cases (1991-1996). *J Vet Intern Med* 13:408–412, 1999.

44. Theon AP, Marks SL, Feldman ES, Griffey S: Prognostic factors and patterns of treatment failure in dogs with unresectable differentiated thyroid carcinomas treated with megavoltage irradiation. *JAVMA* 216:1775–1779, 2000.

45. Brearley MJ, Hayes AM, Murphy S: Hypofractionated radiation therapy for invasive thyroid carcinoma in dogs: a retrospective analysis of survival. *J Small Anim Pract* 40:206–210, 1999.

46. Smith AN, Wright JC, Brawner WR Jr, et al: Radiation therapy in the treatment of canine and feline thymomas: a retrospective study (1985-1999). *J Am Anim Hosp Assoc* 37:489–496, 2001.

47. McCaw DL, Lattimer JC: Radiation and cisplatin for treatment of canine urinary bladder carcinoma: a report of two case histories. *Vet Radiol Ultrasound* 29:264–268, 1998.

48. Turner AI, Hahn KA, King GK, Carreras JK: Mitoxantrone, piroxicam and external-beam radiation therapy in the treatment of canine bladder tumors, 15 cases (2001-2003) [abstract]. *Proc 23rd Annu Conf Vet Cancer Soc* :20, 2003.

49. Poirier VJ, Forrest LJ, Adams WM, Vail DM: Piroxicam, mitoxantrone, and coarse reaction radiotherapy for the treatment of transitional cell carcinoma of the bladder in 10 dogs: A plot sudy. *J Am Anim Hosp Assoc* 40:131–136, 2004.

50. McEntee MC, Page RL, Novotney CA, Thrall DE: Palliative radiotherapy for canine appendicular osteosarcoma. *Vet Radiol Ultrasound* 34:367–370, 1993.

51. Ramirez O III, Dodge RK, Page RL, et al: Palliative radiotherapy of appendicular osteosarcoma in 95 dogs. *Vet Radiol Ultrasound* 40:517–522, 1999.

52. Milner RJ, Dormehl I, Louw WK, Croft S: Targeted radiotherapy with Sm-153-EDTMP in nine cases of canine primary bone tumours. *J S Afr Vet Med Assoc* 69:12–17, 1998.

53. Cooper S, Black AP, Smith BA, et al: Low grade osteosarcoma in a dog. *Aust Vet Pract* 32:104–111, 2002.

54. von Zallinger C, Tempel K: The physiologic response of domestic animals to ionizing radiation: A review. *Vet Radiol Ultrasound* 39:495–503, 1998.

55. Frimberger AE, Ruslander DM, Moore AS, et al: Low-dose whole body irradiation for dogs with chemoresistant lymphoma relapse. *Proc 20th Annu Conf Vet Cancer Soc:* 28, 2000.

56. Laing EJ, Fitzpatrick PJ, Norris AM, et al: Half-body radiotherapy. Evaluation of the technique in normal dogs. *J Vet Intern Med* 3:96–101, 1989.

57. Laing EJ, Fitzpatrick PJ, Binnington AG, et al: Half-body radiotherapy in the treatment of canine lymphoma. *J Vet Intern Med* 3:102–108, 1989.

58. Williams LE, Johnson JL, Hauck ML, et al: Chemotherapy followed by half-body radiation therapy for canine lymphoma. *J Vet Intern Med* 18:703–709, 2004.

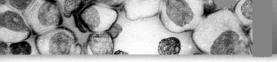

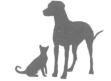

Chapter 22

Surgical oncology

Surgery is the oldest treatment for cancer and, as a single modality, cures more animals and people with cancer than any other therapy. The surgeon has a central role in the prevention, diagnosis, and definitive treatment of neoplastic diseases (figure 22-1). Just as important, the surgeon plays a key roll in palliative and rehabilitative care of cancer patients. Not all surgeons are surgical oncologists but surgeons of all levels of training are key to providing cures for animals with cancer worldwide. A surgical oncologist is unique in that this specialist has completed a post-residency sub-specialty training in surgical oncology that gives him/her unique insights in the understanding of tumor biology. These specialists are trained to know when surgery should be used alone and when to combine it with other modalities such as chemotherapy and radiation therapy to enhance and improve quality of life. This advanced knowledge and training reduces the recurrence rate and mortality rates in the cancer patient, regardless of the species.[1-9] For example, in one study the risk factors for having an incompletely excised soft tissue sarcoma or a mast cell tumor were examined. In that publication, 100 dogs with either soft tissue sarcomas or mast cell tumors were treated with wide excision. The smaller the dog and larger the tumor resulted in a poorer outcome. As one would expect, veterinary surgery residents were at increased risk of incompleteness of excision compared with board certified surgeons and board certified surgeons with additional training in surgical oncology. While it is ideal to have an oncologic surgeon available for each patient with cancer, this is not always possible. It is, however possible for general veterinary surgeons to acquire the skills and knowledge through post graduate education. The very best surgeons are those who do not operate needlessly and, when necessary, refer to others who have better skills or more experience.

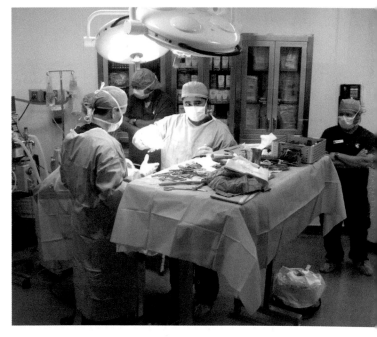

Figure 22-1: The surgeon is vital to diagnose, prevent, and treat cancer or cancer associated disorders and emergencies. The very best surgeons who excel in cancer surgery understand the biological behavior of cancer and the multimodality approach to treat, control, and cure cancer. Ultimately, cancer surgery is only successful if it is done for the patient and client's comfort first and foremost, followed by firm decisive steps to cure or control the cancer.

Key point

The very best surgeons are those who do not operate needlessly and, when necessary, refer to others who have better skills or more experience.

There are a variety of training programs available worldwide to enhance the knowledge of surgeons who remove malignancies. The better programs focus on:

- Recognizing and meeting the nonmedical needs of the client while meeting the medical and surgical needs of the patient.
- Educating the surgeon on the specifics of tumor biology, cellular and molecular cancer medicine, and the mechanisms of cancer growth, survival, and metastasis.
- Giving the surgeon extensive experience in the unique surgical skills associated with the treatment of cancer among surgeons of exceptional skills.
- Empowering the surgeon with the principles and specifics of chemotherapy and radiation therapy.
- Endorsing the team approach to provide comprehensive, compassionate care for the cancer patient.
- Educating the surgeon in the specifics of clinical research including appropriate basic and clinical trial designs and the specifics of appropriate statistical analysis.
- Enhancing awareness of the specific capabilities of diagnostic tests to determine the type and extent of the cancer.

Before a patient is ever treated, the client must be educated and the cancer patient must be fully assessed by physical examination, assessment of hematologic and biochemical findings, tumor type, grade, and the stage of the disease. The surgeon must obtain appropriate tissue samples in such a way to not inhibit the patient's quality of life as well as future efforts to cure or control the cancer. The adverse effects of the cancer and the treatment modality must be known and fully explained to the client in oral and written format. Cure of the cancer must be a top priority, as long as the patient's quality of life is improved in the process. The surgery, if used, must be carefully thought out and all alternative options must be explored with the client. The old adage, "measure twice and cut once" is an important guideline to enhance surgical cures and improve quality of life.

The surgeon must do everything possible to cure the cancer the first time. This not only reduces morbidity and mortality, but it also it decreases the overall cost of care to the client. Untreated tumors tend to have more normal surrounding tissues making the success of the first surgery more likely. When a tumor recurs, it is far more likely to have invaded the tissue planes disrupted by previous surgery, and therefore is likely to be unresectable. Recurrent tumors also have a much higher probability of metastasizing, therefore dramatically reducing the probability for long term tumor control. The most viable tumor is that which is most well vascularized. Leaving behind microscopic tissue that may have greater blood supply causes the cancer to accelerate its rate of growth and potential for metastasis.

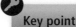

Key point

The surgeon must do everything possible to cure the cancer with the very first surgery.

TYPES OF CANCER SURGERY

Cancer prevention[1-5,9]

Cancer is the most preventable of all chronic diseases in dogs and cats and surgery is one of the most important therapies that increase the success of cancer prevention programs (figure 22-2). Prevention of cancer with ovariohysterectomy and orchiectomy in the dog and cat is well defined. These surgical procedures can be critical to preventing not only tumors (e.g., mammary, uterine, ovarian, and vaginal neoplasia in the female; testicular neoplasia in the male) but also nonneoplastic diseases (e.g., pregnancy, pyometra, prostatomegaly behavioral problems). One has to recognize that in rare circumstances that surgery may increase the risk of developing cancer, such as the placement of surgical implants and the subsequent development of osteosarcoma. Regardless, the roll of the surgeon in preventing cancer is legendary in veterinary medicine.

Staging and diagnosis of cancer[1-5,9]

The staging of a cancer patient includes the use of surgery to determine the location, type, grade, and extent of cancer in the body.[1-4] The methods that the surgeon can use to diagnose the malignant condition or extent of the disease are aspiration biopsy, needle core biopsy, punch, incisional biopsy, and excisional biopsy.[1-4] It is exceedingly important to know the histologic diagnosis of a malignancy before performing definitive procedures. For example, knowing whether a tumor is a benign sebaceous adenoma or a malignant soft tissue sarcoma is extremely important. This is because even though they may have the same outward appearance, the latter requires an extensive surgical resection and additional diagnostic procedures (i.e., abdominal and thoracic radiographs, lymph node aspiration/biopsy to determine the extent of disease. In contrast, a benign adenoma may only require a simple resection.

The first step in successfully managing a patient with cancer is to know which disease is being treated. To determine prognosis, treatment options, and palliative care, one must know the histopathologic diagnosis and, whenever biologically meaningful, the grade of the tumor. This is the key to the successful management of any dog and cat with cancer. A biopsy prior to the definitive procedure is critical in canine and feline oncology because "salvage" procedures are often less successful and usually much more expensive. Consequently, the definitive treatment must be selected correctly the *first time*. The following sections detail the appropriate procedures for obtaining good biopsy samples.

Key point

Before successful cancer therapy can begin, a preoperative biopsy is often ideal to determine the tumor type, biological behavior of the malignancy and the appropriate surgical procedure needed to benefit the patient. The three golden rules in oncology are *biopsy, biopsy,* and *biopsy!*

The biopsy is one of the most important procedures performed when evaluating a dog and cat with cancer. Biopsy results must be interpreted carefully in conjunction with results of other diagnostic procedures such as blood work, radiography, ultrasound, computed tomography (CT), magnetic resonance imaging (MRI), and other imaging modalities. A biopsy specimen is of value only if it is properly collected and prepared and then interpreted by a highly trained pathologist who is willing to use all available clinical information to arrive at an accurate diagnosis.

Each biopsy should be performed with the assumption that the lesion is malignant. Therefore, the procedure should be performed so that the entire surgical field, including all tissues or tissue planes that may have been disturbed and any post-biopsy hemorrhage, seroma, or hematoma, can be removed during subsequent surgery. Second surgeries performed to remove the tumor and surrounding tissues should involve at least one fascial layer below the tumor and all tissues disturbed by previous surgery.

Several types of biopsies exist, including needle core biopsies, punch biopsies, incisional (wedge) biopsies, and excisional biopsies. Examples of many of these are described below. A small core of tissue is obtained with a needle core biopsy, whereas a portion of the tumor is removed with an incisional biopsy. Incisional biopsies are generally taken at the junction of normal and abnormal tissue and are preferred in cases where a punch or needle biopsy cannot provide an adequate tissue sample for analysis. Regardless of the type, the biopsy procedure must be performed correctly to avoid compromising subsequent curative resection. An excisional biopsy, which removes the entire tumor, is preferred in cases in which knowledge of the tissue type will not influence the definitive procedure or treatment plan (e.g., a solitary lung mass or a splenic mass).

As mentioned, the biopsy should be performed prior to definitive therapy if the results will alter the type of therapy to be employed or influence a client's willingness to treat his or her pet. For example, if biopsy results indicate a benign perianal adenoma, the clinician can confidently proceed with a conservative resection and castration if indicated. If, however, the biopsy results reveal that the mass

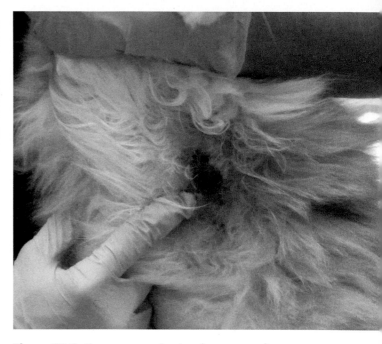

Figure 22-2: Cancer prevention is a key aspect of cancer surgery. Performing an ovariohysterectomy reduces the risk of tumors of the mammary gland dramatically if done before the first estrus. This procedure also reduces the subsequent risk of developing tumors and disorders of the ovaries and uterus.

is a high-grade perianal adenocarcinoma, which is a more aggressive tumor, then wide surgical resection around the periphery of the tumor (after careful evaluation for metastatic disease) is required and adjunctive therapy may be recommended. For financial and/or emotional reasons, some clients may be more willing to treat a dog and cat with a benign tumor than one with a more malignant/aggressive biologic behavior. The following section is a brief introduction to the cornerstone of veterinary oncology: The biopsy!

BIOPSY GUIDELINES

- *When taken appropriately, biopsies do not negatively influence the survival of the patient.* The myth that the biopsy procedure causes cancer cells to spread throughout the dog and cat's body, resulting in early demise of the patient, is not supported in the scientific literature.
- *A biopsy should be performed after consultation with the surgeon who will perform the definitive surgery.* This gives the surgeon the information needed to ensure that the lesion and the entire biopsy "tract" are removed without "spilling" or "seeding" tumor cells into the surgical field. In addition, the biopsy incision should be oriented to cause the least amount of tension on the skin, thereby simplifying any subsequent definitive surgical procedure(s). In

general, the direction of the incision should be made vertically, like the stripes on a tiger, to minimize skin tension and maximize the amount of tissue that can be removed around the tumor. There are, however, some exceptions, such as the presence of odd-shaped tumors in areas where the skin is tight.

- *To assist the pathologist in making a correct diagnosis, as large a sample as possible should be obtained.* With an incisional biopsy, the juncture of normal and abnormal tissue is an ideal site for sampling the tumor. Tumors involving bone, such as osteosarcoma, are exceptions to this rule. When this tumor type is suspected, biopsy specimens should be taken from the center of the tumor because the periphery of the lesion is primarily composed of reactive bone. Ulcerated, necrotic tissue should not be collected unless absolutely necessary because secondary pathologic lesions may obscure the primary diagnosis. In addition, if needle core biopsies are obtained, multiple samples (at least three to five) should be taken throughout the tumor. Regardless of the biopsy technique used, the entire biopsy field must be placed such that the biopsy tracts can be removed with the definitive procedure.
- *The original architecture of the tissue sample should be maintained; therefore, electrocautery, lasers, or surgical instruments that burn, vaporize, crush, or otherwise damage tissues should not be used.*
- *Tissue must be adequately fixed in 10% buffered neutral formalin (one part tissue to 10 parts fixative).* Fresh tissue should be placed in fixative for 24 to 48 hours. Although most pathologists prefer 10% buffered formalin, other fixatives, such as Zenker's or Bouin's, can be used for special purposes (e.g., optic tissue). For best results and to ensure proper exposure to the fixative, tissue samples should not be thicker than 1 cm. If an excisional biopsy is performed and the entire sample is larger than 1 cm, it can be cut like a loaf of bread to allow proper exposure of the tissue to the fixative. The exception to this rule is brain tissue, which can be fixed intact without the bread-loafing technique. Very thin samples should be avoided because the fixation process can distort the tissue architecture. The tissue should not be exposed to heat, cold, or water at any time.
- *Each biopsy specimen should be placed into a separate, properly labeled container.* The container should be labeled on its side rather than on the lid to prevent mix-ups in case the tops are switched. If multiple samples are collected, all containers should be labeled before the procedure to reduce the chance of confusing samples.
- *When possible, all resected tissue should be properly prepared and submitted for appropriate analysis.* This enables the pathologist to examine the tissue for completeness of removal ("clean" or "dirty" margins) and architectural detail. Particularly when

an excisional biopsy is performed, trimming the biopsy specimen or submitting only a small section means that this valuable information may be lost. However, if mailing costs must be reduced, smaller, adequately fixed representative tissue samples can be sent in the minimum amount of formalin to keep them moist. Tissues that are adequately fixed in formalin can be placed in sealable plastic bags with a formalin-saturated paper towel or sponge. If only a portion of the sample is submitted, the original tissue should be kept by the attending clinician in the event that additional samples are needed. Over-fixation may adversely affect future immunohistochemical examination of the tissue. All margins should be marked with ink or suture and submitted to determine the adequacy of surgical excision (figure 22-3). Again, if decreasing the size of sample submission is necessary, margins may be submitted separately.

- *Before the tissue sample is placed in fixative, consideration should be given to submitting portions for culture and sensitivity testing or alternative analysis (e.g., polymerase chain reaction).* For best results, it is essential to plan which types of samples are to be submitted and analyzed before preparing the biopsy sample. Once the tissue is in the formalin, other tests or analyses may not be possible.
- *Biopsy specimens should be submitted to a highly qualified veterinary pathologist who is willing to work with the clinician.* In addition:
  - The pathologist should be given a detailed history and a complete account of all relevant clinical material.
  - When an excisional biopsy is performed, margins should be identified with ink or suture. The pathologist will then have all the information necessary to make an accurate diagnosis.
  - It is important for the clinician and pathologist to work together to help coordinate the clinical picture with the diagnosis. If the two do not match, then the clinician and pathologist should work together to reevaluate all case information, including histopathology. This cooperative interaction is essential for accurate diagnosis and optimum treatment of the dog or cat's disease.
  - Board-certified, anatomic pathologists are best qualified to analyze histopathologic specimens, whereas board-certified clinical pathologists are most appropriate to evaluate cytology, hematology, and biochemical problems.

CONTRAINDICATIONS

The risks and benefits of the biopsy procedure should be evaluated and clearly described to the client. In most cases, risks are minimal. Uncontrollable hemorrhage is the most common (but still rare) complication with all biopsy procedures, except possibly bone marrow aspiration. Therefore, hemostatic abnormalities caused by deficiencies

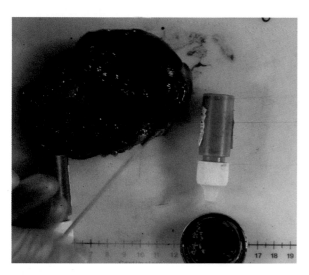

Figure 22-3: The completeness of surgical excision is best determined by the pathologist who can be oriented by the placement of different colored inks on the lateral and deep margins. A detailed history, description of orientation, and the meaning of the different colors is very important to assist the pathologist in creating an informative pathology report.

in platelet numbers and function, or coagulation disorders should be identified and, if possible, corrected before biopsy. Aseptic technique is critical to avoid the uncommon but serious complications of infection at the biopsy site and/or sepsis in the dog and cat. Lastly, a biopsy should not be performed if it could potentially inhibit or jeopardize a definitive procedure. For example, an incisional biopsy of a primary lung tumor or mass on the spleen may contaminate the entire chest or abdominal cavity with tumor cells, which is why primary lung tumors or splenic masses are usually removed during the primary definitive surgical procedure (i.e., an excisional biopsy). Note that diffusely enlarged spleens are most often caused by lymphoma or mast cell tumor and are often diagnosed by transabdominal fine-needle aspiration cytology.

SEDATION AND ANESTHESIA FOR A BIOPSY

Cancer patients are often older and frequently have concurrent medical disorders that must be known before sedation or anesthesia is planned. In addition, since almost every procedure confers some degree of discomfort, an analgesic plan is essential.

- The risks and benefits of the sedation and/or anesthesia and the procedure itself should be carefully outlined with the dog and cat's client prior to obtaining written authorization.
- Each dog and cat should be assessed prior to the procedure by obtaining a history from the client, conducting a physical examination, and

determining pain status. Also, a complete blood count (including platelet count), urinalysis, and biochemical profile, including a blood glucose, alanine transaminase (ALT), alkaline phosphatase (ALP), and blood urea nitrogen (BUN), should be conducted.

- Placing an intravenous catheter is always encouraged. The following guidelines are recommended:
  - The catheter must be placed using aseptic technique, including washing hands and clipping and prepping catheter sites.
  - If the dog or cat is suspected to be or is at risk of being volume contracted and anesthesia will be used, intravenous fluids should be administered via intravenous pumps or drip sets. Mini-drip sets should be used on patients weighing less than 5 kg.
  - Pre-emptive use of analgesics should be considered at this time.
  - If anesthesia is used, continuous monitoring should include evaluation of the following parameters: respiration, heart rate, arterial blood pressure, pulse pressure, palpebral reflex, eye position, jaw tone, and mucous membrane color. In addition, behavioral changes and signs of anxiety and/or pain should be monitored pre- and postoperatively.
  - If sedation is used, respiration, heart rate, mucous membrane color, and respiratory rate must be evaluated every 5 minutes until the patient is alert and responsive.

BIOPSY AS A PRELUDE TO DEFINITIVE THERAPY

A palpable, persistent mass is the most common indication for biopsy as a prelude to definitive therapy. As accuracy and sensitivity of diagnostic tests (e.g., ultrasonography, CT, MRI, positron emission tomography [PET], single-photon emission axial tomography [SPECT]) improve, biopsies are being performed with increasing frequency to clarify the diagnosis of visualized, yet nonpalpable, masses.

When developing a diagnostic strategy for a dog and cat with cancer, the clinician must consider subsequent disease management.[3] Dogs and cats are often diagnosed with advanced malignant disease, and the formulation of an appropriate diagnostic and therapeutic strategy early in the course of the disease is essential. The first step toward diagnosing most palpable lesions is fine-needle aspiration cytology. If the cytologic diagnosis strongly suggests a malignant condition or is highly suggestive of a particular condition (e.g., soft tissue sarcoma), a definitive procedure such as surgical removal can be planned. In addition, this tentative diagnosis can help guide the staging procedure ahead. Fine-needle aspiration cytology can also confirm the presence of a benign process, eliminating the need for further diagnostic steps.

If fine-needle aspiration cytology is not definitive, then an incisional biopsy should be performed or guided by the surgeon who will perform the definitive surgery. Before collecting a biopsy sample, standard diagnostic tests can be performed to identify any concurrent disease or clinically evident metastatic disease.

Staging is accomplished through certain diagnostic tests that determine the extent of the neoplastic disorder. The staging schema differs for each neoplastic disease but should include a history, physical examination, complete blood count, biochemical profile, urinalysis, thoracic radiographs, and cytologic evaluation of regional lymph nodes. Discussions regarding additional diagnostic steps in specific staging schemas are included in the review of each individual disease.

Summary guidelines for obtaining a successful biopsy sample

- Biopsy should be performed only after consultation with a skilled and knowledgeable surgeon who will perform the definitive surgery to formulate a correct plan for the biopsy such that follow-up surgical procedures will not be made more difficult or potentially less successful.
- The risks and benefits of the biopsy procedure should be carefully outlined with the client both verbally and in writing.
- Pre- and post-biopsy analgesia should always be defined prior to the procedure.
- Obtain as large a sample as possible while allowing the definitive therapy to be simple as possible.
- *Do not* use electrocautery, lasers, or any surgical instruments that can potentially crush or otherwise damage tissues.
- Never use lasers to "evaporate" tumors or tumor margins.
- Ensure that the tissue is adequately fixed in a 10% buffered, neutral formalin solution.
- Place each biopsy sample in a separate container and properly label the container (not the lid) of each sample.
- Submit the entire lesion, whenever possible, after it has been resected and properly prepared for fixation.
- Consider submitting portions of the lesion for culture and sensitivity or other analyses prior to placing it in formalin.
- Submit the biopsy to a highly qualified veterinary pathologist. Remember that an anatomic pathologist can best evaluate biopsies and a clinical pathologist can best analyze cytology.

A skin biopsy is essential to diagnose and evaluate potentially malignant skin conditions. *Punch, incisional, excisional,* and *needle core biopsies* are employed.

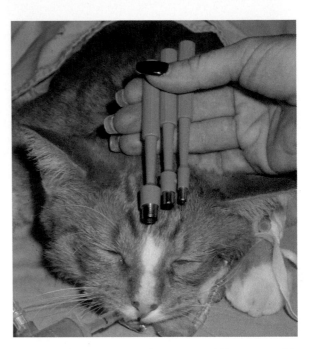

Figure 22-4: Biopsy punches are available as reusable instruments or comparatively inexpensive disposable units that may be reused after appropriate sterilization, until they become dull. Punches are available in diameters ranging from 2 to 6 mm.

PUNCH BIOPSY

Biopsy punches are available as expensive reusable instruments or inexpensive disposable units that may be reused after appropriate sterilization, until they become dull. Punches are available in diameters ranging from 2 to 6 mm (figure 22-4). Generally, taking a larger biopsy specimen is preferred so that the pathologist has an adequate sample from which to make a histologic diagnosis. When possible, multiple samples at the juncture between normal and abnormal tissue should be collected. Punch biopsies are usually inadequate to obtain tissue below the dermis because subcutaneous tissue is rarely obtained in the average punch biopsy of the skin.

Indication

Identification of any dermal or epidermal lesion of unknown etiology.

Contraindications/complications

Coagulopathies; lidocaine toxicities (unlikely).

Benefits

General anesthesia is not required however analgesia is essential; simple outpatient procedure.

Limitation

Small tissue samples obtained may not be diagnostic.

Equipment

Sedation and analgesia should be considered; 2% lidocaine and 8.4% bicarbonate with or without NSAIDs, Tramadol or an opiate; Baker's biopsy instrument; standard surgical instruments; suture material.

Technique (figure 22-5 A-H)

- **Step 1.** Clip the hair and prepare the site with proper aseptic surgical technique.
- **Step 2.** Dilute 2% lidocaine with 8.4% bicarbonate (1 part bicarbonate to 9 parts lidocaine) to reduce stinging on injection. Using a 25-gauge needle, approximately 0.25 to 2 ml of this local anesthetic agent is injected around the lesion to a maximum total dosage of 0.5 mg/kg in the cat and 1 mg/kg in the dog. It is important that injection of lidocaine does not distort or disturb the normal architecture of the tissue to be biopsied.
- **Step 3.** Surgically scrub the biopsy area a final time after the lidocaine is injected.
- **Step 4.** Stretch the skin of the site to be biopsied between the thumb and index finger.
- **Step 5.** Place the biopsy punch instrument at a right angle to the skin surface.
- **Step 6.** Rotate the punch instrument in one direction and, at the same time, apply firm downward pressure until the subcutis is reached.

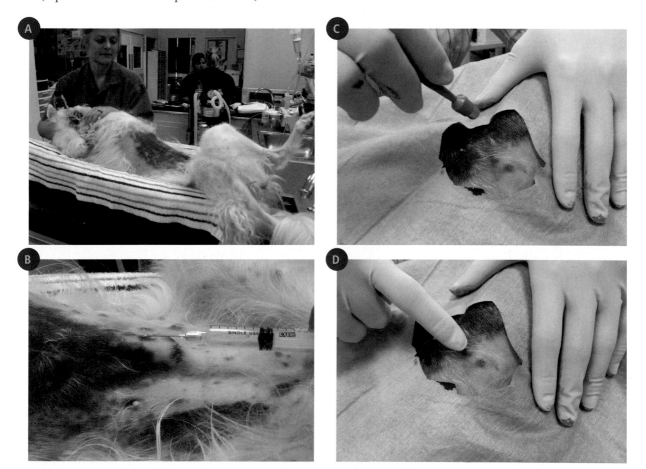

Figure 22-5: The punch biopsy. (A) The patient is placed in a position to allow adequate visualization of the tissue to be biopsied. The region near the area to be biopsied is clipped and prepared with a surgical scrub before and after administering the local anesthetic agent. (B) The local anesthesia is performed by injecting a lidocaine:bicarbonate mixture (1 part bicarbonate to 9 parts lidocaine) to reduce the acidity and thus the discomfort upon injecting the lidocaine (25-gauge needle, 0.25 to 2 ml to a maximum total dosage of 0.5 mg/kg in the cat and 1 mg/kg in the dog). Systemic analgesics are always encouraged. (C) Once the patient is prepared, the skin over the area to be biopsied is stretched between the thumb and index finger and the biopsy punch instrument is placed at a right angle to the skin surface over the area to be sampled. (D) The punch is then rotated in one direction while applying firm downward pressure until the subcutis or the preferred deeper structures are reached. Once the tissue has filled the barrel of the punch, the instrument is placed at a 90 degree angle, almost parallel with the skin while still applying pressure along the long axis of the instrument until the punch to severs at least part of the base of the biopsied tissue.

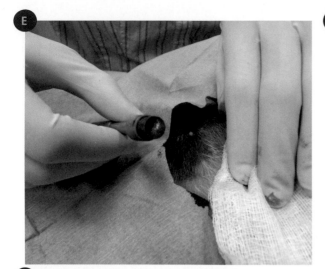

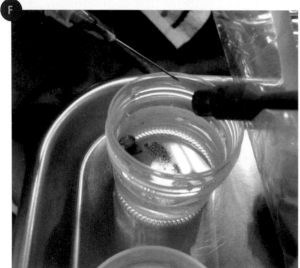

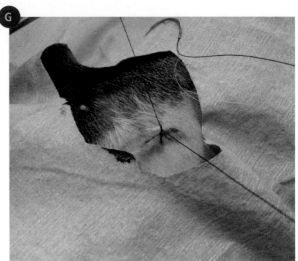

Figure 22-5 (*cont.*): (E) The punch is removed and the biopsied tissue is removed from the barrel with a needle; any remaining strands of tissue that remain at the base are severed with a scalpel blade or a pair of iris scissors. (F) Samples from the tissue are used to make impression smears and to culture, if needed, and then placed into formalin and submitted for histopathology. (G) One or two sutures are used to close the defect, depending on the size of the punch taken. Oral analgesics; periodic cleansing of the surgery site and the use of an Elizabethan collar to prevent self-trauma can be considered.

obtained for histologic diagnosis. In addition, if the lesion is biopsied at the junction of the normal and abnormal tissue, a "wedge" of tissue is obtained that retains a larger section of the tissue's architecture. This makes it easier for the histopathologist to see the characteristics of malignancy, such as invasion into the normal tissue.

- **Step 7.** Angle the punch almost parallel with the skin while still applying pressure along the long axis of the instrument.
- **Step 8.** Rotate the punch to sever at least part, if not all, of the base of the biopsied tissue.
- **Step 9.** Remove the punch instrument and gently elevate the core of tissue with the point of a needle; sever the base that is still attached with a scalpel blade or a pair of iris scissors.
- **Step 10.** Place one or two sutures as needed to close the defect, depending on the size of the punch taken.

Supportive care

Oral analgesics; periodic cleansing of the surgery site; consider the use of an Elizabethan collar to prevent self-trauma.

INCISIONAL BIOPSY

In some cases, an incisional biopsy is preferred to a punch biopsy because larger sections of tissue can be

Indication

Identification of dermal, epidermal, or subcutaneous lesions of unknown etiology.

Contraindications

Coagulopathies; dogs and cats that are at high risk during general anesthesia.

Benefit

Larger tissue sample often results in a more accurate diagnosis.

Limitations

General anesthesia is often needed; not a definitive procedure.

Equipment

General anesthesia; standard surgical instruments; suture material.

Technique (figure 22-6 A-H)

- **Step 1.** Perform routine screening tests to identify problems such as coagulopathies and metabolic disease.
- **Step 2.** Place the dog or cat under general anesthesia.
- **Step 3.** Surgically prepare the area with clipping and strict aseptic technique, then properly drape the site. Make an elliptical or wedge incision at the margin of normal and abnormal tissue. Take care to obtain adequate tissue and to ensure that a subsequent definitive surgery can remove the tumor and the incisional biopsy area successfully.
- **Step 4.** Carefully identify and ligate vessels going to and from the tissue to be biopsied.
- **Step 5.** Lift the specimen and sever the connection at the base with either scissors or a scalpel blade.
- **Step 6.** Suture the incision closed.

Supportive care

Oral or parenteral analgesics for several days to weeks; periodic cleansing of the surgery site.

EXCISIONAL BIOPSY

An excisional biopsy should be performed for the local treatment and histologic diagnosis of a small lesion located in an anatomic location where wide surgical removal is possible but will not compromise

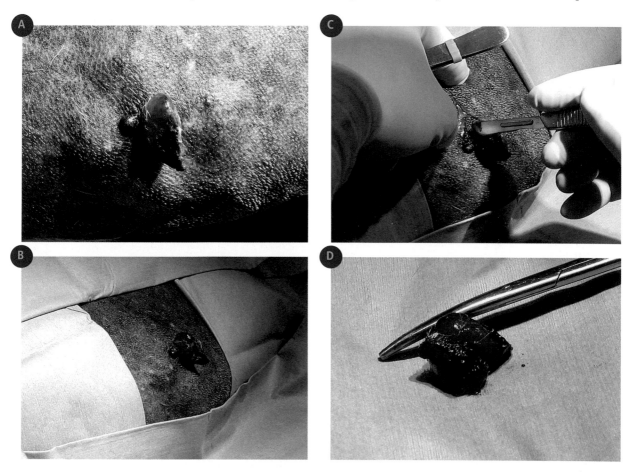

Figure 22-6: The incisional biopsy. (A) After a physical examination and appropriate blood work, the patient is given systemic analgesics, anesthetized and placed in a position to allow adequate visualization of the tissue to be biopsied. The region near the area to be biopsied is clipped and prepared with a surgical scrub before and after administering the local anesthetic agent. (B) The local anesthesia is performed by injecting a lidocaine:bicarbonate mixture (1 part bicarbonate to 9 parts lidocaine) to reduce the acidity and thus the discomfort upon injecting the lidocaine (25-gauge needle, 0.25 to 2 ml to a maximum total dosage of 0.5 mg/kg in the cat and 1 mg/kg in the dog). The area to be biopsied is draped for the surgical procedure. (C) The incision to be made is made in a direction that will create the least amount of tension of the skin. Essentially, incisions should be placed like "stripes on a tiger." Great effort should be made to ensure that the incisional biopsy can be removed with a subsequent definitive wide and deep excision (see below). Once the lesion is biopsied, every effort should be made to ensure there is no bleeding prior to closure. (D)The excised tissue is then used to make impression smears if desired and then tagged with suture or surgical ink prior to placement into formalin. The tagging and subsequent marking will allow the pathologist to identify, examine and report on the biopsy with understanding of its original orientation.

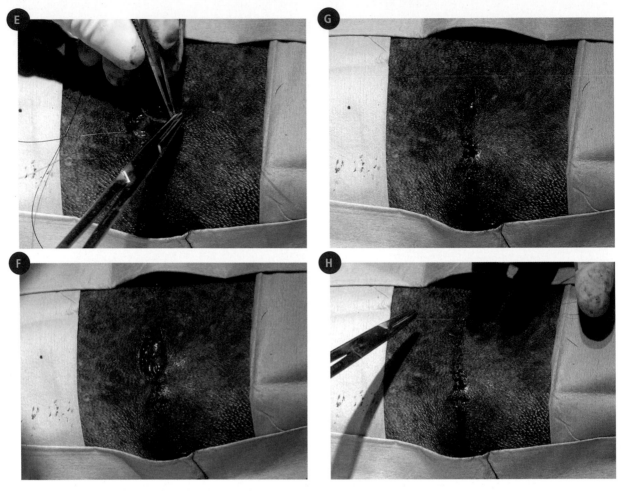

Figure 22-6 (*cont*.): (E-H) Subcutaneous and then subcuticular or dermal sutures are used to close the defect, depending on the size of the biopsy. Oral analgesics, periodic cleansing of the surgery site and the use of an Elizabethan collar to prevent self-trauma are considered.

the normal tissue around it (e.g., a cutaneous, basal cell tumor on the lateral abdominal wall less than 0.5 cm in diameter). The technique is similar to an incisional biopsy except that the tumor, previous incisions and a cuff of normal tissue is removed around the tumor (figure 22-7 A-G). In nearly all dogs and cats, an excisional biopsy is preceded by fine-needle aspiration cytology and/or incisional biopsy to give the surgeon as much information as possible about the characteristics of the tumor prior to removal. For example, a vaccine-associated sarcoma requires wide surgical margins (2 to 3 cm), whereas a benign basal cell tumor can be excised with smaller margins.

Key point

An excisional biopsy should be performed on a lesion that is small enough to be completely excised with adequate wide and deep surgical margins.

Indication

Identification of dermal, epidermal, or subcutaneous lesion of unknown etiology.

Contraindications

Coagulopathies; dogs and cats that are at high risk during general anesthesia.

Benefit

Larger tissue sample often results in a more accurate diagnosis.

Limitation

Requires general anesthesia; may make a definitive second procedure more difficult to achieve.

Equipment

Sedation and general anesthesia; standard surgical instruments; suture material.

Technique

Performed in the same manner as an incisional biopsy except the lesion is excised completely with adequate margins.

Supportive care

Oral or parenteral analgesics for days to weeks; periodic cleansing of the surgery site.

NEEDLE CORE BIOPSY

Needle core biopsy generally is safe and quick and can be performed on an awake, cooperative dog or cat on an outpatient basis when appropriate analgesia and sedation are used. Unless medically contraindicated, analgesics are used before and after the biopsy. Generally, histopathology results are more accurate than those of fine-needle aspiration cytology but are not as accurate as the results of an excisional or incisional biopsy due to the size of tissue sample obtained. Needle core biopsy instruments, especially the spring-loaded models that can be adjusted to obtain tissue from different depths, are preferred (figure 22-8).

Key point

Needle core or spring-loaded needle core biopsy is generally safe and quick and can be performed on an awake, cooperative dog or cat as an outpatient using appropriate analgesia and, when indicated, sedation.

Indication

Identification of a skin or subcutaneous lesion of unexplained etiology.

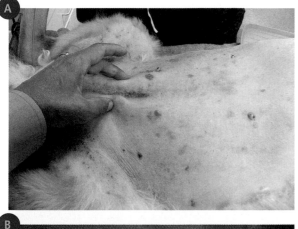

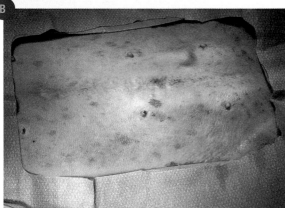

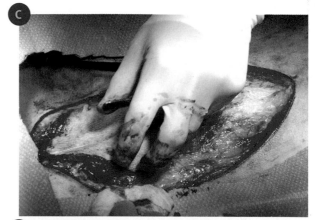

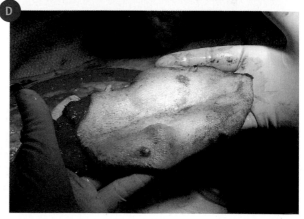

Figure 22-7: The excisional biopsy. (A) The patient with bilateral mammary masses is placed in a dorsal recumbancy after a complete physical examination and appropriate blood work. The goal is to position the patient to allow adequate visualization of the tissue to be completely removed with wide (2-3 cm) and deep (at least one fascial layer) margins. Dogs with mammary tumors should have the associated mammary gland(s) removed during the excision. Cats with mammary tumors should have the entire chain removed with wide margins. (B) The region near the area to be biopsied is clipped and prepared with a surgical scrub before and after administering the local anesthetic agent. The surgical area is draped. (C) The elliptical incision to be made is made around the mammary glands and the tumors within them with 2-3 cm margins laterally. Great effort is made to remove all affected tissue so that the incision will have minimal tension. (D) The incision is made to include at least the deep fascial layer. Hemostasis is managed throughout the entire procedure.

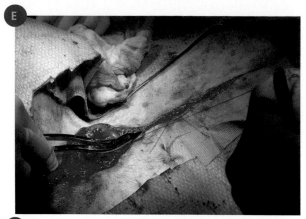

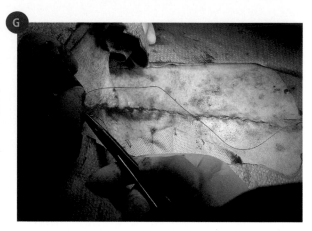

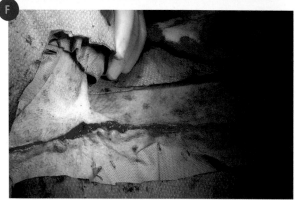

Figure 22-7 (cont.): (E) The deeper fascial layer is removed in one piece with the affected mammary glands and the tumors within them. The orientation of the incision should be retained so that the pathologist can determine if the tumor(s) were removed with wide and deep margins. The margins should be identified with surgical ink or sutures prior to placement into the formalin. (F-G) Subcutaneous and then subcuticular or dermal sutures are used to close the incision, depending on the size of the biopsy. Absorbable monofilament suture should be considered for the subcutaneous and subcuticular sutures. Monofilament nylon should be considered if skin sutures are placed. Oral analgesics, periodic cleansing of the surgery site and the use of an Elizabethan collar to prevent self-trauma should be considered.

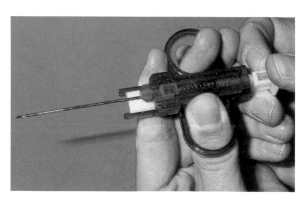

Figure 22-8: Spring-loaded needle core biopsy instruments are preferred as they allow rapid, automatic tissue sampling with minimal effort. They are available in different ganges, needle lengths and sample size options.

Contraindications/complications

Coagulopathies; lidocaine toxicity (unlikely).

Benefit

General anesthesia is not required, so the procedure can be performed on an outpatient basis.

Limitation

The small tissue samples obtained may not be diagnostic.

Equipment

Sedation and analgesia should be considered; No. 11 surgical blade; 2% lidocaine and bicarbonate; needle biopsy instrument.

Technique (figure 22-9 A-D)

- **Step 1.** Immobilize the cutaneous or subcutaneous lesion (usually by an assistant) and prepare the biopsy site with surgical scrub for an aseptic procedure.
- **Step 2.** Dilute 2% lidocaine with 8.4% bicarbonate (1 part bicarbonate to 9 parts lidocaine) to reduce stinging on injection. Using a 25-gauge needle, approximately 0.25 to 2 ml of this local anesthetic agent is injected around the lesion to a maximum total dosage of 0.5 mg/kg in the cat and 1 mg/kg in the dog. It is important that injection of lidocaine does not distort or disturb the normal architecture of the tissue to be biopsied.
- **Step 3.** Using a No. 11 surgical blade, make a stab incision in the skin to allow easy entry of the needle core biopsy instrument.
- **Step 4.** Advance the needle core biopsy instrument through the incision to the outer portion of the lesion to be biopsied. In the case of the skin, the instrument is advanced just into the tissue to be biopsied.
- **Step 5.** Obtain three to five biopsy specimens from the suspect tissue through the same stab incision. This will allow the histopathologist to evaluate a sample of tissue from various portions of the mass, enhancing the probability of making an accurate

diagnosis. These individual biopsies are best obtained by redirecting the needle within the mass.

- **Step 6.** Fix the needle biopsy specimens in 10% buffered formalin, as described previously. A separate container should be used for each lesion that is biopsied and labeled accordingly.
- **Step 7.** Suture the stab incision only if indicated by the size and depth.

Supportive care

Oral analgesics for several days; periodic cleansing of the surgery site.

CUP OR "PINCH" BIOPSY

Cup biopsies are generally safe and quick and can be performed on a dog or cat on an outpatient basis when appropriate analgesia and sedation are used. Unless medically contraindicated, analgesics are used before and after the biopsy. Generally, histopathology results are more accurate than those of fine-needle aspiration cytology but are not as accurate as the results of an excisional or incisional biopsy due to the size of tissue sample obtained. Cup biopsy instruments are easy to operate and can be reused for months to years.

Indication

Identification of any superficial organ, skin or subcutaneous lesion of unexplained etiology.

Contraindications/complications

Coagulopathies; lidocaine toxicity (unlikely).

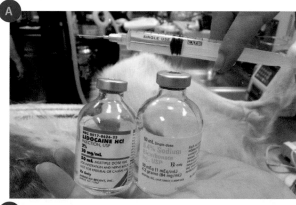
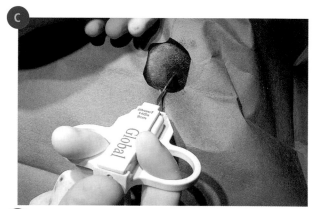
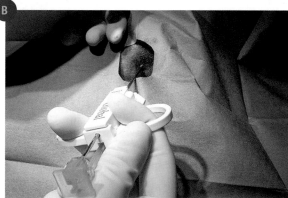
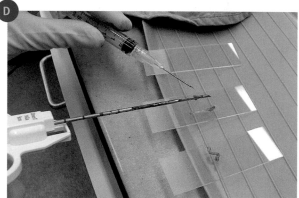

Figure 22-9: Needle core biopsy. (A) The patient is placed in a position to allow adequate visualization of the tissue to be biopsied. The region near the area to be biopsied is clipped and prepared with a surgical scrub before and after administering the local anesthetic agent. The local anesthesia is performed by injecting a lidocaine:bicarbonate mixture (1 part bicarbonate to 9 parts lidocaine) to reduce the acidity and thus the discomfort upon injecting the lidocaine (25-gauge needle, 0.25 to 2 ml to a maximum total dosage of 0.5 mg/kg in the cat and 1 mg/kg in the dog). Systemic analgesics are always encouraged. (B) Using a No. 11 surgical blade, a stab incision is made in the skin nearby or over the tumor to allow easy entry of the needle core biopsy instrument. The needle core biopsy instrument is advanced through the incision to the outer portion of the lesion to be biopsied. In the case of the skin, the instrument is advanced just into the tissue to be biopsied. (C) The inner biopsy stylet that contains a biopsy trough or slot for the tissue to be secured is advanced into the tumor. In the case of the spring loaded biopsy needle, the outer cutting cannula is automatically "fired" thereafter to rapidly cut the tissue sample within the sample trough or slot free of the main tumor. Three to five biopsy specimens from the suspect tissue are obtained through the same stab incision. This will allow the histopathologist to evaluate a sample of tissue from various portions of the mass, enhancing the probability of making an accurate diagnosis. These individual biopsies are best obtained by redirecting the needle within the mass. (D) The needle biopsy specimens are placed on a slide to make impression smears and then in 10% buffered formalin, as described previously. A separate container should be used for each lesion that is biopsied and labeled accordingly.

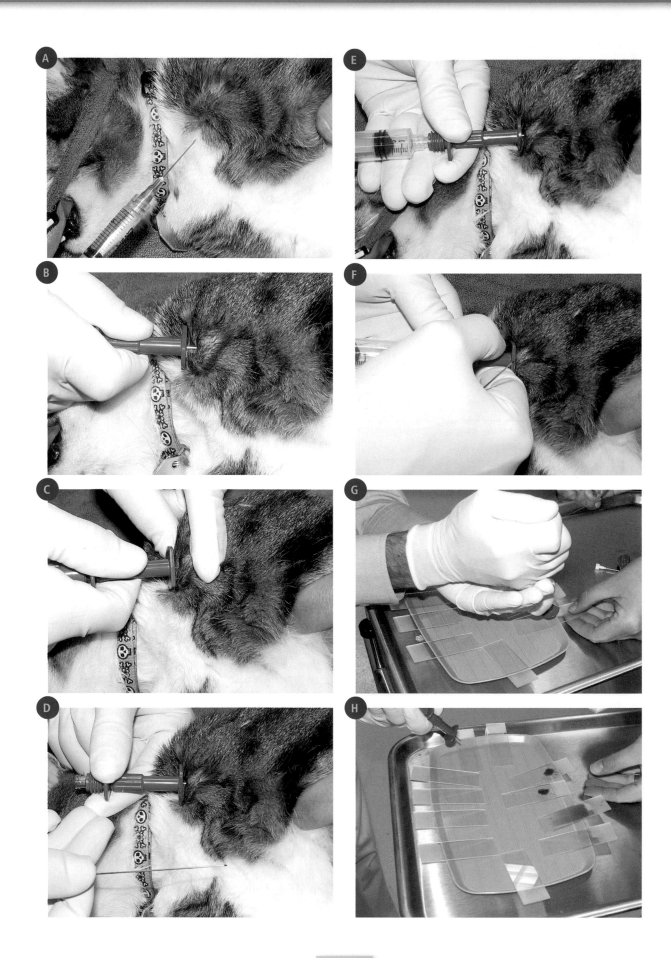

Figure 22-11: Bone marrow aspirate. (A) After a physical examination and appropriate blood work, the patient is given systemic analgesics, anesthetized and placed in a position to allow adequate visualization of the anatomic site that will serve as the site of marrow aspiration. The preferred site in dogs and cats is the proximal anterior non-articular surface of the greater tubercle of the humeral head. If this site is used, the leg is bent so that the humerus is parallel with the spine. The region over the area to be aspirated is clipped and prepared with a surgical scrub before and after administering the local anesthetic agent. The local anesthesia is performed by injecting lidocaine:bicarbonate mixture (1 part bicarbonate to 9 parts lidocaine) to reduce the acidity and thus the discomfort upon injecting the lidocaine (25-gauge needle, 0.25 to 2 ml to a maximum total dosage of 0.5 mg/kg in the cat and 1 mg/kg in the dog). The area to be biopsied is draped for the surgical procedure. A surgical drape may be applied for sterility. (B) The bone marrow site is identified, the skin is stretched between the thumb and index finger, and a small stab incision is made with a No. 11 surgical blade in the area blocked with lidocaine. The bone marrow needle, with the stylet in place, is advanced into the stab incision and through the skin, subcutaneous tissue, and muscle all the way to the bone. Note that the needle is directed down the long axis of the humerus. An 18-gauge (cat or small dog) or 16-gauge (medium to large-sized dog) bone marrow needle is preferred for most dogs and cats. Most find that the disposable needles that have the trochar locked into place are ideal. (C) With the stylet in place, the bone marrow needle is advanced into the bone, using a corkscrew motion. The instrument should not be allowed to wobble and should be fixed firmly into the bone like a nail that has been securely hammered into wood. (D) When the needle is firmly fixed in the bone, the stylet is removed. A 12 cc syringe filled with 3 cc's of air is affixed to the bone marrow needle. Some clinical pathologists suggest rinsing the syringe and bone marrow needle with EDTA before the procedure to reduce clotting of the bone marrow sample. Heparin should never be used. (E) The bone marrow sample is aspirated briskly into the 12-ml syringe; usually 0.25-0.5 ml of marrow is adequate. The aspiration may be accompanied by a few seconds of pain, but this can be prevented by the use of oral or parenteral analgesics such as fentanyl, butorphanol, morphine, NSAID, or other analgesics. If a sample is not obtained, the stylet is replaced in the bone marrow needle, and the instrument is then advanced farther into the bone for a second attempt at aspirating marrow. (F) The syringe and bone marrow needle as a single unit are rapidly removed in preparation for making slides. (G-H) Once marrow has been obtained, smears are prepared. This can be done in a number of ways:
- The marrow and blood are expelled into a small petri dish that contains a few drops of EDTA. The marrow-rich spicules are placed on a slide or coverslip and then spread between slides or coverslips to make a monolayer of cells. The slides must have been cleaned and readied for the sample to be processed, as it will clot quickly.
- A portion of the marrow sample is placed on the proximal portion of the slide; the slide is tipped downward to allow the blood to run down and off the slide. The spicules and heavier nucleated cells do not run off and are used for subsequent slide preparation.
- Marrow can be spread into a monolayer like a routine blood smear as depicted here.
- The first two methods may enhance the ability to evaluate the nucleated cell population of the bone marrow specimen.

- Dorsocranial or lateral aspects of the iliac crest (with the pet in sternal or lateral recumbency).
- Greater trochanter of the femur (pet in lateral recumbency).
- **Step 2.** Dilute 2% lidocaine with 8.4% bicarbonate (1 part bicarbonate to 9 parts lidocaine) to reduce stinging on injection. Using a 25-gauge needle, approximately 0.25 to 2 ml of this local anesthetic agent is injected around the lesion to a maximum total dosage of 0.5 mg/kg in the cat and 1 mg/kg in the dog. Care is taken to inject lidocaine in and around all of the tissue that extends from the skin to the periosteum. The lidocaine will sting less upon injection if it is diluted with bicarbonate.
- **Step 3.** The biopsy area is scrubbed one more time after the lidocaine injection. A surgical drape may be applied for sterility.
- **Step 4.** The bone marrow site is identified, the skin is stretched between the thumb and index finger, and a small stab incision is made with a No. 11 surgical blade in the area blocked with lidocaine.
- **Step 5.** The bone marrow needle, with the stylet in place, is advanced into the stab incision and through the skin, subcutaneous tissue, and muscle all the way to the bone. It is crucial to keep the stylet in place because it has a tendency to back out during the procedure. An 18-gauge (cat or small dog) or 16-gauge (medium to large-sized dog) bone marrow needle is preferred for most dogs and cats. Most find that the disposable needle that has the trochar locked into place is ideal.
- **Step 6.** With the stylet in place, the bone marrow needle is advanced into the bone, using a corkscrew motion. The instrument should not be allowed to wobble and should be fixed firmly into the bone like a nail that has been securely hammered into wood. When the needle is firmly fixed in the bone, the stylet is removed and the syringe is affixed. Many clinical pathologists suggest rinsing the syringe and bone marrow needle with EDTA before the procedure to reduce clotting of the bone marrow sample. Heparin should never be used.
- **Step 7.** The bone marrow sample is aspirated briskly into the 12-ml syringe; usually 0.25-0.5 ml of marrow is adequate. The aspiration may be accompanied by a few seconds of pain, but this can be prevented by the use of oral or parenteral analgesics such as fentanyl, butorphanol, morphine, NSAID, or other analgesics.
- **Step 8.** If a sample is not obtained, the stylet is replaced in the bone marrow needle, and the

instrument is then advanced farther into the bone for a second attempt at aspirating marrow. Once marrow has been obtained, smears are prepared. This can be done in a number of ways:

- The marrow and blood are expelled into a small petri dish that contains a few drops of EDTA. The marrow-rich spicules are placed on a slide or coverslip and then spread between slides or coverslips to make a monolayer of cells. The slides must have been cleaned and readied for the sample to be processed, as it will clot quickly.
- A portion of the marrow sample is placed on the proximal portion of the slide; the slide is tipped downward to allow the blood to run down and off the slide. The spicules and heavier nucleated cells do not run off and are used for subsequent slide preparation.
- Marrow can be spread into a monolayer like a routine blood smear.
- The first two methods may enhance the ability to evaluate the nucleated cell population of the bone marrow specimen.

Bone biopsy

A biopsy of a bone lesion or the bone marrow can be obtained with the bone biopsy needle (figure 22-12). Unlike other biopsies, diagnostic samples are most likely to be diagnostic when obtained through the center of the boney lesion in question.

Indications

Any boney lesion.

Contraindications

Coagulopathies.

Benefits

A bone biopsy can provide tissue to analyze cellularity, architecture, and content; often, this can be done using generalized anesthesia in conjunction with systemic analgesia and/or generalized sedation.

Limitation

A single sample may not be representative of the entire boney lesion.

Equipment

No. 11 surgical blade, 2% lidocaine, bicarbonate, 6- to 12-ml syringe, 14- to 18-gauge bone biopsy needle with a handle as pictured in microscope slides, generalized anesthesia in conjunction with systemic analgesia and/or generalized sedation are preferred.

Technique (figure 22-13 A-H)

- **Step 1.** Analgesics are given and generalized anesthesia is induced. The hair is clipped, the microscope slides are readied for the sample

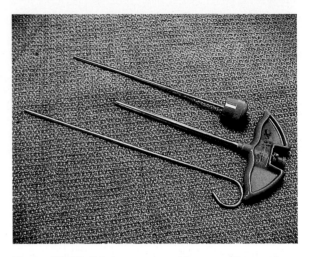

Figure 22-12: This bone marrow biopsy needle contains a trochar, stylet, plastic handle and a wire to push the biopsy specimen out the back of the biopsy needle, not through the slightly narrower tip.

(which will clot quickly) to be processed, and the bone biopsy site is prepared with a surgical scrub
- **Step 2.** Dilute 2% lidocaine with 8.4% bicarbonate (1 part bicarbonate to 9 parts lidocaine) to reduce stinging on injection. Using a 25-gauge needle, approximately 0.25 to 2 ml of this local anesthetic agent is injected around the lesion to a maximum total dosage of 0.5 mg/kg in the cat and 1 mg/kg in the dog. Care is taken to inject lidocaine (2%) in and around all of the tissue that extends from the skin to the periosteum. The lidocaine will sting less upon injection if it is diluted 50:50 with 8.4% bicarbonate.
- **Step 3.** The biopsy area is scrubbed one more time after the lidocaine injection. A surgical drape should be applied for sterility.
- **Step 4.** The bone biopsy site is identified, the skin is stretched between the thumb and index finger, and a small stab incision is made with a No. 11 surgical blade in the area blocked with lidocaine.
- **Step 5.** The bone biopsy needle, with the stylet in place, is advanced into the stab incision and through the skin, subcutaneous tissue, and muscle all the way to the bone. It is crucial to keep the stylet in place. A 14- to 18-gauge bone biopsy needle is preferred for most dogs and cats, depending on their size.
- **Step 6.** With the stylet removed, the bone biopsy needle is advanced into the bone, using a corkscrew motion. The instrument should not be allowed to wobble and should be fixed firmly into the bone like a nail that has been securely hammered into wood. When the needle is firmly fixed in the bone, preferably up to the inner cortex of the opposite side, the needle is then rocked back and forth in an "X" like direction. The purpose of rocking the needle back and forth to sever the sample from

its base. The biopsy instrument is then removed, and a smaller wire obturator is used to retrograde the biopsy piece out of the top end of the biopsy instrument. Bone is sampled for culture and sensitivity, cytology and histopathology.

- **Step 7.** Direct pressure should be applied to the site for several minutes to prevent hematoma formation. The small incision may be sutured or glued closed.
- **Step 8.** Gentle rolling of the biopsy on a glass slide before fixation may provide a good cytologic sample. An adequate sample is 1 cm of cancellous bone.

Supportive care

Oral or parenteral analgesics for hours to days may be indicated.

Bone aspiration

An aspirate of a bone lesion can be obtained with a 14-18-gauge needle (figure 22-14 a-d). Like bone biopsies, aspirates are most likely to be diagnostic when obtained through the center of the boney lesion in question. For most lytic lesions, the needle will drop into the center of the lesion. The probability of getting through the cortex can be enhanced by using diagnostic ultrasound to direct the needle through soft areas into the center of the boney lesion.

Indications

Any boney lesion.

Contraindications

Coagulopathies.

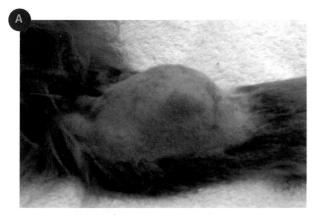

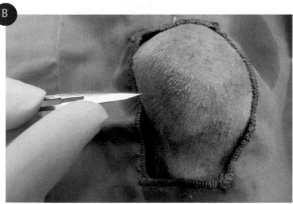

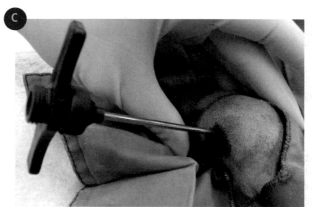

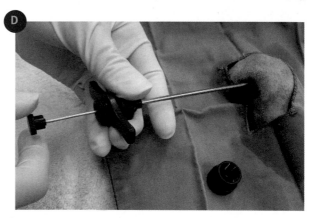

Figure 22-13: Bone biopsy. (A) After a physical examination and appropriate blood work, the patient is given systemic analgesics and the area to be biopsied is clipped. (B) The anesthetized patient is placed in a position to allow adequate visualization of the anatomic site that will serve as the site of the bone biopsy. The region over the area to be biopsied is prepared with a surgical scrub before and after administering the local anesthetic agent. The local anesthesia is performed by injecting lidocaine:bicarbonate mixture (1 part bicarbonate to 9 parts lidocaine) to reduce the acidity and thus the discomfort upon injecting the lidocaine (25-gauge needle, 0.25 to 2 ml to a maximum total dosage of 0.5 mg/kg in the cat and 1 mg/kg in the dog). The area to be biopsied is draped for the surgical procedure. The site is identified, the skin is stretched between the thumb and index finger, and a small stab incision is made with a No. 11 surgical blade in the area blocked with lidocaine. (C) The bone biopsy needle, with the stylet in place, is advanced into the stab incision and through the skin, subcutaneous tissue, and muscle all the way to the bone. An 18-gauge (cat or small dog) or 14-16-gauge (medium to large sized dog) bone biopsy needle is preferred for most dogs and cats. Most find that the disposable needles that have a trochar that can be locked into place is ideal. (D) Once the cortex is encountered, the inner stylet is removed.

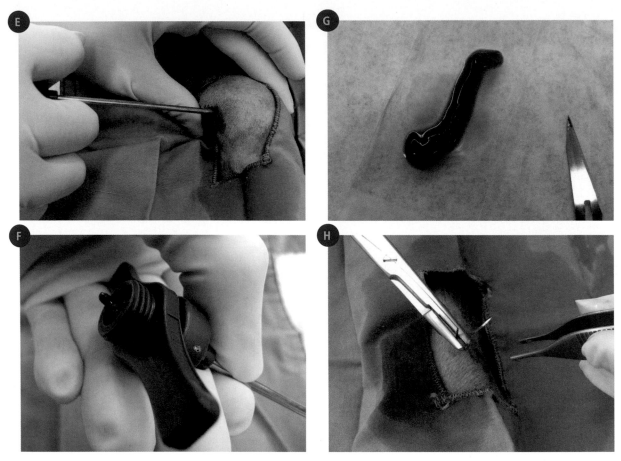

Figure 22-13 (cont.): (E) The biopsy trochar is advanced through the bone, into the marrow and to the opposite cortex. The needle is then moved side to side in an "X" fashion to help sever the base of the biopsy specimen that is now in the needle. (F) The wire is advanced from the narrowed tip to push the biopsy out the back end of the biopsy specimen. (G) Impression smears are taken of the biopsy specimen. (H) The small incision is closed with a suture and analgesics are given for several days.

Benefits

A bone aspirate can provide tissue to analyze cellularity, cytology of the boney lesion. This can be done using generalized anesthesia in conjunction with systemic analgesia.

Limitation

A single sample may not be representative of the entire boney lesion

Equipment

2% lidocaine, bicarbonate, 6- to 12-ml syringe, 14-18-gauge needle with a 12 ml syringe, microscope slides. General anesthesia is preferred with systemic analgesia.

Technique (figure 22-14 A-C)

- **Step 1.** Analgesics are given and generalized anesthesia is induced. The hair is clipped, the microscope slides are readied for the sample (which will clot quickly) to be processed, and the bone aspirate site is prepared with a surgical scrub
- **Step 2.** Dilute 2% lidocaine with 8.4% bicarbonate (1 part bicarbonate to 9 parts lidocaine) to reduce stinging on injection. Using a 25-gauge needle, approximately 0.25 to 2 ml of this local anesthetic agent is injected around the lesion to a maximum total dosage of 0.5 mg/kg in the cat and 1 mg/kg in the dog. Care is taken to inject lidocaine (2%) in and around all of the tissue that extends from the skin to the periosteum. The lidocaine will sting less upon injection if it is diluted with bicarbonate.
- **Step 3.** The area to be aspirated is scrubbed one more time after the lidocaine injection.
- **Step 4.** The bone aspiration site is identified, the skin is stretched between the thumb and index finger, and the area blocked with lidocaine.
- **Step 5.** The needle and the syringe, which are filled with air PRIOR to the sampling, is advanced through the skin, subcutaneous tissue, and muscle

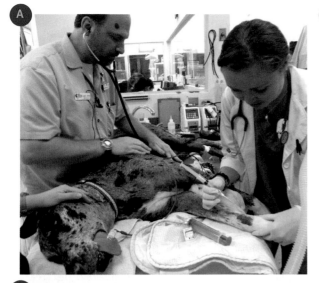

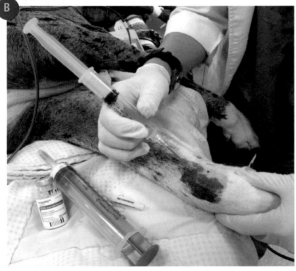

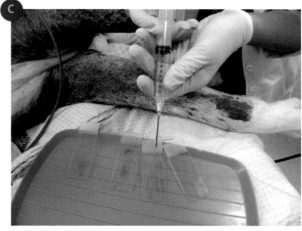

Figure 22-14: Bone aspirate. (A) After a physical examination and appropriate blood work, the patient is given systemic analgesics, anesthetized and placed in a position to allow adequate visualization of the anatomic site that will serve as the site of bone aspiration. The region over the area to be aspirated is clipped and prepared with a surgical scrub before and after administering the local anesthetic agent. The local anesthesia is performed by injecting lidocaine:bicarbonate mixture (1 part bicarbonate to 9 parts lidocaine) to reduce the acidity and thus the discomfort upon injecting the lidocaine (25-gauge needle, 0.25 to 2 ml to a maximum total dosage of 0.5 mg/kg in the cat and 1 mg/kg in the dog). The area to be biopsied is draped for the surgical procedure. (B) The boney site is identified, the skin is stretched between the thumb and index finger, and an 18-gauge (cat or small dog) or 16-gauge (medium to large-sized dog) needle is attached to a 12 ml syringe filled with 6 mls of air. The needle is advanced into the bone, seeking a soft region within the lysis. Ultrasound imaging can help identify a break in the cortex to enter. (C) The syringe and needle as a single unit are rapidly removed in preparation for making slides.

all the way to the bone. Some use the needle alone without the syringe. Others find the air-filled syringe to be a good handle.

- **Step 6.** The bone biopsy needle is advanced repeatedly into the bone with force until it passes through the cortex into the boney lesion. It is ideal to concurrently use diagnostic ultrasound to identify defects in the boney cortex where you can direct the needle. Once the hub of the needle is filled with bone or blood, the material is then expelled for culture and sensitivity, cytology and histopathology.
- **Step 7.** Direct pressure should be applied to the site for several minutes to prevent hematoma formation.

Supportive care

Oral or parenteral analgesics for hours to days may be indicated.

Key point

Bone marrow aspiration and biopsy are essential procedures for determining cytologic and histologic abnormalities of the bone marrow caused by a wide variety of neoplastic, infectious, and myelodysplastic conditions. The accuracy and value of the information from these diagnostics is directly related to the experience and training of the pathologist.

Treatment of cancer

Surgical treatment of cancer can be divided into six areas including definitive or curative surgery, debulking surgery, removal of metastases (metastectomy), surgery for oncologic emergencies, surgery for palliation, as well as surgical intervention for reconstruction and rehabilitation.

Surgical repair of cancer induced fractures can also be of some palliative benefit. In one report,[14] the medical records of 16 dogs with pathologic fractures of the appendicular skeleton due to a bone sarcoma were reviewed. Bone plates or interlocking nails were used for repair in 12 dogs. Limb use immediately after surgery in 13 dogs was good (4), weight-bearing but lame (7) and non-weight bearing (2). Adjunctive therapy was administered in 5 dogs. Survival time ranged from 18 to 897 days; median survival was 166 days. The authors confirmed an improved quality of life due to the palliative surgical procedure.

Surgery for reconstruction and rehabilitation[1–5,9]

Very wide resection of a malignancy is now possible because of the development of plastic surgical techniques, including free flap and microvascular anastomotic methods. These techniques can be used to rehabilitate areas that have been irradiated or areas in which substantial tissue injury is noted. An example would be a vascular flap to cover a defect after a tumor has been surgically removed over a distal extremity.

References

1. Lascelles BDX: Principles of oncological surgery, in Dobson JM, Lascelles BDX: *BSAVA Manual of Canine and Feline Oncology*, ed 2. Gloucester, British Small Animal Veterinary Association, 2003, pp 73–86.

2. Niederhuber JE: Surgical interventions in cancer, in Abeloff MD, Armitage JO, Niederhuber JE, et al: *Clinical Oncology*, ed 3. Philadelphia, Elsevier Churchill Livingstone, 2004, 579–590.

3. Withrow SJ: Surgical oncology, in Withrow SJ, MacEwen EG (eds): *Small Animal Clinical Oncology*, ed 3. Philadelphia, WB Saunders, 2001, pp 70–76.

4. Ogilvie GK, Moore AS: Surgical oncology—Properties, uses, and patient management, in Ogilvie GK, Moore AS. *Feline Oncology: A Comprehensive Guide to Compassionate Care*. Yardley, PA, Veterinary Learning Systems. 2002, pp 88–90.

5. Aiken SW: Principles of surgery for the cancer patient. *Clin Tech Small Anim Pract* 18(2):75–81, 2003.

6. Powers BE, Dernell WS: Tumor biology and pathology. *Clin Tech Small Anim Pract* 13(1):4–9, 1998.

7. Szentimrey D: Principles of reconstructive surgery for the tumor patient. *Clin Tech Small Anim Pract* 13(1):70–76, 1998.

8. Monteiro B, Boston S, Monteith G. Factors influencing complete tumor excision of mast cell tumors and soft tissue sarcomas: a retrospective study in 100 dogs. *Can Vet J*. 52(11):1209-14, 2011.

9. Soderstrom MJ, Gilson SD: Principles of surgical oncology. *Vet Clin North Am Small Anim Pract* 25(1):97–110, 1995.

10. Liptak JM, Brutscher SP, Monnet E, Dernell WS, Twedt DC, Kazmierski KJ, Walter CU, Mullins MN, Larue SM, Withrow SJ. Transurethral resection in the management of urethral and prostatic neoplasia in 6 dogs. *Vet Surg* 33(5):505-516, 2004.

11. Farese JP, Kirpensteijn J, Kik M, Bacon NJ, Waltman SS, Seguin B, Kent M, Liptak J, Straw R, Chang MN, Jiang Y, Withrow SJ. Biologic behavior and clinical outcome of 25 dogs with canine appendicular chondrosarcoma treated by amputation: a Veterinary Society of Surgical Oncology retrospective study. *Vet Surg*. 38(8):914-919, 2009.

12. Hobson HP, Brown MR, Rogers KS. Surgery of metastatic anal sac adenocarcinoma in five dogs. *Vet Surg*. 35(3):267-270, 2006.

13. Lang JM, Schertel E, Kennedy S, Wilson D, Barnhart M, Danielson B. Elective and emergency surgical management of adrenal gland tumors: 60 cases (1999-2006). *J Am Anim Hosp Assoc*. 47(6):428-435, 2011.

14. Boston SE, Bacon NJ, Culp WT, Bhandal J, Bruce C, Cavanaugh RP, Hamilton MH, Lincoln JD, Liptak JM, Scharvogel S. Outcome after repair of a sarcoma-related pathologic fracture in dogs: a Veterinary Society of Surgical Oncology Retrospective Study. *Vet Surg*. 40(4):431-437, 2011.

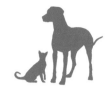

Chapter 23

First commandment: don't let them hurt! Pain management

INTRODUCTION

Compassionate care is the single most important aspect of canine and feline cancer care and pain control is a critical aspect of this caring process. Fortunately, pain control in dogs and cats has recently begun to be prioritized, studied and openly used in veterinary medicine. Canine and feline pain management can be difficult because signs of discomfort may not be recognized by clients and the rest of the veterinary health care team. This is especially true for cats as they often become quiet and secretive when experiencing pain. The key to compassionate pain control is anticipating the onset of discomfort, thereby allowing timely intervention with analgesics. For optimal pain control, analgesics should be given prophylactically, before pain receptors are ever stimulated in a painful process. Educating the entire veterinary health care team, especially veterinary nurses, is key to ensuring that patient comfort is paramount. The "ABCs" of pain management, listed below, must be followed for each case:[1,3]

- Assess each patient for discomfort. Think ahead to anticipate and prevent discomfort from diagnostics, therapeutics, and the disease itself.
- Believe and respond to the client's perception about the pet's pain level and quality of life. Your client's insights about their dog or cat are to be taken seriously at all times.
- Choose optimal analgesics to treat and prevent discomfort or pain. Remember that patients will respond differently to the same analgesic.
- Deliver the drugs in the most appropriate fashion to optimize analgesic effects. The administration of oral analgesics is convenient, and helpful for mild discomfort, but parenteral therapy is often needed for more significant discomfort.
- Empower clients to directly participate in patient care by ensuring they understand as much about the disease, treatment, and philosophy of pain management as the rest of the veterinary health care team.

It is critical to always assume that each patient with cancer has some degree of discomfort. Design a treatment plan for each animal to enhance comfort. In addition, it is important to realize that each pet's need for analgesics is dynamic and that constant assessment by the entire veterinary health care team must be a priority. In many veterinary centers, the nursing team is best at recognizing discomfort and advocating the use of analgesics. Many excellent reviews exist for those seeking additional details of pain prevention, control, and management that are beyond the scope of this section.

Key point

It is critical to always assume that each patient with cancer has some degree of discomfort and to treat for it.

SOURCE OF PAIN FOR THE CANCER PATIENT

Pain can be elicited by the direct destructive effect of the cancer as well as organ swelling and subsequent tissue damage that causes activation of pain receptors.[1–5] Cancer therapeutics can also cause some discomfort. For example, surgery and radiation therapy may ultimately relieve pain and suffering but almost always cause short-term discomfort that must be minimized, hopefully by initiating preventative analgesics. While chemotherapy can help control the underlying malignant process, these drugs can occasionally be associated with discomfort. Cisplatin (warning: never use in cats), vincristine, and vinblastine have caused painful polyneuropathy in a small percentage of human cancer patients that can result in tingling, burning, or numbness. This adverse effect has not been clearly determined to exist in animals however it is suspected to occur in a relatively small number of dogs and cats and can decrease the patient's quality of life. Vincristine can cause ileus that can cause abdominal discomfort that may be helped with promotility drugs such as metoclopramide. Other types of discomfort include:

- Visceral pain that causes a dull, deep, constant, aching pain resulting in pacing, restlessness, vocalization, and anorexia in some pets. Visceral pain is poorly defined; patients with significant visceral pain may respond to opioid or nonopioid analgesics. It is suspected that this type of pain results in decreased activity, anorexia, and behavioral changes in dogs and cats. Metoclopramide may be helpful when ileus is causing pain.
- Inflammatory and somatic pain has been infrequently described in pets with cancer but is localized, constant, and aching and is often caused by bone metastases and tissue damage of muscles, dentition, and skin.[5] Dogs and cats may lick or bite at an area or may exhibit signs of discomfort in subtle ways, such as by decreasing their activity or limping if a limb is affected. Non-steroidal anti-inflammatory agents, palliative radiation, and fatty acids of the n-3 series are often used to treat animals with this type of discomfort. Tramadol and gabapentin can also be used.
- Neuritic pain, also known as neuritis is caused by inflammation of nerves or nerve roots and is either part of a paraneoplastic syndrome or caused by a direct effect of tumor compression. People with this type of pain describe it as a constant, dull, aching pain that may have periods of burning "shock-like" sensations. In dogs and cats, these shock-like sensations can result in sudden, unexplained behavioral changes, such as aggression or scratching and biting at an area, often to the point of self-mutilation. Palliative radiation can be very helpful in those cases where NSAID's, tramadol, gabapentin, and acupuncture are not sufficient.
- Neuropathic pain occurs when a segment of the nervous system that normally transmits pain stimuli is damaged. It arises from metabolic, immunologic, or direct physical effects on the nervous system. Neuropathic pain is difficult to control with standard analgesics however gabapentin, acupuncture, and radiation can be of some help.

RECOGNIZING PAIN

The goal of compassionate cancer care is to prevent pain from occurring and acting rapidly to treat it if it is observed. Cancer patients, regardless of species, do have pain, stress, distress, and discomfort that is directly or indirectly associated with their cancer or the therapy. This pain must be prevented and treated early in the course of the disease. Dogs and cats are quite variable in expressing discomfort. Some hide most outward and measurable manifestations of pain and rarely exhibit signs until discomfort is quite advanced. In these dogs and cats, the only clinical indicator of pain and discomfort may be increased systolic blood pressure, heart rate, or decreased appetite. Other dogs and cats are demonstrative when pain occurs. Experienced practitioners and caregivers watch for subtle changes in activity level, appetite, and movement. Vocalization, while not a specific indicator of pain, is noted in some dogs and cats, especially when discomfort is significant. Some become more reclusive while others pace and may thrash around. Tachypnea,

tachycardia, and dilated pupils can be used to assess pain in dogs and cats, even when they are stuporous.

The best veterinary practitioners anticipate and intervene early rather than waiting for clinical signs associated with discomfort. Caregivers need to be aware of which procedures are likely to cause discomfort, and preemptive analgesia should be practiced when possible.

Comprehensive management of pain involves careful evaluation and treatment of each dog or cat.[1-5] To maximize quality of life, response to therapy, and survival time for canine and feline patients, adequate pain control must be the highest goal for the veterinary practitioner and the associated veterinary health care team. Pain control in veterinary medicine has come to the forefront of attention primarily because of inappropriate attitudes of clinicians and nurses, lack of knowledge about analgesic medications, and lack of skill in assessing pain and appropriate therapeutic methods.[2,3] Client demand has also been an important force in bringing pain control to the forefront of compassionate care. In many cases, analgesics have been withheld because of fear of associated adverse side effects and because research demonstrating the beneficial effects of pain relief in dogs and cats is scant. However, patient needs and client concerns require that pain relief and compassionate care become a priority in veterinary medicine.

Key point

To maximize quality of life, response to therapy, and survival time for canine and feline patients, adequate pain control must be the highest goal for the veterinary practitioner and the associated veterinary health care team.

GENERAL CONCEPTS OF PAIN THERAPY

The choice of analgesics and procedures (table 23-1) to prevent, reduce, and eliminate discomfort will differ depending on the cause, duration of the pain stimulus and the medical condition of the patient (table 23-2). For example, pain control for an abdominal exploratory procedure will differ from management of chronic pain for a dog and cat with metastatic bone disease. Discomfort associated with inflammatory conditions differs from that induced by nerve damage. Other factors that may influence the approach to treating the cancer patient include:[1-3]

- **Body condition:** In obese patients, drugs may be redistributed into fat stores, leading to overdosing. Metabolic derangements associated with cancer cachexia may result in altered pharmacokinetics and analgesic toxicity.
- **Age:** Some analgesics and anxiolytics that affect the central nervous system may have a pronounced sedative or calming effect in very young and old animals.
- **Breed:** Unique breed differences should be considered

when selecting analgesics. For example, Labrador retrievers and other dogs may be more sensitive to a rare hepatopathy associated with the administration of drugs such as carprofen. Doberman pinschers may be more likely to exhibit extrapyramidal side effects of some opiate drugs. Boxers may be very sensitive to the effects of acepromazine and opiates. Collies may have a mutation of the MDR gene that may alter metabolism or action of a number of drugs.

- **Underlying concurrent diseases:** Cancer patients are often older, and they almost always have a metabolic or organ disorder that may influence their degree of, and sensitivity to, discomfort and their response to analgesics. Dogs and cats with renal or hepatic insufficiency should be treated with care because this organ dysfunction will change the toxicity and efficacy profile of drugs metabolized or eliminated by these organs. Long-term use of NSAID's in dogs and cats must be monitored with at least a BUN and serum creatinine. Cats with thyrotoxicosis will metabolize drugs quite differently. Obtaining a minimum database of complete blood count, serum chemistry profile, and urinalysis will help the clinician anticipate any potential problems.

- **Individual variation:** Some patients respond unpredictably to the effect of drugs. Nervous, hyperexcitable, indoor, small pets may be more expressive than sedate Labrador retrievers that are occasionally

used for hunting. Keeping a careful drug history in these patients is critical, especially when many clinicians and nurses are involved in the care of each patient.

- **Duration of discomfort:** The use of a local analgesic agent may be all that is needed for short-term pain management; the same form of analgesia would be inappropriate for long-term chronic pain control.

- **Severity of discomfort:** Mild discomfort is clearly treated differently than severe discomfort.

> **Key point**
>
> Dogs and cats with renal or hepatic insufficiency should be treated with care because this organ dysfunction will change the toxicity and efficacy profile of drugs metabolized or eliminated by these organs.

Recent research has demonstrated that once pain is elicited, the pain response is magnified. Preventive therapy is therefore preferable to suppression of established pain. Premeditated, judicious use of analgesics is likely to increase patient comfort, decrease the need for hospitalization (and the associated costs), and reduce the amount of pain medication needed to achieve the same level of comfort.[3,6]

Table 23-1. General approach to pain management

Degree of pain	Clinical approach[a]
Mild	Nonopioid[b] ± acupuncture
Mild-moderate	Nonopioid + acupuncture + Tramadol + gabapentin + opioids
Moderate	Nonopioid + acupuncture + Tramadol + gabapentin + opioids
Moderate-severe	Nonopioid + acupuncture + Tramadol + gabapentin + opioids (dose escalation, different route of administration) ± anxiolytics
Severe	Nonopioid + acupuncture + Tramadol + gabapentin + opioids (dose escalation, different route of administration) + anxiolytics prn + other palliative procedures (e.g., radiation, surgery)

[a]In each case treat the underlying disease
[b]NSAIDs and acetaminophen. Use with caution in patients with renal disease or at times of hypotension or dehydration.

Table 23-2. Procedures and associated discomfort (and associated pain management)

Degree of pain	Clinical examples
None	Physical examination, restraint, radiographs, bandage change
Mild	Suturing, debridement, fine-needle aspirate, needle core biopsy (nonopioid* ± acupuncture)
Moderate	Abdominal exploratory, skin tumor removal, liver biopsy, laparoscopy, thoracoscopy (nonopioid ± acupuncture + opioids [low-dose] ± anxiolytics)
Severe	Hemipelvectomy, limb-sparing surgery, thoracotomy, chest wall excision, limb amputation, ear canal ablation (nonopioid ± acupuncture + opioids [dose escalation, different route of administration] ± anxiolytics + other palliative procedures [e.g., radiation, surgery])

*NSAIDs and acetaminophen. Use with caution in patients with renal disease.

The management of pain begins with high-quality, compassionate care by every member of the veterinary health care team. Careful nursing care, gentle handling, and provision of a comfortable and relaxing environment are of great benefit to dogs and cats. Local anesthesia and/or acupuncture should be employed to alleviate discomfort, and systemic analgesia should be used when local analgesia may be insufficient.

SELECTION OF MEDICATION TO MANAGE PAIN[5]

Effective selection of analgesics depends on consideration of their mechanism of action, potency, duration of efficacy, effect on the central nervous system, anti-inflammatory effects, toxicity, metabolism, drug interactions, and price. Tables 23-3 and 23-4 list some selected analgesics and their dosing recommendations. The best practitioners gain experience with a select number of drugs, which allows them to prescribe maximum pain control. They educate their clients about realistic expectations as well as the benefits, deficits, and

toxicoses of different pain therapies. They also begin analgesics before the onset of pain and then continually change therapy to meet the pet's needs throughout the course of the disease and its therapy.

Nonopioids

Nonopioids, including nonsteroidal anti-inflammatory drugs (NSAIDs) (e.g., carprofen, etodolac, deracoxib, ketoprofen, piroxicam, meloxicam), provide mild to moderate anti-inflammatory and analgesic effects (figures 23-1 to 23-6). Knowledge about the efficacy and safety in the cat is more limited than in the dog. Some NSAIDs have been approved for long-term use in the cat in some countries, but not the United States. Regardless, the benefits and risks of the long-term use of NSAIDs in the cat have been beautifully reviewed by the American Association of Feline Practitioners and the International Society of Feline Medicine. That excellent review came up with some superb recommendations including the following recommendations on monitoring:[6]
- Based on data from cats and other species, the risk of

Table 23-3. Selected analgesics for the dog

Drug	Dose	Route	Dosing interval
Opioid agonists			
Codeine	0.5–2 mg/kg	PO	6–8 hr
Morphine	0.5–2 mg/kg	PO, IM, SC	2–4 hr
Sustained release	2–5 mg/kg	PO	1–4 hr
Oxycodone	0.1–0.3 mg/kg	PO	8–12 hr
Oxymorphone	0.05–0.4 mg/kg	IV, SC, IM	2–4 hr
Hydromorphone	0.05–0.2 mg/kg	IV, SC, IM	2–6 hr
Methadone	1–1.5 mg/kg	IV, SC, IM	Once
	0.1 mg/kg	IV	3–6 hr
Meperidine	3–5 mg/kg	SC, IM	1–2 hr
Fentanyl	2–5 µg/kg	IV bolus	Prior to CRI*
Postoperative	2–5 µg/kg/hr	CRI	Duration of infusion
Operative	10–45 µg/kg/hr	CRI	Duration of infusion
	(2–3 mg/kg/hr) patch	Dermal application	Replace every 3–5days
Sufentanil	5 µg/kg	IV bolus prior to CRI	2–6 hr
Postoperative	0.1 µg/kg/hr	CRI	Duration of infusion
Remifentanil	4–10 µg/kg	IV bolus prior to CRI	2–6 hr
Postoperative	4–10 µg/kg/hr	CRI	Duration of infusion
Operative	20–60 µg/kg/hr	CRI	Duration of infusion
Opioid agonist-antagonist			
Buprenorphine	0.005–0.02 mg/kg	IV, IM, SC	8–12 hr
Butorphanol	0.1–0.4 mg/kg	IV, IM, SC	1–4 hr
	0.5–2 mg/kg	PO	6–8 hr
Nalbuphine	0.5–1 mg/kg	IV, IM, SC	4 hr
Pentazocine	1–3 mg/kg	IV, IM, SC	2–4 hr

Table 23-3. Selected analgesics for the dog (*cont.*)

Drug	Dose	Route	Dosing interval
NSAIDs			
Ketoprofen	1–2 mg/kg	IV, IM, SC	24 hr
	1 mg/kg	PO	24 hr
Piroxicam	0.3 mg/kg	PO	24–48 hr
Meloxicam	0.1–0.2 mg/kg	IV, IM, SC	24 hr
	0.1 mg/kg	PO	24 hr
Carprofen	2.2 mg/kg	PO	12 hr
Etodolac	10–15 mg/kg	PO	12 hr
Deracoxib	1–2 mg/kg	PO	24 hr
Firocoxib	5 mg/kg	PO	24 hr
Robenacoxib	1–2 mg/kg	PO	24 hr
Tepoxalin	10 mg/kg	PO	24 hr
Tolfenamic acid	4 mg/kg	PO	SC q24h × 3 days, 4 days off
Alpha-2 agonists			
Medetomidine	5–10 µg/kg	IM, SC	Once
	1–4 µg/kg	IV	Once
Romifidine	10–20 µg/kg	IM, SC	Once
Xylazine	0.2–0.5 mg/kg	PO	12 (*cont.*)
Local anesthetics			
Lidocaine	1.5 mg/kg	Intrapleural prior to bupivacaine	1–1.5 hr
	2–4 mg/kg	IV bolus prior to CRI	
	0.02 – 0.05 mg/kg/min	CRI	Duration of infusion
Bupivacaine	1–2 mg/4.5 kg	Local nerve blocks Intrapleural administration prn	2–4 hr
Mepivacaine	1 mg/kg	SQ	1.5–2.5 hr
Ropivacaine	1 mg/kg	SQ	1.5–2.5 hr
Glucocorticoids			
Dexamethasone	0.10–0.20 mg/kg	SQ, PO	24–48 hr
Prednisone	0.25–1.0 mg/kg	PO	24 hr
Other drugs			
Amantadine	3–5 mg/kg	PO	24 hr
Acetaminophen (paracetamol)	5–10 mg/kg	PO	12 hr
Amitriptyline	1–4 mg/kg	PO	24 hr
	1.0–1.5 mg/kg	PO	12–24 hr
Aspirin	10 mg/kg	PO	12 hr
Clomipramine	1–3 mg/kg	PO	24 hr
Gabapentin	5–10 mg/kg	PO	8–24 hr STARTING DOSE
Glucosamine chondroitin	13–15 mg/kg	PO	24 hr
Imipramine	0.5–1.0 mg/kg	PO	8 hr
Ketamine	0.5–1 µg/kg	IM	30 min
	1 µg/kg/min	CRI, IV	Duration of infusion and post-infusion
Methocarbamol	10–40 mg/kg	PO	8–12 hr
Mexiletine	4–10 mg/kg	PO	12 hr
Pamidronate	1 mg/kg	IV slowly	prn every 3–6 weeks with diuresis
Tramadol	2–4 mg/kg	PO	6–8 hr
Zoledronate	0.15–0.25 mg/kg	IV slow in 50mL 0.9% NaCl	q28d

*CRI = constant rate infusion.

Table 23-4. Selected analgesics in cats[2–5]

Drug	Dose	Route	Dosing interval (hr)
Opioid agonists			
Codeine	0.5–1 mg/kg	PO	6–8 hr
Morphine	0.1–0.5 mg/kg	IM, SQ	2–6 hr
	0.05–0.2 mg/kg	IV	1–4 hr
Liquid	0.2–0.5 mg/kg	PO	6–8 hr
Methadone	0.1–0.5 mg/kg	SQ, IM	6 hr
	0.05–0.1 mg/kg	IV	6 hr
Hydromorphone	0.05–0.2 mg/kg	SQ, IM, IV	2–4 hr
Oxymorphone	0.02–0.05 mg/kg	IV	2–4 hr
	0.05–0.2 mg/kg	IM, SQ	2–6 hr
Fentanyl	0.0002–0.05 mg/kg	IV bolus prior to CRI	2–6 hr
	0.001–0.004 mg/kg	CRI	Duration of infusion
	2.5 mg (25 µg) patch	Dermal application	Replace every 3–5days
Opioid agonist-antagonist			
Buprenorphine	0.005–0.01 mg/kg	IV, IM, SQ	4–8 hr
	0.02–0.05 mg/kg	SL	6–12 hr
Butorphanol	0.1–0.4 mg/kg	IV, IM, SQ	1–4 hr
	0.5–2 mg/kg	PO	6–8 hr
NSAIDs			
Ketoprofen	1–2 mg/kg	IV, IM, SQ	24 hr
	1 mg/kg	PO	24 hr
Piroxicam	0.3 mg/kg	PO	48 hr
Carprofen	0.5–2 mg/kg	PO	8–12 hr
	1–2 mg/kg	PO	72 hr
Robenacoxib	1–2.4 mg/kg	PO	24 hr
Tepoxalin	5 mg/kg	PO	q12hr x 3 days, 4 days off
Tolfenamic acid	4 mg/kg	PO	q24hr x 4 days, 3 days off
α_2-adrenergic agonists			
Xylazine	0.5 mg/kg	IV, IM, SQ	0.5–2 hr
Medetomidine	0.001–0.01 mg/kg	IV, IM, SQ	0.5–2 hr
Local anesthetics			
Lidocaine	1.5 mg/kg	Intrapleural prior to bupivacaine	0.3 hr
	1–2 mg/kg	IV bolus prior to CRI	
	0.01 – 0.04 mg/kg/min	CRI	Duration of infusion
Bupivacaine	1–2 mg/4.5 kg	Local nerve blocks	
		Intrapleural administration prn	
Tranquilizers and anxiolytics			
Xylazine	0.05–0.2 mg/kg	IV, IM	15–30 min
Ketamine	0.5–1 mg/kg	IM	30 min
	0.5 mg/kg	IV bolus prior to CRI	
	0.3 -1 mg/kg/hr	CRI	Duration of infusion
Glucocorticoids			
Dexamethasone	0.10–0.20 mg/kg	SC, PO	24–48 hr
Prednisone	0.5–1.5 mg/kg	PO	24 hr

Table 23-4. Selected analgesics in cats[2-5] *(cont.)*

Drug	Dose	Route	Dosing interval (hr)
Other Drugs			
Amantadine	3–5 mg/kg	PO	24 hr
Amitriptyline	2–3 mg/kg	PO	24 hr
Aspirin	10 mg/kg	PO	48–72 hr
Clomipramine	1–5 mg/kg	PO	24 hr
Gabapentin	5–10 mg/kg	PO	8–24 hr STARTING DOSE
Imipramine	2.5–5 mg/kg	PO	12 hr
Methocarbamol	10–40 mg/kg	PO	8–12 hr
Pamidronate	1–1.5 mg/kg	IV slowly	every 3–4 weeks with diuresis
Tramadol	2–5 mg/kg	PO	12–24 hr
Zoledronate	0.15–0.20 mg/kg	IV slow in 25mL 0.9% NaCl	q28d

CRI = constant rate infusion.

acute kidney failure developing during appropriate therapeutic NSAID use in cats is low and not abrogated by the use of COX-selective agents.

- Monitoring serum renal analytes and urine parameters before and after commencement of NSAID therapy is highly recommended as a precaution, in an attempt to recognize acute kidney failure at an early stage, should it occur.

- Risk factors for renal toxicity in humans are presumed to apply to cats. Where an increased risk of renal toxicity is anticipated the lowest effective dose should always be administered (which may be facilitated by the use of adjuvant analgesic therapy) and increased monitoring is prudent.

- NSAIDs should be administered with food, and therapy withheld if food is not eaten. In cats predisposed to dehydration, such as with chronic kidney disease, using a wet rather than dry diet is a sensible precaution to optimize water intake.

- Specific risk factors, such as dehydration and hypovolemia, should always be addressed before therapy is administered, and if analgesia is required in the interim period an alternative such as an opioid can be utilized. Care should be taken to ensure good renal perfusion is also maintained if anesthesia is required during therapy.

- Current data suggest that at least some NSAIDs can be used safely in cats with stable CKD at judicious doses, and that this should not be a reason for withholding analgesic therapy when it is indicated. Further data, particularly in cats with advanced renal disease, would be valuable and such pharmacovigilance studies are vital.

- The combination of cardiac disease and renal disease is problematic – care is urged with the use of NSAIDs in this situation due to the increased risks of acute kidney failure. The exploration of analgesic options other than NSAIDs may be prudent, but the potential risks of exacerbating these diseases should not restrict the use of analgesic therapy where it is needed.

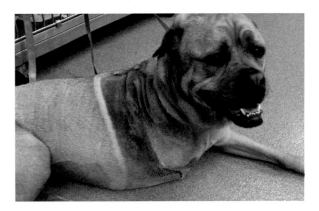

Figure 23-1: Most dogs do very well after amputation for a malignancy of a distal extremity proving that surgery is indeed a powerful tool for providing comfort for the cancer patient. The surgery not only resolves the primary tumor but it is often the greatest gift of comfort for dogs suffering from diseases such as distal radial osteosarcoma. It is a myth that larger dogs do not do as well as smaller dogs post amputation: It matters only that they are neuro-orthopedically sound on the remaining limbs. Regardless, comfort care is important after the post-operative period. Since many older dogs have degenerative joint disease, supplements such as the fatty acid docosahexaenoic acid, glucosamine, chondroitin sulfate along with a non-steroidal anti-inflammatory agent may be indicated. Piroxicam and to a lesser extent, other NSAIDs have an anticancer, anti-inflammatory and an analgesic effect.

- As there is a risk of hyperkalemia developing during NSAID therapy in other species, especially in the face of renal failure or potassium supplementation, potassium monitoring is recommended during therapy.

The older, nonspecific NSAIDs, such as aspirin, ibuprofen, ketoprofen, and piroxicam, may be associated with a greater risk for side effects because they inhibit two cyclooxygenase (COX) enzymes, COX-1 and COX-2.

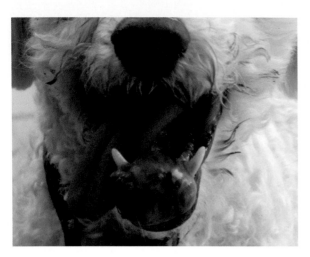

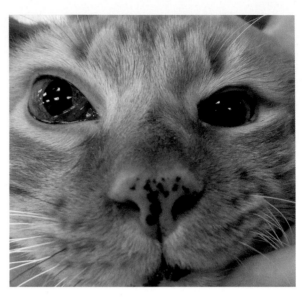

Figure 23-2: This dog has a rostral mandibular squamous cell carcinoma without evidence of distant metastases. A rostral mandibulectomy performed after appropriate systemic analgesia and a bilateral mandibular nerve block or definitive radiation would both likely be quite helpful at providing comfort and controlling the local tumor long term. Palliative radiation, given in a few dosages would likely provide moderate-term comfort and tumor control. A non-steroidal anti-inflammatory agent including piroxicam with or without docosahexaenoic acid tramadol could provide daily comfort if the clients elected not to treat the tumor with surgery or definitive radiation.

Figure 23-4: This retrobulbar lymphoma is causing pressure on the eye and surrounding structures. Chemotherapy, preferably a modified CHOP protocol and/or radiation therapy to the local site has the best chance of alleviating pain and discomfort confirming that chemotherapy can alleviate pain and suffering in the long term. If neither is selected by the client, then prednisone, may help reduce the swelling; buprenorphine may provide additional comfort. The eye should be kept moist and any corneal ulceration diagnosed and treated appropriately.

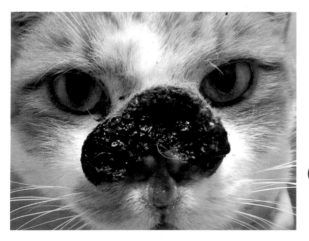

Inhibition of COX-1 can result in serious side effects such as renal failure, gastrointestinal distress and perforation of the upper gastrointestinal tract. However, these drugs are relatively simple to obtain, and their nonselective COX inhibition exerts central analgesic and peripheral anti-inflammatory effects that make them useful in treating pain associated with intrathoracic and intra-abdominal masses and bony metastases.

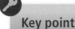

Key point

The older, nonspecific NSAIDs, such as aspirin, ibuprofen, ketoprofen, and piroxicam are at least theoretically associated with a greater risk for side effects because they inhibit two cyclooxygenase (COX) enzymes, COX-1 and COX-2.

Figure 23-3: This cat has a rather unusual form of nasal squamous cell carcinoma. Radiation therapy is likely the best option for tumor control. Oral buprenorphine with or without an oral non steroidal anti-inflammatory agent such as prioxicam or Robenacoxib may provide comfort. Robenacoxib has been very thoroughly investigated in cats and appears extremely effective with a very good safety profile.Carprofen, while not approved for use in cats the United States was the first to be studied specifically in cats and both its pharmacokinetics and pharmacological effects are well described. Clinical studies then demonstrated its efficacy and it is now widely used in many other countries for routine perioperative analgesia.

NSAIDs, especially piroxicam, have been shown to have anticancer effects, especially when used to treat such malignancies as transitional cell carcinoma and squamous cell carcinoma among in the dog and the cat. The mechanisms are complex and largely unknown, however some of the effect is mediated through the COX-2 enzyme. When combined with metronomic cyclophosphamide and/or docosahexaenoic acid, this NSAID-induced anticancer effect may be even more profound.

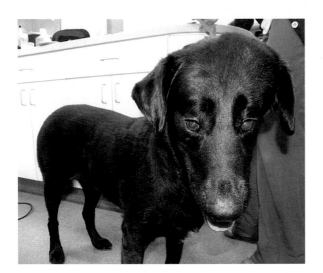

Figure 23-5: This dog has a relatively slow growing boney mass of the skull called multilobular osteochondrosarcoma. This tumor looks like "popcorn balls" on radiographs and often expands inwards as much as it does exteriorly. Surgical excision, if possible is the best treatment. This dog is likely best treated with radiation therapy. A non steroidal anti-inflammatory agent, tramadol, gabapentin and acupuncture may be helpful in these cases. The fatty acid docosahexaenoic acid not only inhibits arachadonic acid and thus, inflammatory mediators, but it also can limit the nephrotoxicity of some renal toxins and has anticancer effects in part mediated through its effect on the COX-2 enzyme.

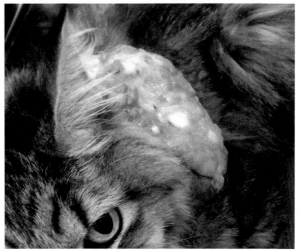

Figure 23-6: This cat is extremely cachectic in part due to an inoperable injection site sarcoma on his back. Nutritional support via appetite stimulants, placement of an esophagostomy tube and management of pain is a good first step of hospice care if euthanasia is not an appropriate at this time. Freedom from the pain and discomfort of hunger is very important for every patient. Palliative radiation may provide comfort. Other options that should be considered include at least a non steroidal anti-inflammatory agent if renal function is normal along with gabapentin, buprenorphine or a fentanyl patch.

The more specific NSAIDs, such as mavacoxib, carprofen, etodolac, and deracoxib, primarily inhibit the COX-2 enzyme and are often associated with fewer side effects (table 23-5). All have unique attributes that distinguish themselves. Mavacoxib is a more recently studied and approved NSAID that has been confirmed to be safe and effective in the dog. It has preferential action on the COX-2 isoform of COX and a long duration of action. The dosage schedule of mavacoxib for clinical use has been determined by integration of owner and veterinary clinical assessments, PK and PD preclinical data and good responses in dogs with osteoarthritis. One recommended schedule is to give the drug at 2 mg/kg once for 14 days, followed by administration at monthly intervals thereafter as needed for discomfort. This dosage regimen has been further confirmed by correlating levels of inhibition of COX isoforms in in vitro whole blood assays with plasma concentrations of mavacoxib achieved in dogs with osteoarthritis. There is in vitro data that serum concentrations of this drug may actually have an anticancer effect. Further clinical studies are warranted. Robenacoxib is the newest FDA approved NSAID for use in cats. This drug is being marketed for the control of post-operative pain associated with inflammation related to orthopaedic surgery, ovariohysterectomy, and castration, and can be given for a maximum of 3 days. This is the first coxib class of drug approved for cats. At clinical doses COX-1 inhibition is minimal and it has a unique pharmacokinetic profile, with a short half-life but long residence time in target tissues. Meloxicam is also marketed for cats, however it has a black label warning due to its known nephrotoxic effects in cats. .

The use of NSAIDs in dogs and cats should always include periodic evaluation of liver and renal function. Some clinicians concurrently prescribe drugs such as misoprostol to reduce the risk of toxicity to the gastrointestinal tract. Acetaminophen, which is believed to block the newly identified COX-3 enzyme, is related to NSAIDs but is not anti-inflammatory; however, it is effective for treating discomfort without the side effects usually associated with NSAIDs. Newer drugs may inhibit only the COX-3 enzyme, resulting in fewer adverse effects.

Prednisone with or without other chemotherapeutic agents have been shown to reduce swelling, edema and to inhibit inflammation and the size and thus the effect of some cancers such as lymphoma and mast cell tumors. The increased appetite and positive feeling of well being is also helpful.

α_2-agonists

α_2-agonists (e.g., clonidine, romifidine, medetomidine, xylazine) provide good to excellent analgesia with moderate to significant sedation and depression. Their short duration of action and tendency to reduce cardiac output and tissue oxygenation may make them an unwise

Table 23-5. Newer coxib class NSAIDs					
Generic	Trade name	COX-1: COX-2	Dose	Injectable	Cat
Mavacoxib	Trocoxil (Pfizer)	COX-2 preferential	Dog: 2 mg/kg monthly	No	No
Firocoxib	Previcox (Merial)	COX-2 selective	Dog: 5 mg/kg q24h	No	No
Robenacoxib	Onsior (Novartis)	COX-2 selective	Dog/Cat: 1 mg/kg q24h	Yes	Yes 6 mg tab
Cimicoxib	Cimalgex (Vetoquinol)	COX-2s elective	Dog: 2 mg/kg q24h	No	No

choice for some frail or infirm patients. When combined with an opioid, they can enhance the analgesic effects of the latter.

Opioids

Opioids (e.g., sustained-release morphine, fentanyl, oxymorphone, codeine) can result in excellent analgesia with low to moderate behavioral changes, such as depression (figures 23-7 to 23-14). These drugs are the most predictable, effective analgesics for use in the cancer patient. They can be administered orally, subcutaneously (SC), intramuscularly (IM), intravenously (IV), or in some cases, transdermally, but the efficacy of oral therapy has yet to be clearly documented in the dog, however oral fentanyl is commonly used in children and is sometimes delivered as a candy. As the severity of discomfort increases, the dosage of the opiates can be increased. Toxicity can include bradycardia, diarrhea, vomiting, constipation, and sedation, although careful dosing can mitigate any problems.

Key point

Opioids (e.g., sustained-release morphine, fentanyl, oxymorphone, codeine) can result in excellent analgesia with low to moderate behavioral changes and are the most predictable, effective analgesics for use to treat pain in the cancer patient.

Oral morphine

Oral morphine is most commonly used for long-term cancer pain management in people despite the fact that it does not penetrate into the central nervous system as rapidly as fentanyl and is often associated with more sedation than some other opiates. Morphine is a natural opioid agonist. On rare occasions, it may produce depression and sedation, or an initial excitement manifested by panting, salivation, nausea, vomiting, urination, defecation, and hypotension when administered to dogs and cats. These reactions arise from activation of the chemoreceptor trigger zone, vagal stimulation, and histamine release.

Oxymorphone

Oxymorphone is a semisynthetic opioid agonist with analgesic properties that are approximately 10 times more potent than those of morphine; its adverse effects on the respiratory, cardiovascular, and gastrointestinal systems are less pronounced. Oxymorphone is indicated for moderate to severe visceral or somatic pain. Lower doses are used for IV administration. When used alone, however,

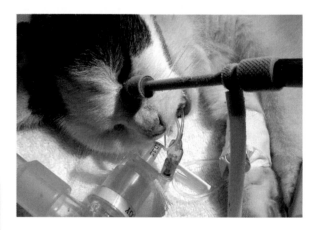

Figure 23-7: Treatment of an eyelid squamous cell carcinoma with cryotherapy can be quite effective. Cryotherapy is the use of liquid nitrogen to rapidly freeze the tumor and the surrounding tissue three times followed by three slow periods of thawing. A local block with lidocaine is mandatory along with systemic analgesia with an drug such as hydromorphone inhalant anesthesia. Analgesics are needed for 5-7 days post treatment. Options include oral NSAIDs and/or butorphanol or buprenorphine. Butorphanol is a mu antagonist which produces analgesia through its kappa agonist activity. It is a weaker analgesic than the pure mu opioids. Butorphanol exhibits a "ceiling" effect after which increasing doses do not produce any further analgesia. Buprenorphine on the other hand is a partial mu agonist. It acts at the mu receptor but its maximal effect is less than that of the pure mu agonists. It has high receptor affinity, resulting in long lasting effect - over 12 hours.. Transmucosal absorption is effective in cats. Buprenorphine has produced better analgesia than morphine and oxymorphone. It is very effective for perioperative pain management in cats as it is easily administered, highly effective, and long acting.

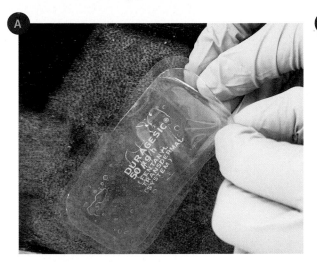

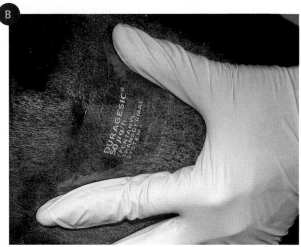

Figure 23-8: Use of the fentanyl patch. (A) The backing of the transdermal fentanyl patch is removed, and (B) the patch is placed on a flat, hairless area of skin where it is unlikely to be removed by the dog or cat. Appropriate gloves should be worn when these patches are handled. The patches are capable of delivering the analgesic over at least a 72-hour period.

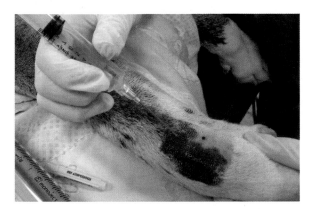

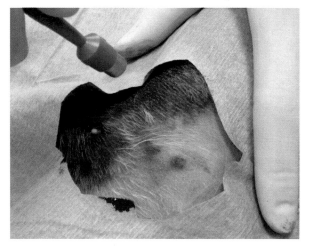

Figure 23-9: Tumors of bone are often diagnosed by obtaining a bone aspirate, assuming the needle is able to penetrate through the bone cortex itself. This can be painful unless an appropriate depth of anesthesia with analgesic properties is used. One example is pre-medication with fentanyl, propofol induction followed by inhalant isoflurane and a local block with lidocaine or bupivacaine. Propofol has almost no analgesic effects.

Figure 23-10: A punch biopsy can be done as an out-patient procedure with our without general anesthesia if a local lidocaine block, a non steroidal anti-inflammatory agent and tramadol are given. NSAIDs are often quite helpful to maintain comfort at home.

oxymorphone may result in excitement or hyperalgesia.[2,3,5] Diazepam given concurrently with oxymorphone may help reduce these side effects.

Fentanyl

Fentanyl is an effective analgesic that can be given IM, SC, or IV as a preanesthetic. It can be administered via an IV bolus, constant-rate infusion, or transdermal patch or a newly approved transdermal solution for long term pain control. Fentanyl can cause respiratory depression, bradycardia, and somnolence at higher dosages. It can also prolong return to normal body temperature during recovery from anesthesia. Fentanyl-

impregnated transdermal patches (25 µg/hr, 75 µg/ hr, and 100 µg/hr) reliably release a controlled amount of fentanyl over a 72-hour period (see figure 23-8). The patches maintain adequate blood levels of fentanyl for 72 hours, but therapeutic levels are not attained for 12 to 24 hours; thus patches may be most effective when used in conjunction with other analgesics or in addition to constant-rate fentanyl infusion during surgery or other painful procedures.

Opioid antagonists

Opioid antagonists (e.g., butorphanol) are generally not as effective as opioids. Butorphanol is a synthetic

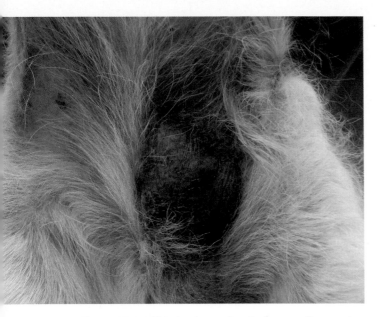

Figure 23-11: This dog has an inguinal mast cell tumor that caused pain by releasing cellular contents of the tumor that induced pain, swelling, inflammation, bruising, bleeding and distant stomach ulcers. Prednisone can help delay release of these cellular chemicals and can reduce the action of inflammatory mediators. An H2 receptor antagonist or a proton pump inhibitor is very helpful for preventing and treating stomach ulcers. Surgery and/or vinblastine chemotherapy and/ or a tyrosine kinase inhibitor such as masitinib or toceranib can eliminate the tumor or reduce its size. While these therapies rarely induce adverse effects, concurrent therapy with metoclopramide, maropitant and metronidazole can prevent or treat the discomfort of nausea, vomiting or diarrhea.

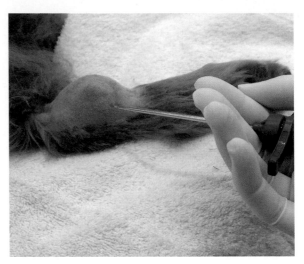

Figure 23-12: Bone biopsies can be done without discomfort if a premedication agent such as hydromorphone is administered prior to propofol induction and inhalant anesthesia. Further comfort is provided with a local block with a 50:50 mixture of lidocaine and bupivacaine is administered at the biopsy site. Lidocaine induces short-term (1-2 hours) local analgesia whereas bupivacaine provides longer-term (2-4 hours) comfort.

opioid agonist-antagonist that has five times the analgesic potency of morphine, but its duration of analgesia is short, approximately 1 to 4 hours. Its sedative effects are, however, 4-6 hours. Adverse effects such as nausea and vomiting are rare, but the drug can induce sedation. Higher dosages are needed for somatic pain, and analgesia lasts only about 2-4 hours. IV butorphanol may result in transient hypotension or bradycardia.[2,3,5] Because butorphanol possesses antagonist properties, it reverses the effects of narcotics. Therefore, butorphanol must not be given within 12 hours of any pre- or intraoperatively administered narcotics. Buprenorphine HCl, an agonist-antagonist, can reverse opioid-induced respiratory depression while maintaining analgesia. Buprenorphine is nearly tasteless and can be absorbed orally and is highly bioavailable when administered by that route, including in cats.

Ketamine

Ketamine is an *N*-methyl-D-aspartate (NMDA) receptor antagonist that is important in the *wind-up phenomenon*, in which pain makes certain nerve receptors even more "sensitive" to subsequent impulses that will be perceived

as a greater degree of discomfort than before. When the drug is administered at microdosages during and up to 24 hours after a painful procedure, the need for additional analgesics is reduced and pain control maximized with few, if any, behavioral or cardiovascular effects (figure 23-15 and see figure 23-13). Typically, a bolus of 0.5 mg/kg IV is administered followed by a constant-rate infusion of 2 µg/kg/min for the first 24 hours after surgery. For simplicity, if an infusion pump is not available, 60 mg of ketamine (0.6 mL) can be mixed in a liter bag of crystalloids. When the fluid is administered at a drip rate of 10 mL/kg/hr, the ketamine is delivered at 10 µg/kg/min. To decrease the dosage to 2 µg/kg/min, the fluid rate should be reduced to 2 mL/kg/hr.

Another option is to use a combination of fentanyl, lidocaine, and ketamine. These three drugs work by different mechanisms with potent anticancer effects. If the fluid rate to be given to a dog is 1-3 ml/kg/hr, the following can be added to a one liter bag of fluids: 50 ml of 2% lidocaine, 1.2 ml ketamine (100 mg/ml), and 1.2 ml fentanyl (15 mg/ml). Cats can have adverse effects to lidocaine; therefore, this option should be reserved for the dog.

Key point

Ketamine is an *N*-methyl-D-aspartate (NMDA) receptor antagonist that is important in the *wind-up phenomenon*, in which pain makes certain nerve receptors even more "sensitive" to subsequent impulses that will be perceived as a greater degree of discomfort than before.

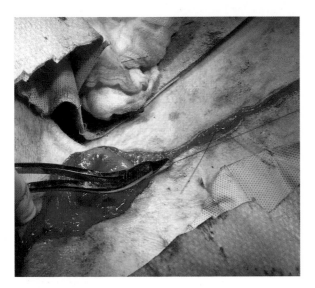

Figure 23-13: The most common malignancy of the intact female dog is a mammary tumor. Fifty percent are malignant and of those, fifty percent metastasize early in the course of the disease. Complete removal of the affected glands cures approximately 75% of all canine mammary tumors, but almost none of those in the cat. The extent of the surgery can induce significant pain that can be prevented with appropriate premedication and a local block of the surgery site followed by oral medication at home (e.g.: NSAID, tramadol and if needed, a fentanyl patch or an oral opiate). The N-methyl d-aspartate (NMDA) receptor is involved in spinal cord sensitization as clinical pain develops. Ketamine is an NMDA antagonist which has been shown to prevent or treat pain. Ketamine is widely used in cats for its anaesthetic properties and has proved an effective analgesic even at sub-anasthetic doses. Ketamine or ketamine containing analgesic protocols have been shown to provide better post operative analgesia than protocols using only barbiturates and volatile anaesthetics. In this case, an extensive resection was required. A constant rate infusion of morphine (or fentanyl), lidocaine and ketamine (MLK or FLK) is an effective option to reduce the amount of analgesics needed intra- and postoperatively by inhibiting the "wind-up" phenomenon.

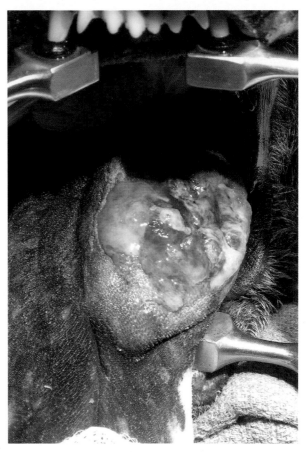

Figure 23-14: This oral malignant melanoma is best treated with a glossectomy. Dogs do quite well after their tongue has been nearly completely removed. Unfortunately, this is not true of cats that require their tongue to eat, drink and groom. If the client decides not to proceed with surgery or radiation therapy, systemic therapy with an NSAID, tramadol and gabapentin is a good first step. Tramadol is a unique non opioid, non NSAID analgesic which acts at least in part via opioid receptors. Oral comfort with "miracle mouthwash" can be achieved with an oral rinse of lidocaine, malox and diphenhydramine with or without tetracycline and nystatin may provide oral comfort.

Tranquilizers

Tranquilizers (e.g., acepromazine, diazepam, midazolam) do not provide analgesia, but their use in management of the cancer patient can be profound because fear, apprehension, and anxiety may magnify the response to pain. To avoid excitation, diazepam and midazolam should only be administered with an opioid in the alert patient.

Tricyclic antidepressants

Tricyclic antidepressants (e.g., amitriptyline, imipramine) have antihistamine effects. They block the reuptake of serotonin and norepinephrine to the central nervous system. They are used at very low dosages to induce analgesic effects and enhance the analgesic effects of opiates.

Gabapentin

This is an anticonvulsant that has pain reducing properties when given alone or preferably when combined with other agents such as NSAIDs and Tramadol (see figures 23-5, 23-6 and 23-14). It is thought to work via the alpha-2 delta portion of the calcium channel and thereby reducing the release of neurotransmitters. It has been found to be useful in both acute and chronic pain. The drug should be started at a low dose (4 mg/kg) and it can be increased gradually to doses as high as 50 mg/kg daily. It may induce drowsiness so the dose can be titrated to minimize this effect.

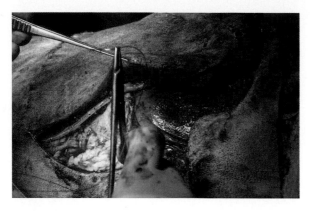

Figure 23-15: This dog is undergoing a chest wall resection for a chondrosarcoma of the rib. General anesthesia with a premedication of an analgesic such as hydromorphone, morphine or fentanyl plus an epidural blockade with lidocaine and/or preservative free morphine may be quite helpful. If morphine or fentanyl are used, then those drugs can be continued with either an MLK o`r FLK infusion. If the fluid rate to be given to this dog is 1-3 ml/kg/hr, the following can be added to a one liter bag of fluids: 50 ml of 2% lidocaine, 1.2 ml ketamine (100 mg/ml), and 1.2 ml fentanyl (15 mg/ml).

Radiation

Palliative radiation is commonly used to reduce discomfort associated with some tumors, especially those involving the skeletal system (see figures 23-2 to 23-4). When combined with low-dosage chemotherapy (doxorubicin or cisplatin), the enhanced effect may be prolonged. The response is related to the severity of the discomfort, the dosage and method of treatment, tumor type and the tissue destruction involved. As a general rule, palliative radiation has the following efficacy: one third of the treated patients have good to excellent results, one third have transient adequate responses, and one third have no noticeable improvement in pain control.

Strontium-89, when administered IV, is taken up in places of active bone turnover. This uptake results in the local release of high quantities of radiation, with enhanced comfort in approximately 50% of cases.

Bisphosphonates

Bisphosphonates may have some efficacy in veterinary medicine to treat primary or metastatic bone disease. Pamidronate and alendronate, given every 3 to 6 weeks, have been associated with enhanced comfort and reossification of lytic sites associated with osteosarcoma, mammary cancer, prostate cancer, and other malignant processes. The author's experience with this analgesic suggests that other options are likely to be more effective. There are some patients in which it works quite well.

Acupuncture

Acupuncture is used to treat many kinds of pain due to cancer or cancer therapy (e.g., surgery, radiation therapy).

It is often used in concert with pharmacologic agents to reduce the dosage and enhance overall wellness. The effect of acupuncture appears to be mediated through opioids. Stimulation of acupuncture points induces the release of endogenous opioids, and opioid antagonists block acupuncture analgesia. Acupuncture analgesia is transferable with cerebrospinal fluid transfer. In human subjects, acupuncture analgesia appears to be most effective against the emotional aspects of pain.[6] Acupuncture can also be helpful for reducing nausea associated with chemotherapy, anesthesia, and the administration of certain antibiotics.

Local anesthesia

Local anesthetic agents (e.g., lidocaine, bupivacaine) can be injected to block sensory or motor nerve fibers (see figures 23-7, 23-9, 23-10, 23-12, 23-13 and 23-15). Lidocaine HCl (2%) administered near an incision provides regional analgesia for about 1 hour. Bupivacaine HCl (0.75%) can be given to provide 6 to 10 hours of regional analgesia for peri-incisional pain. Lidocaine can be administered at or near intercostal nerves proximal to a thoracotomy incision to reduce postsurgical pain. This agent is also frequently administered into the pleural cavity before bupivacaine administration to decrease discomfort associated with thoracotomy. Lidocaine or bupivacaine can be used as a maxillary or mandibular nerve block for oral surgery or in the brachial plexus nerve roots before sectioning during forelimb amputation. Lidocaine can also be administered as a constant-rate infusion to enhance analgesic effect of other drugs while causing depression and anesthesia. The following specific nerve blocks are commonly used to treat the cancer patient.

Intercostal nerve block

The intercostal nerve block can be used to prevent or treat discomfort in the chest and cranial abdomen, including the area of the pancreas:[1]

- A 22-gauge needle attached to extension tubing and that is attached to the syringe filled with the appropriate amount of local anesthesia. The needle is advanced through the surgically prepared skin in each intercostal space. The needle is then advanced from the intercostal space three ribs in front of, to three ribs behind the area in question. The optimal intercostal area is just caudal to the rib, where the nerves are located.
- Aspiration is performed to ensure there is no introduction of lidocaine or bupivacaine IV.
- Lidocaine (canine: 1.5 mg/kg; feline: 1 mg/kg) is administered. The lidocaine can cause short-term discomfort upon injection due to its acidic pH. Some practitioners add injectable bicarbonate to the lidocaine (volume-to-volume ratio of bicarbonate:lidocaine = 10%:90%) to enhance comfort. After the lidocaine is injected, bupivacaine (canine: 1-1.5 mg/kg; feline: 0.5-1 mg/kg) is injected. Bupivacaine, if injected first, can result in discomfort that may last for at least 15 minutes due to the slow onset of local anesthetic effects. Some

practitioners combine the lidocaine and bupivacaine in one syringe. These drugs can also be administered through a chest tube to enhance comfort in the recovery period after a thoracotomy.
- This block can be repeated every 3 to 6 hours.

Infraorbital block

This block is used for analgesia to the rostral maxilla and nearby lip, nose, nasal cavity, and skin ventral to the infraorbital foramen. The infraorbital foramen is palpated rostral and distal to the medial canthus of either eye. A 25-gauge, 2.5-cm needle is inserted through the surgically prepared skin and into the foramen. The attached syringe is aspirated for blood and a small (<1 mL) amount of lidocaine with or without bupivacaine is injected, ideally before any biopsy or surgical procedures.

Mandibular nerve block

The mandibular nerve block is used to provide analgesia of the skin and mucosa at or near the incisors, premolar, and molar teeth on the side to be injected (figure 23-16). This is ideal for surgery to any of this tissue, including mandibulectomy and regional biopsies or tooth extractions.
- The skin overlying the site to be blocked (medial to the mandible) is clipped and prepared as if for surgery. A gloved hand is inserted into the mouth, and the mucosa over the caudal and medial aspect of the mandible under the cheek mucosa is palpated for the mandibular nerve, which can feel like a submucosal thickening or "fibrous band."
- The needle and attached syringe are directed through the skin on the ventromedial aspect of the caudal mandible as directed by the gloved hand. The inserted finger over the nerve is used to guide the needle placement within the tissue next to the nerve. The syringe is aspirated for blood; if none is seen, the local anesthetic is injected to a quantity that should not exceed 1 mL.

Soaker catheter

A soaker catheter is a method of delivering local anesthetic agent(s) to a surgical wound or region of trauma, thereby directing analgesia directly to the site of discomfort. Commercially available soaker catheters or those that are made at the time of surgery are placed through the skin via an incision so that small holes in the catheter will intermittently or continuously deliver lidocaine or other topical analgesics for hours or days. An example of a "home made" soaker catheter is described below:
Required materials:
- 3.5-, 5-, or 8-French red rubber catheter.
- Sterile scissors (Mayo/sharp-blunt).
- Sterile carmalt.
- Heat source, such as a cigarette lighter.
- Sterile 3 and 12 ml syringe.
- Extension set.
- 27- to 22 ga needle.

- Sterile infusion plug.
- Sterile gloves.
- Sterile drape.

Step 1. Seal the distal end of the sterile catheter by first having a non sterile assistant heat the sterile carmault or hemostat and that will then be used to immediately clamp the end of the catheter to melt the it into a closed tube. This can only be done if the tube is sealed above the side holes near the end.

Step 2. Attach a sterile adapter to the proximal end of a red rubber catheter to check for a secure seal by attaching a 3-ml syringe and pushing a small amount of air into the catheter.

Step 3. Use a 27- to 20-ga needle to make holes in the red rubber catheter 5 mm apart the length of the surgical wound to be treated. The needle can go through both sides of the catheter, making two holes with each stick.

Step 4. A stab incision is made with a number 15 blade along side the incision. The sealed tube is pulled through the stab incision so that it extends the entire length of the incision. The holes in the red rubber tube should extend the entire length of the tube within the incision. Ensure that the local anesthetic is coming through the holes before placing the catheter through a stab incision along side the incision to be closed surgically. The incision is sutured closed using standard techniques.

Step 5. Attach the infusion plug to the open end, and preload the catheter with the local anesthetic of choice.

Step 6. Administer lidocaine at 50 ug/kg/min as a constant rate infusion or at 3 mg/kg every 15 minutes.

ROUTES OF ADMINISTRATION[1-5]

The efficacy of a drug, or drug combination, can be enhanced by considering the optimal route of administration. As a general rule, oral analgesics can be effective for mild to moderate discomfort. However, when the degree of discomfort increases efficacy can be increased by administering the same or related drugs IM, SC, or IV. The efficacy can be improved even further by giving the same drug epidurally. A brief discussion of the routes of administration is as follows:
- Oral administration is the easiest and cheapest route and can be performed on an outpatient basis, but it is associated with the lowest level of compliance or efficacy. NSAIDs, tramadol, and gabapentin are most often administered via this route; however, orally administered buprenorphine, codeine, morphine, and sustained-release morphine are also effective for mild to moderate pain.
- IV, IM, and SC administration of drugs is associated with the most predictable efficacy. Injectable NSAIDs, tramadol, and opiates are often very helpful for ensuring comfort. The IV constant-rate infusion technique is optimal. However, this route cannot easily be used in an outpatient setting.
- Epidural or subarachnoid drug therapy can result in good to excellent long-term analgesia. Sterile, preservative-free drugs that have been used in this

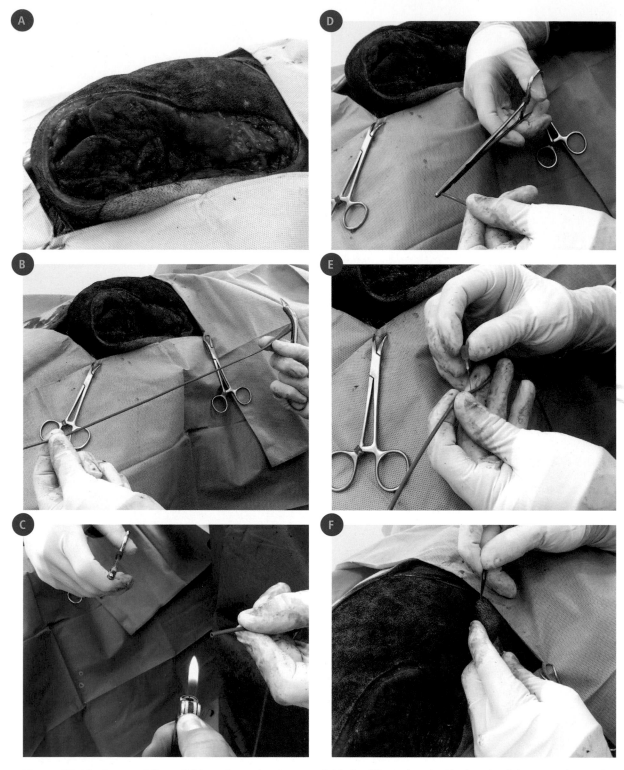

Figure 23-16: Commercially available soaker catheter are available in different lengths. The length of the surgical wound is assessed (A) and a 3.5-, 5-, or 8-French red rubber catheter (B) is selected. The distal end of the sterile catheter is sealed by first having a non sterile assistant heat the sterile carmalt or hemostat (C). This heated instrument will be used to immediately clamp the end of the catheter to melt the catheter into a closed tube (D). This can only be done if the tube is sealed above the side holes near the end. A 22- to 27-ga needle is used to make holes in the red rubber catheter 5 mm apart the length of the surgical wound to be treated (E). The needle can go through both sides of the catheter, making two holes with each stick. A stab incision is made with a number 15 blade along side the incision (F).

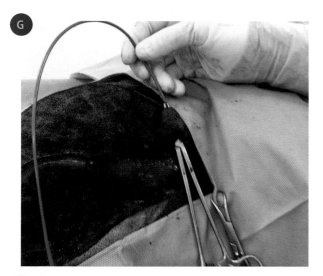

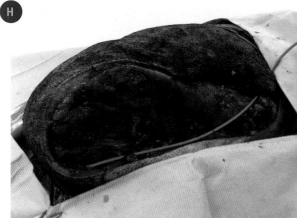

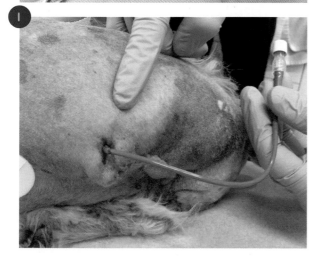

manner include opiates, NSAIDs, ketamine, α_2 agonists, and local anesthetic agents. However, this therapy cannot be performed with the patient as an outpatient.

- Transdermal administration of fentanyl and clonidine, or topical treatment of drugs such as lidocaine, prilocaine, and eutectic mixture of local anesthetics [EMLA] cream, can result in good long-term pain management but is subject to many variables, such as rate of absorption and body condition. Transdermal pain management can be performed as an outpatient therapy.
- Transmucosal therapy with drugs such as fentanyl and buprenorphine may be very helpful in controlling mild discomfort.
- Local nerve blocks provide the precise delivery of local anesthetics directly to the anatomic site of choice with reduced toxicity.

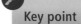

Key point

Oral analgesics can be effective for mild to moderate discomfort however when the degree of discomfort increases, efficacy can be increased by administering the same or related drugs IM, SC, IV, or epidurally.

PREVENTING AND TREATING PAIN AND DISCOMFORT[1]

The best way of managing pain is to prevent it (see tables 23-1 and 23-2). When that is not possible, the discomfort and pain must be treated appropriately and the treatment adjusted continuously as the disease or treatment progresses. Combinations of drugs are most effective and are less likely to result in side effects. Adequate pain therapy can only be achieved by ensuring that the entire team is highly knowledgeable about pain and all the approaches that can be employed to manage discomfort. This includes the client, who is most intimately aware of the patient's quality of life and behavior patterns. The client's perception of the animal's quality of life should be trusted and believed above all.

Pain may be best prevented and treated by dividing it into the categories of acute (e.g.: postoperative) and chronic pain (osteosarcoma of the distal extremity). In most species, severity is far more important than duration of pain with regard to the "memory" of pain. The severity of discomfort at any point in time will result in a repetition of that same degree of discomfort when the same stimulus is applied subsequently. To make the point that preventative analgesia is important, pain is also increased through the wind-up phenomenon. Preventive analgesia helps avoid both the "memory" of pain and the wind-up phenomenon.

Acute pain can be due to the cancer itself, the treatment, or a diagnostic procedure. If discomfort is likely to be inflicted, then a preemptive, immediate, and post-stimulus plan must be designed and implemented. To

Figure 23-16 (cont.): The sealed tube is pulled through the stab incision (G) so that it extends the entire length of the incision (H). The holes in the red rubber tube should extend the entire length of the tube within the incision. The wound is closed normally (I). An adaptor is placed into the open end of the catheter. An extension set attached to the catheter is then hooked to the preload syringe filled with the local anesthetic of choice. Photographs courtesy of Dr. Christian Osmond.

ensure that the plan is effective, the practitioner must determine if the pain to be inflicted is likely to be mild, moderate, or severe and appropriately select the drugs or procedures that are likely to be effective to meet the patient's possible needs.

Chronic pain can also be caused by the cancer (e.g., a metastatic bone lesion in a dog and cat with mammary adenocarcinoma) or, possibly, by a diagnostic or therapeutic procedure, such as chronic infection and implant/plate/screw loosening from a limb-sparing surgery. Unrelenting pain from either cause can last for weeks or months.

Mild pain[1–3,5]

The treatment of mild pain must begin with eliminating the underlying cause and providing general compassionate care, including a comfortable environment, appropriate bedding, and effective bandaging, if indicated. Dogs and cats respond well to gentle comforting, petting, and talking. This is often followed with oral NSAIDs (e.g., robenacoxib, carprofen, deracoxib, etodolac, aspirin, piroxicam, meloxicam, ketoprofen, and, if indicated, local nerve blocks and/or acupuncture. Nonopioids may be used provided that renal and hepatic functions are normal and there is no evidence of gastric inflammation. If NSAIDs are ineffective, an agent from one of the other categories should be selected based on the patient's response.

This type of therapy can include the use of a local lidocaine or bupivacaine nerve block to reduce the local acute discomfort from a needle-core biopsy. An oral NSAID can be given before and after the procedure to manage the relatively minor pain in the hours or few days that follow. That same NSAID can prevent or delay the growth of the primary tumor or metastases, especially if combined with an n-3 polyunsaturated fatty acid like docosahexaenoic acid and metronomic cyclophosphamide. If apprehension is an issue, a tranquillizer such as acepromazine can be used at the time of the procedure.

Key point

The treatment of mild pain must begin with eliminating the underlying cause, providing general compassionate care followed with oral NSAIDs (e.g., robenacoxib, carprofen, deracoxib, etodolac, aspirin, piroxicam, meloxicam, ketoprofen) and, if indicated, local nerve blocks and/or acupuncture and nonopioids provided that renal and hepatic functions are normal.

Moderate pain[1–3, 5]

Moderate pain can be treated by eliminating the cause while providing compassionate care, local analgesia, acupuncture when possible, and nonopioids, including NSAIDs (e.g., robenacoxib, carprofen, etodolac, deracoxib, piroxicam, meloxicam, ketoprofen) in

judicious combination with, tramadol, gabapentin, or amantadine and if needed, opiates. As with all analgesics, the parenteral, continuous administration of these drugs usually results in a more optimal effect than oral therapy. Constant-rate infusion of fentanyl or microdose ketamine is an excellent example. Transdermal delivery of drugs such as fentanyl or lidocaine patches can provide a background of analgesia via a continuous-release delivery system; however, this is rarely adequate alone to prevent perioperative or procedural discomfort. When these therapies are not adequate, an α_2-adrenergic agonist, opioid agonist-antagonist, anxiolytic, or tricyclic antidepressant can be considered.

When an acutely painful procedure is considered, drugs for the cancer patient are often divided into pre-, peri-, and postoperative analgesics.[1,2] Preoperative analgesics often include an opiate such as morphine with or without acepromazine to calm the patient and to relieve anxiety. Atropine or glycopyrrolate are sometimes administered to prevent bradycardia associated with the opiate. Nerve blocks are employed whenever possible. Perioperative therapy is often accomplished by adding fentanyl as a continuous IV infusion. This can decrease the need for additional analgesia and may be combined with microdose ketamine to prevent the wind-up phenomenon, especially when used with fentanyl and lidocaine in an FLK mixture (see above). Pain management in the immediate postoperative period is optimal when local nerve blocks are used in combination with fentanyl and microdose ketamine. Later, acepromazine, diazepam, or midazolam can be used to reduce dysphoria. See the box 23-1 for examples of pre-, peri-, and postoperative analgesia to treat moderate pain.

Key point

Moderate pain can be treated by eliminating the cause while providing compassionate care, local analgesia, acupuncture when possible, nonopioids, including NSAIDs (e.g., robenacoxib, carprofen, etodolac, deracoxib, piroxicam, meloxicam, ketoprofen) in judicious combination with, tramadol, gabapentin, or amantadine and, if needed, opiates. As with all analgesics, the parenteral, continuous administration of these drugs usually results in a more optimal effect than oral therapy.

Severe pain[1,3,6]

Therapy for moderate to severe pain can be emotionally and physically difficult for the entire veterinary health care team and the family. Everyone should be aware of the difficulty of this type of emotional and physical stress and be supported to prevent *compassion fatigue*, which is reviewed elsewhere.

Therapy for severe pain is as outlined for moderate pain (above); however, the dosages of certain drugs, notably the opiates, are continuously adjusted to a balance between maximum efficacy and minimal toxicity. The efficacy of drugs can be maximized by switching to more effective routes of administration such as epidural morphine and constant-rate infusion of fentanyl. When drugs are combined, efficacy is often enhanced and reduction of dosages of individual drugs may be possible; however, the patient must be monitored for additive toxicity. Palliative procedures such as the use of radiation therapy at sites of bone pain can be profoundly beneficial, as can the IV infusion of bisphosphonates. When the degree of discomfort increases, dosages can be escalated for opiates with no ceiling effect (e.g., morphine); changing the route of analgesic administration (e.g., switching from subcutaneous to intravenous administration or to epidural therapy) may also be effective. As with moderate discomfort, sustained-release fentanyl patches or the more recently approved fentanyl sustained release solution or lidocaine patches, which are applied to the skin and slowly release the analgesic over 72 hours, may be helpful. See the box 23-2 for examples of pre-, peri-, and postoperative analgesia to treat severe pain.

Key point

Therapy for severe pain is as outlined for moderate pain, however, the dosages of certain drugs, notably the opiates, are continuously adjusted to a balance between maximum efficacy and minimal toxicity. Quality of life is everything!

SUMMARY

Pain therapy is one of the most important aspects of cancer therapy, not only for the patient and the client, but also for the entire veterinary health care team. Well-thought-out therapeutic approaches are key to the anticipation and prevention of pain. It is the responsibility of the veterinary health care team to stay up-to-date on the many current and emerging pain therapies and to gain experience in the optimal management of the canine and feline cancer patient.

Box 23-1. Treatment of moderate pain associated with invasive procedures for the dog and cat (normal CBC, biochemical profile)

Indication: Simple, minimally painful, short-term procedure (e.g., needle-core biopsy of tumor, small incisional biopsy)
- Preemptive analgesia: oxymorphone SQ or hydromorphone SQ or fentanyl SQ, acepromazine SC plus a local block.
- Anesthesia (as indicated): propofol induction followed by inhalant anesthesia.
- Postoperative analgesia after full recovery and adequate hydration: ketoprofen 2.2 mg/kg SC and/or one of the following: robenacoxib (feline), ketoprofen PO, piroxicam PO, meloxicam PO (canine and in countries that allow it, feline), carprofen PO (canine and in countries that allow it, feline), deracoxib PO (canine), etodolac PO (canine).

Indication: Simple, moderately painful, short-term procedure (e.g., nasal biopsy or bone biopsy in a dog with normal organ and cardiovascular function)
- Preemptive analgesia: Oxymorphone SC or Fentanyl SQ or Hydromorphone SQ
- Anesthesia (as indicated): Propofol induction followed by inhalant anesthesia.
- Postoperative analgesia: Ketoprofen SC.

Indication: Relatively short, simple procedure (e.g., thoracoscopy, laparoscopy, abdominal exploratory, skin biopsy)
- Preemptive analgesia: Hydromorphone SC or Fentanyl SQ, Acepromazine SC
- Anesthesia (as indicated): Propofol induction followed by inhalant anesthesia.
- Postoperative analgesia (one of the following):
  - Morphine SQ
  - Fentanyl SQ
  - Buprenorphine PO
  - Hydromorphone SQ
  - Nalbuphine SC prn
  - Ketoprofen SC
  - Carprofen SC
- Home analgesia (one of the following):
  - Tramadol PO
  - Transdermal Fentanyl if needed and/or one of the following: Robenacoxib (feline), Ketoprofen PO, Piroxicam PO, Meloxicam PO (canine and in countries that allow it, feline), Carprofen PO (canine and in countries that allow it, feline), Deracoxib PO (canine), Etodolac PO (canine)

Box 23-2. Treatment of severe pain associated with invasive procedures in the dog and the cat (normal CBC, biochemical profile)

Indication: Procedure thought to cause moderate to severe discomfort (e.g., maxillectomy, hemipelvectomy, chest wall resection)
- Preemptive analgesia: hydromorphone or buprenorphine SC, acepromazine SC with nerve block, if appropriate to local area. Ketamine microdose constant-rate infusion after an IV bolus of ketamine can reduce the need for analgesics postoperatively.
- Anesthesia (as indicated): propofol or thiopental induction followed by inhalant anesthesia.
- Postoperative analgesia: fentanyl bolus IV followed by fentanyl infusion IV constant-rate infusion by syringe pump or IV pump; bupivacaine nerve block and acupuncture.
- Home analgesia (one or more of of the following):
  - Buprenorphone PO.
  - Transdermal fentanyl may be administered with or without one of the following: Robenacoxib (feline), Ketoprofen PO, piroxicam PO, meloxicam PO (canine and in countries that allow it, feline), carprofen PO (canine and in countries that allow it, feline), deracoxib PO (canine), etodolac PO (canine).

Indication: Procedure thought to cause severe discomfort (e.g., mandibulectomy, laminectomy in combination with hemipelvectomy).
- Preemptive analgesia: hydromorphone SQ with nerve block, if appropriate, to local area (infraorbital block for maxillectomy, for example).
- Anesthesia (as indicated): propofol or thiopental induction followed by inhalant anesthesia.
- Postoperative analgesia: fentanyl bolus followed by fentanyl infusion constant-rate infusion by syringe pump or IV pump; bupivacaine nerve block.
- Home analgesia (one of the following):
  - Buprenorphine PO.
  - Transdermal fentanyl may be administered with or without one of the following: robenacoxib (feline), ketoprofen PO, piroxicam PO, meloxicam PO (canine and in countries that allow it, feline), carprofen PO (canine and in countries that allow it, feline), deracoxib PO (canine), etodolac PO (canine).

Indication: Procedure thought to cause severe discomfort (e.g., such as rear-limb amputation, hemipelvectomy)
- Preemptive analgesia: hydromorphone SC with bupivacaine epidural.
- Anesthesia: propofol induction followed by inhalant anesthesia.
- Postoperative analgesia: fentanyl bolus (SC followed by fentanyl infusion IV constant-rate infusion by syringe pump or IV pump; bupivacaine nerve block.
- Home analgesia: sustained-release morphine PO for dogs only or fentanyl patch (canine or feline) with or without one of the following:
  - Ketoprofen PO or
  - Piroxicam PO or
  - Meloxicam PO (canine and in some countries, feline) or
  - Carprofen PO (canine and in some countries, feline) or
  - Deracoxib PO (canine) or
  - Etodolac PO (canine).

References

1. Gaynor JS, Muir WS (eds): *Handbook of Veterinary Pain Management*. St. Louis, Mosby, 2002 pp 13–447.
2. Tranquilli WK, Grimm KA, Lamont LA (eds): *Pain Management for the Small Animal Practitioner*, Jackson, Wyoming, Teton New Media, 2000, pp 13–69.
3. Lascelles BDX. Relief of chronic cancer pain. In Dobson JM, Lascelles BDX (eds): *BSAVA Manual of Canine and feline and Feline Oncology*. (ed 2) Gloucester, England. British Small Animal Veterinary Association, 2003, pp 137–151.
4. Hellyer P, Rodan I, Brunt J, Downing R, Hagedorn JE, Robertson SA. AAHA/AAFP pain management guidelines for dogs & cats. *J Am Anim Hosp Assoc.* 43(5):235-248, 2007.
5. Hellyer PW, Gaynor JS: Acute postsurgical pain in dogs and cats and cats. *Compend Contin Educ Pract Vet* 20:140–153, 1998.
6. Sparkes AH, Heiene R, Lascelles BD, Malik R, Sampietro LR, Robertson S, Scherk M, Taylor P; ISFM and AAFP. ISFM and AAFP consensus guidelines: long-term use of NSAIDs in cats. *J Feline Med Surg.* 2010 ;12(7):521-538, 2010.

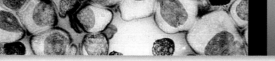

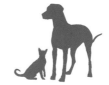

Chapter 24

Second commandment: don't let them vomit (or have diarrhea)! Nausea, vomiting, diarrhea management

Cancer and cancer therapy can be associated with nausea, vomiting, and diarrhea.[1-5] Vomiting can lead to life-threatening problems such as dehydration, severe metabolic imbalances, and wound dehiscence due to increased abdominal pressure. In addition, clients often get the impression that their pet is experiencing unnecessary toxicities, which may result in abandonment of life-saving treatment and subsequent euthanasia. Gastrointestinal problems are common in human cancer patients and thus our clients are often worried this same malady will befall their precious pet. No wonder our clients are so concerned. In one study, seventy five percent of people receiving combination chemotherapy experience vomiting.[1] Fortunately, these problems are much less common in dogs and cats. In fact, in one study completed by the author, clients were asked to enumerate the number of episodes of vomiting and nausea before, during and after receiving five chemotherapeutic agents for the treatment of lymphoma over a 25-week period in 73 dogs. In this study, there was no more nausea or vomiting associated with the administration of any one of the five chemotherapeutic agents. Surprisingly, the clients reported that there was just as much nausea and vomiting before and after receiving chemotherapy as during the 25 week period of receiving chemotherapy. Regardless, risk factors for vomiting include administration of highly emetogenic chemotherapy (e.g.: the rarely used cisplatin), smaller patient size, repetitive administration of chemotherapy, and presence of underlying pathology in the gastrointestinal tract, such as dietary allergies.[2-5] Management of nausea and vomiting is vital to improve the patient's quality of life, which subsequently can enhance response to therapy and increase survival time.

MECHANISM OF VOMITING

Tumor-induced vomiting may be caused by the presence of a tumor that physically obstructs the intestinal tract. Surgical resection or stenting of the tumor is often the only solution to this clinical problem. Chemotherapeutic agents differ in their emetic potential and in the length of time after administration that they cause emesis.[1-8] Unlike humans, animals rarely exhibit any evidence of nausea and vomiting at or shortly after the time drugs are administered, with the exception of patients that receive cisplatin chemotherapy.[4,5] This drug should never be given intravenously to cats. The emetic potential of all chemotherapeutic drugs depends on the sensitivity of each patient as well as the route of administration and the dosage. Drugs associated with low, moderate, and relatively high probabilities of vomiting are listed below (table 24-1).

Chemotherapy may induce nausea and vomiting shortly after administration or as late as 5 to 10 days after administration. In dogs, cisplatin may induce vomiting within 1 to 6 hours, whereas cyclophosphamide may induce vomiting within 4 to 12 hours. Cats may just stop eating. Doxorubicin may induce vomiting in a few patients 4 to 6 hours after treatment whereas others develop nausea 3-5 days when the upper intestinal tract is most sensitive post therapy. All of these chemotherapeutic agents can induce vomiting 3 to 5 days after treatment because of damage to the gastrointestinal tract.

The mechanism of chemotherapy-induced vomiting is complex. The emetic center in the medulla

Table 24-1. Chemotherapeutic agents by probability of inducing nausea or vomiting

Very low[a]	Chlorambucil
	Doxorubicin, liposomal
	L-asparaginase
	Vinblastine
	Vinorelbine
	Steroids
	Bleomycin
Low[a]	Mitoxantrone
	Gemcitabine
	Paclitaxel (Caution in cats)
Moderate[b]	Carboplatin
	Cyclophosphamide
	Doxorubicin
	Methotrexate
	Daunorubicin
	Ifosfamide
High[c]	Dacarbazine
	Nitrogen mustard
Very high[c]	Cisplatin (Not in cats)
	Streptozocin (Caution in cats)

For prevention of emesis:
[a] Very low, to low emetic potential: Metoclopramide and/or Maropitant as needed
[b] Moderate emetic potential: Metoclopramide and Maropitant preventively
[c] High to very high emetic potential: Maropitant or a serotonin antagonist + metoclopramide or butorphanol + steroids preventively

coordinates vomiting and receives input from at least four sources: the chemoreceptor trigger zone (CTZ), peripheral receptors, the cerebral cortex, and the vestibular apparatus. The vestibular apparatus probably does not influence cancer- or chemotherapy-associated vomiting. The CTZ is located in the fourth ventricle of the medulla. It is activated solely by chemical stimuli and plays an important role in chemotherapy-induced nausea and vomiting. Acute nausea and vomiting is mediated by activation of serotonin (5-hydroxytryptamine) type 3 (5-HT-3) receptors in the gastrointestinal tract.1 Peripheral receptors can be triggered either directly by chemotherapeutic agents or indirectly by substances released by the agents' effects on other sites; these impulses arrive at the emetic center via the vagus nerve and other autonomic nerve afferents. Input from higher cognitive centers, a common source of vomiting in humans, is rarely identified in animals. The mechanism of delayed vomiting days to weeks after therapy is unknown. Pharmacologic intervention through any or all of these pathways is important for eliminating vomiting in the cancer patient.

GENERAL CONCEPTS OF EMESIS THERAPY

Most chemotherapeutic agents are unlikely to induce vomiting in animals shortly after administration.[2–5] The exception is cisplatin, which is associated with short lived, self-limiting vomiting within a few hours after treatment.[4,5] Moore and colleagues[5] demonstrated that butorphanol (0.4 mg/kg) administered intramuscularly (IM) at the end of cisplatin infusion was effective for reducing cisplatin chemotherapy–induced vomiting from an incidence of 90% to less than 20%. Another study[4] demonstrated that when vomiting occurred, it was almost always in smaller dogs. If an animal vomited after the first dose of cisplatin, that animal was much more likely than other patients to vomit subsequently, implying that individual animals may be more susceptible to the emetic effects of chemotherapy.

Key point

With the exception of cisplatin, most chemotherapeutic agents are unlikely to induce vomiting in animals shortly after administration.

SELF-LIMITING VOMITING[1–3]

An underlying cause for acute, potentially self-limiting vomiting should be identified and corrected whenever possible. Vomiting should be treated as soon as it is identified as follows:

- Give nothing by mouth until vomiting ceases for at least 12 hours.
- Administer metoclopramide and/or Maropitant or one of the serotonin antagonists to improve quality of life and to speed recovery. Ideally, the antiemetic should initially be administered parenterally. Some serotonin antagonists are available in a rapidly dissolving transmucosal oral delivery system, which is another good route of administration (figure 24-1).
- Subsequently, very small amounts of water (e.g., ice cubes) followed by a bland diet can be offered every 2 to 4 hours.
- Once the animal is able to take in food without vomiting, it can be slowly returned to a normal diet. During this transition period, the food should be soft in consistency, low in fat, and high in carbohydrates. Fat is a complex nutrient that is difficult to digest, can delay gastric emptying, and may induce diarrhea.
- Patients with minimal dehydration can receive fluids subcutaneously (SC); however, intravenous therapy is preferred for significantly dehydrated patients. Many patients improve dramatically shortly after the administration of intravenous fluids.

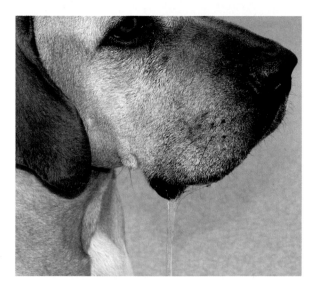

Figure 24-1: Nausea and vomting are an unacceptable consequence of cancer therapy as there are a number of options to delay or prevent this adverse effect. Prevention of nausea and vomiting with acupuncture, maropitant, metoclopramide, ondansetron or mirtazapine is preferable to treating this problem after it occurs. Most nausea is prevented with maropitant alone, however in cases where there is limited peristalsis of the gastrointestinal tract, metoclopramide may be an ideal choice. If nausea precludes the use of drugs that must be swallowed, then these same drugs can be given by injection. Finally, ondansetron and mirtazapine are available as an oral disintegrating tablet that allows the drug to be almost completely absorbed transmucosally.

- Potassium supplementation of intravenous fluids should be provided if hypokalemia is identified (table 24-2).

LIFE-THREATENING VOMITING[1-3, 5]

Clients are often frightened that cancer and cancer therapy will degrade and destroy the quality of life of the cancer patient. Therefore, life-threatening vomiting is not only a serious medical issue but also an emotional 'emergency' for clients. The cause of life-threatening vomiting should be identified and corrected as soon as possible. Specific treatment recommendations include:
- Fluid therapy should be administered to all patients, especially to those that are severely dehydrated (8% to 12% of normal hydration).
- Deficits in fluid and electrolytes secondary to dehydration should be replaced during the first 24 hours. In addition, approximately 66 mL/kg/day of maintenance fluids should be administered. Continued losses, such as from vomiting and diarrhea, should be estimated and replaced.
- As noted previously, potassium chloride (KCl) should be supplemented in the fluids, especially if hypokalemia is identified. Potassium should not be administered at a rate greater than 0.5 mEq/kg/hr

Table 24-2. Intravenous potassium supplementation to correct hypokalemia

Serum potassium (mEq/L)	KCl Maximum added to each liter of fluid (mEq)	Rate of Infusion (mL/kg/hr)*
<2	80	6
2.1–2.5	60	8
2.6–3.0	40	12
3.1–3.5	28	16

* Above this rate the risk of life threatening complications increase.

because this may cause cardiac arrest and death.
- The patient should be monitored for fluid overload using the following parameters: body weight, capillary refill time, skin turgor, chest auscultation, packed cell volume, total solids, and central venous pressure. If vomiting is not likely to subside in a short period, antiemetics such as metoclopramide (constant-rate infusion) and a serotonin antagonist (e.g., ondansetron or dolasetron, especially the oral disintegrating tablets or the intravenous formulation) should be employed; they can be combined for greater efficacy. If vomiting is caused by chemotherapeutic agents, pretreatment with antiemetics is indicated for all future administrations.

Key point

Clients are often frightened that cancer and cancer therapy will degrade and destroy the quality of life of their pet; therefore, life-threatening vomiting is not only a serious medical issue but also an emotional 'emergency' for clients.

ANTIEMETIC AGENTS

Tables 24-3 and 24-4 lists selected antiemetic agents and their recommended dosages for use in dogs and cats.

Maropitant[1-3, 7]

Maropitant works quite well in dogs and in cats as an NK1 receptor antagonist. The drug has been shown to be safe and effective to reduce or prevent acute or delayed vomiting from a wide variety of peripheral and central stimuli that impacts the emetic center, including chemotherapeutic agents. The product comes in an oral and injectable form and can be administered orally, intravenously, intramuscularly and subcutaneously. Given once a day, the drug acts as a ligand for substance P receptors located in the emetic center of the brainstem, particularly the nucleus tractus solitarius. While many believe it is the drug of choice to prevent or delay vomiting, it also prevents motion sickness (in dogs >4 months of age at 8 mg/kg PO) and may have some analgesic and antitussive properties. The dosage to prevent or treat acute vomiting in dogs 4 months of age and older is 1 mg/kg IV over 1-2 minutes or SC q24h for up to 5 consecutive days or at least 2 mg/kg PO til vomiting resolves. The dosage to prevent or treat acute vomiting in cats 4 months of age and older is 1 mg/kg IV over 1-2 minutes or SC q24h for up to 5 consecutive days or 1 mg/kg PO til vomiting resolves.

Metoclopramide[1-3, 7]

Metoclopramide is one of the most commonly administered antiemetics in veterinary medicine. Its antiemetic effect is both central and peripheral. Centrally, metoclopramide is a dopamine antagonist that blocks the CTZ and prevents emesis. Peripherally, it increases the tone of the caudal esophageal sphincter and increases gastric antral contractions by relaxing the pylorus and duodenum, thereby reducing the rate of stomach emptying. Metoclopramide can be given to dogs at a dosage of 0.2 to 0.5 mg/kg IM or SC every 8 hours or at a dosage of 1 to 2 mg/kg as a constant-rate infusion over a 24-hour period by an intravenous pump. This drug should not be given if there is an intestinal obstruction.

Metoclopramide is dispensed at many veterinary health care centers along with maropitant with instructions to administer both drugs before or after chemotherapeutic agents to enhance and improve quality of life. Metoclopramide is relatively safe and inexpensive and readily available. Should nausea and vomiting occur, use of this drug alone or in combination with maropitant a serotonin antagonist such as dolasetron or ondansetron, is recommended. Adverse effects are rare, but can include extrapyramidal effects resulting in odd behavior when very high dosages are used.

Key point

Metoclopramide and Maropitant are dispensed by many veterinary health care professionals with instructions to administer both drugs before or after chemotherapeutic agents to enhance and improve quality of life.

Serotonin antagonists[1-3, 6]

Drugs that inhibit the 5-HT-3 receptor (e.g., ondansetron, dolasetron) constitute a newer and effective class of antiemetics to prevent and treat nausea. These drugs come in oral and intravenous formulations. The oral formulations are standard tablets and a formulation that dissolves and is absorbed transmucosally. Serotonin antagonists

Table 24-3. Selected antiemetics for use in dogs

Generic name	Dosage
Recommended	
Maropitant	1-2 mg/kg q24 hrs IM, SQ, IV, PO
Metoclopramide	1–2 mg/kg constant-rate infusion IV over 24 hr
Ondansetron	0.1-0.5 mg/kg IV, PO 15 min before chemotherapy then daily to bid
Dolasetron	0.1-0.3 mg/kg IV, PO 15 min before chemotherapy then daily to bid
Butorphanol	0.4 mg/kg IM q8h
Less effective	
Chlorpromazine	0.5 mg/kg IM, SC, rectal suppository q6–8h
Prochlorperazine	0.1–0.5 mg/kg IM, SC q6–8h
	1.0 mg/kg rectally q8h
Prochlorperazine- Isopropamide	0.5–0.8 mg/kg IM, SC q12h
Yohimbine	0.25-0.5 mg/kg SC, IM bid
Diphenhydramine	2.0–4.0 mg/kg PO q8h
Dimenhydrinate	8 mg/kg PO q8h
Trimethobenzamide	3 mg/kg IM q8h
Domperidone	0.1–0.3 mg/kg IM, IV bid
Investigational	
Haloperidol	110 µg/kg q 4 days (investigational)
Pimozide	100 µg/kg q 6 days (investigational)
Dexamethasone	1–3 mg IV (investigational)

Table 24-4. Selected antiemetics for use in cats

Generic name	Dosage
Maropitant	1 mg/kg/day IM, SQ, PO
Chlorpromazine	0.5 mg/kg q6–8h IM, SQ
Prochlorperazine	0.1–0.5 mg/kg q6–8h IM, SQ
Diphenhydramine	2.0–4.0 mg/kg q8h PO
Butorphanol	0.1–0.4 mg/kg q1–4h IM, IV, SQ
Dimenhydrinate	8 mg/kg q8h PO
Prochlorperazine	0.5–0.8 mg/kg q12h IM, SQ
Metoclopramide	1–2 mg/kg CRI IV over 24 hours or 0.5 mg/kg PO q6–8h
Ondansetron	0.1–0.3 mg/kg IV 15 min before and 12 hr after chemotherapy or PO q12h
Dolasetron	0.6–3 mg/kg IV q24h
Dexamethasone	1–3 mg IV

are most effective when used in combination with other drugs, such as metoclopramide. Ondansetron and dolasetron are two of the most commonly used antiemetics available. They are equipotent at recommended dosages; however, once the serotonin receptors are fully occupied, increasing the dosage does not enhance efficacy. Serotonin antagonists are effective for reducing vomiting from all chemotherapy agents, including cisplatin in the dog. They appear to be less toxic than other antiemetics, including metoclopramide. Ondansetron and other serotonin antagonists are expensive, but their cost is expected to decline in the future. In addition, early use of these drugs may reduce the need for hospitalization and length of hospital stay, thereby reducing costs. (For dosage recommendations, see tables 24-3 and 24-4.)

Cyproheptadine has some antiserotonin effects, but its efficacy in preventing severe vomiting is poor. It may be a better appetite stimulant.

Narcotic analgesics[1–3]

Butorphanol (0.4 mg/kg IM) is a controlled drug that has been shown to reduce the prevalence of vomiting in response to the administration of cisplatin. The drug also has analgesic properties. For best results, butorphanol should be administered intramuscularly at the end of the cisplatin infusion. This drug has little effect in preventing streptozocin-induced vomiting.

Phenothiazines[1–3]

Phenothiazines (e.g., chlorpromazine, prochlorperazine) block the CTZ and are commonly used as antiemetics

for mild chemotherapy-induced nausea. In human medicine, phenothiazines generally are not effective for reducing efferent gastrointestinal irritation. These drugs can induce vasodilation and therefore should not be used in dehydrated patients or in those with poor cardiac output. In addition, phenothiazines can induce mild depression and make patient monitoring difficult. All phenothiazines can cause seizures in predisposed animals. For these reasons, the author does not recommend their use as first-line therapy. Chlorpromazine can be administered at 0.5 mg/kg IM or SC every 6 to 8 hours; prochlorperazine can be dosed at 0.1 to 0.5 mg/kg IM or SC every 6 to 8 hours. A suppository form (Compazine®, GlaxoSmithKline) is available for use in selected patients.

Antihistamines[1–3]

Antihistamines (e.g., diphenhydramine, dimenhydrinate, trimethobenzamide) are another class of antiemetics. They block input from the vestibular system and work against motion-induced vomiting. Diphenhydramine can be administered at 2 to 4 mg/kg PO every 8 hours; it can cause mild sedation.

Dopamine antagonists and diphenylbutylpiperidine[1–3]

Haloperidol is another dopamine antagonist that blocks the CTZ and can prevent vomiting for up to 4 days in dogs at a dose of 110 μg/kg. Pimozide, a long-acting diphenylbutylpiperidine, can protect dogs and cats from drug-induced vomiting for up to 6 days when given at a dose of 100 μg/kg. Clinical experience with these two drugs in dogs is minimal.

Corticosteroids[1-3]

Dexamethasone has been shown to have antiemetic activity. Its mechanism is unknown. Side effects are few except in patients with diabetes or gastric ulcers. Relatively small (1–3 mg) intravenous doses of dexamethasone are effective in humans; an appropriate dosage in dogs or cats is not known at this time. In human cancer patients, combinations of dexamethasone with serotonin antagonists are very effective. These combinations are therefore are being explored in veterinary oncology.

Cannabinoids[1-3]

Many veterinarians are asked about the antiemetic effects of cannabinoids. Dronabinol is the only orally available formulation commercially available at this time, however, its use and efficacy in the dog is unknown. In human patients, dranabinol is effective for moderate to mild vomiting, but much more effective and less toxic agents exist. The mechanism of cannabinoids is not clearly understood, but it appears to mediate its effects centrally. Until more definitive information is known, cannabinoids are not recommended for routine use in dogs or cats.

Neurokinin-1 receptor antagonists[1-3]

Neurokinin-1 (NK-1) receptor antagonists are the newest antiemetics in human and veterinary medicine and have dramatically reduced vomiting and nausea in the dog and cat with cancer. The NK-1 receptor mediates the centrally-mediated vomiting reflex, and its antagonists have been shown to be very effective in preventing and treating nausea and vomiting. These drugs are quite effective and can be administered IV, SQ, or orally.

Key point

Neurokinin-1 (NK-1) receptor antagonists are the newest antiemetics in human and veterinary medicine that have dramatically reduced vomiting and nausea in the dog and cat with cancer.

DIARRHEA[1-3]

Diarrhea can occur in the cancer patient from a number of causes unrelated to the cancer or cancer therapy, such as inflammatory bowel disease, dietary allergies, food poisoning, bacterial overgrowth, pancreatic disorders and internal parasites or other causes such as:
- A direct effect of the cancer on the gastrointestinal tract,
- An effect of the cancer induced changes in metabolism.
- A direct effect of cancer therapy.

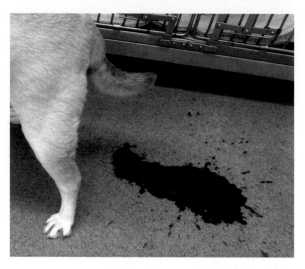

Figure 24-2: Small bowel (large amounts of loose stool, minimal straining, no fresh blood in the stool) or large bowel (small amounts of blood-tinged stool, frequent efforts to strain to defecate) diarrhea can be prevented by limiting rapid changes in the diet, ensuring that there is adequate fiber in the diet, and by administering either metronidazole and/or tylosin.

- A result of acute dietary changes that often occur as our clients do everything they can at home to maintain appetite.

Indeed, lymphoma or solid tumors of the intestinal tract are often associated with large or small bowel diarrhea. Until the underlying cause is resolved, it is highly unlikely that this problem will resolve. Cancer patients often have nutritional deficiencies such as depletion in the serum levels of glutamine, vitamin B$_{12}$ and other nutrients. Supplementing these nutrients may be helpful in some patients. Chemotherapy can cause diarrhea and that lose stool may not be noted for 3-5 days after chemotherapy is administered due to action on the rapidly growing crypt cells that are replacing the senescent enterocytes. Finally, rapid dietary changes can sometimes result in gastrointestinal distress that can be profound.

The first step is to meet the needs of the patient such as providing adequate hydration via intravenous fluids, prescribing appropriate anti-emetics, antibiotics and antidiarrheals such as tylosin and metronidazol. Every attempt should be made to diagnose the underlying cause before prescribing therapy. The first step in this process is to determine if there is small bowel or large bowel diarrhea. The signs are often distinct (table 24-5).

Diagnostics

A minimum database for chronic diarrhea of undisclosed causes includes a complete blood count and biochemistry profile, fecal flotation for ova as well as a fecal saline wet mount for

Table 24-5. Sings of small bowel and large bowel diarrhea

Sign	Small bowel diarrhea	Large bowel diarrhea
Frequency of bowel movement	Usually Normal	Often increased
Volume	Usually increased	Normal or decreased
Blood	Uncommon but if it is present, then it is as black digested blood (melena)	Common (frank blood)
Mucus	Absent	Common
Presence of undigested food	May occur	Absent
Color	Sometimes abnormal	Normal
Steatorrhea	Uncommon	Absent
Weight loss	Common	Rare
Polyphagia	Common	Rare
Urgency	Absent	Common
Straining	Uncommon	Common, small amounts of stool, often with Fresh blood, mucus
Vomiting	Uncommon	Common

protozoa. A serum T_4 test should be run in older cats, and all cats should be evaluated for FeLV and FIV infections. Serial zinc sulfate flotation tests or the ProSpecT® *Giardia* microplate ELISA assay may be helpful for diagnosing Giardia infections. *Cryptosporidium parvum* is a coccidia that can infect people and cats. Diagnosis of this organism is via modified Ziehl-Neelsen or Kinyoun acid-fast staining techniques, immunofluorescence detection or the Alexon ProSpecT® *Cryptosporidium* microplate enzyme immunoassay. *Tritrichomonas foetus* may cause diarrhea in cats and may be identified with light microscopy as a motile flagellated organism, which looks similar to *Giardia*. A PCR for *Tritrichomonas* is more sensitive and exquisitely specific and is the gold standard. Fecal culture may be considered when specific pathogens are to be investigated.

For large bowel diarrhea, cytology from rectal scrapings and Gram stain of prepared slides may be very helpful in achieving a definitive diagnosis in many cases of large bowel diarrhea. Rectal cytology may diagnose bacterial or non-septic suppurative colitis. The presence of clostridial spores with a positive fecal enterotoxin assay can confirm clostridial colitis.

For recurrent or non-resolving small or large bowel diarrhea, diagnostic ultrasound can be helpful for diagnosing a foreign body, intussusceptions, inflammatory or infiltrative disease as well as alterations in hepatic, pancreatic and lymph node structure. Biopsies or aspiration may be performed using ultrasound guidance.

Texas A and M University has a specific GI panel to help diagnose persistent diarrhea. The panel includes serum folate, cobalamin, trypsin-like immunoreactivity (TLI) and pancreatic-like immunoreactivity (PLI) levels for the dog and the cat. If that is not diagnostic, then an endoscopic or surgically obtained biopsy of the upper and/or lower gastrointestinal tract can be quite informative.

Surgically or endoscopically obtained biopsies are required to confirm suspicion of an inflammatory bowel disease and to differentiate IBD from neoplastic disease. Full thickness biopsies may be needed to diagnose the latter group of conditions because superficial histologic changes may be indistinguishable from IBD.

Therapeutics

In recurrent and chronic diarrhea, fluid therapy should be used when dehydration is noted. In general, a highly digestible, low residue diet with moderate protein, low to moderate fat and carbohydrate levels is often helpful. Fiber is important for bowel health and is often used to treat diarrhea. Soluble fiber (oat bran, pectin, beet pulp, vegetable gums, psyllium) are readily digested by bacteria and provide large quantities of short chain fatty acids, beneficial for colonic health. Psyllium (Metamucil) has 79% soluble fiber (with 21% insoluble), oat bran has 50%, wheat bran has 11% and cooked white rice has 0% soluble fiber. Insoluble fibers (cellulose, lignin, wheat bran) are less able to absorb water. They are able to bind toxins, bile acids and may help normalize transit time.

Probiotics have made a great impact in veterinary medicine in the treatment of dogs and cats with diarrhea. Based on the available clinical research in dogs and cats, it appears that certain probiotics shorten recovery time in dogs with acute, non-specific, self-limiting diarrhea. Most of the probiotic research in dogs and cats includes the *Lactobacillus* species, *Bacillus subtilis*, and *Enterococcus faecium* SF68.

More specific dietary therapies are as follows:
- **Gastritis:** Consider a highly digestible, low fat diet such as cooked chicken, turkey, eggs, cooked rice given in small amounts frequently throughout the day.
- **Acute diarrhea:** Consider withholding food initially and then initiating a highly digestible, low fat diet such as cooked chicken, turkey, eggs, cooked rice given in small amounts. A probiotic may be used.
- **Chronic small bowel diarrhea:** Highly digestible, low fat in dogs such as cooked chicken, turkey, eggs and rice. In cats, consider a low carbohydrate diet that such as cooked chicken or turkey. In dogs and cats, probiotics and vitamin B_{12} may also be therapeutic.
- **Chronic large bowel diarrhea:** Consider a diet that has moderate to high amounts of soluble and insoluble sources of fiber. In some cases, a hypoallergenic (hydrolyzed protein/ novel protein) diet and probiotics are quite helpful.

Other therapies that are used in veterinary medicine include:
- Oral protectants such as bismuth subsalicylate may help some patients. Motility modifiers such as loperamide may slow the transit times.
- Metronidazole (10 mg/kg PO q12h) for its immunoregulatory actions; if the patient has concurrent hepatic disease, the dose should be reduced to 7.5 mg/kg PO q12h. At a higher dosage of f 25 mg/kg PO q12h X 5–10 days, this drug can be helpful for treating for *Giardia*.
- Tylosin has been shown to be effective in treating small and large bowel diarrhea in dogs and cats.

It has been reported to increase the proportions of *Enterococcus*-like organisms in the intestine of healthy dogs and possibly cats suggesting that tylosin may indirectly induce a probiotic effect. This makes sense as some enterococci strains are known to have probiotic characteristics that attenuate inflammation on the gut mucosa and normalize the fecal consistency in dogs with diarrhea.
- Anthelmintics should be used when specific parasites have been identified. Given that cancer patients are generally older, parasites are less commonly identified.

Key point

Tylosin has been shown to be effective in treating small and large bowel diarrhea in dogs and cats as this drug has been reported to increase the proportions of *Enterococcus*-like organisms in the intestine of healthy dogs and possibly cats suggesting that tylosin may indirectly induce a probiotic effect.

References

1. Hainsworth JD: Nausea and vomiting, in Abeloff MD, Armitage JO, Niedelhuber JE, et al (eds): *Clinical Oncology*, ed 2. Philadelphia, Elsevier, 2004, pp 759–773.
2. Tams TR: Vomiting, regurgitation and dysphagia, in Ettinger SJ (ed): *Textbook of Veterinary Internal Medicine: Diseases of the Dog and Cat*, ed 3. Philadelphia, WB Saunders, 1989, pp 27–32.
3. Leib MS: Acute vomiting: A diagnostic approach and systematic management, in Kirk RW, Bonagura JD (eds): *Current Veterinary Therapy*. XI. Philadelphia, WB Saunders, 1992, pp 583–587.
4. Ogilvie GK, Moore AS, Curtis CR: Cisplatin-induced emesis in the dog with malignant neoplasia: 115 cases (1984–1987). *JAVMA* 195:1399–1403, 1989.
5. Moore AS, Rand WM, Berg J, L'Heureux DA: A randomized evaluation of butorphanol and cyproheptadine for prevention of cisplatin-induced vomiting in the dog. *JAVMA* 205:441–443, 1994.
6. Ogilvie GK: Dolasetron: A new option for nausea and vomiting. *J Am Anim Hosp Assoc* 36(6):481–483, 2000.
7. Kosecki SM: Metoclopramide. *Compend Contin Educ Pract Vet* 25(11):826–828, 2003.
8. Poirier VJ, Hershey AE, Burgess KE, et al: Efficacy and toxicity of paclitaxel (Taxol) for the treatment of canine malignant tumors. *J Vet Intern Med* 18(2):219–222, 2004.

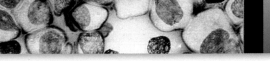

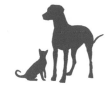

Chapter 25

Third commandment: don't let them starve! Nutritional management

INTRODUCTION

Almost every client who enters our clinics and hospitals are interested in how they can help their dog and cat with cancer or other diseases with nutrition. The value of nutritional management to prevent and treat cancer cannot be underestimated as the nutrients themselves are of profound importance to maintain or regain health and wellness. Just as important is the power of providing the love and care during this process. Indeed, this form of healing is called the mind-body connection.

Specifically formulated diets or dietary supplements to prevent and to treat cancer are evolving rapidly; however, enough information already exists to begin making recommendations to prevent and treat cancer in people and dogs.[1-5] It has been estimated that 30 to 40 percent of all human cancers can be prevented by lifestyle and dietary measures alone.[5] The same may be true in veterinary medicine. The risk of developing cancer, as has been proven, is higher in people who consume excessive refined sugars and simple carbohydrates, low fiber and insufficient essential fatty acids n-3. This factors have already been implicated in augmenting cancer development and progression in dogs, cats, and other animals.[1,2,6-21]

The ideal diet to prevent or treat cancer is, as yet, undiscovered, but based on what we know now, it would likely contain:[3-5]

- Fresh, high quality ingredients that are readily digested and absorbed that maintain normal body mass and that meet or exceed the nutritional requirements for the dog or cat.
- Limited amounts of simple refined sugars or carbohydrates.
- High quality, moderate quantity, highly bioavailable proteins including arginine and glutamine.
- Increased amounts of nucleotides. The best food sources of nucleotides are yeast extract, liver, meat, fish, and mushrooms.
- Limited, but adequate amounts of the conditionally essential n-6 fatty acids often found in red meat fats.
- Increased quantities of the conditionally essential n-3 fatty acids including docosahexaenoic acid derived from fish or some algae.
- Adequate levels of vitamins and minerals including physiologic but not pharmacologic levels of antioxidants, vitamins A, E and C.

Oral or enteral dietary supplementation with nutrients such as arginine, omega 3 fatty acids, and nucleotides known as immunonutrition significantly improve outcomes in patients' quality and length of life, but there is another potential benefit of nutritional care: improving the cost of care. One study was designed to determine the impact on hospital costs of immunonutrition formulas used in human patients undergoing elective surgery for gastrointestinal cancer.[2] The use of dietary supplementation in this study including arginine, omega-3 fatty acids, and nucleotides resulted in savings per patient of $3,300 with costs based on reduction in infectious complication rates or $6,000 with costs based on length of hospital stay. Thus, the use of immunonutrition for patients undergoing elective surgery for gastrointestinal cancer was shown to be an effective and cost-saving intervention. If this same finding is noted in veterinary patients the result is not only an improvement in animal well-being, but fewer euthanasias due to the inability to pay for the cost of care.

This section is presented to assist the clinician in making decisions about nutrition to prevent and treat cancer in dogs and cats.

CANCER, METABOLISM, AND CLINICAL NUTRITION

It is very rare to find a veterinary patient that is thin and debilitated from cancer thanks to sophisticated, compassionate veterinary care and the blessing of euthanasia. Despite this fact, the paraneoplastic syndrome known as cancer cachexia results in profound metabolic changes that occur before weight loss is identified, which increases the need to initiate therapy before weight loss is ever identified.[1,2,6–20] The metabolic alterations that lead to the end stages of cancer cachexia occur early in the course of the disease with profound clinical consequences. The importance of this syndrome cannot be overstated. Humans, dogs, and cats with early to late stage cancer cachexia have a decreased quality of life, decreased response to treatment, and shortened survival time compared to patients who have similar diseases but do not exhibit clinical or biochemical signs associated with this condition (figure 25-1).

The ideal way of treating cancer cachexia is to eliminate the underlying neoplastic condition. Unfortunately, this is not always possible for many veterinary patients due to limited resources, finances, or the advanced state of the disease. Therefore, dietary therapy has been examined as a way to reverse or eliminate cancer cachexia and possibly to treat the cancer itself. Although investigators have demonstrated concern about the possibility of increasing tumor growth by enhancing the nutritional status of the patient, several studies have failed to show this correlation. The benefits that have been shown with dietary support include weight gain and increased response to and tolerance of radiation, surgery, and chemotherapy. Other factors that have been shown to improve with nutritional support include thymic weight, serum albumin, immune responsiveness, and immunoglobulin and complement levels, as well as the phagocytic ability of white blood cells.[1–5] Understanding the alterations in carbohydrate, protein, and lipid metabolism in pets with cancer is essential to knowing what to feed the cancer patient.

Key point

It is very rare to find a veterinary patient that is thin and debilitated from cancer thanks to sophisticated, compassionate veterinary care and the blessing of euthanasia. Despite this fact, the paraneoplastic syndrome known as cancer cachexia results in profound metabolic changes that occur before weight loss is identified, which increases the need to initiate therapy before weight loss is ever identified.

Carbohydrates and cancer

Our society is obsessed with the inclusion of simple carbohydrates in the food and drink of pets and people. This has resulted in an increased consumption of sugars at an alarming rate that has resulted in an epidemic of obesity, insulin dependent diabetes, osteoarthritis, and cancer in dogs, cats, and people. Evidence is mounting that the inclusion of simple carbohydrates may be contraindicated for the nutritional management and prevention of cancer and other disorders in dogs and cats. For example, cancer cells display high rates of aerobic glycolysis, a phenomenon known as the Warburg effect.[21,22] This effect is characterized by the production of large quantities of lactate and pyruvate, the end products of glycolysis, even in the presence of oxygen. It has been found in vivo in human and veterinary cancer patients. Data demonstrating that insulin and lactate levels of dogs with cancer increase above levels in control dogs in response to glucose and a diet-tolerance test[8–11] have been used to suggest that the metabolic alterations in carbohydrate metabolism worsen with the parenteral and enteral administration of simple carbohydrates.

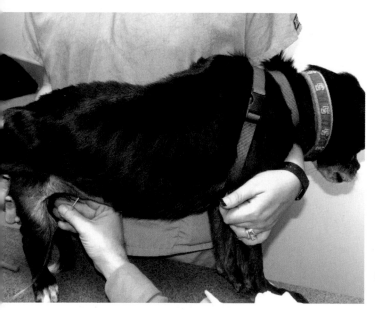

Figure 25-1: Cancer cachexia occurs before any weight loss occurs. Once a debilitated condition is reached, then the prognosis diminishes. Every attempt should be made to support cachectic animals with either esophagostomy, gastrostomy or jejunostomy tube feeding. Appetite stimulants can also be helpful.

Key point

Our society is obsessed with the inclusion of simple carbohydrates in the food of pets and people. This has resulted in an increased consumption of sugars at an alarming rate that has resulted in an epidemic of obesity, insulin dependent diabetes, osteoarthritis, and cancer in dogs, cats, and people.

Research has documented that dogs and likely cats with lymphoma, as well as a wide variety of malignant diseases, have significant alterations in carbohydrate metabolism:[1,2,6–20]

- Dogs with a wide variety of malignant conditions have elevated resting insulin and lactate levels compared to control animals.[8–11,15] It is unknown if the elevated insulin levels are a response to cancer or if they precede and possibly contribute to the development of cancer via stimulation of insulin-like growth-factor (IGF) pathways.

- Elevated lactate and glucose levels do not improve after dogs and cats with cancer are rendered free of disease with chemotherapy and surgery.[8] This suggests that the malignancy causes a fundamental change in metabolism that persists after all clinical evidence of cancer is eliminated.

- Elevated lactate levels can result in inefficient Cori cycle activity to convert lactate back to glucose; this results in a net energy loss by the patient.[8–11,15]

- The administration of lactate-containing parenteral fluids such as lactated Ringer's solution has been shown to increase lactate levels in dogs with lymphoma, suggesting that these types of fluids may place an additional energy burden on the host.[9]

- Before the development of severe malnutrition, human patients with colon, gastric, sarcoma, endometrial, prostate, localized head, neck, or lung cancer have many of the metabolic abnormalities of type II (non–insulin-dependent) diabetes mellitus.[21,22] These metabolic abnormalities include glucose intolerance; an increase in hepatic glucose production, glucose recycling, and insulin resistance; and an increase in anaerobic glycolysis causing increased lactate production. These are essentially the same findings as in dogs and cats with cancer.[1,2,6–20]

The simple carbohydrate concentration of a diet is related to its glycemic potential, which is, in turn, associated with chronically elevated insulin concentrations. These insulin concentrations have been shown to augment the risk of malignancies including the breast cancer risk by stimulating insulin receptor or by affecting insulin-like growth factor I (IGF-I)-mediated mitogenesis.[23–25] For example, one study evaluated the hypothesis that glucose, insulin, and IGFs contribute to breast cancer development in 10,786 women.[23] It was concluded in this research that higher levels of glucose, insulin, and IGF-1 were associated with a higher risk of developing breast cancer and a poorer survival after diagnosis. A separate study involving 603 breast cancer patients was performed to test the hypothesis that excess insulin and related factors are directly related to mortality after a diagnosis of breast cancer.[24] It was confirmed in that study that high levels of insulin were associated with poorer survival for postmenopausal women. In another more recent study performed to further this causal relationship, 11,576 women with invasive breast cancer among 334,849 women were studied.[21] They showed that a diet with a high glycemic load and carbohydrate intake is positively associated with an increased risk of developing estrogen receptor negative and estrogen and progesterone receptor negative breast cancer among postmenopausal women. These findings were further corroborated by Sieri et al[25] who confirmed that in a Mediterranean population characterized by traditionally high and varied carbohydrate intake, a diet high in GL plays a role in the development of breast cancer. While it is unknown if this same relationship exists among dogs and cats, these data and those of other investigators enhance concern over providing diets with high simple carbohydrate concentrations that are in turn associated with a high glycemic potential.

Key point

The simple carbohydrate concentration of a diet is related to its glycemic potential, which is, in turn, associated with chronically elevated insulin concentrations. These insulin concentrations have been shown to augment the risk of malignancies by stimulating insulin receptor or by affecting insulin-like growth factor I (IGF-I)-mediated mitogenesis.

As highlighted earlier, the relative contribution of nutrition-related chronic diseases to the total disease burden of the society and the healthcare costs have risen continuously over the last decades in human medicine and similar concerns have been voiced in veterinary medicine. There is a recent trend in human and veterinary medicine to promote "grain free" diets. The logic of excluding this type of diet is that refined grains often contribute to the glycemic index and therefore increased insulin levels and IGF-mediated mitogenesis. While this logic may be unfounded, most authorities agree that non-refined gains are of great value.

Hauner et al in their research[27] concluded that a high consumption of sugar-sweetened beverages increases the risk of obesity and type 2 diabetes, whereas a high dietary fiber intake, mainly from whole-grain products, reduces the risk of obesity, type 2 diabetes, dyslipidemia, hypertension, coronary heart disease, and colorectal cancer. Goacco et al reviewed the literature and concluded that whole grain consumption can be recommended as one of the features of the diet that may help control body weight but also because is associated with a lower risk of developing type 2 diabetes, cardiovascular diseases, and cancer. There are concerns about using people as a model for animal diseases, but until canine and feline data mature and are available, it seems reasonable to consider appropriate amounts of whole, unrefined grains as part of the diet for the cancer patient in dogs and people. Grains are not part of the normal feline diet therefore they should be excluded.

Dietary recommendations: It seems reasonable with the data before us to consciously limit but not to completely exclude the amount of simple carbohydrates in dogs, cats, and people at high risk of getting or who actually have or are recovering from cancer. Because simple carbohydrates can cause elevated insulin levels, and because hyperinsulinemia has been associated with the development of cancer in some species, a diet lower in carbohydrates may be indicated throughout life, even in healthy dogs and cats. Glickman et al.[26] showed that after adjustment for age, weight, neuter status, and coat color, there was an inverse association between consumption of vegetables at least 3 times per week and risk of developing transitional cell carcinoma in healthy Scottish Terriers. Green leafy vegetables do not have a high glycemic index and thus may be of value for dogs, not cats. A lower-carbohydrate diet may also help maintain a lean body mass and reduce the risks of dental disease and obesity, which may, in turn, enhance wellness by reducing the risk of cancer and metabolic diseases such as diabetes mellitus. As a general rule, inexpensive, extruded dry, and semi-moist commercially available dog and cat foods have the highest carbohydrate content.

Proteins and cancer

Dogs and cats with cancer have alterations in protein metabolism that are very similar to those observed in humans and laboratory animals with cancer.1 For example, there is a significant decrease in a wide variety of amino acids, suggesting that a high-quality, highly bioavailable protein source would be beneficial to the animal and to the tumor. Amino acids of particular importance to patients with cancer are glutamine, cysteine, and arginine.

Glutamine supplementation may enhance the therapeutic index of chemotherapy and radiation by enhancing the efficacy of these treatments while reducing adverse effects such as mucositis, diarrhea, neuropathy, and cardiotoxicity.[27,28] Glutamine is conditionally essential for the health and function of the bowel. At least some of this amino acid is destroyed in the process of making many types of dried and canned pet food.

Cysteine is critically important to replenish the glutathione antioxidant system.[29,30] This system is the principal protective mechanism of the cell and is a crucial factor in the development of the immune response. Cysteine supplementation has been shown to have anticancer activity via the glutathione pathway, the induction of p53 protein in cancer cells, and inhibition of neoangiogenesis.[29,30]

Arginine is a conditionally essential amino acid that is necessary during periods of growth and recovery after injury. Arginine promotes wound healing, prevents nephrotoxicity, has several immunomodulatory effects such as stimulating T- and natural-killer cell activity, and influences proinflammatory cytokine levels.[31] L-arginine is the sole precursor for the multifunctional messenger molecule nitric oxide, which appears to influence tumor initiation, promotion, and progression; tumor-cell adhesion; apoptosis angiogenesis; differentiation; chemosensitivity; radiosensitivity; and tumor-induced immunosuppression.[31] The administration of arginine to human and veterinary cancer patients has resulted in positive outcomes.

Dietary recommendations: Optimally, the cancer patient should be fed a moderate amount of highly bioavailable, digestible protein sources that contain adequate amounts of cysteine, glutamine, and arginine. This is generally not an a problem in the diet is determined to be adequate "for all life stages." Periodically evaluating the patient to ensure maintenance of body weight without the development of hypoalbuminemia is critical. Less expensive, commercially available dog and cat foods, especially those that are extruded dry or semi-moist, are less likely to have highly bioavailable proteins.

Lipids and cancer

There is little doubt in the mind of the health conscious consumer that red meat fats are generally bad for people and that fish or algae source fats are good for health and wellness. It is not difficult to maintain that this same dietary prescription is beneficial for pets. This information is based on a great deal of data in companion animals and in people (as a model for canine and feline health and wellness).

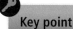
Key point
There is little doubt in the mind of the health conscious consumer that red meat fats are generally bad for people and pets and that fish or algae source fats are good for health and wellness.

Serum lipid profiles were performed in dogs with lymphoma before and after they were put into remission with chemotherapy. These profiles were compared to those of normal dogs before and after they were given the same anticancer drug.[11]
- The dogs with cancer had significantly lower levels of high-density lipoproteins. The total triglyceride levels and very low-density triglycerides of untreated dogs with lymphoma were significantly higher than those of untreated control dogs.[11]
- After a total of five doses of doxorubicin chemotherapy, the total cholesterol level increased in dogs with lymphoma but decreased in treated control dogs.[11]

- All other parameters remained unchanged after doxorubicin therapy, suggesting that lipid abnormalities do not improve significantly, even after a clinical remission is obtained.[11]

Abnormalities in lipid metabolism have been linked to a number of clinical problems, including immunosuppression, which correlates with decreased survival in affected humans.[1-5] The clinical impact of abnormalities in lipid metabolism may be lessened with dietary therapy. In contrast to carbohydrates and proteins, some tumor cells have difficulty using lipids as a fuel source, but host tissues continue to oxidize lipids for energy. This has led to the hypothesis that diets relatively high in fat may be beneficial for animals with cancer compared to diets that are high in simple carbohydrates, assuming that the protein content, caloric density, and palatability remain constant. One study suggested that a high-carbohydrate, low-fat diet induced elevated lactate and insulin levels compared to a diet relatively high in fat and low in carbohydrates.[2,12] It also suggested that a high-fat diet may result in a higher probability of going into remission with chemotherapy as well as a longer survival time. The kind of fat in the diet, rather than the amount, may be the important factor. For example, n-3 polyunsaturated fatty acids (PUFAs) have been shown experimentally to have many beneficial properties.[2,12,16]

Emerging role of polyunsaturated fatty acids (PUFAS): cancer prevention by delay

For the last decade, investigators have searched for dietary lipids that can cause or are associated with a delay in cancer relapse. The use of long-chain polyunsaturated fatty acids (LC-PUFAs), such as docosahexaenoic acid (DHA) and eicosapentaenoic acid (EPA), as adjuvant therapies to enhance the effect of chemotherapy and radiation therapy shows promise. LC-PUFAs have been shown to enhance disease-free interval, survival, and quality of life after surgery by reducing the rate of cancer development or incidence. This concept, known as 'cancer prevention by delay' or clinical cancer chemoprevention, is an important mechanism behind the successes of several therapeutic agents, including tamoxifen, retinoids and interferon-alfa, and nonsteroidal anti-inflammatory drugs.[32]

Cancer prevention by delay is a valuable clinical tool until more effective cancer therapeutics can be developed. Unfortunately, while use of the most effective cancer therapies (i.e., surgery, radiation, and chemotherapy) is effective for improving the disease-free interval of many patients up to a point, it has not increased the cancer cure rate or survival time dramatically in the last 10 years. Therefore, it seems logical to add on relatively nontoxic therapies that can extend the disease-free interval, even if the absolute cure rate is not increased. Tamoxifen, retinoids, and nonsteroidal anti-inflammatory agents are all recognized to improve disease-free interval without necessarily improving the absolute cure rate. Tamoxifen has been shown to significantly diminish the risk of human breast cancer; retinoids and interferon-alfa to reduce the risk of head and neck cancer in dogs, cats, and humans; and nonsteroidal anti-inflammatory drugs to delay or reduce the development of colorectal cancer in humans and transitional cell and squamous cell carcinoma in dogs.

> **Key point**
> Dietary lipids such as DHA and EPA appear to inhibit the growth and metastases of many types of cancer.

Dietary lipids such as DHA and EPA appear to influence the growth of many types of cancer, including breast and prostate cancer.[33-36] A group of investigators in France used adipose tissue sampled during surgery as a biomarker of past dietary intake of PUFAs in a cohort of women treated for localized presentations of breast cancer.[37] They found elevated n-3 PUFAs, especially DHA, to be associated with a higher metastasis-free survival, suggesting that these PUFAs could potentially delay metastasis by decreasing tumor growth or development. Using a case-control approach comparing the fatty acid composition of adipose breast tissue obtained at the time of surgical removal of either malignant or benign breast tumors, they also found α-linoleic acid and docosahexaenoic acid to be positively associated with a decreased risk of having breast cancer.[38]

The French group also explored the role of n-3 PUFAs in mammary tumor growth using the experimental system of N-methylnitrosourea (NMU)-induced mammary tumors in rats. Because PUFAs are substrates for lipid peroxidation processes, the investigators studied the effects of n-3 PUFAs on tumor growth in interaction with anti- or pro-oxidant compounds. They found that dietary n-3 PUFAs, in the form of DHA-containing fish oil, inhibited tumor development. This inhibition was most evident in the absence of the antioxidant vitamin E. Inhibition of tumor growth was even greater when n-3 PUFAs were given in the presence of pro-oxidants.[34] Such effects were not found when the lipid diet was low in PUFAs. These data suggest that oxidized n-3 PUFAs have an inhibiting effect on tumor growth and emphasize the importance of the interaction of anti- and pro-oxidant compounds with n-3 PUFAs.

There is a growing body of data that suggests that the presence of n-3 PUFAs such as DHA and EPA affect several steps of tumor formation. N-3 PUFAs:

- Inhibit tumor vessel formation (angiogenesis).
- Inhibit cell proliferation in several epithelial cell lines.
- Enhance the rate of tumor cell death.
- Induce lipid peroxidation, which enhances the efficacy of radiation- and chemotherapy-induced cancer cell death; this effect is diminished or reduced dramatically with vitamin E.
- Suppress the expression of cyclooxygenase-2 in tumors, thereby decreasing cancer cell proliferation.
- Suppress nuclear factor κB activation and BCL-2 expression, thus allowing apoptosis of cancer cells.

Dietary lipids have been shown to modify the sensitivity of tumors to reactive oxygen species–generating anticancer drugs. For example, when dogs with lymphoma were treated with doxorubicin chemotherapy and a diet supplemented with n-3 PUFAs in the form of fish oils, there was a direct correlation between the level of DHA in the blood and improved disease-free interval.[18] Another study, using the same randomized study design, was used to assess the efficacy of n-3 PUFAs in combination with doxorubicin chemotherapy to improve the disease-free interval in dogs with hemangiosarcoma, a highly metastatic, rapidly fatal malignancy. There was a statistically significant positive correlation between the n-3 PUFA levels in the serum and disease-free interval.[39] A similar approach was used in rats bearing autochthonous, NMU-induced mammary tumors. It was found that dietary supplementation with fish oil or DHA increased the sensitivity of mammary tumors to anthracyclines, compared with dietary supplementation with saturated fatty acids.[39]

DHA is the most polyunsaturated of the PUFAs. Lipoperoxidation is a likely molecular mechanism implicated in the enhancement of the response of cancer cells to many cytotoxic drugs. Therefore, DHA is a very important adjuvant for the treatment of certain cancers. Addition of vitamin E to the diet provided to rats with mammary tumors abolished the enhancing effect of DHA on tumor sensitivity to anthracyclines.[39] In all studies done to date, there has been no clinically significant toxicity other than transient gastrointestinal (GI) distress linked to the dietary change.[17,18] Therefore, based on the safety and efficacy profile of n-3 PUFAs, it seems reasonable to further define the efficacy of n-3 PUFAs, especially DHA, for the treatment of spontaneously occurring cancer in dogs, with the intent to provide evidence for their use in randomized human clinical trials.

Key point

DHA is the most polyunsaturated of the PUFAs. Lipoperoxidation is a likely molecular mechanism implicated in the enhancement of the response of cancer cells to many cytotoxic drugs. Therefore, DHA is a very important adjuvant for the treatment of certain cancers.

DHA and EPA also augment the efficacy of chemotherapy and radiation therapy, potentially enhancing the efficacy of traditional cancer therapies. Radiation therapy is currently the most effective treatment for many localized malignancies. Research is under way to identify methods to maximize its efficacy while minimizing the adverse effects associated with it. Among the agents being evaluated to minimize the damage to normal tissue are n-3 LC-PUFAs, which are readily incorporated into cell membranes and ameliorate inflammation and carbohydrate dyshomeostasis. In one study, 12 dogs with histologically confirmed malignant carcinomas of the nasal cavity were randomized to receive isocaloric amounts of a diet supplemented with menhaden fish oil, including DHA (experimental diet), or an otherwise identical diet supplemented with corn oil (control diet). Megavoltage radiation was delivered to all dogs. The data in this study suggest that feeding a diet supplemented with fish oil and arginine is associated with decreased concentrations of inflammatory mediators involved with radiation damage in skin and mucosa and with improved performance scores in dogs with malignant nasal tumors.[41]

Key point

DHA and EPA also augment the efficacy of chemotherapy and radiation therapy, potentially enhancing the efficacy of traditional cancer therapies.

The ability of PUFAs to sensitize tumors to radiation has been investigated. Vartak et al[42,43] studied the in vitro response of a chemically induced rat malignant astrocytoma cell line to radiation after the cell culture medium was supplemented with γ-linoleic acid (GLA) or n-3 LC-PUFAs. They found that n-3 PUFAs enhanced radiation-induced cell cytotoxicity. In a separate study, Colas et al44 documented enhanced radiosensitivity of rat autochthonous mammary tumors after administration of dietary DHA.

Whether use of dietary n-3 PUFAs can enhance sensitivity of tumor tissue in the absence of a similar increase in the radiosensitivity of nontumor tissue remains a critical issue. Several studies have suggested that PUFAs do not sensitize normal tissue to radiation. For example, because ionizing radiation generates reactive oxygen species, we initiated a study to determine whether dietary DHA might sensitize mammary tumors to irradiation using a model in which mammary tumors were induced by NMU in Sprague-Dawley rats. In the study, we showed that dietary DHA sensitized mammary tumors to radiation. The addition of vitamin E inhibited the beneficial effect of DHA, suggesting that this effect might be mediated by oxidative damage to the peroxidizable lipids.[44]

Dietary recommendations: N-3 LC-PUFAs may be beneficial for preventing and treating cancer in dogs and cats. Therefore, n-3 PUFAs, such as DHA, should be used as dietary supplements. The addition of antioxidants such as vitamin A, E, or C is important to keep the PUFAs from oxidizing; however, excessive amounts may reduce or eliminate the beneficial effects of PUFAs.

Nutritional and water needs and cancer

Our knowledge of the nutrient and water needs of dogs and cats is primarily based on work done years ago or extrapolated from research in rodents or humans. Most data concerning energy and water requirements in dogs and cats may be overestimated.[45,46] It has been determined that the resting energy expenditure, which is an estimate of the nutrient and water needs of normal dogs, is lower than data previously published implied.[46] In addition, one study showed that dogs with lymphoma and dogs that have undergone surgery for various problems have resting energy requirements that are lower than those of normal animals.[45] This is in stark contrast to publications that suggest that cancer and surgery result in dramatic increases in the nutrient and water requirements of animals. This is of critical value for practicing veterinarians who are attempting to meet the nutrient and fluid needs of normal and ill patients. It also may be of great importance for our clients.

Key point

Most published data concerning energy and water requirements in dogs and cats may overestimate the needs of this population as a whole.

Dietary recommendations: The caloric needs of each cancer patient should be monitored carefully by evaluating body weight and serum albumin levels. Many dogs and cats with cancer do not have dramatically elevated caloric needs compared with the normal patient. Similarly, because the fluid needs of dogs and cats are directly related to the number of kilocalories consumed on a basis of 1 mL of water to 1 kcal, the fluid needs of the cancer patient may be more conservative than once anticipated.

Vitamins, minerals, and enzymes and cancer

Vitamins

Retinoids, β-carotene, and vitamins C, D, and E may influence the growth and metastasis of cancer cells via a variety of mechanisms. These vitamins increase and decrease in popularity based on the results of select studies and the lay press. However, recent data confirm that pharmacologic levels of vitamins may be associated with an increased risk of developing cancer and may actually inhibit the treatment of cancer. This is considered by many as hearsay, but the published literature confirms this observation.

Retinoids (vitamin A)

Retinoids are not used as a mainstay of cancer therapy; however, there is a growing body of knowledge about the anticancer effect of vitamin A in humans and animals.[47–50] In humans, 13-cis retinoic acid prevents secondary tumors in patients treated for squamous cell carcinoma of the head and neck[47–50] and can reverse the effects of cervical human papillomavirus infection. Retinoic acid, when used in the adjuvant treatment of retinoblastoma (a childhood cancer), leads to translocation of bound receptor-vitamin complexes to the nucleus, which results in the regulation of the neuroblastoma gene.[48] Melanoma in mice has been successfully treated with retinoids.[49]

The efficacy of retinoids is not confined to rodents and people. A study was completed to evaluate the synthetic retinoids isotretinoin and etretinate in treating dogs with intracutaneous cornifying epithelioma, other benign skin neoplasias, and cutaneous lymphoma.[50] This study showed reduction in the size of some tumors and elimination of others.

Vitamin C

Vitamin C has been studied continuously over the last several decades as an antioxidant and an agent that can effectively treat conditions such as colds, cardiovascular disease, and cancer. There have been some data suggesting that vitamin C may be of value for the prevention and treatment of certain types of cancers.[51,52] Water-soluble vitamin C has been widely reported to inhibit nitrosation reactions and prevent chemical induction of cancers of the esophagus and stomach.[52] Processed foods high in nitrates and nitrites, such as bacon and sausage, are often supplemented with vitamin C to reduce the carcinogenic capability of the resultant nitrosamines.

Vitamin E

Lipid-soluble vitamin E, or α-tocopherol, can also inhibit nitrosation reactions, but vitamin E also has a broad capacity to inhibit mammary tumor and colon carcinogenesis in rodents.[52–54] In addition to its chemopreventive properties, vitamin E possesses antiproliferative activity that may convey potential therapeutic efficacy against certain malignancies.[52–54] As mentioned above, antioxidants may inhibit the effect of n-3 PUFAs, making it difficult to know how to administer these vitamins.

Key point

The effects of vitamins are not always positive. Indeed, data exist that show that pharmacologic levels of vitamins A, E and C may be associated with an increased prevalence of disease and a poorer quality of life. Similarly, antioxidants may diminish the efficacy of some cancer therapies.

The effects of vitamins are not always positive. A meta-analysis of the dose-response relationship between vitamin E supplementation and total mortality was performed using data from 135,967 human participants in 19 randomized, controlled clinical trials.[55] A dose-response analysis showed a statistically significant relationship between vitamin E dosage and all-cause mortality, with increased risk in dosages greater than 150 IU/day. The study concluded that high-dosage (≥400 IU/day) vitamin E supplements may increase all-cause mortality and should be avoided. Another study documented that higher dosages of β-carotene caused a poorer outcome in people who smoked and had lung cancer.[56] Thus, vitamins have a complex role in the treatment and prevention of cancer, and more must be known about the impact of their dosage and form before they can be used effectively in the treatment of cancer.

Dietary recommendations: Moderate, physiologic dosages of antioxidant vitamins are recommended for the cancer patient; however, megadosages of vitamins are not encouraged at this time.

Minerals

Minerals that have been suggested to have chemopreventative or anticancer effects and that are of value as nutrients include selenium, copper, zinc, magnesium, calcium, chromium, lead, iron, potassium, sodium, arsenic, iodine, and germanium. Zinc, chromium, and iron have been shown to be reduced in dogs with spontaneously occurring cancer.[19] Selenium is one of the most heavily studied minerals associated with the development of cancer.[57–60] Low serum selenium levels have been seen in human patients with prostate and gastrointestinal cancer.[57] In rodents, dietary supplementation of selenium has been shown to inhibit colon, mammary gland, and stomach carcinogenesis.[57–60] Additional study is essential to determine whether alteration of selenium levels would be of value for the treatment of veterinary or human cancer patients. Selenium may be toxic at high levels and thus should not be supplemented without first seeking advice from a veterinary nutritionist.

Dietary recommendations: Care should be taken to ensure that the diet contains adequate levels of minerals for all life stages. Specific care should be taken to ensure that there are adequate amounts zinc, chromium, and iron in the diet. Selenium supplementation should be done cautiously and without inducing selenium toxicity.

Therapeutic enzymes

Enzymes have therapeutic potential but limited approval in the United States. L-asparaginase is probably the most valuable therapy for the treatment of lymphoma and leukemia in animals and humans.61 Oral enzyme preparations are used for the treatment of chronic pancreatic insufficiency and disaccharidase deficiency. Several enzyme preparations, including Wobenzyme™ and Musal™, are available in Europe for oral adjuvant treatment of cancer and other diseases. Although manufacturers of these preparations note the efficacy of therapeutic enzymes in the treatment of cancer patients, the mechanism by which they act is not precisely known. One hypothesis is that these enzymes eliminate pathogenic immune complexes. Therefore, enzymes may be of value for the adjuvant treatment of cancer.

Information suggests that soybean-derived Bowman-Birk inhibitor (BBI) can inhibit or suppress carcinogenesis in vivo and in vitro.[62–66] Extracts of BBI have been shown to inhibit carcinogenesis in several animal model systems, including colon- and liver-induced carcinogenesis in mice, anthracene-induced cheek pouch carcinogenesis in hamsters, lung tumorigenesis in mice, and esophageal carcinogenesis in rats.[62–66] BBI concentration has been shown to inhibit metastasis and weight loss associated with radiation-induced thymic lymphoma in mice.[63] Irradiated rodents treated with dietary BBI concentration have fewer deaths, lower average grade of lymphoma, and larger fat stores than controls. Therefore, this protease inhibitor may be important as an adjunct to cancer chemotherapy protocols and in the prevention of secondary cancers.

NUTRITIONAL CANCER PREVENTION AND THERAPY

The following general recommendations for cancer prevention and therapy are based on the above information. These recommendations should be revised as new knowledge is gained.

Prevention

Dogs and cats generally eat the same diet for long periods of time; therefore, that diet should be designed to prevent the development of cancer. Until a special cancer prevention diet is developed, existing data can be employed to potentially reduce the risk of cancer in dogs and cats eating commercially available food. Avoidance of obesity seems to be a basic preventive measure. As noted earlier, Glickman et al.[26] showed that after adjustment for age, weight, neuter status, and coat color, there was an inverse association between consumption of vegetables at least 3 times per week and risk of developing transitional cell carcinoma in healthy Scottish Terriers. In addition, a lifetime study of restricted daily food intake was done in 48 Labrador retriever dogs from seven litters.[67,68] The dogs were paired; in each pair, the restricted-fed dog received 25% less food than the control-fed dog. The median life span of the restricted-fed dogs was significantly longer. While the prevalence of cancer between the groups was similar, dogs that received the restricted diet lived an average of 2 years longer before dying of cancer.

EPA and DHA have consistently been shown to inhibit the proliferation of breast and prostate cancer cell lines in vitro and to reduce the risk and progression of these tumors in many species.[69,70] Adding these LC-PUFAs to the diet may be useful in preventing some types of cancer.

The following are basic dietary recommendations to prevent cancer in dogs and cats:

- Restrict daily intake to maintain a low body weight throughout life.
- Minimize simple carbohydrates in the diet to reduce insulin levels and obesity; this may reduce the risk of a number of diseases.
- Feed a balanced diet specifically for dogs and cats, with possible consideration of the use of n-3 PUFAs.

Therapy

The ideal anticancer diet in dogs and cats that already have cancer is unknown. However, as noted above, it may be logical to use a diet that contains 30% to 50% of nonprotein calories as fat, particularly n-3 PUFAs; a highly bioavailable protein source that has adequate amounts of glutamine, cysteine, and arginine; and a relatively low percentage of carbohydrates.[1–4] This type of diet may slow tumor growth and decrease glucose intolerance and fat loss. Glucose-containing fluids may result in increased lactate production, which may cause an energy drain on the host.

Enteral nutrition

As a general rule, mature dogs and cats with functional GI tracts that have a history of inadequate nutritional intake for 5 to 7 days or that have lost at least 10% of their body weight over a 1- to 2-week period are candidates for enteral nutritional therapy. All methods to encourage food consumption should be attempted. These include warming the food to just below body temperature; providing a selection of palatable, aromatic foods; and providing comfortable, stress-free surroundings. When these simple procedures fail, such chemical stimulants as benzodiazepine derivatives (e.g., diazepam, oxazepam) and antiserotonin agents (mirtazapine, cyproheptadine and pizotifen) can be used. Propofol at 1 mg/kg IV can also enhance the appetite in many hospitalized cancer patients. Megestrol acetate (2.5 mg PO daily for 4 days, then every 2–3 days thereafter) and diazepam (0.05–0.5 mg/kg IV) are effective for enhancing appetite. Dogs and cats may have improved appetite when metoclopramide, Maropitant, ondansetron, or dolasetron is given orally to decrease nausea associated with chemotherapy or surgery. When all these measures fail, enteral nutritional support, designed to deliver nutrients to the GI tract by various methods, should be considered because it is practical, cost-effective, physiologic, and safe.[1–4]

Key point

Dogs and cats with functional GI tracts that have a history of inadequate nutritional intake for 5 to 7 days or that have lost at least 10% of their body weight over a 1- to 2-week period are candidates for enteral nutritional therapy. Patients that lose weight often have a very difficult time regaining weight and often have increased toxicity from therapy.

Calculating contents and volumes

Calculation of the nutritional requirements for enteral feeding is essentially the same as for parenteral feeding,[1,2] which is relatively straightforward.[1–4] Parenteral feeding is discussed separately below. Although recent research suggests that animals with cancer do not have increased nutritional requirements, the following method is still in use:

- The basal energy requirement (BER, in kcal/day) is calculated by multiplying the animal's weight in kg$^{0.75}$ by 70. This value is then multiplied by different factors to derive the maintenance energy requirement (MER) or illness energy requirement (IER).
- The standard guidelines state that to calculate the MER for normal dogs and cats that are at rest in a cage, the BER is multiplied by a factor of 1.25. For dogs and cats that have undergone recent surgery or that are recovering from trauma, the IER equals the BER multiplied by 1.2 to 1.6. To calculate the IER for dogs and cats that are septic or have major burns, the BER is multiplied by 1.5 to 2.0.

Box 25-1. Homemade canine cancer food

Recipe 1

The following recipe will make 3 days' worth of food for a 25- to 30-lb dog. The diet is nutritionally complete for the cat, however

Ingredients	Amount
Lean ground beef, fat drained	454 grams (1 pound)
Brown rice, cooked	227 grams (1 1/3 cups)
Liver, beef	138 grams (1/3 pound)
Vegetable oil	63 grams (4½ Tbsp)
Fish oil or algae source DHA (preferred)	9 grams fish oil or 4 grams DHA
Calcium carbonate	3.3 grams**
Dicalcium phosphate***	2.9 grams (3/4 tsp)
Salt substitute (potassium chloride)	1.9 grams (1/3 tsp)

* Note: Clients are encouraged to feed the highest fish or, preferably, DHA oil dose tolerated by the dog and cat.

** Calcium carbonate is available as oyster shell calcium tablets or Tums® tablets (0.5 g in regular Tums®, 0.75 g in Tums Extra®, and 1.0 g in Tums Ultra®, GlaxoSmithKline).

*** Bone meal can be used in place of dicalcium phosphate.

Directions: Cook the rice with salt substitute added to the water. Cook the ground beef and drain the fat. Cook the liver and dice or finely chop into small pieces. Pulverize the calcium carbonate and vitamin/mineral tablets. Mix the vegetable oil, fish oil (break open capsules), and supplements with the rice; add the cooked ground beef and liver. Mix well, cover, and refrigerate. Feed approximately one third of this mixture each day to a 25- to 30-lb dog. Palatability will be increased if the daily portion is heated to approximately body temperature. (Caution: when using a microwave to reheat, avoid "hot spots," which can burn the mouth.)

Nutrient profile (% dry matter basis)	
Protein	35.3
Fat	41.6
Carbohydrate	17.8
Calcium	0.65
Phosphorus	0.54
Sodium	0.36
Potassium	0.68
Magnesium	0.05
Energy	1,989 kcal/kg as fed

Recipe 2

Generic cancer diet for dogs by Susan G. Wynn, DVM, CVA, CVCH, RH (AGH)[71]

This recipe makes a batch of about 800 grams, supplying about 1000 kcal which is enough for an active 45 lb dog.

Ingredients	Amount
Chicken breast, no skin, broiled, baked or stewed	1 lb
Vegetables*	1½ cup
Calcium carbonate powder	¾ teaspoon
Salmon oil	5 teaspoons
Centrum Adult Multi Vitamin & Mineral	2 tablets
Choline bitartrate, 500mg/tablet	½ tablet

*Use a variety of vegetables of all colors, and be sure to include cruciferous types. Choose mostly from broccoli, cabbage, carrots, bok choy, kale, red/yellow bell peppers, shiitake or maitake mushroom, etc.

Table 25-1. Specifics of diets for the feline cancer patient

Product	Caloric content (kcals/ml)	Protein content g/100 kcal-g/ml	Fat content (g/100 kcal)	Osmolarity (mOsm/kg)
Feline a/d	1.30	8.06-0.105	5.07	
Feline p/d*	0.8	10.89-0.087	7.13	
Feline k/d**	0.64	5.62-0.036	7.88	
Feline c/d**	0.62	9.02-0.56	6.04	
Canine nd	0.62	7.2-0.056	5.9	
Jevity	1.06	4.20-0.045	3.48	310
Osmolite HN	1.06	4.44-0.047	3.68	310
Vital HN	1.0	4.17-0.042	1.08	460
Vivonex HN	1.0	4.60-0.046	0.90	810
Clinicare Feline	1.0	8.60-0.086	5.30	235

*Blenderize ½ can (225 g) + ¾ cup (170 ml) water
**Blenderize ½ can (224 g) + 5/4 cup (284 ml) water

Table 25-2. Examples of commercial diets for cats with cancer

Cat's BW (pounds/kg)	5/2.3	8/3.6	10/4.5	12/5.5	15/6.8
kcal/day	170	215	250	280	330
Canine/Feline a/d® can **Protein=45.7, Fat=28.7, Nitrogen Free Extract=16.5***					
Arginine, mg/d	631	798	928	1,039	1,224
Arginine to add, mg**	294	399	432	484	571
Total n-3, mg/d	806	1,019	1,185	1,327	1,564
Feline Growth® dry **Protein=37.1, Fat=26.5, Nitrogen Free Extract=28.5***					
Arginine, mg/d	755	955	1,110	1,243	1,465
Arginine to add, mg**	170	242	250	280	330
Total n-3, mg/d	100	127	148	165	195
Fish oil caps to add***	2	3	3.5	4	4.5
Feline Maintenance® Seafood can **Protein=45.1, Fat=25.4, Nitrogen Free Extract=20.1***					
Arginine, mg/d	1,097	1,387	1,613	1,806	2,129
Arginine to ad d, mg**	0	0	0	0	0
Total n-3, mg/d	318	402	468	524	617
Fish oil caps to add***	1.5	2	2.5	2.5	3

*Nutrients expressed as %DM.
**Amount of arginine to add to this product (L-arginine is usually available as 500- and 1000-mg tablets).
***Number of fish oil capsules to add to this product.
Note: Algae source or fish oil capsules should be given with each meal and/or broken open and mixed with food.

• The IER (kcal/day as nonprotein calories) has not been determined for dogs and cats with cancer but is reported to be quite high, even in animals without sepsis, burns, trauma, or surgery. Work[9,10] suggests that the energy requirement of dogs and cats with cancer may not exceed those of normal dogs and cats. Until this is confirmed, it may be better to overestimate, rather than underestimate, nutrient requirements of the cancer patient.

Key point

Recent research suggests that animals with cancer do not have increased nutritional requirements, however this may or may not pertain to any one patient as an individual. Therefore, feed each patient to his or her own needs and requirements.

Some patients have a very high energy expenditure that may exceed that seen in animals with infections, sepsis, or burns. Other research suggests that the energy needs of most cancer patients do not exceed those of a healthy animal. Dogs and cats with renal or hepatic insufficiency should not be given high protein loads (<3 g/100 Kcal in dogs). Because most high-quality pet foods can be put through a blender to form a gruel that can be passed through a large feeding tube, the IER of the animal is divided by the caloric density of the canned pet food in order to determine the amount of food to feed. The same calculation can be done with human enteral feeding products; the volume fed may need to be increased if the enteral feeding product is diluted to ensure it is approximately iso-osmolar before administration.

Suggested diets: There is one commercially prepared cancer diet, Hill's Prescription Diet n/d. The recipe for a homemade alternative is provided in the box.

Routes of enteral feeding

Esophagostomy tubes. Recently, esophagostomy tube feeding has gained great popularity because the tube can be placed easily without special equipment, can be removed at any time, and requires no waiting time before feeding begins (figures 25-2 and 25-3).[1-3,5] Fourteen to twenty French (Fr) tubes are used in dogs whereas much smaller tubes (8-12 French) are used in cats. Esophagostomy tubes can be placed percutaneously with the use of a curved Rochester-Carmalt forceps or hemostat. Complications include local cellulitis and, occasionally, a dissecting abscess of the cervical tissues; these complications are rare and heal shortly after the tube is removed and the local reaction treated appropriately.

Many practitioners prefer to place esophagostomy tubes rather than gastrostomy tubes. Esophagostomy tubes should be considered when the patient has a functional upper GI tract, including the absence of esophageal motility disorders, such as megaesophagus. Esophagostomy tubes are easier to place, maintain, and remove than gastrostomy tubes. Many caregivers seem to accept esophagostomy tubes over gastrostomy tubes.

Gastrostomy tubes. Gastrostomy tubes are used frequently in veterinary practice for animals that need nutritional support for more than 7 days.[1,2] These tubes can be placed surgically or with endoscopic guidance. A 5-mL balloon-tipped urethral catheter (e.g., Foley catheter, Bardex, Murray Hill, NJ) can be placed surgically, as can a mushroom-tipped Pezzer proportionate head urologic catheter (Bard Urological Catheter, Bard Urological Division, Covington, GA). For smaller dogs and cats, an 18- to 24-Fr catheter is used; larger dogs require a 26- to 30-Fr tube. Commercially available low-profile gastrostomy tubes are also available for use. The procedure is as follows:

• Before placement of the tube, the left paracostal area just below the paravertebral epaxial musculature is clipped and prepared for surgery. A 2- to 3-cm incision is made just caudal to the last rib through the skin and subcutaneous tissue to allow blunt dissection through the musculature into the abdominal cavity.

• The stomach is inflated through a tube placed down the esophagus to allow the surgeon to easily locate the stomach through the opening in the abdominal wall. Stay sutures are placed to temporarily fix the stomach against the abdominal wall; these stay sutures are used later to help close the muscular wall.

• Two concentric purse string sutures of 2-0 non-absorbable nylon suture are then placed deep in the stomach wall; the first purse string is deeper than the second to allow a two-layered closure.

• The feeding tube is placed into the lumen of the stomach through a stab incision in the middle of the purse string sutures. The tip of the catheter is usually clipped off to allow easy introduction of food through the tube and into the stomach.

• If a balloon-tipped catheter is used, the balloon is inflated with water once the tube is in place. The Pezzer catheter has an expanded head that flattens and then returns to its normal shape when a stylet is extended and then removed in the catheter lumen during placement through the stab incision into the stomach.

• With the tube in place, the purse strings are tied to cause the stomach to invert in the region adjacent to the tube. The free ends of the purse strings are then used to close the lateral abdominal musculature and subcutaneous tissue.

• The skin is closed before the tube is secured to the abdominal skin by sutures. To prevent the animal from removing the tube, an abdominal wrap and an Elizabethan collar are recommended.

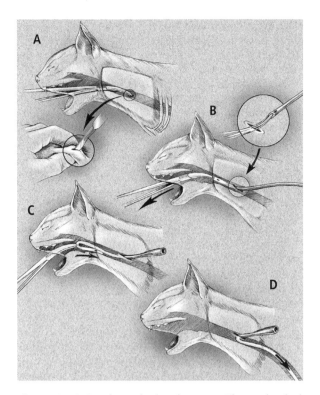

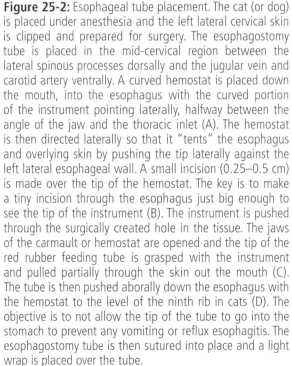

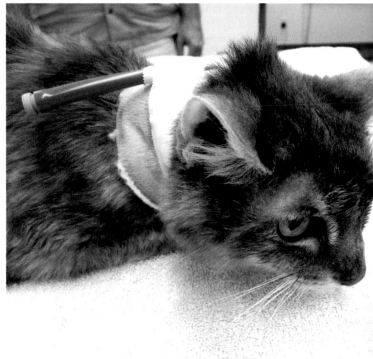

Figure 25-2: Esophageal tube placement. The cat (or dog) is placed under anesthesia and the left lateral cervical skin is clipped and prepared for surgery. The esophagostomy tube is placed in the mid-cervical region between the lateral spinous processes dorsally and the jugular vein and carotid artery ventrally. A curved hemostat is placed down the mouth, into the esophagus with the curved portion of the instrument pointing laterally, halfway between the angle of the jaw and the thoracic inlet (A). The hemostat is then directed laterally so that it "tents" the esophagus and overlying skin by pushing the tip laterally against the left lateral esophageal wall. A small incision (0.25–0.5 cm) is made over the tip of the hemostat. The key is to make a tiny incision through the esophagus just big enough to see the tip of the instrument (B). The instrument is pushed through the surgically created hole in the tissue. The jaws of the carmault or hemostat are opened and the tip of the red rubber feeding tube is grasped with the instrument and pulled partially through the skin out the mouth (C). The tube is then pushed aborally down the esophagus with the hemostat to the level of the ninth rib in cats (D). The objective is to not allow the tip of the tube to go into the stomach to prevent any vomiting or reflux esophagitis. The esophagostomy tube is then sutured into place and a light wrap is placed over the tube.

Feeding can begin soon after the animal has recovered from anesthesia. The tube should be checked daily to ensure proper placement and should be flushed with warm water after each feeding to maintain patency. After 7 to 10 days, an adhesion will form, allowing the tube to be removed or replaced

Figure 25-3: An esophagostomy tube can be removed within hours after placing or it can remain in place for months. The wrap should be changed and the site examined for any evidence of infection every few weeks. Oral feeding can proceed as per normal along with the assisted tube feeding.

as needed. The fistula generally heals within a week after the tube is removed permanently.

The percutaneous placement of a gastrostomy tube by endoscopic guidance is quick, safe, and effective.[1,2] In this procedure, a specialized 20-Fr tube (e.g., Dobbhoff PEG, Biosearch, Summerville, NJ, or Bard Urological Catheter, Bard Urological Division, Covington, GA) is used.

- As described previously, an area of skin is clipped and surgically prepared. The stomach is distended with air from an endoscope that is placed into the stomach.
- Once the stomach is distended to the point that it is in apposition with the body wall, a finger is used to depress an area just caudal to the last left rib below the transverse processes of the lumbar vertebrae. The area of depression is located by the person viewing the stomach lining by endoscopy.
- A polyvinyl chloride (PVC) over-the-needle IV catheter is placed through the skin and into the stomach in the area previously located by the endoscopist. The stylet is removed to allow the introduction of the first portion of a 5-ft piece of 8-lb test-weight nylon filament or suture.
- A biopsy snare passed through the endoscope

51. Block KI, Mead MN: Vitamin C in alternative cancer treatment: Historical background. Integr Cancer Ther 2(2):147–154, 2003.

52. Branda RF: Effects of folic acid deficiency on tumor cell biology, in Jacobs MM (ed): Vitamins and Minerals in the Prevention and Treatment of Cancer. Boca Raton, FL, CRC Press, 1991, pp 167–185.

53. Kline K, Sanders BG: Modulation of immune suppression and enhanced tumorigenesis in retrovirus tumor challenged chickens treated with vitamin E. In Vivo 3:161–185, 1989.

54. Kline K, Cochran GS, Sanders BG: Growth inhibitory effects of vitamin E succinate on retrovirus-transformed tumor cells in vitro. Nutr Cancer 14:27–35, 1990.

55. Miller ER 3rd, Pastor-Barriuso R, Dalal D et al: Meta-analysis: High-dosage vitamin E supplementation may increase all-cause mortality. Ann Intern Med 142(1):37–46, 2005; Epub 2004 Nov 10.

56. Paolini M, Abdel-Rahman SZ, Cantelli-Forti G, Legator MS: Chemoprevention or antichemoprevention? A salutary warning from the beta-carotene experience. J Natl Cancer Inst 93(14):1110–1101, 2001.

57. Shamberger RJ, Rukovena E, Longfield AK et al: Antioxidants and cancer. I. Selenium in the blood of normals and cancer patients. J Natl Cancer Inst 50:863–870, 1973.

58. Ip C: Factors influencing the anticarcinogenic efficacy of selenium in dimethylbenzanthracene-induced mammary tumorigenesis in rats. Cancer Res 41:2638–2644, 1981.

59. Jacobs MM, Jansson B, Griffin AC: Inhibitory effects of selenium on 1,2-dimethylhydrazine and methylazoxymethanol acetate induction of colon tumors. Cancer Lett 2:133–2144, 1977.

60. Jacobs MM, Griffin AC: Effects of selenium on chemical carcinogenesis: Comparative effects on antioxidants. Biol Trace El Res 1:2–21, 1979.

61. Asselin BL, Ryan D, Frantz CN et al: In vitro and in vivo killing of acute lymphoblastic leukemia cells by l-asparaginase. Cancer Res 49:4363–4369, 1989.

62. Weed H, McGandy RB, Kennedy AR: Protection against dimethylhydrazine induced adenomatous tumors of the mouse colon by the dietary addition of an extract of soybeans containing the Bowman-Birk protease inhibitor. Carcinogenesis 6:1239–1241, 1985.

63. Messadi DV, Billings P, Shklar G, Kennedy AR: Inhibition of oral carcinogenesis by a protease inhibitor. J Natl Cancer Inst 76:447–452, 1986.

64. St. Clair W, Billings P, Carew J et al: Suppression of DMH-induced carcinogenesis in mice by dietary addition of the Bowman-Birk protease inhibitor. Cancer Res 50:580–586, 1990.

65. Kennedy AR: Effects of protease inhibitors and vitamin E in the prevention of cancer, In Prasad KN, Meyskens FL (eds): Nutrients and Cancer Prevention. The Humana Press, Inc. 1990, pp 79–98.

66. Witschi H, Kennedy AR: Modulation of lung tumor development in mice with the soybean-derived Bowman-Birk protease inhibitor. Carcinogenesis 10:2275–2277, 1989.

67. Kealy RD, Lawler DF, Ballam JM et al: Influence of diet restriction on life span and age-related changes in Labrador retrievers. JAVMA 220:1315–1320, 2002.

68. Lawler DF, Evans RH, Larson BT et al: Influence of lifetime food restriction on causes, time, and predictors of death in dogs. JAVMA 226(2):225–231, 2005.

69. Terry PD, Rohan TE, Wolk A: Intakes of fish and marine fatty acids and the risks of cancers of the breast and prostate and of other hormone-related cancers: A review of the epidemiologic evidence. Am J Epidemiol 141(4):352–359, 1995.

70. Sonnenschein EG, Glickman LT, Goldschmidt MH, McKee LJ: Body conformation, diet, and risk of breast cancer in pet dogs: A case-control study. Am J Epidemiol 133(7):694–703, 1991.

71. http://www.vin.com/members/cms/document/default.aspx?id=4574504&pid=373&catid=&said=1

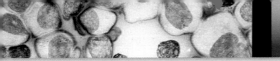
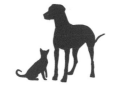

Chapter 26

Canine lymphoma

Clinical presentation

- Common, generally not painful, and very responsive to therapy and associated with a good quality of life.
- Generalized peripheral lymphadenopathy common (clinical stage III, see table 26-1).
- Non nodal lymphomas (e.g.: nasal cavity, bone, etc) can be localized.
- Diffuse large or intermediate cell, immunoblastic lymphoma, and small lymphocytic lymphoma common types.
- B-cell immunophenotype more common than T-cell.
- Indolent lymphoma is becoming more recognized as an important clinical type, often with a slow growth rate.
- All breeds, middle-aged; systemic disease.
- Causation includes association with specific environmental factors.

> **Key point**
> Genetic and environmental factors have been associated with an increased risk of lymphoma. Breed selection and avoiding certain environmental contaminants may decrease that risk.

Staging and diagnosis

- Minimun data base (MDB): includes a CBC, biochemical profile, urinalysis, diagnosis by cytology and/or biopsy, and three-view thoracic radiographs or computerized tomography of the chest.
- Molecular biological testing: PPAR vs. flow cytometry.
  - PPAR is a molecular biological test to determine if the disorder is a clonal expansion, and thus a malignancy, vs. reactive lymphoid cells, and if it is of T or B-cell origin, including plasma cells.

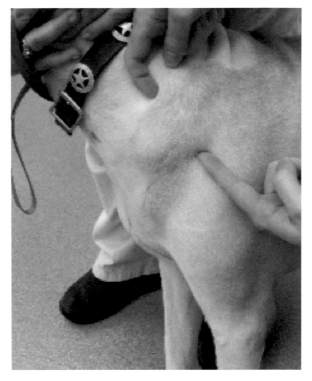

Figure 26-1: Most dogs with lymphoma present with generalized lymphadenopathy with or without liver and spleen involvement (stage III or IV lymphoma). Occasionally they will have bone marrow involvement despite a normal hemogram. Lymphoma is generally considered a non-painful malignancy that responds very well to therapy. Combination chemotherapy, especially when containing doxorubicin, is generally the most effective. Monoclonal antibodies and an n-3 long chain fatty acid, docosahexaenoic acid (DHA), can be used in addition to the chemotherapy to enhance and improve quality of life as well as progression-free and overall survival times. A key point is that clients should be made aware that lymphoma is best treated as a sequence of remissions. Bone marrow transplantation, while not universally available, is also being used to improve response to therapy. Most clients show a high degree of satisfaction when they treat their dogs.

Table 26-1. Clinical stages of canine lymphoma (WHO)[26]

Clinical Stage*	Criteria
Stage I	Involvement limited to single node or lymphoid tissue in single organ (excluding the bone marrow)
Stage II	Regional involvement of many lymph nodes, with or without involvement of the tonsils
Stage III	Generalized lymph node involvement
Stage IV	Involvement of liver and/or spleen, with or without generalized lymph node involvement
Stage V	Involvement of blood, bone marrow, and/or other organs

*Stages are further classified to clinical substage a (no clinical signs) or b (with clinical signs). For example, stage IIIa describes a dog with generalized lymphadenopathy and no clinical signs.

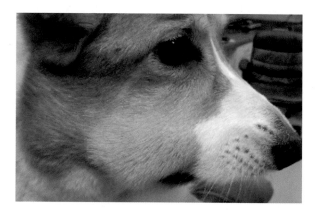

Figure 26-2: Some dogs with lymphoma present with swelling of the head and neck due to decreased lymphatic and venous drainage secondary to enlarged cervical or mediastinal lymph nodes. Treatment usually results in normalization of this condition within a week's time.

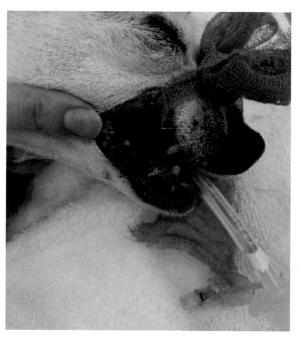

Figure 26-4: Dogs with mycosis fungoides present with flat to proliferative lesions of the skin, often around mucocutaneous sites such as the oral cavity, eyes and anus. A review of a histologic biopsy by a highly competent pathologist is necessary to make a specific diagnosis. Treatment with CCNU-based protocols with vitamin A analogs can improve quality of life for dogs with this condition.

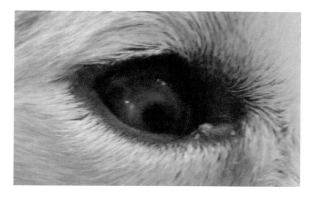

Figure 26-3: Some dogs with lymphoma will present for hyphema, anterior uveitis and iritis. The corneas of these dogs are usually cloudy, the iris color is usually darker than normal and the patient exhibits photophobia and discomfort to each eye. If hyphema is present, fresh blood may be noted, making the eyes appear red as in this image. Without a rapid diagnosis and therapy, blindness can result. This therapy involves treatment of the lymphoma and using topical and systemic steroids. If there is evidence of glaucoma, then aggressive therapy for this disorder is essential.

- Flow cytometry of neoplastic cells from blood, lymph nodes, or aspirates of spleen, liver, lymph nodes or other tissue can confirm neoplasia by ascertaining if the cells are a homogeneous expansion of a single cell, and can determine if there is an abnormal phenotype, which is critical for diagnosis, prognostication and for directing therapy.
- Canine B-cell lymphomas that express low levels of class II MHC have a worse prognosis than B-cell lymphomas with high class II MHC.[37]

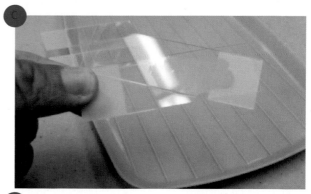

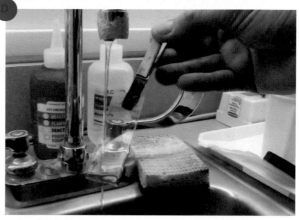

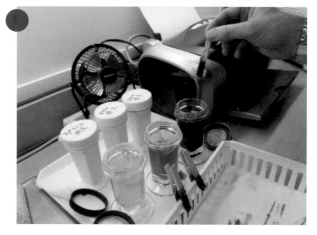

Figure 26-5: Lymphoma is best staged by doing a complete blood count, biochemical profile, urinalysis, chest radiographs, abdominal ultrasound, a biopsy, flow cytometry and/or cytology of involved tissue and a bone marrow aspirate. This chest radiograph confirms the presence of a mediastinal mass anterior to the heart. This finding is periodically associated with the presence of an elevated ionized calcium, which is commonly seen in dogs with T-cell lymphoma. The elevated ionized calcium can cause nephrotoxicity, which can be more dangerous to the patient than the lymphoma itself. Therefore, swift treatment to support renal health with fluid therapy may be warranted along with definitive chemotherapy for the lymphoma. Imaging courtesy of Lenore Anderson Mohammadian, DVM, MSpVM, Diplomate ACVR.

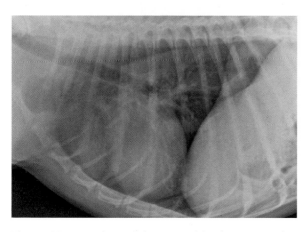

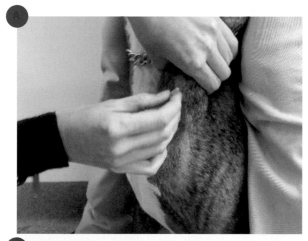

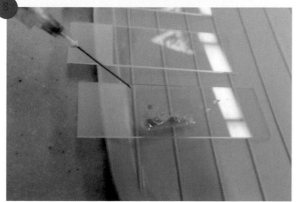

Figure 26-6: Lymphoma is one of the most successfully treated malignancies in veterinary medicine. Obtaining an appropriate cytologic diagnosis is extremely important. The first step is to insert a 20-gauge needle into the enlarged lymph node and redirect it throughout the tissue (A) in order to fill the needle with cells. The syringe is then filled with air before it is attached to the needle. The contents of the needle are then expelled onto a clean slide (B). Because lymphoma cells are extremely fragile, the expelled sample is treated with great gentleness by putting one clean slide on top of another; the two are gently slid one upon the other to pull them apart to make two mirror images of the lymph node tissue (C). One representative slide is then stained by Diff-Quick or other suitable stain exactly as per manufacturer's instructions (D) and then gently rinsed (d) and dried before examining on the microscope (E).

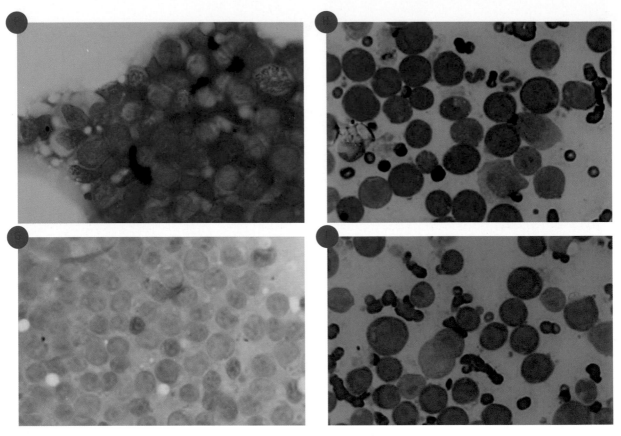

Figure 26-6 (cont.): The other slide is submitted for review by a board certified pathologist. When examining the cells under the microscope, find the cells that are not piled one on another. Lymphoma (F-I) is best described as being composed of cells that are composed of a monotonous population of small to large, poorly differentiated lymphoid cells with scant blue cytoplasm, dense nuclear margins, and round to slightly irregularly shaped nuclei with generally at least one nucleolus. Some lymphoma cells may have azurophilic granules upon staining. Lymphoma cells usually resemble lymphoblasts, although in many cases they can be very well differentiated and resemble normal lymphocytes.

- Measure all lymph nodes and extranodal sites.
- Abdominal ultrasonography or radiographs.
- Bone marrow aspirate cytology if indicated.

Key point

Immunophenotype is one of the strongest indicators of prognosis for a dog with lymphoma. Flow cytometry is a key and important diagnostic procedure to help the clinician understand the type of lymphoma to direct therapy, therefore improving response to therapy.

Key point

The cause of hypercalcemia in the dog should be identified as soon as possible so that supportive care can be initiated and the underlying cause eliminated. Lymphoma is one of the most common causes of hypercalcemia in the dog and most of these patients have mediastinal masses. A chest radiograph may be important.

Prognostic factors

Negative prognostic indicators:
- T-cell, major histocompatibility complex (MHC-), large cell size, as determined by flow cytometry.
- CD34+ leukemias, as determined by flow cytometry, have a much poorer prognosis (median survival 16 days) when compared with all other types of lymphoproliferative disorders involving peripheral blood.
- Substage b (clinically ill).
- Higher stage.
- Hypercalcemia (may reflect T-cell immunophenotype; often associated with a mediastinal mass).
- Increasing grade of malignancy, proliferative indices (AgNORs only).
- Presence of multidrug resistance protein.
- Pretreatment corticosteroids.
- Low serum albumin.
Positive prognostic indicators:
- B-cell, MHC+, intermediate cell size, as determined by flow cytometry.
- T-cell chronic lymphocytic leukemia (CLL) has a significantly better prognosis than B-cell CLL.

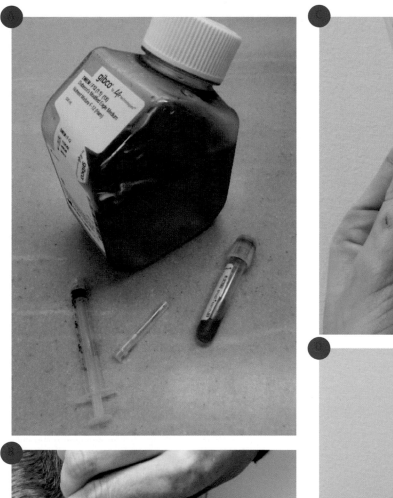

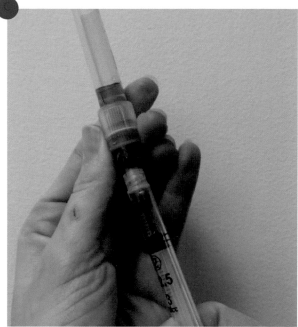

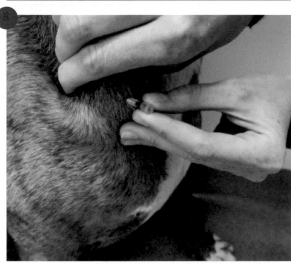

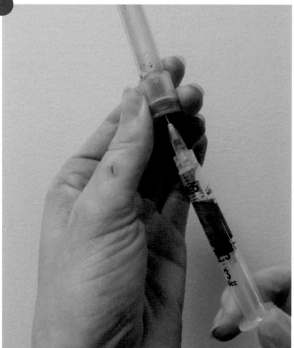

Figure 26-7: Flow cytometry is an important diagnostic test performed on live, viable cells that provides the clinician with a number of pieces of data including but not limited to a confirmation of a diagnosis of lymphoma, the cell type involved (T vs B vs indolent), if it is positive or negative for major histocompatibility complex (MHC+ or -), and the cell size involved (large, intermediate and small cell). Each laboratory should be consulted to determine their preferred method of sample preparation. In this example, either tissue culture media or sterile saline with 10% by volume of the patient's own serum or fetal calf serum is used (A). The needle is repeatedly inserted into the tissue that likely contains the lymphoma (B) and then the contents of the needle is expelled into a sterile tube that contains the media or saline with the serum additive (C). The contents of the tube are then withdrawn into the syringe and then expelled again into the tube (D), put on ice and sent overnight to the laboratory that does the test. Flow cytometry or peroxisome proliferator-activated receptors (PPAR) can also be done on blood submitted in a lavender top tube for analysis. PPAR are a group of nuclear receptor proteins that function as transcription factors regulating the expression of genes that can be used to confirm the presence of lymphoma.

Table 26-2. COP PROTOCOL[64]

Vincristine is administered at 0.75 mg/m² IV. Cyclophosphamide* is given at 250 mg/m² PO or 200 mg/m² IV. The dose for prednisone is 1 mg/kg PO daily for 7 days, then PO every other day.

Week	Vincristine	Cyclophosphamide*	Prednisone
1	•	•	↓
2	•		
3	•		
4	•	•	
5			
6			
7	•	•	
10	•	•	
	↓	↓	
		Every 3 weeks	

*If hemorrhagic cystitis occurs, chlorambucil is substituted on the same schedule at 15 mg/m² PO daily for 4 consecutive days (or 6 to 8 mg/m² PO daily continuously).

Table 26-3. VELCAP-S PROTOCOL[10]

Vincristine is administered at 0.75 mg/m² IV. Cyclophosphamide* is given at 250 mg/m² PO. The dose for L-asparaginase is 10,000 IU/m² IM (maximum treatment dose = 10,000 IU). Doxorubicin is administered at 25 mg/m² IV. Prednisone is given at 40 mg/m² PO sid for 7 days, then every other day.

Week	Vincristine	Cyclophosphamide*	L-asparaginase	Doxorubicin
1	•			
2	•			•
3	•			
4				•
5				
6				
7	•	•	•	
8			•	
9			•	
12	•	•		

*If hemorrhagic cystitis occurs, chlorambucil is substituted on the same schedule at 15 mg/m² PO daily for 4 consecutive days (or 6 to 8 mg/m² PO daily continuously.

Table 26-4. Modified CHOP protocol for the treatment of canine lymphoma

Week 1	Vincristine 0.7 mg/m² IV L-asparaginase 400 IU/kg IM Prednisone 2 mg/kg PO once daily
Week 2	Cyclophosphamide 250 mg/m² IV L-asparaginase 400 IU/kg IM Prednisone 1.5 mg/kg PO once daily
Week 3	Vincristine 0.7 mg/m² IV Prednisone, 1.0 mg/kg PO once daily
Week 4	Doxorubicin 30 mg/m² IV Prednisone 0.5 mg/kg PO once daily

Table 26-4. Modified CHOP protocol for the treatment of canine lymphoma (*cont.*)	
Week 6	Vincristine 0.7 mg/m² IV
Week 7	Cyclophosphamide 250 mg/m² IV
Week 8	Vincristine 0.7 mg/m² IV
Week 9	Doxorubicin 30 mg/m² IV
Week 11	Vincristine 0.7 mg/m² IV
Week 13	Cyclophosphamide 250 mg/m² IV
Week 15	Vincristine 0.7 mg/m² IV
Week 17	Doxorubicin 30 mg/m² IV
Week 19	Vincristine 0.7 mg/m² IV
Week 21	Cyclophosphamide 250 mg/m² IV
Week 23	Vincristine 0.7 mg/m² IV
Week 25	Doxorubicin 30 mg/m² IV

- Low body weight (<15 kg).
- Complete response to therapy.
- Toxicity to chemotherapy.
- Low-grade lymphoma.
- Diet (limited amounts of simple carbohydrates and n-6 polyunsaturated fatty acids; moderate amounts of high quality protein; enhanced amounts of n-3 polyunsaturated fatty acids).
- Trisomy chromosome 13.

Treatment

> **Key point**
>
> Doxorubicin is considered the most effective single agent in the treatment of canine lymphoma, especially B-cell lymphoma.

The goal is to have a series of remissions with the BEST protocol given first. This section is divided into three options:

- Comfort for those who want to improve quality of life.
- Comfort and control for those who want to improve quality of life while trying to provide some control of the tumor.
- Comfort and longer-term control for those who want to improve quality of life while trying to maximize the chance of controlling the tumor.

Comfort

- Therapy to enhance comfort and freedom from nausea, vomiting, diarrhea and lack of appetite plus prednisone alone (1 mg/kg/day), or in combination

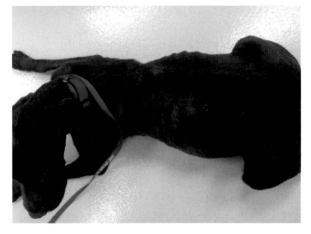

Figure 26-8: There are many prognostic factors that can predict response to therapy and duration of remission including the type, stage and extent of lymphoma, initial response to therapy, and the presence of hypercalcemia and illness. The dog depicted here is exhibiting advanced signs of cancer cachexia. A poor response to therapy is likely unless the patient receives aggressive supportive care including but not limited to fluid therapy, analgesics, antiemetics (e.g.: maropitant, metoclopramide), antidiarrheals (e.g.: tylosin, metronidazole) and nutritional support (e.g.: mirtazapine). Regardless, all dogs with lymphoma should be given medications to delay or prevent adverse effects associated with the administration of chemotherapy or the actual lysis of tumor cells due to the treatment. The first three weeks of cancer therapy for lymphoma is the most likely to be associated with nausea, vomiting, discomfort and lack of appetite due to either the therapy or, more likely, the presence of lysed tumor cells within the body. Quality of life can only be assured by educating each client on the steps that they can and should take to mitigate any adverse effects.

with chlorambucil (6 mg/m² PO every other day), may provide palliation with few risks of side effects. A CBC should be collected every 2 to 3 weeks to make sure that myelosuppression is not occurring.
• 30-50% in PR or CR for 1 to 3 months.

> **Key point**
>
> Dogs with advanced lymphoma, particularly if they are clinically ill, have a poor prognosis compared to healthy dogs with limited disease. Ill animals should be given supportive care with chemotherapy to minimize adverse effects and maximize quality of life and response to therapy.

Comfort and control (first remission)

Above mentioned therapy for comfort plus:
• Cyclophosphamide, vincristine, prednisone (COP, see table 26-2): 70% in CR for median 5 months.
• Doxorubicin as a single agent every three weeks for 5 treatments (30 mg/m² for dogs >10 kg and 1 mg/kg for dogs < 10 kg): 60%–75% in CR for median 6 to 8 months.
• CCNU as a single agent every three weeks for 5 treatments (lomustine, 60-70 mg) plus Denamarin for a median duration of remission of 40 days.
  • Supportive care if the patient is ill (substage b).

> **Key point**
>
> Combination chemotherapy with or without immunotherapy is the treatment of choice for most dogs with lymphoma.

Comfort and longer-term control (first remission)

Above mentioned therapy for comfort plus:
• Modified CHOP protocol (80-92.5% in PR or CR for median first remission of 11-12 months) +/- monoclonal antibody therapy directed to T or B-cell epitopes (see tables 26-3 and 26-4).
• Enhance alkylating agents if T-cell.
• Use appropriate supportive care if substage b.

Comfort and longer-term control (emerging therapies)

Above mentioned therapy for comfort and the modified CHOP protocol plus:
• Chemotherapy and radiation: CR for median 16 months.
• Autologous bone marrow transplant post radiation and/or chemotherapy: CR for median 12.5 months; 57% 1-year remission.

Rescue protocols

These treatment protocols are used to attain second and third and occasionally fourth remissions. The choice of protocols depends on the response to the prior protocol. If, for example, the patient has a long, durable remission to a modified CHOP protocol, that protocol can be repeated. If the patient has a poor response to the modified CHOP protocol, then it would be important to choose a protocol or a single agent that does not contain the previously used protocols. In general, the duration of remission for a rescue protocol is half the duration of the previous remission. Options include, but are not limited to:
• Single agents: Lomustine, DTIC, mitoxantrone, actinomycin D and doxorubicin.
• MOPP: Mechlorethamine, vincristine, procarbazine and prednisone.
• DMAC: Dexamethasone, melphalan, actinomycin D and cytosine arabinoside.
• BOPP: Carmustine, vincristine, procarbazine and prednisone.
• LOPP—Lomustine, vincristine, procarbazine and prednisone.
• MOMP: Mechlorethamine, vincristine, melphalan and prednisone.
CR = complete remission (complete disappearance of all clinical evidence of lymphoma).
PR = partial remission (>50% reduction in clinical disease parameters, no new lesions, but < CR).

References

1. Weiss DJ. A retrospective study of the incidence and the classification of bone marrow disorders in the dog at a veterinary teaching hospital (1996-2004). *J Vet Intern Med.* 20(4):955-961, 2006.
2. Schneider R: Comparison of age- and sex-specific incidence rate patterns of the leukemia complex in the cat and the dog. *J Natl Cancer Inst* 70:971–977, 1983.
3. Teske E: Canine malignant lymphoma: A review and comparison with human non-Hodgkin's lymphoma. *Vet Q* 16:209–219, 1994.
4. Dobson JM, Samuel S, Milstein H, et al: Canine neoplasia in the UK: Estimates of incidence rates from a population of insured dogs. *J Small Anim Pract* 43:240–246, 2002.
5. Clancy E, McConnell W, Patronek G, Moore A: Epidemiological study of canine lymphoma in New England. *Proc 19th Ann Conf Vet Cancer Soc* 71. 1999.
6. Priester WA: Canine lymphoma: Relative risk in the boxer breed. *J Natl Cancer Inst* 39:833–845, 1967.
7. Lurie DM, Lucroy MD, Griffey SM, et al: T-cell-derived malignant lymphoma in the boxer breed. *Vet Comp Oncol* 2:171–175, 2004.
8. Onions DE: A prospective survey of familial canine lymphosarcoma. *J Natl Cancer Inst* 72:909–912, 1984.
9. Edwards DS, Henley WE, Harding EF, et al: Breed incidence of lymphoma in a UK population of insured dogs. *Vet Comp Oncol* 1:200–206, 2003.
10. Moore AS, Cotter SM, Rand WM, et al: Evaluation of a discontinuous treatment protocol (VELCAP-S) for canine lymphoma. *J Vet Intern Med* 15:348–354, 2001.
11. Zemann BI, Moore AS, Rand WM, et al: A combination chemotherapy protocol (VELCAP-L) for dogs with lymphoma. *J Vet Intern Med* 12:465–470, 1998.
12. Jagielski D, Lechowski R, Hoffmann-Jagielska M, Winiarczyk S: A retrospective study of the incidence and prognostic factors of multicentric lymphoma in dogs (1998-2000). *J Vet Med A Physiol Pathol Clin Med* 49:419–424, 2002.
13. Teske E, de Vos JP, Egberink HF, Vos JH: Clustering in canine malignant lymphoma. *Vet Q* 16:134–136, 1994.
14. Onions D: RNA-dependent DNA polymerase activity in canine lymphosarcoma. *Eur J Cancer* 16:345–350, 1980.
15. Tomley FM, Armstrong SJ, deSouza PN: Retrovirus particles associated with canine lymphosarcoma and leukemia. *Brit J Cancer* 45:644, 1982.

16. O'Brien DJ, Kaneene JB, Getis A, et al: Spatial and temporal distribution of selected canine cancers in Michigan, USA, 1964-1994. *Prev Vet Med* 42:1–15, 1999.

17. Gavazza A, Presciuttini S, Barale R, et al: Association between canine malignant lymphoma, living in industrial areas, and use of chemicals by dog owners. *J Vet Intern Med* 15:190–195, 2001.

18. Hayes HM, Tarone RE, Cantor KP, et al: Case-control study of canine malignant lymphoma: positive association with dog owners use of 2,4-dichlorophenoxyacetic acid herbicides. *J Natl Cancer Inst* 83:1226–1231, 1991.

19. Reynolds PM, Reif JS, Ramsdell HS, Tessari JD: Canine exposure to herbicide-treated lawns and urinary excretion of 2,4-dichlorophenoxyacetic acid. *Cancer Epidemiol Biomarkers Prev* 3:233–237, 1994.

20. Carlo GL, Cole P, Miller AB, et al: Review of a study reporting an association between 2,4-dichlorophenoxyacetic acid and canine malignant lymphoma: Report of an expert panel. *Regul Toxicol Pharmacol* 16:245–252, 1992.

21. Kaneene JB, Miller R: Re-analysis of 2,4-D use and the occurrence of canine malignant lymphoma. *Vet Human Toxicol* 41:164–170, 1999.

22. Hayes HM, Tarone RE, Cantor KP: On the association between canine malignant lymphoma and opportunity for exposure to 2,4-dichlorophenoxyacetic acid. *Environ Res* 70:119–125, 1995.

23. Reif JS, Lower KS, Ogilvie GK: Residential exposure to magnetic fields and risk of canine lymphoma. *Am J Epidemiol* 141:352–359, 1995.

24. Keller ET: Immune-mediated diseases as a risk factor for canine lymphoma. *Cancer* 70:2334–2337, 1992.

25. Day MJ, Whitbread TJ: Pathological diagnoses in dogs with lymph node enlargement. *Vet Rec* 136:72–73, 1995.

26. Owen L M: TNM classification of tumours in domestic animals. Geneva: *World Health Organization*. 1st. 1980.

27. Keller ET, MacEwen EG, Rosenthal RC, et al: Evaluation of prognostic factors and sequential combination chemotherapy with doxorubicin for canine lymphoma. *J Vet Intern Med* 7:289–295, 1993.

28. Burnett RC, Vernau W, Modiano JF, et al: Diagnosis of canine lymphoid neoplasia using clonal rearrangements of antigen receptor genes. *Vet Pathol* 40:32–41, 2003.

29. Krohne SG, Henderson NM, Richardson RC, Vestre WA: Prevalence of ocular involvement in dogs with multicentric lymphoma: prospective evaluation of 94 cases. *Vet Comp Ophthalmology* 4:127–135, 1994.

30. Wyatt KM, Robertson ID: Canine lymphosarcoma: A West Australian perspective. *Aust Vet Pract* 28:63–66, 1998.

31. Ackerman N, Madewell BR: Thoracic and abdominal radiographic abnormalities in the multicentric form of lymphosarcoma in dogs. *JAVMA* 176:36–40, 1980.

32. Sauerbrey ML1, Mullins MN, Bannink EO, et al: Lomustine and prednisone as a first-line treatment for dogs with multicentric lymphoma: 17 cases (2004-2005). *JAVMA* 15;230(12):1866-1869, 2007.

33. Skorupski KA, Hammond GM, Irish AM, Kent MS, et al:. Prospective randomized clinical trial assessing the efficacy of Denamarin for prevention of CCNU-induced hepatopathy in tumor-bearing dogs. *J Vet Intern Med* 25(4):838-845, 2011.

34. Steyn PF, Ogilvie G: 99m Tc-methoxy-isobutyl-isonitrile (sestamibi) imaging of malignant canine lymphoma. *Vet Radiol Ultrasound* 36:411–416, 1995.

35. Avery PR1, Burton J, Bromberek JL, et al: Flow cytometric characterization and clinical outcome of CD4+ T-cell lymphoma in dogs: 67 cases. *J Vet Intern Med* 28(2):538-46, 2014.

36. Raskin RE, Krehbiel JD: Histopathology of canine bone marrow in malignant lymphoproliferative disorders. *Vet Pathol* 25:83–88, 1988.

37. Rao S, Lana S, Eickhoff J, et al: Class II major histocompatibility complex expression and cell size independently predict survival in canine B-cell lymphoma. *J Vet Intern Med* 25(5):1097-1105, 2011.

38. Comazzi S, Gelain ME, Martini V, et al: Immunophenotype predicts survival time in dogs with chronic lymphocytic leukemia. *J Vet Intern Med* 25(1):100-106, 2011.

39. Morrison-Collister KE, Rassnick KM, Northrup NC, et al: A combination chemotherapy protocol with MOPP and CCNU consolidation (Tufts VELCAP-SC) for the treatment of canine lymphoma. *Vet Comp Oncol* 1:180–190, 2003.

40. Rosol TJ, Nagode LA, Couto CG, et al: Parathyroid hormone (PTH)-related protein, PTH, and 1,25-dihydroxyvitamin D in dogs with cancer-associated hypercalcemia. *Endocrinology* 131:1157–1164, 1992.

41. Lemmens P, De Bruin A, De Meulemeester J, et al: Paraneoplastic pemphigus in a dog. *Vet Dermatol* 9:127–134, 1998.

42. Anderson RK, Carpenter JL: Severe pruritus associated with lymphoma in a dog. *JAVMA* 207:455–456, 1995.

43. Nelson RW, Hager D, Zanjani ED: Renal lymphosarcoma with inappropriate erythropoietin production in a dog. *JAVMA* 182:1396–1397, 1983.

44. Mayhew PD, Bush WW, Glass EN: Trigeminal neuropathy in dogs: A retrospective study of 29 cases (1991-2000). *JAAHA* 38:262–270, 2002.

45. Fournel-Fleury C, Magnol JP, Bricaire P, et al: Cytohistological and immunological classification of canine malignant lymphomas: Comparison with human non-Hodgkin's lymphomas. *J Comp Pathol* 117:35–59, 1997.

46. Vail DM, Kravis LD, Kisseberth WC, et al: Application of rapid CD3 immunophenotype analysis and argyrophilic nucleolar organizer region (AgNOR) frequency to fine needle aspirate specimens from dogs with lymphoma. *Vet Clin Pathol* 26:66–69, 1997.

47. Fisher DJ, Naydan D, Werner LL, Moore PF: Immunophenotyping lymphomas in dogs: a comparison of results from fine needle aspirate and needle biopsy samples. *Vet Clin Pathol* 24:118–123, 1995.

48. Caniatti M, Roccabianca P, Scanziani E, et al: Canine lymphoma: Immunocytochemical analysis of fine-needle aspiration biopsy. *Vet Pathol* 33:204–212, 1996. 49. Dobson JM, Blackwood LB, McInnes EF, et al: Prognostic variables in canine multicentric lymphosarcoma. *J Small Anim Pract* 42:377–384, 2001.

50. Appelbaum FR, Sale GE, Storb R, et al: Phenotyping of canine lymphoma with monoclonal antibodies directed at cell surface antigens: Classification, morphology, clinical presentation and response to chemotherapy. *Hematol Oncol* 2:151–168, 1984.

51. Ruslander DA, Gebhard DH, Tompkins MB, et al: Immunophenotypic characterization of canine lymphoproliferative disorders. *In Vivo* 11:169–172, 1997.

52. Williams LE, Johnson JL, Hauck ML, et al: Chemotherapy followed by half-body radiation therapy for canine lymphoma. *J Vet Intern Med* 18:703–709, 2004.

53. Teske E, Wisman P, Moore PF, van Heerde P: Histologic classification and immunophenotyping of canine non-Hodgkin's lymphomas: Unexpected high frequency of T-cell lymphomas with B-cell morphology. *Exp Hematol* 22:1179–1187, 1994.

54. Alvarez-Berger FJ, Chavez-Gris G, Aburto-Fernandez E, Aristi-Urista G: Histopathologic and immunophenotypic study of lymphoma in Mexico. *Proc 23rd Ann Conf Vet Cancer Soc* 28, 2003.

55. Kiupel M, Teske E, Bostock D: Prognostic factors for treated canine malignant lymphoma. *Vet Pathol* 36:292–300, 1999.

56. Ponce F, Magnol JP, Ledieu D, et al: Prognostic significance of morphological subtypes in canine malignant lymphomas during chemotherapy. *Vet J* 167:158–166, 2004.

57. Gibson D, Aubert I, Woods JP, et al: Flow cytometric immunophenotype of canine lymph node aspirates. *J Vet Intern Med* 18:710–717, 2004.

58. Baskin CR, Couto CG, Wittum TE: Factors influencing first remission and survival in 145 dogs with lymphoma: a retrospective study. *JAAHA* 36:404–409, 2000.

59. Garrett LD, Thamm DH, Chun R, et al: Evaluation of a 6-month chemotherapy protocol with no maintenance therapy for dogs with lymphoma. *J Vet Intern Med* 16:704–709, 2002.

60. Valerius KD, Ogilvie GK, Mallinckrodt CH, Getzy DM: Doxorubicin alone or in combination with asparaginase, followed by cyclophosphamide, vincristine, and prednisone for treatment of multicentric lymphoma in dogs: 121 cases (1987-1995). *JAVMA* 210:512–516, 1997.

61. MacEwen EG, Hayes AA, Matus RE, Kurzman I: Evaluation of some prognostic factors for advanced multicentric lymphosarcoma in the dog: 147 cases (1978-1981). *JAVMA* 190:564–568, 1987.

62. Greenlee PG, Filippa DA, Quimby FW, et al: Lymphomas in dogs. A morphologic, immunologic, and clinical study. *Cancer* 66:480–490, 1990.

63. Theilen GH, Worley M, Benjamini E: Chemoimmunotherapy for canine lymphosarcoma. *JAVMA* 170:607–610, 1977.

64. Cotter SM: treatment of lymphoma and leukemia with cyclophosphamide, vincristine and prednisone: I. treatment of dogs. *JAAHA* 19:159–165, 1983.

65. Squire RA, Bush M, Melby EC, et al: Clinical and pathologic study of canine lymphoma: Clinical staging, cell classification, and therapy. *J Natl Cancer Inst* 51:565–574, 1973.

66. MacEwen EG, Brown NO, Patnaik AK, et al: Cyclic combination chemotherapy of canine lymphosarcoma. *JAVMA* 178: 1178–1181, 1981.

67. Carter RF, Harris CK, Withrow SJ, et al: Chemotherapy of canine lymphoma with histopathological correlation: Doxorubicin alone compared to COP as first treatment regimen. *JAAHA* 23:587–596, 1987.

68. Weller RE, Theilen GH, Madewell BR: Chemotherapeutic responses in dogs with lymphosarcoma and hypercalcemia. *JAVMA* 181:891–893, 1982.

69. Rosenberg MP, Matus RE, Patnaik AK: Prognostic factors in dogs with lymphoma and associated hypercalcemia. *J Vet Intern Med* 5:268–271, 1991.

70. Price GS, Frazier DL: Use of body surface area (BSA)-based dosages to calculate chemotherapeutic drug dose in dogs: I. Potential problems with current BSA formulae. *J Vet Intern Med* 12:267-271, 1998.

71. Teske E, van Heerde P: Diagnostic value and reproducibility of fine-needle aspiration cytology in canine malignant lymphoma. *Vet Q* 18:112–115, 1996.

72. Hahn KA, Richardson RC, Teclaw RF, et al: Is maintenance chemotherapy appropriate for the managment of canine malignant lymphoma? *J Vet Intern Med* 6:3–10, 1992.

73. Kiupel M, Bostock D, Bergmann V: The prognostic significance of AgNOR counts and PCNA-positive cell counts in canine malignant lymphomas. *J Comp Pathol* 119:407–418, 1998.

74. Fournel-Fleury C, Ponce F, Felman P, et al: Canine T-cell lymphomas: A

Chapter 27

Canine bone marrow neoplasias

CANINE MYELODYSPLASIA

Clinical presentation

- Uncommon, yet new diagnostics are making diagnosis more common. Generally not painful.
- Clinical signs due to cytopenias (e.g., fever and neutropenia, petechiation and thrombocytopenia).
- Differentiated from leukemia by <30% blasts in dysplastic bone marrow.
- No age, gender, or breed predilection known.
- May progress to an acute leukemia.

Staging and diagnosis

> **Key point**
> A bone marrow aspirate is often necessary to diagnose bone marrow neoplasia. Occasionally, a bone marrow core biopsy and/or flow cytometry may be needed to determine the specific type of marrow neoplasia present.

- Minimum data base (MDB): includes a CBC, biochemical profile, urinalysis, diagnosis by cytology and/or biopsy, flow cytometry and/or PPAR and three-view thoracic radiographs.
- Bone marrow aspirate and biopsy.

> **Key point**
> Myelodysplasia is characterized by bone marrow that contains abnormalities in cellular maturation but less than 30% blast cells.

> **Key point**
> Dogs with multiple myeloma have a monoclonal gammopathy, however the total globulins may not be elevated. An electrophoresis is essential to diagnose the gammopathy.

Prognostic factors

- None identified.

Treatment

This section is divided into two options:
- Comfort for those who want to improve quality of life.
- Comfort and control for those who want to improve quality of life while trying to provide some control of the tumor.

> **Key point**
> Dogs with chronic lymphocytic leukemia usually begin improving shortly after therapy begins, however the lymphocyte count may not decrease significantly for 3-4 months.

Comfort

- Therapy to enhance comfort and freedom from nausea, vomiting, diarrhea and lack of appetite.
- Erythropoietin and if needed, blood transfusions, granulocyte colony-stimulating factor and corticosteroids may minimize clinical signs and cause remission in some dogs with myelodysplastic syndrome with refractory anemia.

Comfort and control

Above mentioned therapy for comfort plus:
- Differentiating agents and/or cytosine arabinoside. Retinoids are under investigation.

CANINE ACUTE MYELOID OR MYELOMONOCYTIC LEUKEMIA

Clinical presentation

- Uncommon, yet new diagnostics are making diagnosis more common. Generally not painful.
- Nonspecific, lethargy and weight loss; clinical signs also result from cytopenias.
- Females, large breeds, all ages; median age is 6 years.
- Rapidly progressive, terminating in pancytopenia due to myelophthisis.

Staging and diagnosis

- Minimum data base (MDB): includes a CBC, biochemical profile, urinalysis, diagnosis by cytology and/or biopsy, flow cytometry and three-view thoracic radiographs or computerized tomography of the chest.
- Bone marrow aspirate.
- Immunostaining and/or flow cytometry.
- Multiple subtypes/subclassifications are recognized, myelomonocytic (M4) is most common.
- Dogs with any subtype have a poor prognosis.

Prognostic factors

- None identified. The prognosis for this disease and probability for response to therapy is poor.

Treatment

This section is divided into two options:
- Comfort for those who want to improve quality of life.
- Comfort and control for those who want to improve quality of life while trying to provide some control of the tumor.

Comfort

- Therapy to enhance comfort and freedom from nausea, vomiting, diarrhea and lack of appetite.
- Erythropoietin and, if needed, blood transfusions, recombinant granulocyte colony-stimulating factor and corticosteroids may minimize clinical

signs and cause remission in some dogs with myelodysplastic syndrome with refractory anemia.

Comfort and control

Above mentioned therapy for comfort plus:
- Differentiating agents and/or cytosine arabinoside. Retinoids are under investigation.

CANINE ACUTE LYMPHOBLASTIC LEUKEMIA

Clinical presentation

- Acute onset lethargy, weight loss, and anorexia; splenomegaly common; mild lymphadenopathy.
- Generally not painful.
- Clinical signs also result from cytopenias.
- No age or gender predilection; large-breed dogs.
- Rapidly progressive; pancytopenia due to myelophthisis.

Staging and diagnosis

- Minimum data base (MDB): includes a CBC, biochemical profile, urinalysis, diagnosis by cytology and/or biopsy, flow cytometry and/or PPAR and three-view thoracic radiographs or computerized tomography of the chest.
- Bone marrow aspirate.

Prognostic factors

- Neutropenia is a negative prognostic indicator.

Treatment

This section is divided into three options:
- Comfort for those who want to improve quality of life.
- Comfort and control for those who want to improve quality of life while trying to provide some control of the tumor.
- Comfort and longer-term control for those who want to improve quality of life while trying to maximize the chance of controlling the tumor.

Comfort

- Therapy to enhance comfort and freedom from nausea, vomiting, diarrhea and lack of appetite, plus antibiotics and transfusions of blood and blood products as needed.
- Single agent prednisone.

Comfort and control

Above mentioned therapy for comfort plus:
- Use minimally myelosuppressive chemotherapy agents, at least initially (e.g., vincristine, prednisone, L-asparaginase), until normal neutrophil counts are obtained, then use standard lymphoma protocols.

Comfort and control

Above mentioned therapy for comfort plus:
- Phlebotomy.
  - Periodic removal eventually induces iron deficiency and microcytic cells that may assist in palliation.
- Chemotherapy.
  - Hydroxyurea gives long-term control.

CANINE MULTIPLE MYELOMA

Clinical presentation

- Anemia and secondary infections due to myelophthisis.
- Lameness and pain from bone lytic lesions.
- Polyuria and polydipsia from hypercalcemia, renal disease, and paraproteinuria.
- Hemorrhage and retinal lesions due to hyperviscosity.
- Median age is 8 to 9 years; most cases occur in purebred dogs.

Staging and diagnosis

- Minimum data base (MDB): includes a CBC, biochemical profile, urinalysis, diagnosis by cytology and/or biopsy, flow cytometry, PPAR and three-view thoracic radiographs or computerized tomography of the chest.
- Bone marrow aspirate.
- Radiographs of ribs, spine, and any painful sites.
- Serum protein electrophoresis and immunoelectrophoresis.
- Urine Bence-Jones protein test (or urine immunoelectrophoresis).

Prognostic factors

- Dogs with hypercalcemia have a worse prognosis.
- Dogs with extensive bone lysis have a worse prognosis.
- Dogs with light-chain (Bence-Jones) proteinuria have a worse prognosis.

Treatment

This section is divided into two options:
- Comfort for those who want to improve quality of life.
- Comfort and control for those who want to improve quality of life while trying to provide some control of the tumor.

Comfort

- Therapy to enhance comfort and freedom from nausea, vomiting, diarrhea and lack of appetite. Radiation therapy and/or bisphosphonates have been shown to be palliative for localized bone lesions.

Comfort and control

Above mentioned therapy for comfort plus:
- Prednisone alone only palliative; median survival is 220 days.
- Melphalan and prednisone causes complete remission in 40% and partial remission in 50% of dogs, for median survival of 540 days.
- Cyclophosphamide or chlorambucil may also be effective.
- GS-9219/VDC-1101, a prodrug of the acyclic nucleotide PMEG, has antitumor activity in spontaneous canine multiple myeloma.

References

1. Weiss DJ, Aird B: Cytologic evaluation of primary and secondary myelodysplastic syndromes in the dog. *Vet Clin Pathol* 30:67–75, 2001.
2. Weiss DJ, Raskin R, Zerbe C: Myelodysplastic syndrome in two dogs. *JAVMA* 187:1038–1040, 1985.
3. Jain NC, Blue JT, Grindem CB, et al: Proposed criteria for classification of acute myeloid leukemia in dogs and cats. *Vet Clin Pathol* 20:63–82, 1991.
4. Seed TM, Kaspar LV: Acquired radioresistance of hematopoietic progenitors (granulocyte/monocyte colony-forming units) during chronic radiation leukemogenesis. *Cancer Res* 52:1469–1476, 1992.
5. Raskin RE: Myelopoiesis and myeloproliferative disorders. *Vet Clin North Am Small Anim Pract* 26:1023–1042, 1996.
6. McManus PM, Hess RS: Myelodysplastic changes in a dog with subsequent acute myeloid leukemia. *Vet Clin Pathol* 27:112–115, 1998.
7. Gorman NT, Evans RJ: Myeloproliferative disease in the dog and cat: Clinical presentations, diagnosis and treatment. *Vet Rec* 121:490–496, 1987.
8. Couto CG, Kallet AJ: Preleukemic syndrome in a dog. *JAVMA* 184:1389–1392, 1984.
9. Tolle DV, Cullen SM, Seed TM, Fritz TE: Circulating micromegakaryocytes preceding leukemia in three dogs exposed to 2.5 R/day gamma radiation. *Vet Pathol* 20:111–114, 1983.
10. Boone LI, Knauer KW, Rapp SW, et al: Use of human recombinant erythropoietin and prednisone for treatment of myelodysplastic syndrome with erythroid predominance in a dog. *JAVMA* 213:999–1001, 1998.
11. Ide K, Momoi Y, Minegishi M, et al: A severe hepatic disorder with myelodysplastic syndrome, treated with cytarabine ocfosate, in a dog. *Aust Vet J* 81:47–49, 2003.
12. MacLeod JN, Tetreault JW, Lorschy KA, Gu DN: Expression and bioactivity of recombinant canine erythropoietin. *Am J Vet Res* 59:1144–1148, 1998.
13. Weiss DJ: New insights into the physiology and treatment of acquired myelodysplastic syndromes and aplastic pancytopenia. *Vet Clin North Am Small Anim Pract* 33:1317–1334, 2003.
14. Graves TK, Swenson CL, Scott MA: A potentially misleading presentation and course of acute myelomonocytic leukemia in a dog. *J Am Anim Hosp Assoc* 33:37–41, 1997.
15. Grindem CB, Stevens JB, Perman V: Cytochemical reactions in cells from leukemic dogs. *Vet Pathol* 23:103–109, 1986.
16. Couto CG: Clinicopathologic aspects of acute leukemias in the dog. *JAVMA* 186:681–685, 1985.
17. Grindem CB: Cytogenetic analysis of leukaemic cells in the dog: A report of 10 cases and a review of the literature. *J Comp Pathol* 96:623–635, 1986.
18. Jain NC, Madewell BR, Weller RE, Geissler MC: Clinicalpathological findings and cytochemical characterization of myelomonocytic leukaemia in 5 dogs. *J Comp Pathol* 91:17–31, 1981.
19. Grindem CB, Stevens JB, Perman V: Morphological classification and clinical and pathological characteristics of spontaneous leukemia in 17 dogs. *J Am Anim Hosp Assoc* 21:219–226, 1985.
20. Grindem CB, Steven JB, Brost DR, Johnson DD: Chronic myelogenous leukaemia with meningeal infiltration in a dog. *Compar Haematol Int* 2:170–174, 1992.
21. Rohrig KE: Acute myelomonocytic leukemia in a dog. *JAVMA* 182:137–141, 1983.
22. Colbatzky F, Hermanns W: Acute megakaryoblastic leukemia in one cat and two dogs. *Vet Pathol* 30:186–194, 1993.
23. Messick J, Carothers M, Wellman M: Identification and

characterization of megakaryoblasts in acute megakaryoblatic leukemia in a dog. *Vet Pathol* 27:212–214, 1990.

24. Bolon B, Buergelt CD, Harvey JW, et al: Megakaryoblastic leukemia in a dog. *Vet Clin Pathol* 18:69–72, 2003.
25. Cain GR, Feldman BF, Kawakami TG, Jain NC: Platelet dysplasia associated with megakaryoblastic leukemia in a dog. *JAVMA* 188:529–530, 1986.
26. Miyamoto T, Hachimura H, Amimoto A: A case of megakaryoblastic leukemia in a dog. *J Vet Med Sci* 58:177–179, 1996.
27. Facklam NR, Kociba GJ: Cytochemical characterization of leukemic cells from 20 dogs. *Vet Pathol* 22:363–369, 1985.
28. Grindem CB: Ultrastructural morphology of leukemic cells from 14 dogs. *Vet Pathol* 22:456–462, 1985.
29. Canfield PJ, Watson ADJ, Begg AP, Dill-Macky E: Myeloproliferative disorder in four dogs involving derangements of erythropoiesis, myelopoiesis and megakaryopoiesis. *J Small Anim Pract* 27:7–16, 1986.
30. Weiss DJ: Evaluation of proliferative disorders in canine bone marrow by use of flow cytometric scatter plots and monoclonal antibodies. *Vet Pathol* 38:512–518, 2001.
31. Fernandes PJ, Modiano JF, Wojcieszyn J, et al: Use of the cell-Dyn 3500 to predict leukemic cell lineage in peripheral blood of dogs and cats. *Vet Clin Pathol* 31:167–182, 2002.
32. Vernau W, Moore PF: An immunophenotypic study of canine leukemias and preliminary assessment of clonality by polymerase chain reaction. *Vet Immunol Immunopathol* 69:145–164, 1999.
33. Cooper BJ, Watson AD: Myeloid neoplasia in a dog. *Aust Vet J* 51:150–154, 1975.
34. Alroy J: Basophilic leukemia in a dog. *Vet Pathol* 9:90–95, 1972.
35. Holscher MA, Collins RD, Cousar JB, et al: Megakaryocytic leukemia in a cat. *Fel Pract* 13:8–12, 1983.
36. Capelli JL: Érythroleucémie chez un chien. *J Pratique Medicale & Chirurgicale de l'Animal de Compagnie* 26:337–340, 1991.
37. Mori T, Kadosawa T, Okada Y, et al: Acute respiratory failure caused by leukaemic infiltration of the lung of a dog. *J Small Anim Pract* 42:349–351, 2001.
38. Matus RE, Leifer CE, MacEwen EG: Acute lymphoblastic leukemia in the dog: A review of 30 cases. *JAVMA* 183:859–862, 1983.
39. Henry CJ, Lanevschi A, Marks SL, et al: Acute lymphoblastic leukemia, hypercalcemia, and pseudohyperkalemia in a dog. *JAVMA* 208:237–239, 1996.
40. Ruslander DA, Gebhard DH, Tompkins MB, et al: Immunophenotypic characterization of canine lymphoproliferative disorders. *In Vivo* 11:169–172, 1997.
41. McDonough SP, Moore PF: Clinical, hematologic, and immunophenotypic characterization of canine large granular lymphocytosis. *Vet Pathol* 37:637–646, 2000.
42. Moldovanu G: Continuing long-term remission after cyclophosphamide (NSC-26271) therapy for canine leukemia. *Cancer Chemother Rep* 53:223–227, 1969.
43. MacEwen EG, Patnaik AK, Hayes AA, et al: Temporary plasma-induced remission of lymphoblastic leukemia in a dog. *Am J Vet Res* 42:1450–1452, 1981.
44. Hodgkins EM, Zinkl JG, Madewell BR: Chronic lymphocytic leukemia in the dog. *JAVMA* 177:704–707, 1980.
45. Leifer CE, Matus RE: Chronic lymphocytic leukemia in the dog: 22 cases (1978–1984). *JAVMA* 189:214–217, 1986.
46. Kristensen AT, Klausner JS, Weiss DJ, et al: Spurious hyperphosphatemia in a dog with chronic lymphocytic leukemia and an IgM monoclonal gammopathy. *Vet Clin Pathol* 20:45–48, 1998.
47. Olivry T, Atlee BA: Leucemie lymphoide chronique avec ulcerations buccales chez un chien. *J Pratique Medicale & Chirurgicale de l'Animal de Compagnie* 27:177–181, 1992.
48. Harvey JW, Terrell TG, Hyde DM, Jackson RI: Well-differentiated lymphocytic leukemia in a dog: Long-term survival without therapy. *Vet Pathol* 18:37–47, 1981.
49. Couto GC, Sousa C: Chronic lymphocytic leukemia with cutaneous involvement in a dog. *J Am Anim Hosp Assoc* 22:374–379, 1986.
50. Comazzi S, Gelain ME, Martini V, et al: Immunophenotype predicts survival time in dogs with chronic lymphocytic leukemia. *J Vet Intern Med* 25(1):100-106, 2011.
51. Fujino Y, Sawamura S, Kurakawa N, et al: treatment of chronic lymphocytic leukaemia in three dogs with melphalan and prednisolone. *J Small Anim Pract* 45:298–303, 2004.
52. Leporrier M, Chevret S, Cazin B et al: Randomized comparison of fludarabine, CAP, and ChOP in 938 previously untreated stage B and C chronic lymphocytic leukemia patients. *Blood* 98:2319–2325, 2001.
53. Leifer CE, Matus RE, Patnaik AK, MacEwen EG: Chronic myelogenous leukemia in the dog. *JAVMA* 183:686– 689, 1983.
54. Thomsen MK, Jensen AL, Skak-Nielsen T, Kristensen F: Enhanced granulocyte function in a case of chronic granulocytic leukemia in a dog. *Vet Immunol Immunopathol* 28:143–156, 1991.

55. Ndikuwera J, Smith DA, Obwolo MJ, Masvingwe C: Chronic granulocytic leukaemia/eosinophilic leukaemia in a dog? *J Small Anim Pract* 33:553–557, 1992.
56. Mears EA, Raskin RE, Legendre AM: Basophilic leukemia in a dog. *J Vet Intern Med* 11:92–94, 1997.
57. MacEwen EG, Drazner FH, McClelland AJ, Wilkins RJ: treatment of basophilic leukemia in a dog. *JAVMA* 166:376–380, 1975.
58. Jensen AL, Nielsen OL: Eosinophilic leukaemoid reaction in a dog. *J Small Animal Pract* 33:337–340, 1992.
59. Perkins M, Watson A: Successful treatment of hypereosinophilic syndrome in a dog. *Aust Vet J* 79:686–689, 2001.
60. Degen MA, Feldman BF, Turrel JM, et al: Thrombocytosis associated with a myeloproliferative disorder in a dog. *JAVMA* 194:1457–1459, 1989.
61. Fine DM, Tvedten HW: Chronic granulocytic leukemia in a dog. *JAVMA* 214:1809–1812, 1791, 1999.
62. Tarrant JM, Stokol T, Blue JT, et al: Diagnosis of chronic myelogenous leukemia in a dog using morphologic, cytochemical, and flow cytometric techniques. *Vet Clin Pathol* 30:19–24, 2001.
63. Ehninger G, Schuler U, Renner U, et al: Use of a water-soluble busulfan formulation—pharmacokinetic studies in a canine model. *Blood* 85:3247–3249, 1995.
64. Favier RP, van Leeuwen M, Teske E: Essential thrombocythaemia in two dogs. *Tijdschr Diergeneeskd* 129:360–364, 2004.
65. Hopper PE, Mandell CP, Turrel JM, et al: Probable essential thrombocythemia in a dog. *J Vet Intern Med* 3:79–85, 1989.
66. Dunn JK, Heath MF, Jefferies AR, et al: Diagnostic and hematologic features of probable essential thrombocythemia in two dogs. *Vet Clin Pathol* 28:131–138, 1999.
67. Smith M, Turrel JM: Radiophosphorus (32P) treatment of bone marrow disorders in dogs: 11 cases (1970–1987). *JAVMA* 194:98–102, 1989.
68. Kammermann-Luscher B: Polycythaemia vera beim hund. *Schweiz Arch Tierheilk* 117:557–568, 1975.
69. Bass MC, Schultze AE: Essential thrombocythemia in a dog: Case report and literature review. *JAAHA* 34:197–203, 1998.
70. McGrath CJ: Polycythemia vera in dogs. *JAVMA* 164:1117–1122, 1974.
71. Quesnel AD, Kruth SA: Polycythemia vera and glomerulonephritis in a dog. *Can Vet J* 33:671–672, 1992.
72. Peterson ME, Randolph JF: Diagnosis of canine primary polycythemia and management with hydroxyurea. *JAVMA* 180:415–418, 1982.
73. Gray HE, Weigand CM, Cottrill NB, et al: Polycythemia vera in a dog presenting with uveitis. *JAAHA* 39:355–360, 2003.
74. Cook SM, Lothrop CD Jr: Serum erythropoietin concentrations measured by radioimmunoassay in normal, polycythemic, and anemic dogs and cats. *J Vet Intern Med* 8:18–25, 1994.
75. Meyer HP, Slappendel RJ, Greydanus-van der Putten SW: Polycythaemia vera in a dog treated by repeated phlebotomies. *Vet Q* 15:108–111, 1993.
76. Carb AV: Polycythemia vera in a dog. *JAVMA* 154:289–297, 1969.
77. Lester SJ, Mesfin GM: A solitary plasmacytoma in a dog with progression to a disseminated myeloma. *Can Vet J* 21:284–286, 1980.
78. Walton GS, Gopinath C: Multiple myeloma in a dog with some unusual features. *J Small Anim Pract* 13:703–708, 1972.
79. Matus RE, Leifer CE, MacEwen EG, Hurvitz AI: Prognostic factors for multiple myeloma in the dog. *JAVMA* 188:1288–1292, 1986.
80. Osborne CA, Perman V, Sautter JH, et al: Multiple myeloma in the dog. *JAVMA* 153:1300–1319, 1968.
81. Stone RW: The unexpected diagnosis of multiple myeloma in a Shiba Inu incidental to warfarin intoxication. *Canine Pract* 18:26–28, 1993.
82. Orr CM, Higginson J, Baker JR, Jones DR: Plasma cell myeloma with IgG paraproteinemia in a bitch. *J Small Anim Pract* 22:31–37, 1981.
83. Pechereau D, Lanore D, Martel PH: Le mylome multiple: Mise au point a partir de neuf cas. *Prat Med Chirurgicale* 26:369–378, 1991.
84. Lautzenhiser SJ, Walker MC, Goring RL: Unusual IgM secreting multiple myeloma in a dog. *JAVMA* 223:645–648, 636, 2003.
85. MacEwen EG, Patnaik AK, Huruitz AI, et al: Non-secretory multiple myeloma in two dogs. *JAVMA* 184:1283–1286, 1984.
86. Oduye OO, Losos GJ: Multiple myeloma in a dog. *J Small Anim Pract* 13:257–263, 1972.
87. Breuer W, Colbatzky F, Platz S, Hermanns W: Immunoglobulin-producing tumours in dogs and cats. *J Comp Pathol* 109:203–216, 1993.
88. Maeda H, Ozaki K, Abe T, et al: Bone lesions of multiple myeloma in three dogs. *Zentralbl Veterinarmed A* 40:384–392, 1993.
89. Cayzer J, Jones BR: IgA multiple myeloma in a dog. *N Z Vet J* 39:139–144, 1991.
90. Finnie JW, Wilks CR: Two cases of multiple myeloma in the dog. *J Small Anim Pract* 23:19–27, 1982.
91. Day MJ, Penhale WJ, McKenna RP, et al: Two cases of IgA multiple myeloma in the dog. *J Small Anim Pract* 28:147–156, 1987.
92. Zinkl JG, LeCouteur RA, Davis DC, Saunders GK: "Flaming" plasma cells in a dog with IgA multiple myeloma. *Vet Clin Pathol* 12:15–19, 1998.

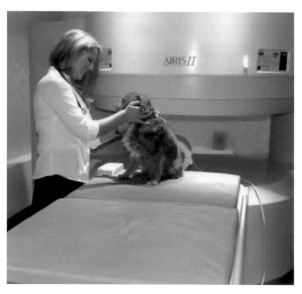

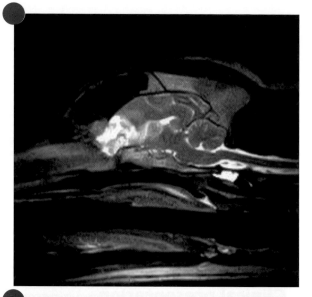

Figure 28-1: Tumors of the brain in MRI. Dogs with brain tumors can present for subtle neurologic signs to full blown seizures. The first step in evaluating these patients is to do a complete physical examination including a detailed assessment of the brain, spinal cord, as well as cranial and peripheral nerves. The second step is to rule in or out any metabolic diseases or other disorders that may be mimicking or indirectly causing changes in the neurologic system. Once these have been excluded, then a direct assessment of the brain, spinal cord or peripheral nerves is indicted, while supporting and comforting the patient.

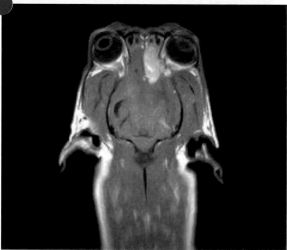

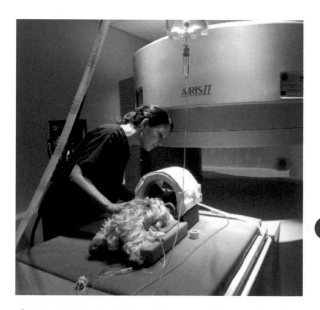

Figure 28-3: Sagittal (A) and transverse (B) images of a dog with a tumor of the cerebrum that is causing a herniation of that portion of the brain and disturbances of the surrounding tissues. Because this dog has evidence of increased intracranial pressure, a CNS tap was not acquired. Imaging courtesy of Lenore Anderson Mohammadian, DVM, MSpVM, Diplomate ACVR.

Key point

Treatment of brain tumors is often dictated by the location and extent of the disease as well as the clinical state of the patient. Surgery and radiation have each been confirmed to be quite effective in improving quality of life and survival time.

Figure 28-2: An MRI or CT scan with or without an analysis of the cerebral spinal fluid is recommended for those dogs that may have a lesion within the brain or spinal cord. If an MRI is performed, a coil is placed around the area to be imaged to receive signals from the MRI.

• Comfort and longer-term control for those who want to improve quality of life while trying to maximize the chance of controlling the tumor.

Comfort

- Therapy to enhance comfort and freedom from nausea, vomiting, diarrhea and lack of appetite. Prednisone and mannitol may help reduce edema in the central nervous system. Anticonvulsants may also be indicated in select patients.

Comfort and control

Above mentioned therapy for comfort plus:
- Palliative radiation (e.g.: 2-5 dosages of radiation) to first enhance comfort, second, to reduce the rate of growth and third, occasionally to reduce the size of the tumor.
  - Median survival has been reported to be 69 days, however dogs with supratentoral tumors tend to respond better.[13]
- Possible role for carmustine (BCNU) or lomustine (CCNU).

Comfort and longer-term control

Above mentioned therapy for comfort plus:
- Surgery and/or definitive radiation therapy (e.g: 16-19 dosages of radiation) may be beneficial for brain tumors including meningiomas and some gliomas
  - When definitive, three-dimensional conformal radiation therapy was used with or without surgery for the treatment of meningiomas of the brain, the median overall survival was 577 days when all deaths were considered, and 906 days when only dogs dying due to meningioma were considered.[14]
  - Median survival time was 2,104 days for dogs with forebrain meningiomas surgically removed with endoscopic assistance, and 702 days for dogs with caudal brain meningiomas.[15]
  - When dogs with pituitary tumors treated with definitive radiation, a median survival time was not reached, however the mean survival time was 1,405 days. Untreated dogs in this study had a median survival of 359 days.[17]
- Stereotactic body radiation therapy (SBRT) or CyberKnife robotic radiosurgery (e.g.: 1-3 dosages) can be used for ultraprecise treatments to enhance tumor control while minimizing normal tissue injury.

CANINE TUMORS OF THE SPINE

Clinical presentation

- Relatively uncommon.
- May be painful; ataxia and paresis.
- May be primary tumors of the spine or metastatic lesions involving the spine.
- Extradural tumors most common; vertebral body affected.
- Large-breed dogs, young to middle-aged.
- Locally invasive.

Staging and diagnosis

- Minimum data base (MDB): includes a CBC, biochemical profile, urinalysis, biopsy and three-

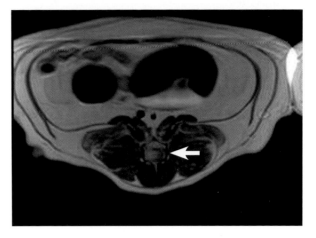

Figure 28-4: Dogs with spinal cord tumors often present with acute, chronic or progressive weakness, paresis or paralysis. Standard radiography has been used for decades to determine the cause of these lesions. Despite this, computerized tomography or magnetic resonance imaging is the best option for assessing these lesions. This transverse magnetic resonance image of this dog was used to characterize the destructive lesion involving the lumbar spinal cord.

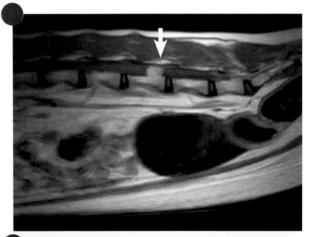

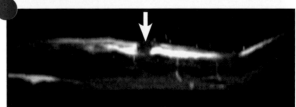

Figure 28-5: The sagittal MRI image of this dog defines a well-defined mass-like lesion of the lumbar vertebrae (A). The mass is further imaged (B) to define a lesion compressing the spinal cord. The image was used to direct a biopsy that confirmed the tumor was a sarcoma. The lesion was surgically decompressed and then treated with radiation, with excellent results. Imaging courtesy of Lenore Anderson Mohammadian, DVM, MSpVM, Diplomate ACVR.

view thoracic radiographs or computerized tomography of the chest.
- Plain radiographs of spine may show vertebral lysis.
- Myelogram may be helpful in localizing the lesion.
- CT or MRI of the spine is preferred.

Prognostic factors

- None identified.

Treatment

This section is divided into three options:
- Comfort for those who want to improve quality of life.
- Comfort and control for those who want to improve quality of life while trying to provide some control of the tumor.
- Comfort and longer-term control for those who want to improve quality of life while trying to maximize the chance of controlling the tumor.

Key point

Surgery to decompress the spinal cord and to make a specific diagnosis is often needed in patients with tumors of the spinal cord. Radiation therapy may be helpful in some patients. The greatest clinical responses are seen in those animals that are ambulatory and that have limited clinical signs.

Comfort

- Therapy to enhance comfort and freedom from nausea, vomiting, diarrhea and lack of appetite. Prednisone and mannitol may help reduce edema in the spinal cord.

Comfort and control

Above mentioned therapy for comfort plus:
- Palliative radiation (e.g.: 2-5 dosages of radiation) to first enhance comfort, second, to reduce the rate of growth and third, occasionally to reduce the size of the tumor.
- Possible role for carmustine (BCNU) or lomustine (CCNU).

Comfort and longer-term control

Above mentioned therapy for comfort plus:
- Surgery and/or definitive radiation therapy (e.g.: 16-19 dosages of radiation) may be beneficial for spinal cord tumors that are extradural or intradural extramedullary.
- Stereotactic body radiation therapy (SBRT) or CyberKnife robotic radiosurgery (e.g.: 1-3 dosages) can be used for ultraprecise treatments to enhance tumor control while minimizing normal tissue injury.

CANINE TUMORS OF THE PERIPHERAL NERVES

Clinical presentation

- Moderately uncommon.
- May be painful, especially if involving the brachial plexus.
- Slowly progressive lameness.
- Neurofibrosarcoma most common.
- Large-breed dogs, middle-aged (average age is 7 years).
- Local disease, rare metastasis.

Key point

Dogs with nerve root tumors often have localized muscle atrophy and/or nerve deficits associated with the involved nerve. Many present with focal pain that is often difficult to localize.

Staging and diagnosis

- Minimum data base (MDB): includes a CBC, biochemical profile, urinalysis, biopsy and three-view thoracic radiographs or computerized tomography of the chest.
- Myelogram may be helpful in localizing lesion that is invading nerve root.
- MRI of the spine and nerve roots.

Key point

Tumors of nerve roots causing a "root signature" often extend into the vertebral foramen and into the spinal cord. MRI and/or CT is needed to diagnose the location and extent of disease of these tumors.

Prognostic factors

- None identified.

Treatment

This section is divided into three options:
- Comfort for those who want to improve quality of life.
- Comfort and control for those who want to improve quality of life while trying to provide some control of the tumor.
- Comfort and longer-term control for those who want to improve quality of life while trying to maximize the chance of controlling the tumor.

Comfort

- Therapy to enhance comfort and freedom from nausea, vomiting, diarrhea and lack of appetite.

> **Key point**
>
> Surgery to decompress the spinal cord and to make a specific diagnosis is often need in patients with tumors of the spinal cord. Radiation therapy may be helpful in some patients. The greatest clinical responses are seen in those animals that are ambulatory and that have limited clinical signs.

Comfort and control

Above mentioned therapy for comfort plus:

- Palliative radiation (e.g.: 2-5 dosages of radiation) to first enhance comfort, second, to reduce the rate of growth and third, occasionally to reduce the size of the tumor.

Comfort and longer-term control

Above mentioned therapy for comfort plus:

- Surgery and/or definitive radiation therapy (e.g.: 16-19 dosages of radiation) may be beneficial for some patients and may include amputation. Involvement of the spinal cord may require decompressive surgery and/or radiation.
- Stereotactic body radiation therapy (SBRT) or CyberKnife robotic radiosurgery (e.g.: 1-3 dosages) can be used for ultraprecise treatments to enhance tumor control while minimizing normal tissue injury.

References

1. Heidner GL, Kornegay JN, Page RL, et al: Analysis of survival in a retrospective study of 86 dogs with brain tumors. *J Vet Intern Med* 5:219–226, 1991.
2. Foster ES, Carrillo JM, Patnaik AK: Clinical signs of tumors affecting the rostral cerebrum in 43 dogs. *J Vet Intern Med* 2:71–74, 1988.
3. Snyder JM, Lipitz L, Skorupski KA, et al: Secondary intracranial neoplasia in the dog: 177 cases (1986-2003). *J Vet Intern Med* 22(1):172-177, 2008.
4. Kube SA, Bruyette DS, Hanson SM: Astrocytomas in young dogs. *JAAHA* 39:288–293, 2003.
5. Uchida K, Nakayama H, Endo Y, et al: Ganglioglioma in the thalamus of a puppy. *J Vet Med Sci* 65:113–115, 2003.
6. Porter B, de Lahunta A, Summers B: Gliomatosis cerebri in six dogs. *Vet Pathol* 40:97–102, 2003.
7. Lipsitz D, Higgins RJ, Kortz GD, et al: Glioblastoma multiforme: Clinical findings, magnetic resonance imaging, and pathology in five dogs. *Vet Pathol* 40:659–669, 2003.
8. Dickinson PJ. Advances in diagnostic and treatment modalities for intracranial tumors. *J Vet Intern Med* 28(4):1165-185, 2014.
9. Young BD, Fosgate GT, Holmes SP, et al: Evaluation of standard magnetic resonance characteristics used to differentiate neoplastic, inflammatory, and vascular brain lesions in dogs. *Vet Radiol Ultrasound* 55(4):399-406, 201410. Axlund 10. TW, McGlasson ML, Smith AN: Surgery alone or in combination with radiation therapy for treatment of intracranial meningiomas in dogs: 31 cases (1989-2002). *JAVMA* 221:1597–1600, 2002.
11. Ródenas S, Pumarola M, Gaitero L, et al: Magnetic resonance imaging findings in 40 dogs with histologically confirmed intracranial tumours. *Vet J* 187(1):85-91, 2011.
12. Mamelak AN, Owen TJ, Bruyette D. Transsphenoidal surgery using a high definition video telescope for pituitary adenomas in dogs with pituitary dependent hypercortisolism: methods and results. *Vet Surg* 43(4):369-379, 2014
13. Rossmeisl JH Jr, Jones JC, Zimmerman KL et al: Survival time following hospital discharge in dogs with palliatively treated primary brain tumors. *J Am Vet Med Assoc* 242(2):193-198, 2013.
14. Keyerleber MA, McEntee MC, Farrelly J, et al: Three-dimensional conformal radiation therapy alone or in combination with surgery for treatment of canine intracranial meningiomas. *Vet Comp Oncol* doi: 10.1111/vco.12054, 2013.
15. Klopp LS, Rao S. Endoscopic-assisted intracranial tumor removal in dogs and cats: long-term outcome of 39 cases. *J Vet Intern Med.* 23(1):108-115, 2009.
16. Van Meervenne S, Verhoeven PS, de Vos, J et al: Comparison between symptomatic treatment and lomustine supplementation in 71 dogs with intracranial, space-occupying lesions. *Vet Comp Oncol* 12(1):67-77, 2014.
17. Kent MS, Bommarito D, Feldman E, Theon AP. Survival, neurologic response, and prognostic factors in dogs with pituitary masses treated with radiation therapy and untreated dogs. *J Vet Intern Med* 21(5):1027-1033, 2007.
18. Steiss JE, Cox NR, Knecht CD: Electroencephalographic and histopathologic correlations in eight dogs with intracranial mass lesions. *Am J Vet Res* 51:1286–1291, 1990.
19. Wolf M, Pedroia V, Higgins RJ, et al: Intracranial ring enhancing lesions in dogs: A correlative CT scanning and neuropathologic study. *Vet Radiol Ultrasound* 36:16–20, 1995.
20. Bergman R, Jones J, Lanz O, et al: Post-operative computed tomography in two dogs with cerebral meningioma. *Vet Radiol Ultrasound* 41:425–432, 2000.
21. Kraft SL, Gavin PR: Intracranial neoplasia. *Clin Techn Small Anim Pract* 14:112–123, 1999.
22. Hathcock JT: Low field magnetic resonance imaging characteristics of cranial vault meningiomas in 13 dogs. *Vet Radiol Ultrasound* 37:257–263, 1996
23. Thomas WB, Wheeler SJ, Kramer R, Kornegay JN: Magnetic resonance imaging features of primary brain tumors in dogs. *Vet Radiol Ultrasound* 37:20–27, 1996.
24. Kraft SL, Gavin PR, DeHaan C, et al: Retrospective review of 50 canine intracranial tumors evaluated by magnetic resonance imaging. *J Vet Intern Med* 11:218–225, 1997.
25. Garosi LS, Dennis R, Penderis J, et al: Results of magnetic resonance imaging in dogs with vestibular disorders: 85 cases (1996-1999). *JAVMA* 218:385–391, 2001.
26. Koblik PD, LeCouteur RA, Higgins RJ, et al: CT-guided brain biopsy using a modified Pelorus Mark III stereotactic system: Experience with 50 dogs. *Vet Radiol Ultrasound* 40: 434–440, 1999.
27. Moissonnier P, Blot S, Devauchelle P, et al: Stereotactic CT guided brain biopsy in the dog. *J Small Anim Pract* 43:115–123, 2002.
28. Platt SR, Alleman AR, Lanz OI, Chrisman CL: Comparison of fine-needle aspiration and surgical-tissue biopsy in the diagnosis of canine brain tumors. *Vet Surg* 31:65–69, 2002.
29. Ribas JL: Application of immunohistochemistry in canine neuro-oncology. *Schweiz Arch Tierheilk* 132:463–464, 1990.
30. Barnhart KF, Wojcieszyn J, Storts RW: Immunohistochemical staining patterns of canine meningiomas and correlation with published immunophenotypes. *Vet Pathol* 39:311–321, 2002.
31. Kaldrymidou E, Polizopoulou ZS, Papaioannou N, et al: Papillary meningioma in the dog: A clinicopathological study of two cases. *J Comp Pathol* 124:227–230, 2001.
32. Schulman FY, Carpenter JL, Ribas JL, Brum DE: Cystic papillary meningioma in the sella turcica of a dog. *JAVMA* 200:67–69, 1992.
33. Kitagawa M, Kanayama K, Sakai T: Cystic meningioma in a dog. *J Small Anim Pract* 43:272–274, 2002.
34. Bagley RS, Kornegay JN, Lane SB, et al: Cystic meningiomas in 2 dogs. *J Vet Intern Med* 10:72–75, 1996.
35. Bagley RS, Silver GM, Gavin PR: Cerebellar cystic meningioma in a dog. *JAAHA* 36:413–415, 2000.
36. Mandara MT, Ricci G, Rinaldi L, et al: Immunohistochemical identification and image analysis quantification of oestrogen and progesterone receptors in canine and feline meningioma. *J Comp Pathol* 127:214–218, 2002.
37. Adamo PF, Cantile C, Steinberg H: Evaluation of progesterone and estrogen receptor expression in 15 meningiomas of dogs and cats. *Am J Vet Res* 64:1310–1318, 2003.
38. Thèon AP, LeCouteur RA, Carr EA, Griffey SM: Influence of tumor cell proliferation and sex-hormone receptors on effectiveness of radiation therapy for dogs with incompletely resected meningiomas. *JAVMA* 216:701–707, 2000.
39. Schulman FY, Ribas JL, Carpenter JL, et al: Intracranial meningioma with pulmonary metastasis in three dogs. *Vet Pathol* 29:196–202, 1992.
40. Schmidt P, Geyer C, Hafner A, et al: Malignes meningeommit lungenmetastastasen bei einem Boxer. [Malignant meningioma with lung metastases in a Boxer] *Tierarztl Prax* 19:315–319, 1991.
41. Turrel JM, Fike JR, LeCouteur RA, et al: Radiotherapy of brain tumors in dogs. *JAVMA* 184:82–86, 1984.
42. Bagley RS, Harrington ML, Pluhar GE, et al: Acute, unilateral transverse sinus occlusion during craniectomy in seven dogs with space-occupying intracranial disease. *Vet Surg* 26: 195–201, 1997.
43. Higgins RJ, LeCouteur RA, Vernau KM, et al: Granular cell tumor

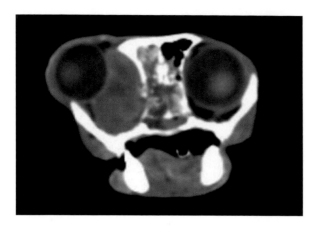

Figure 29-4: Retrobulbar tumors. This patient has a retrobulbar adenocarcinoma that was diagnosed via fine needle aspiration and cytology. This computerized tomography demonstrates that the tumor is compressing and deviating the eye laterally and dorsally. There is intranasal involvement. Palliative radiation therapy normalized this finding and enhanced and improved quality of life. Imaging courtesy of Lenore Anderson Mohammadian, DVM, MSpVM, Diplomate ACVR

- Comfort for those who want to improve quality of life.
- Comfort and control for those who want to improve quality of life while trying to provide some control of the tumor.
- Comfort and longer-term control for those who want to improve quality of life while trying to maximize the chance of controlling the tumor.

Comfort

- Therapy to enhance comfort and freedom from nausea, vomiting, diarrhea and lack of appetite.

Comfort and control

Above mentioned therapy for comfort plus:
- Palliative radiation (e.g.: 2-5 dosages of radiation) to first enhance comfort, second, to reduce the rate of growth and third, occasionally to reduce the size of the tumor.

Comfort and longer-term control

Above mentioned therapy for comfort plus:
- Orbital exenteration may be curative for small tumors. Definitive radiation therapy if surgical margins are not clean may be helpful (e.g.: 16-19 dosages of radiation).
  - Tumor resection by orbitectomy has been reported to provide a local disease-free interval of more than 1 year in more than 50% of patients and a survival rate for the first year of 70.4%.[41]
- Stereotactic body radiation therapy (SBRT) or CyberKnife robotic radiosurgery (e.g.: 1-3 dosages) can be used for ultraprecise treatments to enhance tumor control while minimizing normal tissue injury in those tumors that have defined margins.

CANINE TUMORS OF THE EAR CANAL

Clinical presentation

- Chronic, recurring suppurative to pyogranulomatous otitis externa.
- Adenomas and adenocarcinomas (particularly ceruminous gland) are most common. Squamous cell carcinoma and mast cell tumors are among the other histologic types.
  - Usually older animals, cocker spaniels predisposed breed.

Table 29-1. Types of tumors in the ear canals of 81 dogs[42]

Benign	Number of dogs	Malignant	Number of dogs
Polyp	8	Ceruminous adenocarcinoma	23
Papilloma	6	Undifferentiated carcinoma	9
Sebaceous adenoma	5	Squamous cell carcinoma	8
Basal cell tumor	5	Round cell tumor	3
Ceruminous adenoma	4	Sarcoma	2
Histiocytoma	2	Melanoma	2
Plasmacytoma	1	Hemangiosarcoma	1
Fibromas	1		
Melanoma	1		
Total	**33**		**48**

Table 29-2. Tumors in the ear canals of 81 dogs[42]

	Benign % of dogs	Malignant % of dogs
Clinical signs		
Mass	63	72
Discharge	50	82
Odor	25	34
Pruritus	25	26
Pain	19	26
Neurologic signs (facial nerve paralysis, head tilt, circling)	0	13
Clinical appearance		
Raised	55	42
Pedunculated	52	0
Irregular	30	0
Ulcerated	18	29
Broad-based	0	23
Location		
Vertical canal	52	29
Horizontal canal	36	35
Canal and bulla	0	23
Bulla	3	4

Key point

Almost all tumors of the ear canal are associated with chronic, refractory otitis externa. Imaging, bacterial culture, and biopsy are essential to confirm the diagnosis.

Staging and diagnosis

- Minimum data base (MDB): includes a CBC, biochemical profile, urinalysis, biopsy and three-view thoracic radiographs or computerized tomography of the chest.
- Aural examination.
- CT or MRI to evaluate middle ear and bulla.
- Biopsy (may require surgery).
- Malignant tumors are locally aggressive, however metastases are rare. If they occur, they are primarily via the lymphatics to parotid and mandibular lymph nodes.

Prognostic factors

- None identified.

Treatment

This section is divided into three options:
- Comfort for those who want to improve quality of life.
- Comfort and control for those who want to improve quality of life while trying to provide some control of the tumor.
- Comfort and longer-term control for those who want to improve quality of life while trying to maximize the chance of controlling the tumor.

Key point

Ear canal ablation may be effective alone to treat these tumors if they are localized, however incomplete removal can be treated with definitive radiation therapy, with excellent results.

Comfort

- Therapy to enhance comfort and freedom from nausea, vomiting, diarrhea and lack of appetite.

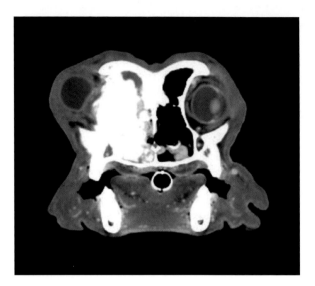

Figure 30-2: Nasal tumor. Dogs with nasal tumors often have partial or complete obstruction of at least one side of the nasal cavity. Directing a biopsy instrument up the nostril to the mass is generally quite helpful at securing appropriate tissue to make a diagnosis. Imaging courtesy of Lenore Anderson Mohammadian, DVM, MSpVM, Diplomate ACVR.

Treatment

This section is divided into three options:
- Comfort for those who want to improve quality of life.
- Comfort and control for those who want to improve quality of life while trying to provide some control of the tumor.
- Comfort and longer-term control for those who want to improve quality of life while trying to maximize the chance of controlling the tumor.

> **Key point**
>
> Palliative or definitive radiation therapy is commonly employed to treat dogs with nasal tumors, often with great success. Survival approaching or exceeding one year has been reported.

Comfort

- Therapy to enhance comfort and freedom from nausea, vomiting, diarrhea and lack of appetite.
- Possibly a feeding tube.
- Topical eye care, pain relief, and topical skin treatments as needed.
- Antibiotics for secondary infections.
- Neurologic signs: corticosteroids and anticonvulsants.
  - In one study, dogs that were not treated survived an overall median survival time of 95 days.[15]

Table 30-1. Clinical signs associated with primary lung tumors in dogs

Clinical signs	Frequency
Cough	52%
Dyspnea	24%
Lethargy	18%
Weight loss	12%
Tachypnea	5%
Pyrexia	6,4%
Lameness	3,8%

Comfort and control

Above mentioned therapy for comfort plus:
- Palliative radiation (e.g.: 2-5 dosages of radiation) to first enhance comfort, second, to reduce the rate of growth and third, occasionally to reduce the size of the tumor.
  - The response of 38 dogs treated with a course fractionated, palliative radiation protocol based on CT-based 3D treatment planning revealed an overall median progression-free interval of 10 months.[42]
  - When dogs with histologically confirmed, previously untreated nasal carcinomas were treated with a selective COX-2 inhibitor (firocoxib) and palliative radiation therapy, or palliative radiation therapy alone, the overall survival times were 335 days and 244 days, respectively. The NSAID-treated group had an improved quality of life.[43]

Comfort and longer-term control

Above mentioned therapy for comfort plus:
- Definitive radiation therapy may be helpful (e.g.: 16-19 dosages of radiation).
  - Median survival range from 8 to 23 months.
  - Dogs with nasal sarcomas treated with daily-fractionated radiation therapy protocols; Monday, Wednesday and Friday fractionated radiation therapy protocols; and palliative radiation therapy protocols had median survival times of 641, 347, and 305 days, respectively.[44]
- Chemotherapy with platinum and/or doxorubicin drugs may improve survival and local control.
  - Dogs with nasal tumors treated with alternating dosages of doxorubicin and carboplatin had a median survival of 7 months.[45]
- Stereotactic body radiation therapy (SBRT) or CyberKnife robotic radiosurgery (e.g.: 1-3 dosages) can be used for ultraprecise treatments to enhance tumor control while minimizing normal tissue injury in those tumors that have defined margins.

CANINE LUNG TUMORS

Clinical presentation

- Moderately common.
- Usually not painful.
- Often present without clinical signs, however as the disease progresses, may present with a chronic non-productive cough, dyspnea, lethargy, lameness (hypertrophic osteopathy), and weight loss; some dogs are asymptomatic.
- Most common tumor type is a carcinoma, followed by papillary adenocarcinoma, bronchoalveolar carcinoma, adenosquamous carcinoma and squamous cell carcinoma.[49] Chemotherapy is quite helpful for the treatment of dogs with another lung tumor that may be a precursor to lymphoma, pulmonary lymphomatoid granulomatosis.
- Older, large-breed dogs.
- Occasionally these tumors can metastasize to the brain and cause neurologic signs. Therefore,

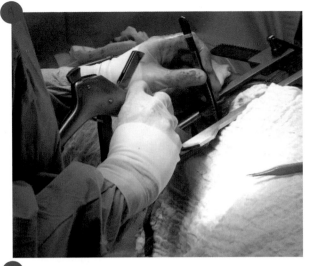

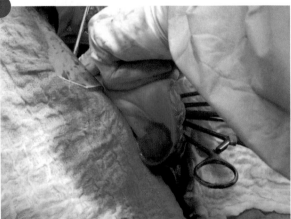

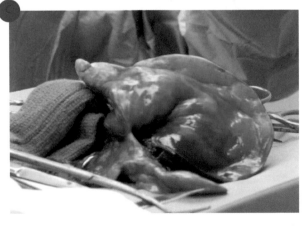

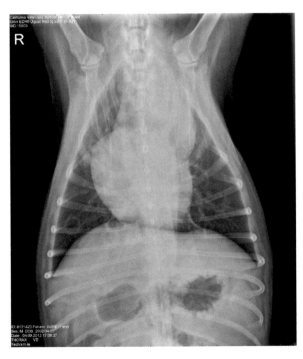

Figure 30-3: Lung masses can occur in any lobe, however primary lung tumors occur more commonly in the right caudal lung lobe than elsewhere. The image above shows a mass in the left cranial lung lobe that was confirmed to be a primary lung tumor. Animals with primary lung tumors may be asymptomatic or they may present for lethargy, anorexia, weight loss and coughing. They can metastasize within the chest and to distant sites such as toes or brain. Patients with evidence of hilar lymph node involvement generally have a worse prognosis. Imaging courtesy of Lenore Anderson Mohammadian, DVM, MSpVM, Diplomate ACVR.

Figure 30-4: Primary lung tumors are most expeditiously removed by making an intercostal incision and placing a retractor to optimize the surgical field. The lung with the tumor is excised by placing surgical stapling device proximal to the mass to ensure the mass and associated lung is removed with a wide margin (A). The device is used to staple and therefore seal the normal lung while excising the abnormal lung with the tumor (B). The lung is then submitted for histopathology and the patient is recovered once the incision is closed and a chest tube is used to evacuate air from the chest cavity (C).

49. Dorn CR, Taylor DO, Schneider R, et al: Survey of animal neoplasms in Alameda and Contra Costa Counties, California. II. Cancer morbidity in dogs and cats from Alameda County. *J Natl Cancer Inst* 40:307–318, 1968.

50. Saegusa S, Yamamura H, Morita T, Hasegawa A: Pulmonary neuroendocrine carcinoma in a four-month-old dog. *J Comp Pathol* 111:439–443, 1994.

51. Ogilvie GK, Weigel RM, Haschek WM, et al: Prognostic factors for tumor remission and survival in dogs after surgery for primary lung tumor: 76 cases (1975-1985). *JAVMA* 195:109–112, 1989.

52. Nielsen SW, Horava A: Primary pulmonary tumors of the dog. A report of sixteen cases. Am *J Vet Res* 21:813–830, 1960.

53. Reif JS, Dunn K, Ogilvie GK, Harris CK: Passive smoking and canine lung cancer risk. *Am J Epidemiol* 135:234–239, 1992.

54. McNiel EA, Ogilvie GK, Powers BE, et al: Evaluation of prognostic factors for dogs with primary lung tumors: 67 cases (1985-1992). *JAVMA* 211:1422–1427, 1997.

55. Dallman MJ, Martin RA, Roth L: Pneumothorax as the primary problem in two cases of bronchioloalveolar carcinoma in the dog. *J Am Anim Hosp Assoc* 24:710–714, 1988.

56. Puerto DA, Brockman DJ, Lindquist C, Drobatz K: Surgical and nonsurgical management of and selected risk factors for spontaneous pneumothorax in dogs: 64 cases (1986-1999). *JAVMA* 220:1670–1674, 2002.

57. Bailiff NL, Norris CR: Clinical signs, clinicopathological findings, etiology, and outcome associated with hemoptysis in dogs: 36 cases (1990-1999). *J Am Anim Hosp Assoc* 38:125–133, 2002.

58. Madewell BR, Nyland TG, Weigel JE: Regression of hypertrophic osteopathy following pneumonectomy in a dog. *JAVMA* 172:818–821, 1978.

59. Mariani CL, Shelton SB, Alsup JC: Paraneoplastic polyneuropathy and subsequent recovery following tumor removal in a dog. *J Am Anim Hosp Assoc* 35:302–305, 1999.

60. Sharkey LC, Rosol TJ, Grone A, et al: Production of granulocyte colony-stimulating factor and granulocyte-macrophage colony-stimulating factor by carcinomas in a dog and a cat with paraneoplastic leukocytosis. *J Vet Intern Med* 10:405–408, 1996.

61. Meinkoth JH, Rochat MC, Cowell RL: Metastatic carcinoma presenting as hind-limb lameness: diagnosis by synovial fluid cytology. *J Am Anim Hosp Assoc* 33:325–328, 1997.

62. Reichle JK, Wisner ER: Non-cardiac thoracic ultrasound in 75 feline and canine patients. *Vet Radiol Ultrasound* 41:154–162, 2000.

63. Paoloni MC, Dubielzig RR, O'Brien RT, et al: Use of CT imaging for lymph node assessment in dogs with primary lung tumors. *Proc 22rd Ann Conf Vet Cancer Soc* 37, 2002.

64. Tidwell AS, Johnson KL: Computed tomography-guided percutaneous biopsy in the dog and cat: Description of technique and preliminary evaluation in 14 patients. *Vet Radiol Ultrasound* 35:445–446, 1994.

65. Tidwell AS, Johnson KL: Computed tomography-guided percutaneous biopsy: Criteria for accurate needle tip identification. *Vet Radiol Ultrasound* 35:440–444, 1994.

66. Davies DR, Lucas J: Actinomyces infection in a dog with pulmonary carcinoma. *Aust Vet J* 81:132–135, 2003.

67. Mehlhaff CJ, Leifer CE, Patnaik AK, Schwarz PD: Surgical treatment of primary pulmonary neoplasia in 15 dogs. *J Am Anim Hosp Assoc* 20:799–803, 1984.

68. Gressus JC, Debray B: Surgical treatment of a primary chondrosarcoma of the lung in a dog. *Pract Med Chirurgicale de L'animal Compagnie* 37:69–79, 2002.

69. Poulson JM, Vujaskovic Z, Gillette SM, et al: Volume and dose-response effects for severe symptomatic pneumonitis after fractionated irradiation of canine lung. *Int J Radiat Biol* 76:463–468, 2000.

70. de Boer WJ, Mehta DM, Timens W, Hoekstra HJ: The short and long-term effects of intraoperative electron beam radiotherapy (IORT) on thoracic organs after pneumonectomy an experimental study in the canine model. *Int J Radiat Oncol Biol Phys* 45:501–506, 1999.

71. Hayata Y, Kato H, Konaka C, et al: Fiberoptic bronchoscopic photoradiation in experimentally induced canine lung cancer. *Cancer* 51:50–56, 1983.

72. Poirier VJ, Burgess KE, Adams WM, Vail DM: Toxicity, dosage, and efficacy of vinorelbine (Navelbine) in dogs with spontaneous neoplasia. *J Vet Intern Med* 18:536–539, 2004.

73. Baum B, Winkenwerder F, Nolte I, Hewicker-Trautwein M: Lymphomatoid granulomatosis in a Borzoi. *Teirartzl Prax* 30:427–431, 2002.

74. Postorino NC, Wheeler SL, Park RD, et al: A syndrome resembling lymphomatoid granulomatosis in the dog. *J Vet Intern Med* 3:15–19, 1989.

75. Berry CR, Moore PF, Thomas WP, et al: Pulmonary lymphomatoid granulomatosis in seven dogs (1976-1987). *J Vet Intern Med* 4:157–166, 1990.

76. Fitzgerald SD, Wolf DC, Carlton WW: Eight cases of canine lymphomatoid granulomatosis. *Vet Pathol* 28:241–245, 1991.

77. Calvert CA, Mahaffey MB, Lappin MR, Farrell RL: Pulmonary and disseminated eosinophilic granulomatosis in dogs. *J Am Anim Hosp Assoc* 24:311–320, 1988.

78. Moore PF: Utilization of cytoplasmic lysozyme immunoreactivity as a histiocytic marker in canine histiocytic disorders. *Vet Pathol* 23:757–762, 1986.

79. Smith KC, Day MJ, Shaw SC, et al: Canine lymphomatoid granulomatosis: An immunophenotypic analysis of three cases. *J Comp Pathol* 115:129–138, 1996.

80. McKay LW, Levy JK, Thompson MS: What is your diagnosis? Pulmonary lymphoma. *JAVMA* 224:1587–1588, 2004.

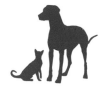

Chapter 31

Canine cardiac tumors

Clinical presentation

- Uncommon or under-recognized.
- Generally not painful, but most present with pericardial effusion and signs of cardiac failure.
- Most common tumor type is hemangiosarcoma; next most common is chemodectoma. Other tumor types are rare.

Key point

Clinical signs may be vague or they may be associated with cardiac abnormalities resulting in exercise intolerance, coughing, syncope and difficulty breathing.

Staging and diagnosis

- Minimal database (MDB): includes a CBC, biochemical profile, urinalysis, and three-view thoracic radiographs.
- Cardiac ultrasonography and biopsy, which may require surgery.

Key point

Cardiac ultrasound and chest radiographs have allowed clinicians to more easily diagnose tumors of the heart. The result is that they appear to be more common than ever before and they are being identified earlier in the course of the disease, making treatment more effective.

Figure 31-1: Tumors that arise from or that are involving the heart often cause pericardial effusion that can reduce cardiac output and in some case be a greater immediate threat than the mass itself. Pericardiocentesis can transiently help alleviate clinical signs in some patients.

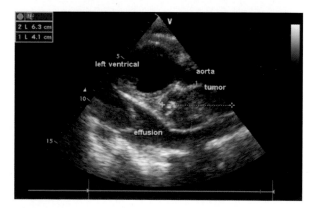

Figure 31-2: The tumor involving the heart depicted here was treated with palliative radiation therapy and adjuvant chemotherapy. The dog had improved clinical signs, reduced pericardial effusion and reduction of the size of the mass for over one year. While this great success is not seen in all patients, attending clinicians should be aware that options do exist and that a diagnosis of a tumor involving the heart is not necessarily a death sentence.

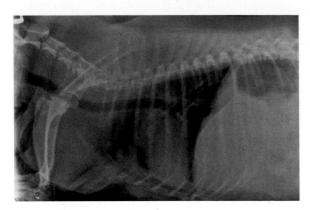

Figure 31-3: Most dogs with tumors of the auricle of the heart do not have distinct visible lesions as noted on this thoracic radiograph. This dog had a localized hemangiosarcoma that was treated with a pericardectomy and removal of the tumor via an auriculectomy followed by doxorubicin chemotherapy. The patient did well long term. Imaging courtesy of Lenore Anderson Mohammadian, DVM, MSpVM, Diplomate ACVR.

Prognostic factors

- Pericardectomy improves survival for dogs with chemodectoma.

Treatment

This section is divided into three options:
- Comfort for those who want to improve quality of life.
- Comfort and control for those who want to improve quality of life while trying to provide some control of the tumor.
- Comfort and longer-term control for those who want to improve quality of life while trying to maximize the chance of controlling the tumor.

Key point

Treating any cardiac dysfunction or failure is essential. Some tumors may respond to surgical removal, radiation therapy, or to medical management.

Comfort

- Therapy to enhance comfort and freedom from nausea, vomiting, diarrhea and lack of appetite.

Comfort and control

Above mentioned therapy for comfort plus:
- Palliative radiation (e.g.: 2-5 dosages of radiation) to first enhance comfort, second, to reduce the rate of growth and third, occasionally to reduce the size of the tumor. This can be done regardless of the tumor type as long as it is localized.

Comfort and longer-term control

Above mentioned therapy for comfort plus:
- Surgical resection of the tumor(s) if possible with evaluation and biopsy of regional lymph nodes. Definitive radiation therapy may be helpful.
  - Surgical removal of chemodectoma is difficult.
  - Carotid body tumors may be resected.
  - Surgery for hemangiosarcomas may provide short-term palliation; however, doxorubicin chemotherapy is recommended postoperatively.
- Doxorubicin chemotherapy can be used alone (1 dosage, every 3 weeks for 5-7 treatments).
  - Partial and complete remission rate of 41% for 2-4 months.
- Tyrosine kinase inhibitors, metronomic cyclophosphamide, piroxicam and docosahexaenoic acid may be helpful.

References

1. Girard C, Helie P, Odin M: Intrapericardial neoplasia in dogs. *J Vet Diagn Invest* 11:73–78, 1999.
2. Ware WA, Hopper DL: Cardiac tumors in dogs: 1982-1995. *J Vet Intern Med* 13:95–103, 1999.
3. Kirsch JA, Dhupa S, Cornell KK: Pericardial effusion associated with metastatic disease from an unknown primary tumor in a dog. *J Am Anim Hosp Assoc* 36:121-124, 2000
4. Ogilvie GK, Brunkow CS, Daniel GB, Haschek WM: Malignant lymphoma with cardiac and bone involvement in a dog. *JAVMA* 194:793–796, 1989.
5. MacGregor JM, Faria MLE, Moore AS, Tobias AH, Brown DJ, Morais HSA. Primary cardiac lymphoma causing pericardial effusion in dogs: 12 Cases (1997-2004). *J Am Vet Med Assoc* in press.
6. Simpson DJ, Hunt GB, Church DB, Beck JA: Benign masses in the pericardium of two dogs. *Aust Vet J* 77:225–229, 1999.
7. Vicari ED, Brown DC, Holt DE, Brockman DJ: Survival times of and prognostic indicators for dogs with heart base masses: 25 cases (1986-1999). *JAVMA* 219:485–487, 2001.
8. Ehrhart N, Ehrhart EJ, Willis J, et al: Analysis of factors affecting survival in dogs with aortic body tumors. *Vet Surg* 31:44–48, 2002.
9. Hayes HM: An hypothesis for the aetiology of canine chemoreceptor system neoplasms, based upon an epidemiological study of 73 cases among hospital patients. *J Small Anim Pract* 16:337–343, 1975.
10. Cho KO, Park NY, Park IC, et al: Metastatic intracavitary cardiac aortic body tumor in a dog. *J Vet Med Sci* 60:1251–1253, 1998.
11. Brown PJ, Rema A, Gartner F: Immunohistochemical characteristics of canine aortic and carotid body tumours. *J Vet Med A Physiol Pathol Clin Med* 50:140–144, 2003.
12. Wykes PM, Rouse GP, Orton EC: Removal of five canine cardiac tumors using a stapling instrument. *Vet Surg* 15:103–106, 1986.
13. Blackmore J, Gorman NT, Kagan K, et al: Neurologic complications of a chemodectoma in a dog. *JAVMA* 184:475–478, 1984.
14. Patnaik AK, Liu SK, Hurvitz AI, McClelland AJ: Canine chemodectoma (extra-adrenal paragangliomas)—a comparative study. *J Small Anim Pract* 16:785–801, 1975.
15. Kerstetter KK, Krahwinkel DJ Jr, Millis DL, Hahn K: Pericardiectomy in dogs: 22 cases (1978-1994). *JAVMA* 211:736–740, 1997.
16. Jackson J, Richter KP, Launer DP: Thoracoscopic partial pericardiectomy in 13 dogs. *J Vet Intern Med* 13:529–533, 1999.
17. Dean MJ, Strafuss AC: Carotid body tumors in the dog: a review and report of four cases. *JAVMA* 166:1003–1006, 1975.
18. Obradovich JE, Withrow SJ, Powers BE, Walshaw R: Carotid body tumors in the dog. Eleven cases (1978–1988). *J Vet Intern Med* 6:96–101, 1992.
19. Sander CH, Whitenack DL: Canine malignant carotid body tumor. *JAVMA* 156:606–610, 1970.
20. Fife W, Mattoon J, Drost WT, et al: Imaging features of a presumed carotid body tumor in a dog. *Vet Radiol Ultrasound* 44:322–325, 2003.
21. Mansfield CS, Callanan JJ, McAllister H: Intra-atrial rhabdomyoma causing chylopericardium and right-sided congestive heart failure in a dog. *Vet Rec* 147:264–267, 2000.
22. Albers TM, Alroy J, Garrod LA, et al: Histochemical and

ultrastructural characterization of primary cardiac chondrosarcoma. *Vet Pathol* 34:150–151, 1997.

23. Greenlee PG, Liu SK: Chondrosarcoma of the mitral leaflet in a dog. *Vet Pathol* 21:540–542, 1984.

24. Southerland EM, Miller RT, Jones CL: Primary right atrial chondrosarcoma in a dog. *JAVMA* 203:1697–1698, 1993.

25. Machida N, Kobayashi M, Tanaka R, et al: Primary malignant mixed mesenchymal tumour of the heart in a dog. *J Comp Pathol* 128:71–74, 2003.

26. Callanan JJ, McCarthy GM, McAllister H: Primary pulmonary artery leiomyosarcoma in an adult dog. *Vet Pathol* 37:663–666, 2000.

27. Pérez J, Pérez-Rivero A, Montoya A, et al: Right-sided heart failure in a dog with primary cardiac rhabdomyosarcoma. *J Am Anim Hosp Assoc* 34:208–211, 1998.

28. Briggs OM, Kirberger RM, Goldberg NB: Right atrial myxosarcoma in a dog. *J S Afr Vet Assoc* 68:144–146, 1997.

29. Krotje LJ, Ware WA, Niyo Y: Intracardiac rhabdomyosarcoma in a dog. *JAVMA* 197:368–371, 1990.

30. Camy G: Tumeur intracardiaque (rhabdomyosarcoma). *Pract Med Chirurgicale de L'animal Compagnie* 21:229–230, 1986.

31. Gonin-Jmaa D, Paulsen DB, Taboada J: Pericardial effusion in a dog with rhabdomyosarcoma in the right ventricular wall. *J Small Anim Pract* 37:193–196, 1996.

32. Foale RD, White RA, Harley R, Herrtage ME: Left ventricular myxosarcoma in a dog. *J Small Anim Pract* 44:503–507, 2003.

33. Machida N, Hoshi K, Kobayashi M, et al: Cardiac myxoma of the tricuspid valve in a dog. *J Comp Pathol* 129:320–324, 2003.

34. Ghaffari S, Pelio DC, Lange AJ, et al: A retrospective evaluation of doxorubicin-based chemotherapy for dogs with right atrial masses and pericardial effusion. *J Small Anim Pract* 2014 May;55(5):254-257, 2014.

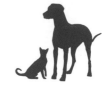

Chapter 32

Canine tumors of the gastrointestinal tract

CANINE ORAL AND LINGUAL TUMORS

Clinical presentation

- Oral mass, halitosis, bleeding from the mouth, and dysphagia.
- Most common benign tumor types include fibromatous epulis, acanthomatous ameloblastomas (previously known as acanthomatous epulis; may invade bone, and therefore not strictly benign), ossifying epulis and giant cell epulis.
  - Do not metastasize.
  - All ages.
- Malignant melanoma.
  - High metastatic rate.
  - Older dogs.
- Squamous cell carcinoma (SCC).
  - Moderately metastatic.
  - Tonsillar SCC is highly metastatic.
  - Older dogs.
  - Locally invasive.
  - May originate from the tonsil with a high probability of metastases.
- Oral papillary SCC in younger dogs.
- Fibrosarcoma.
  - Lower metastatic rate.
  - Younger dogs.
- Tumors of the tongue are most often squamous cell carcinomas and malignant melanomas.

Key point

Oral or lingual tumors, regardless of cause and degree of malignancy, often cause malodorous breath, ptyalism and prehension problems, which may cause weight loss and anorexia.

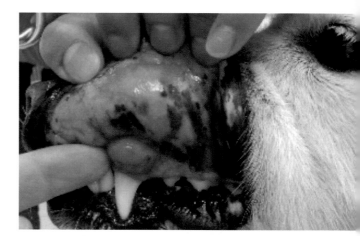

Figure 32-1: Oral tumors may be benign or malignant. A biopsy and appropriate staging to assess the extent of the disease and general health are essential for each oral tumor. In this case, the patient had a biopsy proven acanthomatous ameloblastoma. This type of epulis is likely to invade bone as did this tumor. This tumor was completely excised and was cured. The fibromatous epulis, acanthomatous ameloblastomas (previously known as acanthomatous epulis), ossifying epulis and giant cell epulis can each be cured with complete excision. Radiation therapy is another excellent option.

Staging and diagnosis

- Minimum data base (MDB): includes a CBC, biochemical profile, urinalysis, biopsy and three-view thoracic radiographs or computerized tomography of the chest.
- Lymph node assessment.
- Fine-detail radiographs or preferably computerized tomography of affected area of mouth.
  - CT preferred if radiation therapy planned.

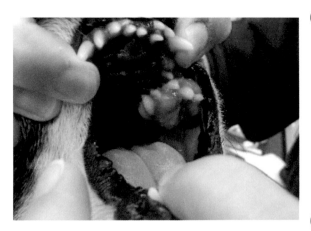

Figure 32-2: This Boston terrier has a maxillary epulis that was imaged by computerized tomography to define the extent of disease followed by a curative surgical excision.

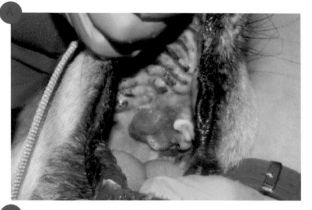

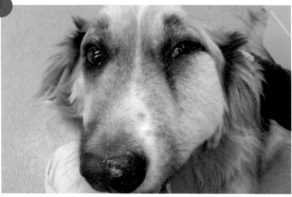

Figure 32-4: Dogs with maxillary tumors may present for difficulty eating and chewing (A) or facial deformity (B) or both as in this dog with a fibrosarcoma. The client chose Comfort and some control for this dog, therefore analgesia and palliative radiation was given with excellent results for 9 months.

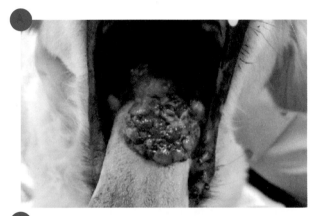

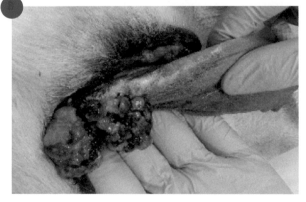

Figure 32-3: This dog presented unconscious and cyanotic as he had inhaled his tumor that resulted in complete respiratory obstruction. As soon as the tongue was pulled out, the black mass that was subsequently determined to be a malignant melanoma came out of the trachea (A) and the dog recovered uneventfully after cardiopulmonary resuscitation. The tumor was determined to be on the edge of the tongue (B). It was subsequently resected after no metastatic disease was detected.

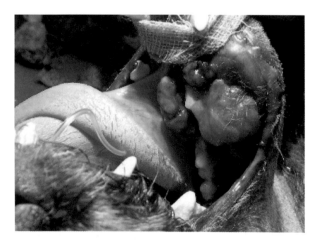

Figure 32-5: Some dogs will not have any clinical signs relating to their tumor other than a protruding lump as with this dog with a mandibular fibrosarcoma. The tumor was confined to the rostral half of the mandible that was treated with a mandibulectomy with excellent results and long term control that was measured in years.

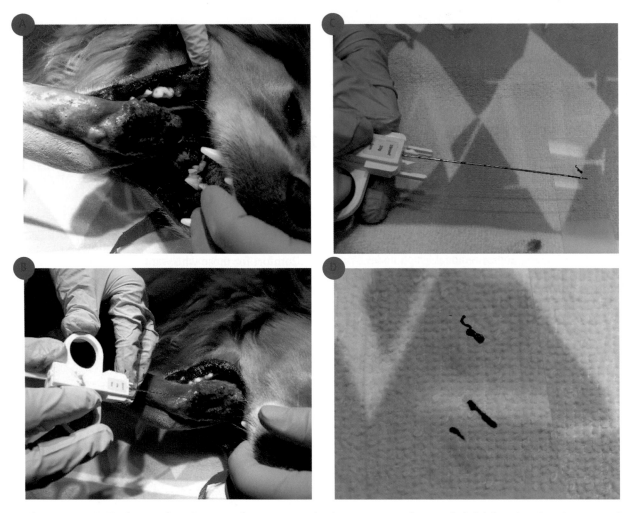

Figure 32-12: Understanding the type of tumor on or in the tongue can be very helpful for planning therapy and giving a prognosis. This is especially true when the tumor is rather large and located in a portion of the tongue that might require the removal of significant portions of the tongue (A). A needle core biopsy of the tongue (B) is very helpful at obtaining multiple pieces of tissue to be submitted for cytology and histopathology (C). The dark black tissue noted in this case was highly suggestive of malignant melanoma (D).

- Comfort and longer-term control for those who want to improve quality of life while trying to maximize the chance of controlling the tumor.

> **Key point**
> Cryotherapy is most effective for the treatment of tumors <2 cm in diameter.

Comfort

- Therapy to enhance comfort and to ensure adequate nutritional intake despite the oral tumor and its treatment is vital.

Comfort and control

Above mentioned therapy for comfort plus:

- Palliative radiation for mandibular or maxillary tumors can be done (e.g.: 2-5 dosages of radiation) to first enhance comfort, second, to reduce the rate of growth and third, occasionally to reduce the size of the tumor.
- Cryotherapy may be quite helpful for controlling or curing small, superficial benign or malignant tumors. The cryotherapy should be done three times, each with a rapid deep freeze to include all aspects of the tumor and surrounding tissue, followed by a slow, complete thaw.

Comfort and longer-term control

Above mentioned therapy for comfort plus:
- Surgical resection of the tumor(s) with evaluation and biopsy of regional lymph nodes.
  - Complete local excision may be curative for ossifying and fibromatous epulides.

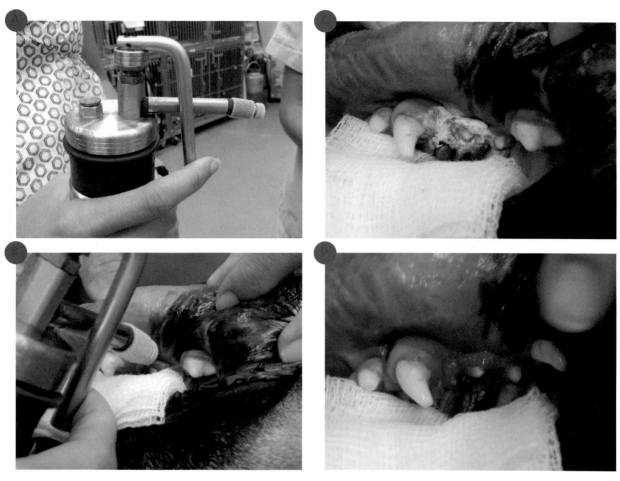

Figure 32-13: Small (<3 cm) oral tumors with limited amount of invasion into surrounding tissues can be treated effectively with three quick freezes and three slow thaws using cryotherapy. The patient is given local and systemic analgesia before he or she is anesthetized. The tumor is localized and surrounding tissues protected (A) before the container filled with liquid nitrogen (B) is used to either spray (C) or place a metal applicator (-70 degrees) directed from the cryotherapy "gun." Once the tumor and a "cuff" of normal tissue deep and wide are frozen, the tissue is allowed to slowly thaw before the subsequent treatment under anesthesia and appropriate analgesia is employed. A minimum of three treatments is given for each site.

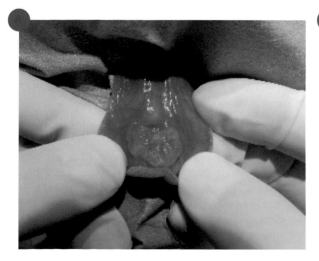
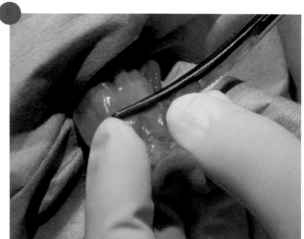

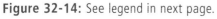

Figure 32-14: See legend in next page.

Comfort and control

Above mentioned therapy for comfort plus:

- Palliative radiation (e.g.: 2-5 dosages of radiation) to first enhance comfort, second, to reduce the rate of growth and third, occasionally to reduce the size of the tumor.
- Toceranib has been shown to have efficacy for the treatment of this tumor, including those with hypercalcemia.

Comfort and longer-term control

Above mentioned therapy for comfort plus:

- Surgical resection of the tumor(s) with evaluation and removal of all regional (e.g.: external iliac) lymph nodes. Note that longer-term benefit can be realized if regrowth is recognized and resected.
- Radiation therapy and/or chemotherapy may be helpful to delay or prevent tumor recurrence or metastases. If radiation is employed, caution should be taken to prevent damage to bladder or colon and/or chemotherapy is recommended.
  - Median survival range from 8 to 26 months.
  - Chemotherapy with carboplatin, mitoxantrone, doxorubicin or melphalan and/or a tyrosine kinase inhibitor can be employed as they have been reported to be effective at improving progression-free interval.
- Best treatment combination of surgery, radiation and chemotherapy.
  - Median overall survival has been reported to be 956 days.[179]

References

1. Verstraete FJ, Kass PH, Terpak CH: Diagnostic value of fullmouth radiography in dogs. *Am J Vet Res* 59:686–691, 1998.
2. Poulet FM, Valentine BA, Summers BA: A survey of epithelial odontogenic tumors and cysts in dogs and cats. *Vet Pathol* 29:369–380, 1992.
3. Dubielzig RR, Goldschmidt MH, Brodey RS: The nomenclature of peridontal epulides in dogs. *Vet Pathol* 16:209–214,1979.
4. Thrall DE: Orthovoltage radiotherapy of acanthomatous epulides in 39 dogs. *JAVMA* 184:826–829, 1984.
5. Gorman NT, Bright RM, Mays MB, Thrall DE: Chemotherapy of a recurrent acanthomatous epulis in a dog. *JAVMA* 184:1158–1160, 1984.
6. Yoshida K, Yanai T, Iwasaki T, et al: Clinicopathological study of canine oral epulides. *J Vet Med Sci* 61:897–902, 1999.
7. Yoshida K, Yanai T, Iwasaki T, et al: Proliferative potential of canine oral epulides and malignant neoplasms assessed by bromodeoxyuridine labeling. *Vet Pathol* 36:35–41, 1999.
8. Theon AP, Rodriguez C, Griffey S, Madewell BR: Analysis of prognosis factors and patterns of failure in dogs with periodontal tumors treated with megavoltage irradiation. *JAVMA* 210:785–788, 1997.
9. McEntee MC, Page RL, Theon A, et al: Malignant tumor formation in dogs previously irradiated for acanthomatous epulis. *Vet Radiol Ultrasound* 45:357–361, 2004.
10. Kühnel S, Kessler M. [Prognosis of canine oral (gingival) squamous cell carcinoma after surgical therapy. A retrospective analysis in 40 patients]. *Tierarztl Prax Ausg K Kleintiere Heimtiere* 42(6):359-366, 2014.
11. Coyle VJ, Rassnick KM, Borst LB, et al: Biological behaviour of canine mandibular osteosarcoma. A retrospective study of 50 cases (1999-2007). *Vet Comp Oncol* doi: 10.1111/vco.12020, 2013.
12. Tuohy JL, Selmic LE, Worley DR, et al: Outcome following curative-intent surgery for oral melanoma in dogs: 70 cases (1998-2011). *JAVMA* 245(11):1266-1273, 2014.
13. Culp WT, Ehrhart N, Withrow SJ, et al: Results of surgical excision and evaluation of factors associated with survival time indogs with lingual neoplasia: 97 cases (1995-2008). *JAVMA* 242(10):1392-1397, 2013.
14. Werner RE Jr: Canine oral neoplasia: A review of 19 cases. *JAAHA* 17:67–69, 1981.
15. Ishikawa T, Yamamoto H: Case of calcifying epithelial odontogenic tumour in a dog. *J Small Anim Pract* 37:597–599, 1996.
16. Delverdier M, Guire F, Van Harverbeke G: Les tumeurs de la cavite buccale du chien: Etude anatomoclinique a partir de 117 cas. *Revue Med Vet* 142:811–816, 1991.
17. Todoroff RJ, Brodey RS: Oral and pharyngeal neoplasia in the dog: A retrospective study of 361 cases. *JAVMA* 175: 567–571, 1979.
18. von Reiswitz A, Hörsting N, Meyer-Lindenberg A, et al: Orale und pharyngeale umfangsvermehrungen des hundeseine retrospektive kasuistische und pathohistologische untersuchung. *Kleintierpraxis* 45:745–759, 2000.
19. Schwarz PD, Withrow SJ, Curtis CR, et al: Partial maxillary resection as a treatment for oral cancer in 61 dogs. *JAAHA* 27:617–624, 1991.
20. Schwarz PD, Withrow SJ, Curtis CR, et al: Mandibular resection as a treatment for oral cancer in 81 dogs. *JAAHA* 27:601–610, 1991.
21. Lascelles BD, Thompson MJ, Dernell WS, et al: Combined dorsolateral and intraoral approach for the resection of tumors of the maxilla in the dog. *JAAHA* 39:294–305, 2003.
22. Lascelles BD, Henderson RA, Seguin B, et al: Bilateral rostral maxillectomy and nasal planectomy for large rostral maxillofacial neoplasms in six dogs and one cat. *AAHA* 40: 137–146, 2004.
23. Frazier SA, Johns SM, Ortega J, et al: Outcome in dogs with surgically resected oral fibrosarcoma (1997-2008). *Vet Comp Onco* 10(1):33-43, 2012.
24. Mas A, Blackwood L, Cripps P, et al: Canine tonsillar squamous cell carcinoma -- a multi-centre retrospective review of 44 clinical cases. *J Small Anim Pract* 52(7):359-364, 2011.
25. Fox LE, Geoghegan SL, Davis LH, et al: Owner satisfaction with partial mandibulectomy or maxillectomy for treatment of oral tumors in 27 dogs. *JAAHA* 33:25–31, 1997.
26. Kessler M: Mandibulectomy and maxillectomy for treatment of bone invasive oral neoplasia in the dog: A retrospective analysis in 31 patients. *Kleintierpraxis* 48:289–300, 2003.
27. Wallace J, Matthiesen DT, Patnaik AK: Hemimaxillectomy for the treatment of oral tumors in 69 dogs. *Vet Surg* 21:337–341, 1992.
28. Evans SM, Shofer F: Canine oral nontonsillar squamous cell carcinoma: Prognostic factors for recurrence and survival following orthovoltage radiation therapy. *Vet Radiol Ultrasound* 29:133–137, 1998.
29. Beck ER, Withrow SJ, McChesney AE, et al: Canine tongue tumors: A retrospective review of 57 cases. *JAAHA* 22:525–532, 1996.
30. Ogilvie GK, Sundberg JP, O'Banion K, et al: Papillary squamous cell carcinoma in three young dogs. *JAVMA* 192:933–936, 1988.
31. Bradley RL, MacEwen EG, Loar AS: Mandibular resection for removal of oral tumors in 30 dogs and 6 cats. *JAVMA* 184:460–463, 1984.
32. Théon AP, Rodriguez C, Madewell BR: Analysis of prognostic factors and patterns of failure in dogs with malignant oral tumors treated with megavoltage irradiation. *JAVMA* 210:778–784, 1997.
33. Salisbury SK, Lantz GC: Long-term results of partial mandibulectomy for treatment of oral tumors in 30 dogs. *JAAHA* 24:285–294, 1988.
34. LaDue-Miller T, Price S, Page RL, Thrall DE: Radiotherapy of canine non-tonsillar squamous cell carcinoma. *Vet Radiol Ultrasound* 37:74–77, 1996.
35. Salisbury SK, Richardson DC, Lantz GC: Partial maxillectomy and premaxillectomy in the treatment of oral neoplasia in the dog and cat. *Vet Surg* 15:16–26, 1986.
36. Withrow SJ, Nelson AW, Manley PA, Biggs DR: Premaxillectomy in the dog. *JAAHA* 21:45–55, 1985.
37. Buhles WC Jr, Theilen GH: Preliminary evaluation of bleomycin in feline and canine squamous cell carcinoma. *Am J Vet Res* 34:289–291, 1973.
38. Himsel CA, Richardson RC, Craig JA: Cisplatin chemotherapy for metastatic squamous cell carcinoma in two dogs. *JAVMA* 189:1575–1578, 1986.
39. Knapp DW, Richardson RC, Bonney PL, Hahn K: Cisplatin therapy in 41 dogs with malignant tumors. *J Vet Intern Med* 2:41–46, 1988.
40. Shapiro W, Kitchell BE, Fossum TW, et al: Cisplatin for treatment of transitional cell and squamous cell carcinomas in dogs. *JAVMA* 193:1530–1533, 1988.

41. Ogilvie GK, Obradovich JE, Elmslie RE, et al: Efficacy of mitoxantrone against various neoplasms in dogs. *JAVMA* 198:1618–1621, 1991.

42. Schmidt BR, Glickman NW, DeNicola DB, et al: Evaluation of piroxicam for the treatment of oral squamous cell carcinoma in dogs. *JAVMA* 218:1783–1786, 2001.

43. Boria PA, Murry DJ, Bennett PF, et al: Evaluation of cisplatin combined with piroxicam for the treatment of oral malignant melanoma and oral squamous cell carcinoma in dogs. *JAVMA* 224:388–394, 2004.

44. de Vos JP, Burm AG, Focker BP, et al: Results of the combined treatment with piroxicam and carboplatin in canine oral non-tonsillar squamous cell carcinoma. *Proc 24th Annu Conf Vet Cancer Soc*:62. 2004.

45. MacMillan R, Withrow SJ, Gillette EL: Surgery and regional irradiation for treatment of canine tonsillar squamous cell carcinoma: Retrospective review of eight cases. *JAAHA* 18: 311–314, 1982.

46. Brooks MB, Matus RE, Leifer CE, et al: Chemotherapy versus chemotherapy plus radiotherapy in the treatment of tonsillar squamous cell carcinoma in the dog. *J Vet Intern Med* 2:206–211, 1988.

47. Withers FW: Squamous-celled carcinoma of the tonsil in the dog. J Pathol Bact 49:429–432, 1939.

48. Wyers M, Irgens K, Parodi A-L: Le cancer de l'amygdale dans l'espece canine. *Rec Méd Vét* XX:333–351, 1969.

49. Cotchin E: Some tumours of dogs and cats of comparative veterinary and human interest. *Vet Rec* 71:1040–1054, 1959.

50. Ragland WL 3rd, Gorham JR: Tonsillar carcinoma in rural dogs. *Nature* 214:925–926, 1967.

51. Reif JS, Cohen D: The environmental distribution of canine respiratory tract neoplasms. *Arch Environ Health* 22:136–140,1971.

52. Bostock DE, Curtis R: Comparison of canine oropharyngeal malignancy in various geographical locations. *Vet Rec* 114:341–342, 1984.

53. Brewer WG Jr, Turrel JM: Radiotherapy and hyperthermia in the treatment of fibrosarcomas in the dog. *JAVMA* 181:146–150, 1982.

54. Thrall DE: Orthovoltage radiotherapy of oral fibrosarcomas in dogs. *JAVMA* 179:159–162, 1981.

55. Ciekot PA, Powers BE, Withrow SJ, et al: Histologically lowgrade, yet biologically high-grade, fibrosarcomas of the mandible and maxilla in dogs: 25 cases (1982–1991). *JAVMA* 204:610–615, 1994.

56. Forrest LJ, Chun R, Adams WM, et al: Postoperative radiotherapy for canine soft tissue sarcoma. *J Vet Intern Med* 14:578–582, 2000.

57. McChesney SL, Withrow SJ, Gillette EL, et al: Radiotherapy of soft tissue sarcomas in dogs. *JAVMA* 194:60–63, 1989.

58. McChesney SL, Gillette EL, Dewhirst MW, Withrow SJ: Influence of WR 2721 on radiation response of canine soft tissue sarcomas. *Int J Radiat Oncol Biol Phys* 12:1957–1963, 1986.

59. Theon AP, Madewell BR, Ryu J, Castro J: Concurrent irradiation and intratumoral chemotherapy with cisplatin: A pilot study in dogs with spontaneous tumors. *Int J Radiat Oncol Biol Phys* 29:1027–1034, 1994.

60. Dvorak LD, Beaver DP, Ellison GW, et al: Major glossectomy in dogs: A case series and proposed classification system. *JAAHA* 40:331–337, 2004.

61. Rallis TS, Tontis DK, Soubasis NH, et al: Immunohistochemical study of a granular cell tumor on the tongue of a dog. *Vet Clin Pathol* 30:62–66, 2001.

62. Giles RC Jr, Montgomery CA Jr, Izen L: Canine lingual granular cell myoblastoma: A case report. *Am J Vet Res* 35:1357–1359, 1974.

63. Lascelles BD, McInnes E, Dobson JM, White RA: Rhabdomyosarcoma of the tongue in a dog. *J Small Anim Pract* 39:587–591, 1998.

64. Patnaik AK: Histologic and immunohistochemical studies of granular cell tumors in seven dogs, three cats, one horse, and one bird. *Vet Pathol* 30:176–185, 1993.

65. Schoofs SH: Lingual hemangioma in a puppy: A case report and literature review. *JAAHA* 33:161–165, 1997.

66. Karbe E, Schiefer B: Primary salivary gland tumors in carnivores. *Can Vet J* 8:212–215, 1967.

67. pangler WL, Culbertson MR: Salivary gland disease in dogs and cats: 245 cases (1985–1988). *JAVMA* 198:465–469, 1991.

68. Carberry CA, Flanders JA, Harvey HJ, Ryan AM: Salivary gland tumors in dogs and cats: A literature and case review. *JAAHA* 24:561–567, 1988.

69. Koestner A, Buerger L: Primary neoplasms of the salivary glands in animals compared to similar tumors in man. *Path Vet* 2:201–226, 1965.

70. Thomsen BV, Myers RK: Extraskeletal osteosarcoma of the mandibular salivary gland in a dog. *Vet Pathol* 36:71–73, 1999.

71. Bindseil E, Madsen JS: Lipomatosis causing tumour-like swelling of a mandibular salivary gland in a dog. *Vet Rec* 140:583584, 1997.

72. Hammer A, Getzy D, Ogilvie G, et al: Salivary gland neoplasia in the dog and cat: Survival times and prognostic factors. *JAAHA* 37:478–482, 2001.

73. Louw GJ, van Schouwenburg SJ: A case of a highly invasive carcinoma of a salivary gland in a crossbred dog. *J S Afr Vet Assoc* 55:131–132, 1984.

74. Habin DJ, Else RW: Parotid salivary gland adenocarcinoma with bilateral ocular and osseous metastases in a dog. *J Small Anim Pract* 36:445–449, 1995.

75. Valentini S, Spinella G, Negrini S, Fedrigo M: Ultrasonography of the salivary glands in dogs and cats. *Summa* 20:51–56, 2003.

76. Leifer CE, Peterson ME, Matus RE, Patnaik AK: Hypoglycemia associated with nonislet cell tumor in 13 dogs. *JAVMA* 186:53–55, 1985.

77. Evans SM, Thrall DE: Postoperative orthovoltage radiation therapy of parotid salivary gland adenocarcinoma in three dogs. *JAVMA* 182:993–994, 1983.

78. Ratto A, Peiffer RL Jr, Peruccio C, Rossi L: Zygomatic salivary gland adenocarcinoma in a dog. *Vet Comp Ophthal* 1:59–62, 1991.

79. Ridgeway RL, Suter PF: Clinical and radiographic signs in primary and metastatic esophageal neoplasms of the dog. *JAVMA* 174:700–704, 1979.

80. Frost D, Lasota J, Miettinen M: Gastrointestinal stromal tumors and leiomyomas in the dog: a histopathologic, immunohistochemical, and molecular genetic study of 50 cases. *Vet Pathol* 40:42–54, 2003.

81. Ranen E, Lavy E, Aizenberg I, et al: Spirocercosis-associated esophageal sarcomas in dogs. A retrospective study of 17 cases (1997–2003). *Vet Parasitol* 119:209–221, 2004.

82. Lobetti RG: Survey of the incidence, diagnosis, clinical manifestations and treatment of *Spirocerca lupi* in South Africa. *J S Afr Vet Assoc* 71:43–46, 2000.

83. Berry WL: *Spirocerca lupi* esophageal granulomas in 7 dogs: Resolution after treatment with doramectin. *J Vet Intern Med* 14:609–612, 2000.

84. Matros L, Jergens AE, Miles KG, Kluge JP: Megaesophagus and hypomotility associated with esophageal leiomyoma in a dog. *JAAHA* 30:15–19, 1994.

85. Wilson RB, Holscher MA, Laney PS: Esophageal osteosarcoma in a dog. *JAAHA* 27:361–363, 1991.

86. Nohara H: Fibrosarcoma arising from the thoracic part of the esophagus in a dog. *J Jan Vet Med Assoc* 44:227–229, 1991.

87. Randolph JF, Center SA, Flanders JA, Diters RW: Hypertrophic osteopathy associated with adenocarcinoma of the esophageal glands in a dog. *JAVMA* 184:98–99, 1984.

88. Jacobs TM, Rosen GM: Photodynamic therapy as a treatment for esophageal squamous cell carcinoma in a dog. *JAAHA* 36:257–261, 2000.

89. Hamilton TA, Carpenter JL: Esophageal plasmacytoma in a dog. *JAVMA* 204:1210–1211, 1994.

90. Ranen E, Shamir MH, Shahar R, Johnston DE: Partial esophagectomy with single layer closure for treatment of esophageal sarcomas in 6 dogs. *Vet Surg* 33:428–434, 2004.

91. Murray M, Robinson PB, McKeating FJ, et al: Primary gastric neoplasia in the dog: a clinico-pathological study. *Vet Rec* 91:474–479, 1972.

92. Patnaik AK, Hurvitz AI, Johnson GF: Canine gastrointestinal neoplasms. *Vet Pathol* 14:547–555, 1977.

93. Sautter JH, Hanlon GF: Gastric neoplasms in the dog: a report of 20 cases. *JAVMA* 166:691–696, 1975.

94. Albers TM, Alroy J, McDonnell JJ, Moore AS: A poorly differentiated gastric carcinoid in a dog. *J Vet Diagn Invest* 10:116–118, 1998.

95. Fonda D, Gualtieri M, Scanziani E: Gastric carcinoma in the dog: a clinicopathological study of 11 cases. *J Small Anim Pract* 30:353–360, 1989.

96. Scanziani E, Giusti AM, Gualtieri M, Fonda D: Gastric carcinoma in the Belgian shepherd dog. *J Small Anim Pract* 32:465–469, 1991.

97. Patnaik AK, Hurvitz AI, Johnson GF: Canine gastric adenocarcinoma. *Vet Pathol* 15:600–607, 1978.

98. Sullivan M, Lee R, Fisher EW, et al: A study of 31 cases of gastric carcinoma in dogs. *Vet Rec* 120:79–83, 1987.

99. Frank JD, Reimer SB, Kass PH, et al: Clinical outcomes of 30 cases (1997-2004) of canine gastrointestinal lymphoma. *J Am Anim Hosp Assoc* 43(6):313-321, 2007.

100. Kolbjornsen O, Press CM, Landsverk T: Gastropathies in the Lundehund. II. A study of mucin profiles. *APMIS* 102:801–809, 1994.

101. Kolbjornsen O, Press CM, Landsverk T: Gastropathies in the Lundehund. I. Gastritis and gastric neoplasia associated with intestinal lymphangiectasia. *APMIS* 102:647–661, 1994.

102. Sano T, Kobori O, Kuroki S, et al: Effect of experimental

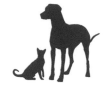

Chapter 33

Canine melanomas

CANINE ORAL MELANOMA

Clinical presentation

- Friable, often pigmented oral lesion in older dogs.

> **Key point**
> Oral melanomas can be non-pigmented and thus can masquerade clinically as another tumor type.

Staging and diagnosis

- Minimum data base (MDB): includes a CBC, biochemical profile, urinalysis, biopsy and three-view thoracic radiographs and abdominal ultrasound or computerized tomography of the chest and abdomen.
- Regional lymph node cytology, even if the lymph nodes palpate normally.
- Metastasis common, usually regional lymph nodes and/or lungs.

> **Key point**
> Lymph node metastases are common, even if the lymph nodes are not enlarged. Cytology or histopathology is recommended to rule in or out regional lymph node metastases.

Prognostic factors

- Melanoma of the lip may have longer survival.
- Mitotic index not as predictive of behavior as for other sites.
- Size: small tumors have a better prognosis.
- Location: caudal is worse.
- Staging: higher stage is worse.
- Histopathologic grade correlates with survival.

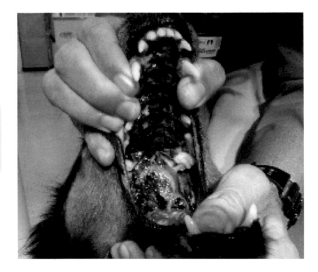

Figure 33-1: Melanoma of the oral cavity is essentially always malignant with a relatively high metastatic rate, most often to the regional lymph nodes (even if the lymph nodes palpate normally) and lungs. Evaluation of both sites is strongly encouraged. Local disease control with either surgery or radiation followed by the DNA xenogeneic melanoma vaccine is often indicated. In this case, the tumor was too large to completely excise, therefore six treatments of coarse fractionated photon beam radiation therapy were given over three weeks followed by the vaccine.

Treatment

This section is divided into three options:
- Comfort for those who want to improve quality of life.
- Comfort and control for those who want to improve quality of life while trying to provide some control of the tumor.
- Comfort and longer-term control for those who want to improve quality of life while trying to maximize the chance of controlling the tumor.

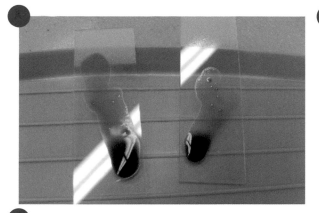

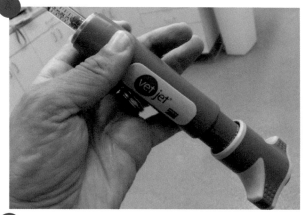

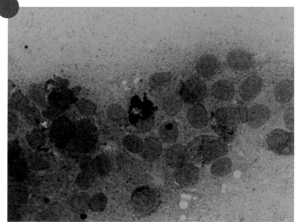

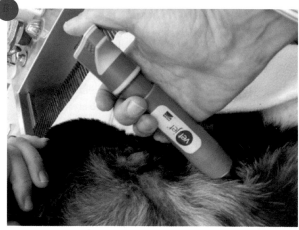

Figure 33-2: Aspirates of melanoma can often result in dark brown to black fluid (A) that is represented on cytology as black charcoal-like dust or larger particles that can at times obscure the nucleus (B).

Figure 33-3: When the primary oral malignant melanoma is under control, the DNA xenogeneic melanoma vaccine is given with a unique needle-less device (A) that administers the vaccine in the medial aspect of the hind leg (B).

> **Key point**
> Surgery and/or coarse fractionated radiation therapy is often recommended along with appropriate adjuvant immunotherapy using a DNA xenogeneic melanoma vaccine and/or a tyrosine kinase inhibitor.

Comfort

- Therapy to enhance comfort and freedom from nausea, vomiting, diarrhea and lack of appetite.

Comfort and control

Above mentioned therapy for comfort plus:
- Coarse fractionated radiation (e.g.: 6 dosages of radiation given twice weekly) to first enhance comfort, second, to reduce the rate of growth and third, occasionally to reduce the size of the tumor or wide and deep surgical removal of the tumor.
- The DNA xenogeneic melanoma vaccine or carboplatin may be helpful to delay or prevent recurrence or metastases.

Comfort and longer-term control

Above mentioned therapy for comfort plus:
- Surgical resection of the tumor(s) with evaluation and if indicated removal of regional lymph nodes. Radiation therapy may be helpful (e.g.: 16-19 dosages of radiation).
- The DNA xenogeneic melanoma vaccine or carboplatin may be helpful to delay or prevent recurrence or metastases.

CANINE CUTANEOUS MELANOMA

Clinical presentation

- Moderately common.
- Darkly pigmented epidermal lesion in adult to aged dogs.
- Usually raised but not ulcerated.
- Usually not painful.
- Most tumors of haired skin are well differentiated (benign), non-painful and slowly growing.

7. Voros K, Vrabely T, Papp L, et al: Correlation of ultrasonographic and pathomorphological findings in canine hepatic diseases. *J Small Anim Pract* 32:627–634, 1991.

8. Feeney DA, Johnston GR, Hardy RM: Two-dimensional, grayscale ultrasonography for assessment of hepatic and splenic neoplasia in the dog and cat. *JAVMA* 184:68–81, 1984.

9. Biller DS, Kantrowitz B, Miyabayashi T: Ultrasonography of diffuse liver disease. A review. *J Vet Intern Med* 6:71–76, 1992.

10. Roth L: Comparison of liver cytology and biopsy diagnoses in dogs and cats: 56 cases. *Vet Clin Pathol* 30:35–38, 2001.

11. Cole TL, Center SA, Flood SN, et al: Diagnostic comparison of needle and wedge biopsy specimens of the liver in dogs and cats. *JAVMA* 220:1483–1490, 2002.

12. Center SA, Baldwin BH, Erb HN, Tennant BC: Bile acid concentrations in the diagnosis of hepatobiliary disease in the dog. *JAVMA* 187:935–940, 1985.

13. Clifford CA, Pretorius ES, Weisse C, et al: Magnetic resonance imaging of focal splenic and hepatic lesions in the dog. *J Vet Intern Med* 18:330–338, 2004.

14. Morrell CN, Volk MV, Mankowski JL: A carcinoid tumor in the gallbladder of a dog. *Vet Pathol* 39:756–758, 2002.

15. Brömel C, Smeak DD, Léveillé R: Porcelain gallbladder associated with primary biliary adenocarcinoma in a dog. *JAVMA* 213:1137–1139, 1998.

16. Lowseth LA, Gillett NA, Chang IY, et al: Detection of serum alpha-fetoprotein in dogs with hepatic tumors. *JAVMA* 199:735–741, 1991.

17. Yamada T, Fujita M, Kitao S, et al: Serum alpha-fetoprotein values in dogs with various hepatic diseases. *J Vet Med Sci* 61:657–659, 1999.

18. Martin de las Mulas J, Gomez-Villamandos JC, Perez J, et al: Immunohistochemical evaluation of canine primary liver carcinomas: distribution of alpha-fetoprotein, carcinoembryonic antigen, keratins and vimentin. *Res Vet Sci* 59:124–127, 1995.

19. Duran ME, Ezquerra J, Roncero V, et al: Acute necrotizing myelopathy associated with a hepatocarcinoma. *Progress Vet Neurol* 3:35–38, 1998.

20. Krotje LJ, Fix AS, Potthoff AD: Acquired myasthenia gravis and cholangiocellular carcinoma in a dog. *JAVMA* 197:488-490, 1990.

21. Ramos-Vara JA, Miller MA, Johnson GC: Immunohistochemical characterization of canine hyperplastic hepatic lesions and hepatocellular and biliary neoplasms with monoclonal antibody hepatocyte paraffin 1 and a monoclonal antibody to cytokeratin 7. *Vet Pathol* 38:636–643, 2001.

22. Liptak JM, Dernell WS, Monnet E, et al: Massive hepatocellular carcinoma in dogs: 48 cases (1992–2002). *JAVMA* 225:1225–1230, 2004.

23. Fahie MA, Martin RA: Extrahepatic biliary tract obstruction: A retrospective study of 45 cases (1983–1993). *J Am Anim Hosp Assoc* 31:478–482, 1995.

24. Patnaik AK, Hurvitz AI, Lieberman PH, Johnson GF: Canine bile duct carcinoma. *Vet Pathol* 18:439–444, 1981.

25. Patnaik AK, Lieberman PH, Hurvitz AI, Johnson GF: Canine hepatic carcinoids. *Vet Pathol* 18:445–453, 1981.

26. McDonald RK, Helman RG: Hepatic malignant mesenchymoma in a dog. *JAVMA* 188:1052–1053, 1986.

27. Haines DM, Doige CE, Matte G, Wilkinson AA: Multifocal telangiectatic osteosarcoma and malignant mixed hepatic tumor in a dog. *JAAHA* 23:509–513, 1987.

28. Weisse C, Clifford CA, Holt D, Solomon JA: Percutaneous arterial embolization and chemoembolization for treatment of benign and malignant tumors in three dogs and a goat. *JAVMA* 221:1430–1436, 1419, 2002.

29. Cave TA, Johnson V, Beths T, et al: Treatment of unresectable hepatocellular adenoma in dogs with transarterial iodized oil and chemotherapy with and without an embolic agent: A report of two cases. *Vet Comp Oncol* 1:191–199, 2003.

30. Fry PD, Rest JR: Partial hepatectomy in two dogs. *J Small Anim Pract* 34:192–195, 1993.

31. Ginn PE: Immunohistochemical detection of P-glycoprotein in formalin-fixed and paraffin-embedded normal and neoplastic canine tissues. *Vet Pathol* 33:533–541, 1996.

32. Ogilvie GK, Obradovich JE, Elmslie RE, et al: Efficacy of mitoxantrone against various neoplasms in dogs. *JAVMA* 198:1618–1621, 1991.

33. Moore AS, Kitchell BE: New chemotherapy agents in veterinary medicine. *Vet Clin North Am Small Anim Pract* 33:629–649, viii, 2003.

34. Spangler WL, Kass PH: Pathologic factors affecting postsplenectomy survival in dogs. *J Vet Intern Med* 11:166–171, 1997.

35. Weinstein MJ, Carpenter JL, Schunk CJ: Nonangiogenic and nonlymphomatous sarcomas of the canine spleen: 57 cases (1975–1987). *JAVMA* 195:784–788, 1989.

36. Day MJ, Lucke VM, Pearson H: A review of pathological diagnoses made from 87 canine splenic biopsies. *J Small Anim Pract* 36:426–433, 1995.

37. Hendrick MJ, Brooks JJ, Bruce EH: Six cases of malignant fibrous histiocytoma of the canine spleen. *Vet Pathol* 29:351– 354, 1992.

38. Wrigley RH, Park RD, Knode LJ, Lebel JL: Ultrasonographic features of splenic hemangiosarcoma in dogs: 18 cases (1980–1986). *JAVMA* 192:1113–1117, 1988.

39. Spangler WL, Culbertson MR, Kass PH: Primary mesenchymal (nonangiomatous/nonlymphomatous) neoplasms occurring in the canine spleen: Anatomic classification, immunohistochemistry, and mitotic activity correlated with patient survival. *Vet Pathol* 31:37–47, 1994.

40. Kapatkin AS, Mullen Hs, Matthiesen DT, Patnaik AK: Leiomyosarcoma in dogs: 44 cases (1983–1988). *JAVMA* 201:1077–1079, 1992.

41. Kircher CH, Nielsen SW: Tumours of the pancreas. *Bull World Health Organ* 53:195–202, 1976.

42. Rowlatt U: Spontaneous epithelial tumours of the pancreas of mammals. *Br J Cancer* 21:82–107, 1967.

43. Anderson NV, Johnson KH: Pancreatic carcinoma in the dog. *JAVMA* 150:286–295, 1967.

44. Brown PJ, Mason KV, Merrett DJ, et al: Multifocal necrotising steatitis associated with pancreatic carcinoma in three dogs. *J Small Anim Pract* 35:129–132, 1994.

45. Xu FN: Ultrastructural examination as an aid to the diagnosis of canine pancreatic neoplasms. *Aust Vet J* 62:197–198, 1985.

46. Ditchfield J, Archibald J: Carcinoma of the pancreas in small animals. A report of two cases. *Small Anim Clin* 1:173–176, 1961.

47. Northrup NC, Rassnick KM, Gieger TL, et al: Prospective evaluation of biweekly streptozotocin in 19 dogs with insulinoma. *J Vet Intern Med* 27(3):483-490, 2913.

48. Polton GA, White RN, Brearley MJ, et al: Improved survival in a retrospective cohort of 28 dogs with insulinoma. *J Small Anim Pract.* 48(3):151-156, 2007.

49. Bennett PF, Hahn KA, Toal RL, Legendre AM: Ultrasonographic and cytopathological diagnosis of exocrine pancreatic carcinoma in the dog and cat. *JAAHA* 37:466–473, 2001.

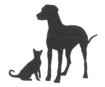

Chapter 35

Canine tumors of blood and lymph vessels

CANINE SPLENIC HEMANGIOSARCOMA

Clinical presentation

- Common, usually not painful.
- Hemangiosarcoma can originate from or metastasize to anywhere in the body.
- Average age of affected dogs is 10 years.
- German shepherd dogs predisposed.
- Metastases are often confined to abdominal cavity if no concurrent right atrial lesion exists.

> **Key point**
> Most dogs with splenic hemangiosarcoma present for acute signs associated with intra-abdominal pain or blood loss due to a ruptured spleen.

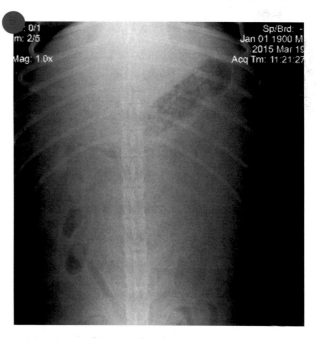

Figure 35-1: The dog with a splenic tumor often presents with a hemoabdomen that is visualized on abdominal radiographs with loss of abdominal detail (A and B). These masses, regardless of cause can and do rupture. No imaging can or should be used to determine the histologic diagnosis of the splenic mass. Because hemangiosarcoma of the spleen is a common cause of these splenic disorders, full staging to identify metastases is warranted. Staging includes but is not necessarily limited to a chest radiograph, ultrasound of the heart, abdominal ultrasound, complete blood count, biochemical profile and urinalysis. Transfusions are often needed in association with aggressive fluid therapy to combat volume depletion, therefore cross matches and blood typing is also commonly done. Once the patient is stable and appropriately staged, then a lifesaving splenectomy should be done. Imaging courtesy of Lenore Anderson Mohammadian, DVM, MSpVM, Diplomate ACVR.

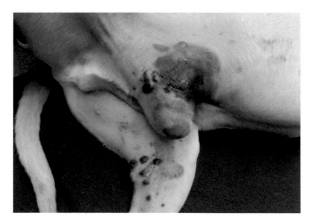

Figure 35-3: Multiple dark red to black masses are seen on or around this dog's ventrum and on the inside of the medial aspect of the left rear leg that were confirmed to be low grade hemangiosarcomas. These tumors are very common on dogs that spend significant time in the sun. Many of these tumors are noted in lightly haired regions. The metastatic rate is generally low, however chest radiographs, abdominal and cardiac ultrasound are always good ideas before resecting these lesions. In this case, the larger one was treated with a penile and preputial resection with a perineal urethrostomy. The smaller lesions were resected or treated with a biopsy and cryotherapy. Sun avoidance, sunscreen, non-steroidal anti-inflammatory drugs such as piroxicam and docosahexaenoic acid were encouraged for comfort and to hopefully reduce the frequency of the development of new lesions.

- Comfort and control for those who want to improve quality of life while trying to provide some control of the tumor.
- Comfort and longer-term control for those who want to improve quality of life while trying to maximize the chance of controlling the tumor.

> **Key point**
>
> Unresectable disease of the heart may be appropriately treated with radiation. Hemangiosarcoma of the heart can metastasize and cause pericardial effusion. Pericardial taps or creating a pericardial window is often required. As with splenic hemangiosarcoma, the risk of distant metastatic disease is high, and therefore systemic therapy to include, but not necessarily limited to, doxorubicin, Coriolus Versicolor (Mycelia) with polysaccharopeptide, and Yunnan Baiyao should be employed.

Comfort

- Therapy to enhance comfort and freedom from nausea, vomiting, diarrhea and lack of appetite. A transfusion may be needed in some patients. Pericardiocentesis if indicated.

Comfort and control

Above mentioned therapy for comfort plus:
- Palliative radiation (e.g.: 2-5 dosages of radiation) to first enhance comfort, second, to reduce the rate of growth and third, occasionally to reduce the size of the tumor and/or
- Doxorubicin chemotherapy (median survival time, 116 days).
- Drugs that suppress angiogenesis such as select tyrosine kinase inhibitors plus metronomic therapy have been suggested to be beneficial.

CANINE CUTANEOUS HEMANGIOSARCOMA

Clinical presentation

- Raised, red lesion; often in skin that is lightly pigmented and sun exposed.
- Usually not painful.
- Average age is 10 years.
- Whippets and other dogs with lightly pigmented, lightly haired skin are predisposed.

Staging and diagnosis

Treatment

This section is divided into two options:
- Comfort for those who want to improve quality of life.
- Comfort and control for those who want to improve quality of life while trying to provide some control of the tumor.

Comfort

- Therapy to enhance comfort and freedom from nausea, vomiting, diarrhea and lack of appetite. Sun avoidance, sunscreen, and/or body suits.

Comfort and control

Above mentioned therapy for comfort plus:
- Surgical resection of the tumor(s) with evaluation and biopsy of regional lymph nodes.
- Doxorubicin should be reserved for grade II or III tumors or if the tumors are located in part or entirely in the subcutaneous space.

CANINE LYMPHANGIOMA AND LYMPHANGIOSARCOMA

Clinical presentation

- Uncommon, usually not painful unless extensive.
- Most often in skin.
- May be a sequel to chronic lymphatic obstruction.
- Average age is 7 years; may occur in very young animals.
- Beagles may be predisposed.

Key point

Patients with this neoplastic disorder have a non-painful swelling that changes over time.

Staging and diagnosis

- Minimum data base (MDB): includes a CBC, biochemical profile, urinalysis, biopsy and three-view thoracic radiographs or computerized tomography of the chest and abdomen and/or, ultrasound of the abdomen.
- Check regional lymph nodes.
- Metastasis is uncommon; most reported tumors are benign.

Prognostic factors

- None reported.

Treatment

This section is divided into three options:
- Comfort for those who want to improve quality of life.
- Comfort and control for those who want to improve quality of life while trying to provide some control of the tumor.
- Comfort and longer-term control for those who want to improve quality of life while trying to maximize the chance of controlling the tumor.

Key point

Margins are difficult to determine, therefore wide and deep surgical excision or radiation therapy should be performed with this in mind.

Comfort

- Therapy to enhance comfort and freedom from nausea, vomiting, diarrhea and lack of appetite.

Comfort and control

Above mentioned therapy for comfort plus:
- Palliative radiation (e.g.: 2-5 dosages of radiation) to first enhance comfort, second, to reduce the rate of growth and third, occasionally to reduce the size of the tumor.

Comfort and longer-term control

Above mentioned therapy for comfort plus:
- Surgical resection of the entire tumor(s) with evaluation and biopsy of regional lymph nodes.
- Definitive radiation therapy may be helpful (e.g.: 16-19 dosages of radiation) if the margins are incomplete or questionable.
- Doxorubicin based chemotherapy likely helpful.

References

1. Srebernik N, Appleby EC: Breed prevalence and sites of haemangioma and haemangiosarcoma in dogs. *Vet Rec* 129:408–409, 1991.
2. Ng CY, Mills JN: Clinical and haematological features of haemangiosarcoma in dogs. *Aust Vet J* 62:1–4, 1985.
3. Prymak C, McKee LJ, Goldschmidt MH, Glickman LT: Epidemiologic, clinical, pathologic, and prognostic characteristics of splenic hemangiosarcoma and splenic hematoma in dogs: 217 cases (1985). *JAVMA* 193:706–712, 1988.
4. Sorenmo K, Duda L, Barber L, et al: Canine hemangiosarcoma treated with standard chemotherapy and minocycline. *J Vet Intern Med* 14:395–398, 2000.
5. Spangler WL, Culbertson MR: Prevalence, type, and importance of splenic diseases in dogs: 1,480 cases (1985–1989). *JAVMA* 200:829–834, 1992.
6. Popper H, Thomas LB, Telles NC, et al: Development of hepatic angiosarcoma in man induced by vinyl chloride, thorotrast, and arsenic. Comparison with cases of unknown etiology *Am J Pathol* 92:349–369, 1978.
7. Johnson KA, Powers BE, Withrow SJ, et al: Splenomegaly in dogs. Predictors of neoplasia and survival after splenectomy. *J Vet Intern Med* 3:160–166, 1989.
8. Sorenmo KU, Jeglum KA, Helfand SC: Chemotherapy of canine hemangiosarcoma with doxorubicin and cyclophosphamide. *J Vet Intern Med* 7:370–376, 1993.
9. Wruck M: Milzhämatom bei einem rauhaardackel. *Kleintierpraxis* 44:773–779, 1999.
10. Maruyama H, Miura T, Sakai M, et al: The incidence of disseminated intravascular coagulation in dogs with malignant tumor. *J Vet Med Sci* 66:573–575, 2004.
11. Wrigley RH, Park RD, Konde LJ, Lebel JL: Ultrasonographic features of splenic hemangiosarcoma in dogs: 18 cases (1980–1986). *JAVMA* 192:1113–1117, 1988.
12. Waters DJ, Caywood DD, Hayden DW, Klausner JS: Metastatic pattern in dogs with splenic haemangiosarcoma: Clinical implications. *J Small Anim Pract* 29:805–814, 1988.
13. Wandera JG, Kamuau JA, Ngatia TA, et al: Haemangiosarcoma in dogs: Morphological and clinical findings. *Bull Anim Health Prod Afr* 38:301–308, 1990.
14. Vail DM, MacEwen EG, Kurzman ID, et al: Liposomeencapsulated muramyl tripeptide phosphatidylethanolamine adjuvant immunotherapy for splenic hemangiosarcoma in the dog: A randomized multi-institutional clinical trial. *Clin Cancer Res* 1:1165–1170, 1995.
15. O'Keefe DA, Couto CG: Fine-needle aspiration of the spleen as an aid in the diagnosis of splenomegaly. *J Vet Intern Med* 1:102–109, 1987.
16. Ferrer L, Fondevila D, Rabanal RM, Vilafranca M: Immunohistochemical detection of CD31 antigen in normal and neoplastic canine endothelial cells. *J Comp Pathol* 112:319–326, 1995.
17. Hayden DW, Bartges JW, Bell FW, Klausner JS: Prostatic hemangiosarcoma in a dog: Clinical and pathologic findings. *J Vet Diagn Invest* 4:209–211, 1992.
18. Clifford CA, Hughes D, Beal MW, et al: Plasma vascular endothelial growth factor concentrations in healthy dogs and dogs with hemangiosarcoma. *J Vet Intern Med* 15:131–135, 2001.
19. Hammer AS, Couto CG, Filppi J, et al: Efficacy and toxicity of VAC chemotherapy (vincristine, doxorubicin, and cyclophosphamide) in dogs with hemangiosarcoma. *J Vet Intern Med* 5:160–166, 1991.
20. Sorenmo KU, Baez JL, Clifford CA, et al: Efficacy and toxicity of a dose-intensified doxorubicin protocol in canine hemangiosarcoma. *J Vet Intern Med* 18:209–213, 2004.
21. Spangler WL, Kass PH: Pathologic factors affecting postsplenectomy survival in dogs. *J Vet Intern Med* 11:166–171, 1997.
22. Ogilvie GK, Powers BE, Mallinckrodt CH, Withrow SJ: Surgery and doxorubicin in dogs with hemangiosarcoma. *J Vet Intern Med* 10:379–384, 1996.
23. Wood CA, Moore AS, Gliatto JM, et al: Prognosis for dogs with stage I or II splenic hemangiosarcoma treated by splenectomy alone: 32 cases (1991–1993). *JAAHA* 34:417–421, 1998.
24. Keyes ML, Rush JE, Autran B, et al: Ventricular arrhythmias in dogs with splenic masses. *Vet Emerg Critical Care* 3:33–38, 1994.
25. Vail DM, Kravis LD, Cooley AJ, et al: Preclinical trial of doxorubicin entrapped in sterically stabilized liposomes in dogs with spontaneously arising malignant tumors. *Cancer Chemother Pharmacol* 39:410–416, 1997.
26. Rassnick KM, Frimberger AE, Wood CA, et al: Evaluation of ifosfamide for treatment of various canine neoplasms. *J Vet Intern Med* 14:271–276, 2000.
27. Mallinckrodt MJ, Gottfried SD. Mass-to-splenic volume ratio and spleen weight as a percentage of body weight in dogs with malignant and benign splenic masses: 65 cases (2007-2008). *JAVMA* 239(10):1325-1327, 2011.

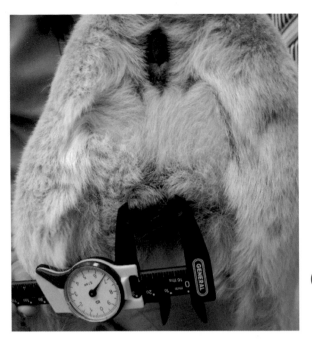

Figure 37-1: There are many different types of vaginal tumors. Those that begin in the vulva like vaginal leiomyoma, leiomyosarcoma or lymphoma, those that involve the vulva but that originate within the vulva or urethra such as transitional cell carcinoma, and those tumors surrounding the vulva that eventually grow to involve the vulva like this dog with the vulvar mast cell tumor. Each should be staged to ensure they have not spread. In this case, the dog was evaluated with abdominal ultrasound and aspirates of liver, spleen, lymph node and bone marrow. Since there was no evidence of spread, the tumor and the vulva was removed via a vulvovaginectomy. Since the margins were clean and the tumor was relatively low grade, no additional therapy was required.

Treatment

This section is divided into two options:
- Comfort for those who want to improve quality of life.
- Comfort and control for those who want to improve quality of life while trying to provide some control of the tumor.

Comfort

- Therapy to enhance comfort and freedom from nausea, vomiting, diarrhea and lack of appetite. Methimazole may help control clinical signs associated with thyrotoxicosis.

Comfort and control

Above mentioned therapy for comfort plus:
- Surgery that is usually curative.
- Metastatic lesions respond well to definitive or palliative radiation therapy with or without carboplatin, cisplatin or bleomycin chemotherapy.

CANINE TESTICULAR TUMORS

Clinical presentation

- Uncommon except where orchiectomy is uncommon.
- Generally not painful.
- Palpable mass in normal or atrophic testis.
- Tumors are seminomas, Sertoli cell tumors, and interstitial cell tumors.
- Many are not palpable.
- Feminization changes with some Sertoli cell tumors and seminomas.
- Seminomas and Sertoli cell tumors have a high incidence in retained testes.
- Older dogs; no breed predilection.

> **Key point**
> Dogs with one clinically evident testicular tumor often have a tumor on the contralateral side.

Staging and diagnosis

- Minimum data base (MDB): includes a CBC, biochemical profile, urinalysis, biopsy and three-view thoracic radiographs or computerized tomography of the chest and abdomen and/or ultrasonography.
- Metastasis rare, usually regional lymph nodes.

Prognostic factors

- Histologically diffuse seminomas may be more likely to metastasize.
- Seminomas with high AgNOR counts may be more likely to metastasize.

Treatment

This section is divided into two options:
- Comfort for those who want to improve quality of life.
- Comfort and control for those who want to improve quality of life while trying to provide some control of the tumor.

Comfort

- Therapy to enhance comfort and freedom from nausea, vomiting, diarrhea and lack of appetite.

Comfort and control

Above mentioned therapy for comfort plus:
- Surgical resection of the testicular tumor(s) with evaluation and biopsy of regional lymph nodes.
- Radiation therapy may achieve long-term

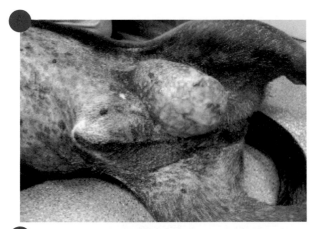

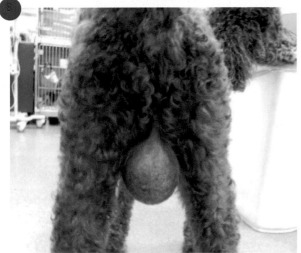

Figure 37-2: Testicular tumors (seminomas, Sertoli cell tumors, and interstitial cell tumors), especially those that produce sex hormones, may cause signs of feminization and, in some cases, serious changes in the hemogram. Seminomas and Sertoli cell tumors are more likely to occur in cryptorchid testicles (A), however they may also be seen in descended testes (B). Removal of these tumors is important. A significant percentage of dogs with a tumor in one testicle will have a tumor in the contralateral testicle.

control for metastatic seminoma to sublumbar nodes.
• Cisplatin, carboplatin and bleomycin chemotherapy may be effective for metastatic tumors.

CANINE PROSTATIC TUMORS

Clinical presentation

• Tenesmus, constipation, dyschezia, and (less commonly) dysuria and hematuria.
• Carcinoma arises from ducts; most prostatic tumors are transitional cell carcinoma and many of these cases concurrently involve the urethra and bladder.

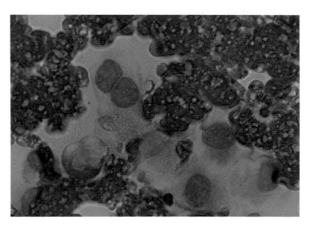

Figure 37-3: Most tumors of the prostate are actually transitional cell carcinomas that involve the prostate and as such, often involve the urethra or bladder. Performing a transcutaneous biopsy or aspirate is generally contraindicated as the tumor cells can be transplanted during either procedure throughout the tract formed by the needle or biopsy instrument. Plugs of tissue can be obtained by placing a red rubber catheter within the urethra to the level of the prostatic mass and applying negative pressure via a syringe while repeatedly moving the catheter 3-4 cm back and forth. Essentially, the negative pressure aspirates plugs of tissue into the side ports of the catheter that are then torn free from the tumor via the in and out movement. The tissue is submitted for histopathology and impression smears are submitted for cytopathology. Note the very large round cells forming clumps or small sheets. The nucleus of many cells have a nucleoli and there is a difference in nuclear:cytoplasmic ratio. Piroxicam can be used to enhance comfort, reduce inflammation and improve clinical signs if the patient has normal renal function. The addition of mitoxantrone, carboplatin and/or radiation therapy can provide greater comfort and control for most patients.

• Equal frequency in castrated and uncastrated dogs regardless of age at castration.
• Older dogs (median age, 10 years).

> **Key point**
>
> The most common tumor of the canine prostate is transitional cell carcinoma, which often concurrently involves the urethra and bladder. A rectal examination is important to help determine if the urethra is thickened, suggesting extension of the tumor into that structure.

Staging and diagnosis

• Minimum data base (MDB): includes a CBC, biochemical profile, urinalysis, biopsy and three-view thoracic radiographs or computerized tomography of the chest and abdomen and/or ultrasonography. Evaluate carefully for metastasis to regional lymph nodes and bone.

> **Key point**
>
> Prostatic carcinomas are often fixed or adherent to the pelvic tissues and may metastasize or invade the lumbar vertebrae, causing back pain, stranguria and hematuria. Radiographs of the abdomen may be helpful, however CT of the chest and abdomen is preferred to determine the extent of disease.

Prognostic factors

- May be more aggressive in castrated dogs (but highly malignant in both castrated and uncastrated).

Treatment

This section is divided into three options:
- Comfort for those who want to improve quality of life.
- Comfort and control for those who want to improve quality of life while trying to provide some control of the tumor.
- Comfort and longer-term control for those who want to improve quality of life while trying to maximize the chance of controlling the tumor.

> **Key point**
>
> Radiation, either palliative or definitive, is the treatment of choice. Stereotactic radiosurgery is ideal for those well-defined, localized, discrete tumors of the prostate. Adjuvant treatment with mitoxantrone chemotherapy and piroxicam is often recommended.

Comfort

- Therapy to enhance comfort and freedom from nausea, vomiting, diarrhea and lack of appetite. Piroxicam may be helpful at reducing discomfort and may provide anticancer effect.

Comfort and control

Above mentioned therapy for comfort plus:
- Cystoscopic laser therapy may improve clinical signs.
- Palliative radiation (e.g.: 2-5 dosages of radiation) to first enhance comfort, second, to reduce the rate of growth and third, occasionally to reduce the size of the tumor.

Comfort and longer-term control

Above mentioned therapy for comfort plus:
- Surgical resection of the tumor(s) and or sites of metastases with evaluation and biopsy of regional lymph nodes usually not helpful unless very localized.

- Stereotactic body radiation therapy (SBRT) or CyberKnife robotic radiosurgery (e.g.: 1-3 dosages) can be used for ultraprecise treatments to enhance tumor control while minimizing normal tissue injury in those tumors that have defined margins.
- Mitoxantrone, carboplatin or cisplatin chemotherapy may be helpful adjuvantly.

CANINE TRANSMISSIBLE VENEREAL TUMOR

Clinical presentation

- Bleeding mass on external genitalia.
- Spread by coitus and canine social behavior; females more susceptible than males.
- Spontaneous regression in most cases after months, but not in immunosuppressed animals.
- Metastasis rare.

Staging and diagnosis

- Minimum database and lymph node evaluation.
- Metastasis rare, usually in immunosuppressed animals.

Prognostic factors

- Increase in the ratio of AgNOR area to nuclear area may correlate with poor prognosis.
- Resistance to chemotherapy is heralds a poor prognosis.
- Presence of metastases suggests a poor prognosis.

Treatment

This section is divided into three options:
- Comfort for those who want to improve quality of life.
- Comfort and control for those who want to improve quality of life while trying to provide some control of the tumor.
- Comfort and longer-term control for those who want to improve quality of life while trying to maximize the chance of controlling the tumor.

Comfort

- Therapy to enhance comfort and freedom from nausea, vomiting, diarrhea and lack of appetite.

Comfort and control

Above mentioned therapy for comfort plus:
- Radiation (e.g.: 2-5 dosages of radiation) to first enhance comfort, second, to reduce the rate of growth and third, occasionally to reduce or eliminate the size of the tumor.

Comfort and longer-term control

Above mentioned therapy for comfort plus:
- Surgical resection of the tumor(s) with evaluation and biopsy of regional lymph nodes.

- Chemotherapy with vincristine (0.5 mg/m^2) is treatment of choice. Other drugs such as doxorubicin or cyclophosphamide may also be used.

References

1. Patnaik AK, Greenlee PG: Canine ovarian neoplasms: a clinicopathologic study of 71 cases, including histology of 12 granulosa cell tumors. *Vet Pathol* 24:509–514, 1987.
2. Patnaik AK, Saigo PE, Lieberman PH, Greenlee PG: Morphology of canine ovarian Sertoli–Leydig cell neoplasms. A report of 12 cases. *Cancer* 62:577–584, 1988.
3. Ervin E, Homans P: Giant ovarian cyst in a bitch. *Compend Contin Educ Pract Vet* 8:698–700, 1986.
4. Faulkner RT, Johnson SE: An ovarian cyst in a West Highland white terrier. *Vet Med* 75:1375–1377, 1980.
5. Diez-Bru N, Garcia-Real I, Martinez EM, et al: Ultrasonographic appearance of ovarian tumors in 10 dogs. *Vet Radiol Ultrasound* 39:226–233, 1998.
6. Pluhar GE, Memon MA, Wheaton LG: Granulosa cell tumor in an ovariohysterectomized dog. *JAVMA* 207:1063–1065, 1995.
7. Sivacolundhu RK, O'Hara AJ, Read RA: Granulosa cell tumour in two spayed bitches. *Aust Vet J* 79:173–176, 2001.
8. Seaman WJ: Canine ovarian fibroma associated with prolonged exposure to mibolerone. *Toxicol Pathol* 13:177–180, 1985.
9. Jergens AE, Knapp DW, Shaw DP: Ovarian teratoma in a bitch. *JAVMA* 191:81–83,1987.
10. Cheng N: Aberrant behavior in a bitch with a granulosatheca cell tumor. *Aust Vet J* 70:71–72, 1992.
11. Greenlee PG, Patnaik AK: Canine ovarian tumors of germ cell origin. *Vet Pathol* 22:117–122, 1985.
12. Fernández T, Díez-Bru N, Ríos A, et al: Intracranial metastases from an ovarian dysgerminoma in a 2-year-old dog. *JAAHA* 37:553–556, 2001.
13. Yamini B, VanDenBrink PL, Refsal KR: Ovarian steroid cell tumor resembling luteoma associated with hyperadrenocorticism (Cushing's disease) in a dog. *Vet Pathol* 34:57–60, 1997.
14. Jackson ML, Mills JHL, Fowler JD: Ovarian dysgerminoma in a bitch. *Can Vet J* 26:285–287, 1985.
15. Wilson RB, Cave JS, Copeland JS, Onks J: Ovarian teratoma in two dogs. *JAAHA* 21:249–253, 1985.
16. Nagashima Y, Hoshi K, Tanaka R, et al: Ovarian and retroperitoneal teratomas in a dog. *J Vet Med Sci* 62:793–795, 2000.
17. McCormick AE, McEntee M: Analyzing and unusual canine ovarian mass. *Vet Med* 83:368–373, 1988.
18. Moore AS, Kirk C, Cardona A: Intracavitary cisplatin chemotherapy experience with six dogs. *J Vet Intern Med* 5:227–231, 1991.
19. Olsen J, Komtebedde J, Lackner A, Madewell BR: Cytoreductive treatment of ovarian carcinoma. *J Vet Intern Med* 8:133–135, 1994.
20. McKee WM: Granulosa cell tumor and attempted chemotherapy in a 17 month old bitch. *Vet Rec* 117:501–502, 1985.
21. Greene JA, Richardson RC, Thornhill JA, Boon GD: Ovarian papillary cystadenocarcinoma in a bitch: Case report and literature review. *JAAHA* 15:351–356, 1979.
22. Brodey RS, Roszel JF: Neoplasms of the canine uterus, vagina and vulva: a clinicopathologic survey of 90 cases. *JAVMA* 151:1294–1307, 1967.
23. Münnic A, Grüssel T, Celzner J, Walter J: Untersuchungen zum auftreten von scheidenerkrankungen bei der hündin. *Kleintierpraxis* 44:831–842, 1999.
24. Kydd DM, Burnie AG: Vaginal neoplasia in the bitch: a review of forty clinical cases. *J Small Anim Pract* 17:255–263, 2004.
25. Thacher C, Bradley RL: Vulva and vaginal tumors in the dog: a retrospective. *JAVMA* 183:690–692, 1983.
26. Salomon JF, Deneuche A, Viguier E: Vaginectomy and urethroplasty as a treatment for non-pedunculated vaginal tumours in four bitches. *J Small Anim Pract* 45:157–161, 2004.
27. Bilbrey SA, Withrow SJ, Klein MK, et al: Vulvovaginectomy and perineal urethrostomy for neoplasms of the vulva and vagina. *Vet Surg* 18:450–453, 1989.
28. Hill TP, Lobetti RG, Schulman ML: Vulvovaginectomy and neo-urethrostomy for treatment of haemangiosarcoma of the vulva and vagina. *J S Afr Vet Assoc* 71:256–259, 2000.
29. Peavy GM, Rettenmaier MA, Berns MW: Carbon dioxide laser ablation combined with doxorubicin hydrochloride treatment for vaginal fibrosarcoma in a dog. *JAVMA* 201:109–110, 1992.
30. Murakami Y, Uchida K, Yamaguchi R, Tateyama S: Diffuse bilateral hemangiosarcoma of the uterus in a dog. *J Vet Med Sci* 63:191–193, 2001.
31. Sailasuta A, Tateyama S, Yamaguchi R, et al: Adenomatous papilloma of the uterine tube (oviduct) fimbriae in a dog. *Jpn J Vet Sci* 51:632–633, 1989.
32. Minoccheri F, Meluzzi A: Su di un tumore adenomatoide primitivo della salpinge. *Arch Vet Ital* 30:90–95, 1979.
33. Payne-Johnson CE, Kelly DF, Davies PT: Endometrial carcinoma in a young dog. *J Comp Pathol* 96:463–467, 1986.
34. Cave TA, Hine R, Howie F, et al: Uterine carcinoma in a 10-month-old golden retriever. *J Small Anim Pract* 43:133–135, 2002.
35. Vos JH: Uterine and cervical carcinomas in five dogs. J Vet Med 35:385–390, 1988.
36. Boisclair J, Dore M: Uterine angiolipoleiomyoma in a dog. *Vet Pathol* 38:726–728, 2001.
37. Patnaik AK: A clinicopathologic, histologic and immunohistochemical study of mixed germ cell-stromal tumors of the testis in 16 dogs. *Vet Pathol* 30:287–295, 1993.
38. Nielson SW, Lein DH: Tumours of the testis. *Bull World Health Organ* 50:71–78, 1992.
39. Hayes HM, Pendergrass TW: Canine testicular tumors. Epidemiologic features of 410 dogs. *Int J Cancer* 18:482–487, 1976.
40. Nieto JM, Pizarro M, Balaguer LM, Romano J: Canine testicular tumors in descended and cryptorchid testes. *Dtsch Tierarztl Wochenschr* 96:186–189, 1989.
41. Reif JS, Brodey RS: The relationship between cryptorchidism and canine testicular neoplasia. *JAVMA* 155:2005–2010, 1969.
42. Yates D, Hayes G, Heffernan M, Beynon R: Incidence of cryptorchidism in dogs and cats. *Vet Rec* 152:502–504, 2003.
43. Hayes HM Jr, Wilson GP, Pendergrass TW, Cox VS: Canine cryptorchism and subsequent testicular neoplasia: case-control study with epidemiologic update. *Teratology* 32:51–56, 1985.
44. Hayes HM, Tarone RE, Casey HW, Huxsoll DL: Excess of seminomas observed in Vietnam service U.S. military working dogs. *J Natl Cancer Inst* 82:1042–1046, 1990.
45. Suess RP Jr, Barr SC, Sacre BJ, French TW: Bone marrow hypoplasia in a feminized dog with an interstitial cell tumor. *JAVMA* 200:1346–1348, 1992.
46. Sanpera N, Masot N, Janer M, et al: Oestrogen-induced bone marrow aplasia in a dog with a Sertoli cell tumour. *J Small Anim Pract* 43:365–369, 2002.
47. HogenEsch H, Whiteley HE, Vicini DS, Helper LC: Seminoma with metastases in the eyes and the brain in a dog. *Vet Pathol* 24:278–280, 1987.
48. Takiguchi M, Iida T, Kudo T, Hashimoto A: Malignant seminoma with systemic metastases in a dog. *J Small Anim Pract* 42:360–362, 2001.
49. Spugnini EP, Bartolazzi A, Ruslander D: Seminoma with cutaneous metastases in a dog. *JAAHA* 36:253–256, 2000.
50. Barrand KR, Scudamore CL: Canine hypertrophic osteoarthropathy associated with a malignant Sertoli cell tumour. *J Small Anim Pract* 42:143–145, 2001.
51. Inoue M, Wada N: Immunohistochemical detection of p53 and p21 proteins in canine testicular tumours. *Vet Rec* 146: 370–372, 2000.
52. Golubeva VA, Kuz'mina ZV, Gershtein ES, et al: [Steroid hormone receptors in spontaneous testicular tumors in dogs]. *Vopr Onkol* 38:464–469, 1986.
53. De Vico G, Papparella S, Di Guardo G: Number and size of silver-stained nucleoli (Ag-NOR clusters) in canine seminomas: correlation with histological features and tumour behaviour. *J Comp Pathol* 110:267–273, 1994.
54. Sarli G, Benazzi C, Preziosi R, Marcato PS: Proliferative activity assessed by anti-PCNA and Ki67 monoclonal antibodies in canine testicular tumours. *J Comp Pathol* 110:357–368, 1994.
55. Restucci B, Maiolino P, Paciello O, et al: Evaluation of angiogenesis in canine seminomas by quantitative immunohistochemistry. *J Comp Pathol* 128:252–259, 2003.
56. Johnston GR, Feeney DA, Johnston SD, O'Brien TD: Ultrasonographic features of testicular neoplasia in dogs: 16 cases (1980-1988). *JAVMA* 198:1779–1784, 1991.
57. England GC: Ultrasonographic diagnosis of non-palpable Sertoli cell tumor in infertile dogs. *J Small Anim Pract* 36: 476–480, 1995.
58. McDonald RK, Walker M, Legendre AM, et al: Radiotherapy of metastatic seminoma in the dog: case reports. *J Vet Intern Med* 2:103–107, 1988.
59. Dhaliwal RS, Kitchell BE, Knight BL, Schmidt BR: treatment of aggressive testicular tumors in four dogs. *JAAHA* 35: 311–318, 1999.
60. Kast VA: Probleme der präputial- und Zervixkarzinome bei tieren. *Geburtshilfe Frauenheilkd* 19:1080–1086, 1959.
61. Patnaik AK, Matthiesen DT, Zawie DA: Two cases of canine penile neoplasm: Squamous cell carcinoma and mesenchymal chondrosarcoma. *JAAHA* 24:403–406, 1988.
62. Wakui S, Furusato M, Nomura Y, et al: Testicular epidermoid cyst and penile squamous cell carcinoma in a dog. *Vet Pathol* 29:543–545, 1992.
63. Leav I, Schelling KH, Adams JY, et al: Role of canine basal cells in postnatal prostatic development, induction of hyperplasia, and sex hormone-stimulated growth; and the ductal origin of carcinoma. *Prostate* 48:210–224, 2001.
64. Cornell KK, Bostwick DG, Cooley DM, et al: Clinical and pathologic aspects of spontaneous canine prostate carcinoma: A retrospective analysis of 76 cases. *Prostate* 45:173–183, 2000.

65. Sorenmo KU, Goldschmidt M, Shofer F, et al: Immunohistochemical characterization of canine prostatic carcinoma and correlation with castration status and castration time. *Vet Comp Oncol* 1:48–56, 2003.
66. LeRoy BE, Nadella MV, Toribio RE, et al: Canine prostate carcinomas express markers of urothelial and prostatic differentiation. *Vet Pathol* 41:131–140, 2004.
67. Leav I, Ling GV: Adenocarcinoma of the canine prostate. *Cancer* 22:1329–1345, 1968.
68. Hargis AM, Miller LM: Prostatic carcinoma in dogs. *Compend Contin Educ Pract Vet* 5:647–653, 1983.
69. O'Shea JD: Studies on the canine prostate gland II. Prostatic neoplasms. *J Comp Pathol* 73:244–252, 1963.
70. Weaver AD: Fifteen cases of prostatic carcinoma in the dog. *Vet Rec* 109:71–75, 1981.
71. Bell FW, Klausner JS, Hayden DW, et al: Clinical and pathological features of prostatic adenocarcinoma in sexually intact and castrated dogs: 31 cases (1970–1987). *JAVMA* 199:1623–1630, 1991.
72. Teske E, Naan EC, van Dijk EM, et al: Canine prostate carcinoma: epidemiological evidence of an increased risk in castrated dogs. *Mol Cell Endocrinol* 197:251–255, 2002.
73. Waters DJ, Bostwick DG: Prostatic intraepithelial neoplasia occurs spontaneously in the canine prostate. *J Urol* 157:713–716, 1997.
74. Madewell BR, Gandour-Edwards R, deVere White RW: Canine prostatic intraepithelial neoplasia: is the comparative model relevant? *Prostate* 58:314–317, 2004.
75. Aquilina JW, McKinney L, Pacelli A, et al: High-grade prostatic intraepithelial neoplasia in military working dogs with and without prostate cancer. *Prostate* 36:189–193, 1998.
76. Obradovich JE, Walshaw R, Goulland E: The influence of castration of the development of prostatic carcinoma in the dog: 43 cases (1978–1985). *J Vet Intern Med* 1:183–187, 1987.
77. Teske E, Nickel RF: Zur aussagekraft der zytologie bei der diagnostik des prostatakarzinoms beim hund. *Kleintierpraxis* 41:239–247, 1996.
78. Durham SK, Deitze AE: Prostatic adenocarcinoma with and without metastasis to bone in dogs. *JAVMA* 188:1432–1436, 1986.
79. Swinney GR: Prostatic neoplasia in five dogs. *Aust Vet J* 76:669–674, 1998.
80. Rohleder JJ, Jones JC: Emphysematous prostatitis and carcinoma in a dog. *JAAHA* 38:478–481, 2002.
81. Nickel RF, Teske E: Diagnosis of canine prostatic carcinoma. *Tijdschr Diergeneeskd* 117 Suppl 1:32S, 1992.
82. Barsanti JA, Finco DR: Evaluation of techniques for diagnosis of canine prostatic diseases. *JAVMA* 190:48–52, 1987.
83. Bell FW, Klausner JS, Hayden DW, et al: Evaluation of serum and seminal plasma markers in the diagnosis of canine prostatic disorders. *J Vet Intern Med* 9:149–153, 1995.
84. Rogers L, Lopez A, Gillis A: Priapism secondary to penile metastasis in a dog. *Can Vet J* 43:547–549, 2002.
85. Feeney DA, Johnston GR, Klausner J, et al: Canine prostatic disease—comparison of radiographic appearance with morphologic and microbiology findings in 30 cases (1981–1985). *JAVMA* 190:1018–1026, 1987.
86. Feeney DA, Johnston GR, Klausner JS, et al: Canine prostatic disease—comparison of ultrasonographic appearance with morphologic and microbiologic findings: 30 cases (1981–1985). *JAVMA* 190:1027–1034, 1987.
87. Hayden DW, Klausner JS, Waters DJ: Prostatic leiomyosarcoma in a dog. *J Vet Diagn Invest* 11:283–286, 1999.
88. Cromeens DM, Johnson DE, Price RE: Transurethral canine prostatectomy with the Nd:YAG laser. *J Invest Surg* 6:97–103, 1993.
89. Liptak JM, Brutscher SP, Monnet E, et al: Transurethral resection in the management of urethral and prostatic neoplasia in 6 dogs. *Vet Surg* 33:1–12, 2004.
90. Turrel JM: Intraoperative radiotherapy of carcinoma of the prostate gland in ten dogs. *JAVMA* 190:48–52, 1987.
91. Mann FA, Barrett RJ, Henderson RA: Use of a retained urethral catheter in three dogs with prostatic neoplasia. *Vet Surg* 21:342–347, 1992.
92. Proulx DR, Ruslander DM, Hauck ML, et al: Canine prostatic neoplasia: a retrospective analysis of 10 dogs treated with external beam radiation (1989–2001). *Proc 22nd Ann Conf Vet Cancer Soc*:40, 2002.
93. Anderson CR, McNiel EA, Gillette EL, et al: Late complications of pelvic irradiation in 16 dogs. *Vet Radiol Ultrasound* 43:187–192, 2002.
94. Lucroy MD, Bowles MH, Higbee RG, et al: Photodynamic therapy for prostatic carcinoma in a dog. *J Vet Intern Med* 17:235–237, 2003.
95. Sorenmo KU, Goldschmidt MH, Shofer FS, et al: Evaluation of cyclooxygenase-1 and cyclooxygenase-2 expression and the effect of cyclooxygenase inhibitors in canine prostatic carcinoma. *Vet Comp Oncol* 2:13–23, 2004.
96. Karlson AG, Mann FC: The transmissible venereal tumor of dogs: observations on forty generations of experimental transfers. *Ann N Y Acad Sci* 54:1197–1213, 1952.
97. Boscos C: Canine transmissible venereal tumor: clinical observations and treatment. *Anim Fam* 3:10–15, 1988.
98. Rogers KS, Walker MA, Dillon HB: Transmissible venereal tumor: A retrospective study of 29 cases. *JAAHA* 34:463–470, 1998.
99. Yang TJ: Immunolobiology of a spontaneously regressive tumor, the canine transmissible venereal sarcoma (review). *Anticancer Res* 8:93–96, 1988.
100. Yang TJ, Palker TJ, Harding MW: Tumor size, leukocyte adherence inhibition and serum levels of tumor antigen in dogs with the canine transmissible venereal sarcoma. *Cancer Immunol Immunother* 33:255–262, 1991.
101. Batamuzi EK, Kristensen F: Urinary tract infection: the role of canine transmissible venereal tumour. *J Small Anim Pract* 37:276–279, 1996.
102. Harmelin A, Zuckerman A, Nyska A: Correlation of Ag-NOR protein measurements with prognosis in canine transmissible venereal tumour. *J Comp Pathol* 112:429–433, 1995.
103. Amber EI, Henderson RA: Canine transmissible venereal tumor: evaluation of surgical excision of primary and metastatic lesions in Zaria-Nigeria. *JAAHA* 1882:350–352, 1982.
104. Thrall DE: Orthovoltage radiotherapy of canine transmissible venereal tumors. *Vet Radiol* 23:217–219, 1998.
105. Calvert CA, Leifer CE, MacEwen EG: Vincristine for treatment of transmissible venereal tumor in the dog. *JAVMA* 181:163–164, 1982.
106. Ferreira AJ, Jaggy A, Varejao AP, et al: Brain and ocular metastases from a transmissible venereal tumour in a dog. *J Small Anim Pract* 41:165–168, 2000.
107. Pereira JS, Silva AB, Martins AL, et al: Immunohistochemical characterization of intraocular metastasis of a canine transmissible venereal tumor. *Vet Ophthalmol* 3:43–47, 2000.
108. Amber EI, Henderson RA, Adeyanju JB, Gyang EO: Single-drug chemotherapy of canine transmissible venereal tumor with cyclophosphamide, methotrexate or vincristine. *J Vet Intern Med* 4:144–147, 1990.
109. Wasecki A, Mazur O: Zastosowanie preparatu vinblastin w leczeniu gozow Stickera. *Med Weter* 33:142–143, 1977.
110. Singh J, Rana JS, Sood N, et al: Clinico-pathological studies on the effect of different anti-neoplastic chemotherapy regimens on transmissible venereal tumours in dogs. *Vet Res Commun* 20:71–81, 1996.
111. Gobello C, Corrada Y: Effects of vincristine treatment on semen quality in a dog with a transmissible venereal tumour. *J Small Anim Pract* 43:416–417, 2002.

Chapter 38

Canine mammary neoplasias

Clinical presentation

- Presence of a mass in the mammary chain, especially in an intact female dog or one spayed later in life.
- 50% of tumors are multiple.
- Approximately 50% are benign (e.g., fibroadenomas, simple adenomas, benign mixed mammary tumors).
- Approximately 50% are malignant (e.g., solid carcinomas, tubular or papillary adenocarcinomas, rarely inflammatory carcinomas).
- Most common neoplasm in females. Usually not painful.
- Average age, 10 to 11 years.
- Poodles, terriers, Cocker spaniels, and German shepherd dogs are overrepresented.
- Early ovariohysterectomy protective for mammary tumors, however there is evidence the surgery may increase the risk of other diseases, tumors or disorders.

> **Key point**
> Many dogs with mammary tumors do not have clinical signs and are either intact or spayed later in life.

Staging and diagnosis

- Minimum data base (MDB): includes a CBC, biochemical profile, urinalysis, and thoracic radiographs (three views) or helical CT of the chest. Fine needle aspiration cytology or preoperative biopsy may be performed.
- Lungs and lymph nodes are most common sites of metastasis.

> **Key point**
> Metastases to regional lymph nodes (axillary or inguinal) or the lung are important to evaluate in patients with mammary tumors.

Prognostic factors

- Poor prognosis:
  - Stage (increasing tumor size).
  - Metastasis.
  - Ulceration.
  - Degree of invasion.
  - Increasing degree of malignancy, proliferative indices, solid or ductular tumors.
  - Histologic margins.
  - Inflammatory carcinomas.
  - Lack of hormone receptors.
- No effect on prognosis:
  - Diet (fat and protein).
  - Ovariectomy status.
  - Type of surgery.
  - Number of tumors.
  - Tumor location.
  - History of parity, estrus cycles.

Treatment

This section is divided into three options:
- Comfort for those who want to improve quality of life.
- Comfort and control for those who want to improve quality of life while trying to provide some control of the tumor.
- Comfort and longer-term control for those who want to improve quality of life while trying to maximize the chance of controlling the tumor.

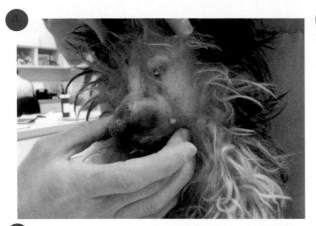

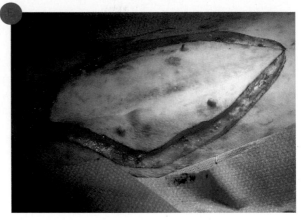

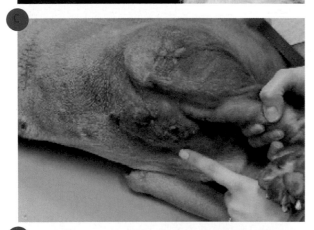

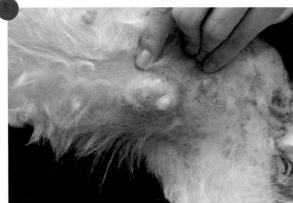

Figure 38-1: The three patients presented here (A-C) show the diversity of types of mammary tumors. While mammary tumors can and do occur in male dogs, this tumor is the most common tumor of the intact female dog. They can be multifocal with in the mammary tissue. The malignant forms of the disease occur in approximately 50% of all dogs with mammary tumors with approximately half of the more aggressive tumors metastasizing. The most common site of metastases include regional lymph nodes and lung. Therefore, staging should include at least blood work, chest radiographs and assessment of the regional lymph nodes. Cytology can be performed (D) and may confirm the presence of a carcinoma as depicted here. Note the large cells forming sheets and the presence of malignant characteristics such as varying nuclear to cytoplasmic ratios and the lack of uniformity between cells. Regardless of the cell type, wide and deep removal (2-3 cm and 1 facial layer deep) of the tumor and the surrounding tissue is mandatory (E). If the tumor has recurred, then the mass and the entire previous surgical site must be removed with 2-3 cm margins laterally and one facial layer deep. Note the misplaced incision in figure C. It would be very difficult to remove that previous surgical scar with wide and deep margins due to its placement against the long axis of the patient.

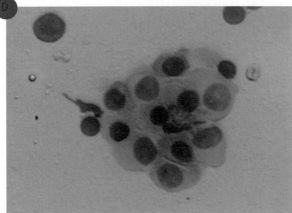

Key point

A complete, wide removal of the mammary tumor and a "cuff" of normal tissue around the mass with or without the regional lymph node is important. Performing an ovariohysterectomy at the time of tumor removal may help reduce the risk of recurrence in a subset of these patients.

Comfort

- Therapy to enhance comfort and freedom from nausea, vomiting, diarrhea and lack of appetite.
- Docosahexaenoic acid has been shown to delay or prevent recurrence in a number of species.
- Piroxicam has been shown to be helpful for at least dogs with highly malignant inflammatory mammary carcinoma.

- Dogs with inflammatory mammary carcinoma treated with piroxicam had with mean and median progression-free survival of 171 and 183 days, respectively.[83]

Comfort and control

Above mentioned therapy for comfort plus:
- Regional surgical resection of tumor is as effective as mastectomy of the entire chain for localized tumor(s); removal of lymph node may be of prognostic value; ovariohysterectomy may be of value for preventing recurrence.
  - Ovariohysterectomy performed at the time of benign mammary tumor excision reduced the risk of new tumors by about 50%.[80]
  - In one study[81], surgery was performed to remove mammary tumors in 134 dogs, resulting in an overall survival time of 1113 days. Median survival in benign, grade 1 and grade 2 malignant tumors was 1319, 670, and 406 days, respectively.
  - A study done[82] in dogs that had a regional mastectomy of a single mammary tumor revealed that 58% of dogs developed a new tumor in the remaining mammary glands of the ipsilateral chain. This should be taken into account when deciding on the surgical management (radical or regional mastectomy) in dogs with single mammary tumors.

Comfort and longer-term control

Above mentioned therapy for comfort plus:
- Doxorubicin- or mitoxantrone-based chemotherapy protocols post-surgery +/- ovariectomy may be effective in some cases. Taxanes emerging as effective agents. Randomized studies are needed to affirm efficacy.
- Dogs with inflammatory mammary carcinoma treated with piroxicam had with mean and median progression-free survival of 171 and 183 days, respectively.[83]

References

1. Dorn CR, Taylor DO, Schneider R, et al: Survey of animal neoplasms in Alameda and Contra Costa Counties, California. II Cancer morbidity in dogs and cats from Alameda county. *J Natl Cancer Inst* 40:307–318, 1968.
2. Priester WA, Mantel N: Occurrence of *tumors in domestic animals*. Data from 12 United States and Canadian colleges of veterinary medicine. *J Natl Cancer Inst* 47:1333–1344, 1971.
3. Kurzman ID, Gilbertson SR: Prognostic factors in canine mammary tumors. *Semin Vet Med Surg (Small Anim)* 1:25–32, 1986.
4. Misdorp W: Canine mammary tumours: Protective effect of late ovariectomy and stimulating effect of progestins. *Vet Quarterly* 10:26–33, 1988.
5. Bender AP, Dorn RC, Schneider R: An epidemiological study of canine multiple primary neoplasia involving the female and male reproductive systems. *Preventive Vet Med* 2: 715–731, 1984.
6. Morris JS, Dobson JM, Bostock DE, O'Farrell E: Effect of ovariohysterectomy in bitches with mammary neoplasms. *Vet Rec* 142:656–658, 1998.
7. Wey N, Kohn B, Gutberlet K, et al: Mammatumore bei der hündin: klinische verlaufsstudie (1995–1997). *Kleintierpraxis* 44:565–578, 1999.
8. Alenza DP, Rutteman GR, Peña L, et al: Relationship between habitual diet and canine mammary tumors in a case-control study. *J Vet Intern Med* 12:132–139, 1998.
9. Brodey RS, Fidler IJ, Howson AE: The relationship of estrous irregularity, pseudopregnancy, and pregnancy to the development of canine mammary neoplasms. *JAVMA* 149: 1049, 1966.
10. Allen SW, Mahaffey EA: Canine mammary neoplasia: Prognostic indications and response to surgical therapy. *JAAHA* 25:540–546, 1989.
11. Schneider R, Dorn CR, Taylor DO: Factors influencing canine mammary cancer development and postsurgical survival. *J Natl Cancer Inst* 43:1249–1261, 1969.
12. Frank DW, Kirton KT, Murchison TE, et al: Mammary tumors and serum hormones in the bitch treated with medroxyprogesterone acetate or progesterone for four years. *Fertil Steril* 31:340–346, 1979.
13. Stovring M, Moe L, Glattre E: A population-based case-control study of canine mammary tumours and clinical use of medroxyprogesterone acetate. *APMIS* 105:590–596, 1997.
14. Sonnenschein EG, Glickman LT, Goldschmidt MH, McKee LJ: Body conformation, diet, and risk of breast cancer in pet dogs: A case-control study. *Am J Epidemiol* 133:694–703, 1991.
15. Philibert JC, Snyder PW, Glickman LT, et al: Influence of host factors on survival in dogs with malignant mammary gland tumors. *J Vet Intern Med* 17:102–106, 2003.
16. Schafer KA, Kelly G, Schrader R, et al: A canine model of familial mammary gland neoplasia. *Vet Pathol* 35:168–177, 1998.
17. Muto T, Wakui S, Takahashi H, et al: p53 Gene mutations occurring in spontaneous benign and malignant mammary tumors of the dog. *Vet Pathol* 37:248–253, 2000.
18. Mayr B, Dressler A, Reifinger M, Feil C: Cytogenetic alterations in eight mammary tumors and tumor-suppressor gene p53 mutation in one mammary tumor from dogs. *Am J Vet Res* 59:69–78, 1998.
19. Tiemessen I: Thoracic metastases of canine mammary gland tumors. A radiographic study. *Vet Radiol* 30:249–252, 1989.
20. Yamagami T, Kobayashi T, Takahashi K, Sugiyama M: Prognosis for canine malignant mammary tumors based on TNM and histologic classification. *J Vet Med Sci* 58:1079–1083, 1996.
21. Gonzalez de Bulnes A, Garcia Fernandez P, Mayenco Aguirre AM, Sanchez dela Muela M: Ultrasonographic imaging of canine mammary tumours. *Vet Rec* 143:687–689, 1998.
22. Allen SW, Prasse KW, Mahaffey EA: Cytologic differentiation of benign from malignant canine mammary tumors. *Vet Pathol* 23:649–655, 1986.
23. Stockhaus C, Kohn B, Rudolph R, et al: Correlation of haemostatic abnormalities with tumour stage and characteristics in dogs with mammary carcinoma. *J Small Anim Pract* 40:326–331, 1999.
24. Sartin EA, Barnes S, Kwapien RP, Wolfe LG: Estrogen and progesterone receptor status of mammary carcinomas and correlation with clinical outcome in dogs. *Am J Vet Res* 53: 2196–2200, 1992.
25. MacEwen EG, Patnaik AK, Harvey HJ, Panko WB: Estrogen receptors in canine mammary tumors. *Cancer Res* 42: 2255–2259, 1982.
26. Rutteman GR, Misdorp W, Blankenstein MA, Van den Brom WE: Oestrogen (ER) and progestin receptors (PR) in mammary tissue of the female dog: Different receptor profile in non-malignant and malignant states. *Br J Cancer* 58:594–599, 1988.
27. Wey N, Gutberlet K, Kohn B, et al: Mammatumore bei der hündin: hormonelle abhängigkeit unter besonderer berücksichtigung von 17ß-östradiol und progesteron. *Kleintierpraxis* 45:19–31, 2000.
28. Donnay I, Rauis J, Devleeschouwer N, et al: Comparison of estrogen and progesterone receptor expression in normal and tumor mammary tissues from dogs. *Am J Vet Res* 56:1188–1194, 1995.
29. Nieto A, Peña L, Pérez-Alenza MD, et al: Immunohistologic detection of estrogen receptor alpha in canine mammary tumors: Clinical and pathologic associations and prognostic significance. *Vet Pathol* 37:239–247, 2000.
30. Geraldes M, Gartner F, Schmitt F: Immunohistochemical study of hormonal receptors and cell proliferation in normal canine mammary glands and spontaneous mammary tumours. *Vet Rec* 146:403–406, 2000.
31. Ogilvie GK, Allhands RV, Reynolds HA: Use of radionuclide imaging to identify malignant mammary tumor bone metastases in dogs. *JAVMA* 195:220–222, 1989.
32. Pumarola M, Balasch M: Meningeal carcinomatosis in a dog. *Veterinary Record* 138:523–524, 1996.
33. Sorenmo KU, Shofer FS, Goldschmidt MH: Effect of spaying and timing of spaying on survival of dogs with mammary carcinoma. *J Vet Intern Med* 14:266–270, 2000.

34. Pérez-Alenza MD, Peña L, del Castillo N, Nieto AI: Factors influencing the incidence and prognosis of canine mammary tumours. *J Small Anim Pract* 41:287–291, 2000.

35. Peña L, Nieto AI, Pérez-Alenza MD, et al: Immunohistochemical detection of Ki-67 and PCNA in canine mammary tumors: relationship to clinical and pathologic variables. *J Vet Diagn Invest* 10:237–246, 1998.

36. Mellin A, Simon D, Wasielewski RV, et al: Different criteria and their prognostic relevance for malignant canine mammary tumors. *Proc 21st Ann Conf Vet Cancer Soc.*2, 2001.

37. Fidler IJ, Brodey RS: A necropsy study of canine malignant mammary neoplasms. *JAVMA* 151:710–715, 1967.

38. MacEwen EG, Harvey HJ, Patnaik AK, et al: Evaluation of effects of levamisole and surgery on canine mammary cancer. *J Biol Response Mod* 4:418–426, 1985.

39. Löhr CV, Teifke JP, Failing K, Weiss E: Characterization of the proliferation state in canine mammary tumors by the standardized AgNOR method with postfixation and immunohistologic detection of Ki-67 and PCNA. *Vet Pathol* 34:212–221, 1997.

40. Hellmen E, Bergstrom R, Holmberg L, et al: Prognostic factors in canine mammary tumors: A multivariate study of 202 consecutive cases. *Vet Pathol* 30:20–27, 1993.

41. Shofer FS, Sonnenschein EG, Goldschmidt MH, et al: Histopathologic and dietary prognostic factors for canine mammary carcinoma. *Breast Cancer Res Treat* 13:49–60, 1989.

42. Misdorp W, Hart AA: Canine mammary cancer. I. Prognosis. *J Small Anim Pract* 20:385–394, 1979.

43. Fowler EH, Wilson GP, Koestner A: Biologic behavior of canine mammary neoplasms based on a histogenetic classification. *Vet Pathol* 11:212–229, 1974.

44. Gilbertson SR, Kurzman ID, Zachrau RE, et al: Canine mammary epithelial neoplasms: Biologic implications of morphologic characteristics assessed in 232 dogs. *Vet Pathol* 20:127–142, 1983.

45. Bostock DE: The prognosis following the surgical excision of canine mammary neoplasms. *Eur J Cancer* 11:389–396, 1975.

46. Benjamin SA, Lee AC, Saunders WJ: Classification and behavior of canine mammary epithelial neoplasms based on lifespan observations in beagles. *Vet Pathol* 36:423–436, 1999.

47. Gama A, Alves A, Gartner F, Schmitt F: p63: A novel myoepithelial cell marker in canine mammary tissues. *Vet Pathol* 40: 412–420, 2003.

48. Griffey SM, Verstraete FJM, Kraegel SA, et al: Computerassisted image analysis of intratumoral vessel density in mammary tumors from dogs. *Am J Vet Res* 59:1238–1242, 1998.

49. Zuccari DA, Santana AE, Cury PM, Cordeiro JA: Immunocytochemical study of Ki-67 as a prognostic marker in canine mammary neoplasia. *Vet Clin Pathol* 33:23–28, 2004.

50. Funakoshi Y, Nakayama H, Uetsuka K, et al: Cellular proliferative and telomerase activity in canine mammary gland tumors. *Vet Pathol* 37:177–183, 2000.

51. Bratulic M, Grabarevic Z, Artukovic B, Capak D: Number of nucleoli and nucleolar organizer regions per nucleus and nucleolus—prognostic value in canine mammary tumors. *Vet Pathol* 33:527–532, 1996.

52. Saba CF, Rogers KS, Mauldin GE, Vail DM: Mammary tumors in male dogs: A retrospective study. *Proc 23rd Ann Conf Vet Cancer Soc.*27, 2003.

53. Withrow SJ: Symposium on surgical techniques in small animal practice. Surgical management of canine mammary tumors. *Vet Clin North Am* 5:495–506, 1975.

54. Yamagami T, Kobayashi T, Takahashi K, Sugiyama M: Influence of ovariectomy at the time of mastectomy on the prognosis for canine malignant mammary tumours. *J Small Anim Pract* 37:462–464, 1996.

55. Misdorp W, Hart AA: Canine mammary cancer. II. Therapy and causes of death. *J Small Anim Pract* 20:395–404, 1979.

56. Johnston SD: Reproductive systems. In Slatter D (ed): *Textbook of Small Animal Surgery*, ed 2. Philadelphia, WB Saunders, 1993, pp 2177–2200.

57. Simon D, Knebel JW, Baumgärtner W, et al: In vitro efficacy of chemotherapeutics as determined by 50% inhibitory concentrations in cell cultures of mammary gland tumors obtained from dogs. *Am J Vet Res* 62:1825–1830, 2001.

58. Yamashita A, Maruo K, Suzuki K, et al: Experimental chemotherapy against canine mammary cancer xenograft in SCID mice and its prediction of clinical effect. *J Vet Med Sci* 63:831–836, 2001.

59. Karayannopoulou M, Kaldrymidou E, Constantinidis TC, Dessiris A: Adjuvant post-operative chemotherapy in bitches with mammary cancer. *J Vet Med A Physiol Pathol Clin Med* 48:85–96, 2001.

60. Ogilvie GK, Reynolds HA, Richardson RC, et al: Phase II evaluation of doxorubicin for treatment of various canine neoplasms. *JAVMA* 195:1580–1583, 1989.

61. Hahn KA, Richardson RC, Knapp DW: Canine malignant mammary neoplasia: Biological behavior, diagnosis, and treatment alternatives. *JAAHA* 28:251–256, 1992.

62. Simon D, Schoenrock D, Nolte I, Baumgartner W: Adjuvant treatment of canine malignant invasive mammary gland tumors with doxorubicin and docetaxel. *J Vet Intern Med* 18:790–791, 2004.

63. Ogilvie GK, Obradovich JE, Elmslie RE, et al: Efficacy of mitoxantrone against various neoplasms in dogs. *JAVMA* 198:1618–1621, 1991.

64. Poirier VJ, Hershey AE, Burgess KE, et al: Efficacy and toxicity of paclitaxel (Taxol) for the treatment of canine malignant tumors. *J Vet Intern Med* 18:219–222, 2004.

65. Dore M, Lanthier I, Sirois J: Cyclooxygenase-2 expression in canine mammary tumors. *Vet Pathol* 40:207–212, 2003.

66. Heller DA, Clifford CA, Goldschmidt MH, et al: COX-2 expression in canine hemangiosarcoma, histiocytic sarcoma, mast cell tumor and mammary carcinoma. *Proc 23rd Ann Conf Vet Cancer Soc.*10, 2003.

67. Knapp DW, Richardson RC, Bottoms GD, et al: Phase I trial of piroxicam in 62 dogs bearing naturally occurring tumors. *Cancer Chemother Pharmacol* 29:214–218, 1992.

68. Morris JS, Dobson JM, Bostock DE: Use of tamoxifen in the control of canine mammary neoplasia. *Veterinary Record* 133: 539–542, 1993.

69. Schmidt I, Allgoewer I, Walter J, et al: Laser-induzierte thermotherapie (LITT) an mammatumoren von hunden - invitro-und in-vivo-untersuchungen. *Kleintierpraxis* 41:871–880, 1996.

70. Parodi AL, Misdorp W, Mialot JP, et al: Intratumoral BCG and *Corynebacterium parvum* therapy of canine mammary tumours before radical mastectomy. *Cancer Immunol Immunother* 15:172–177, 1983.

71. Teske E, Rutteman GR, vd Ingh TS, et al: Liposome-encapsulated muramyl tripeptide phosphatidylethanolamine (LMTP-PE): A randomized clinical trial in dogs with mammary carcinoma. *Anticancer Res* 18:1015–1019, 1998.

72. Visonneau S, Cesano A, Jeglum KA, Santoli D: Adoptive therapy of canine metastatic mammary carcinoma with the human MHC non-restricted cytotoxic T-cell line TALL-104. *Oncol Rep* 6:1181–1188, 1999.

73. London CA, Hannah AL, Zadovoskaya R, et al: Phase I dose-escalating study of SU11654, a small molecule receptor tyrosine kinase inhibitor, in dogs with spontaneous malignancies. *Clin Cancer Res* 9:2755–2768, 2003.

74. Yazawa M, Setoguchi A, Hong SH, et al: Effect of an adenoviral vector that expresses the canine p53 gene on cell growth of canine osteosarcoma and mammary adenocarcinoma cell lines. *Am J Vet Res* 64:880–888, 2003.

75. Susaneck SJ, Allen TA, Hoopes J, et al: Inflammatory mammary carcinoma in the dog. *JAAHA* 19:971–976, 1983.

76. Pérez-Alenza MD, Tabanera E, Peña L: Inflammatory mammary carcinoma in dogs: 33 cases (1995–1999). *JAVMA* 219:1110–1114, 2001.

77. Ginel PJ, Perez J, Lucena R, Mozos E: Vesiculopustular dermatitis associated with cutaneous metastases of an inflammatory mammary carcinosarcoma in a bitch. *Vet Rec* 147: 550–552, 2000.

78. Peña L, Pérez-Alenza MD, Rodriguez-Bertos A, Nieto A: Canine inflammatory mammary carcinoma: histopathology, immunohistochemistry and clinical implications of 21 cases. *Breast Cancer Res Treat* 78:141–148, 2003.

79. Peña L, Silvan G, Pérez-Alenza MD, et al: Steroid hormone profile of canine inflammatory mammary carcinoma: A preliminary study. *J Steroid Biochem Mol Biol* 84:211–216, 2003.

80. Kristiansen VM, Nødtvedt A, Breen AM, et al: Effect of ovariohysterectomy at the time of tumor removal in dogs with benign mammary tumors and hyperplastic lesions: a randomized controlled clinical trial. *J Vet Intern Med.* 27(4):935-942, 2013.

81. Betz D, Schoenrock D, Mischke R, et al: Postoperative treatment outcome in canine mammary tumors. Multivariate analysis of the prognostic value of pre- and postoperatively available information. *Tierarztl Prax Ausg K Kleintiere Heimtiere* 40(4):235-242, 2012.

82. Stratmann N, Failing K, Richter A, Wehrend A. Mammary tumor recurrence in bitches after regional mastectomy. *Vet Surg* 37(1):82-86, 2008.

83. de M Souza CH, Toledo-Piza E, Amorin R, Barboza A, Tobias KM. Inflammatory mammary carcinoma in 12 dogs: clinical features, cyclooxygenase-2 expression, and response to piroxicam treatment. *Can Vet J* 50(5):506-510, 2009.

Chapter 39

Canine tumors of the urinary tract

CANINE RENAL TUMORS

Clinical presentation

- Often not painful with no clinical signs; hematuria with tumors of the renal pelvis.
- Most commonly carcinomas and adenocarcinomas.
- Older dogs, usually males; nephroblastoma in young dogs.
- German shepherd dogs often present for dermatologic disorders as they develop cystoadenocarcinomas and nodular dermatofibrosis on an inherited basis.

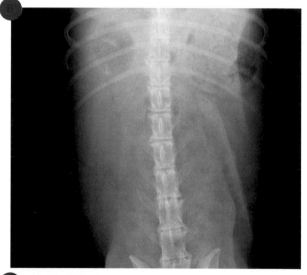

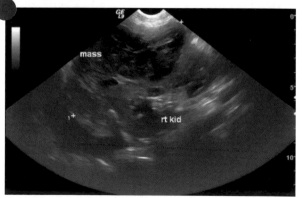

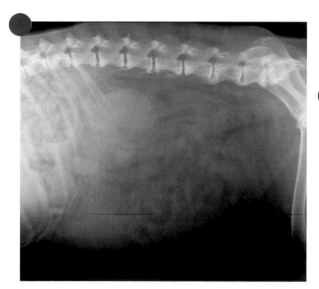

Figure 39-1: Patients with renal mass may present with or without biochemical evidence of renal disease such as an elevated BUN, creatinine and serum phosphorus with a fixed urine specific gravity. Many dogs have abdominal effusion and some have ill-defined pain. Radiographs (A and B) are often quite helpful for helping to localize a mass and to define if there is abdominal effusion as illustrated in these radiographs. Ultimately, abdominal ultrasound (C) or computerized tomography are considered the optimal diagnostic tests for defining the primary or metastatic tumor and for localizing any intra-abdominal metastases. If the disease is localized and the contralateral kidney is normal, then a nephrectomy can be considered. Imaging courtesy of Lenore Anderson Mohammadian, DVM, MSpVM, Diplomate ACVR.

culture during the course of treatment. Dogs with urethral involvement were significantly more likely to have at least 1 positive culture than dogs without urethral involvement (75% versus 30%).

Comfort and control

Above mentioned therapy for comfort plus:
- Palliative radiation (e.g.: 2-5 dosages of radiation) to first enhance comfort, second, to reduce the rate of growth and third, occasionally to reduce the size of the tumor. May be combined with medical therapy (see below).
- Cystoscopic laser therapy may improve clinical signs.
  - In one study[121] evaluating ultrasound-guided endoscopic diode laser ablation for palliative management of urinary tract obstruction due to transitional cell carcinoma, the median survival time for all dogs was 380 days.

Comfort and longer-term control

Above mentioned therapy for comfort plus:
- Chemotherapy post radiation therapy or alone is mostly palliative; best results with combination of mitoxantrone and piroxicam. Responses also seen to piroxicam alone, cisplatin, carboplatin, and possibly doxorubicin and cyclophosphamide in combination.
  - A prospective open-label phase III randomized study was conducted[121] in which either mitoxantrone or carboplatin was administered every 3 weeks concurrently with piroxicam for the treatment of transitional cell carcinoma. No difference was seen between groups with progression-free intervals, however dogs with prostatic involvement experienced a shorter survival (median, 109 days) compared to dogs with urethral, trigonal, or apically located tumors; this difference was significant (median 300, 190, and 645 days, respectively).
- Toceranib has been suggested as an effective therapy for transitional cell carcinomas.
- Surgery may be quite helpful if the tumor is located in the apex of the bladder, however transitional cell carcinomas often involve the entire bladder.
  - In one study[122] involving ten dogs with transitional cell carcinomas of the bladder, a total cystectomy and ureteral transplantation to the prepuce or vagina was performed with an estimated median survival time was 385 days.

References

1. Hayes HM Jr, Fraumeni JF Jr: Epidemiological features of canine renal neoplasms. *Cancer Res* 37:2553–2556, 1977. 2. Baskin GB, De Paoli A: Primary renal neoplasms of the dog. *Vet Pathol* 14:591–605, 1977.
3. Klein MK, Cockerell GL, Harris CK, et al: Canine primary renal neoplasms: A retrospective review of 54 cases. *JAAHA* 24:443–452, 1988.
4. Diters RW, Wells M: Renal interstitial cell tumors in the dog. *Vet Pathol* 23:74–76, 1986.
5. Picut CA, Valentine BA: Renal fibroma in four dogs. *Vet Pathol* 22:422–423, 1985.
6. Zwicker GM, Cronin NS: Naturally occurring renal neurofibroma in a laboratory beagle. *Toxicol Pathol* 20:112–114, 1992.
7. Buergelt CD, Adjiri-Awere A: Bilateral renal oncocytoma in a Greyhound dog. *Vet Pathol* 37:188–192, 2000.
8. Rudd RG, Whitehair JG, Leipold HW: Spindle cell sarcoma in the kidney of a dog. *JAAHA* 198:1023–1024, 1991.
9. Konde LF, Wrigley RH, Park RD: Sonographic appearance of renal neoplasia in the dog. *Vet Radiol* 26:74–81, 1985.
10. Widmer WR, Carlton WW: Persistent hematuria in a dog with renal hemangioma. *JAVMA* 197:237–239, 1990.
11. Lappin MR, Latimer KS: Hematuria and extreme neutrophilic leukocytosis in a dog with renal tubular carcinoma. *JAVMA* 192:1289–1292, 1988.
12. Mott JC, McAnulty JF, Darien DL, Steinberg H: Nephron sparing by partial median nephrectomy for treatment of renal hemangioma in a dog. *JAVMA* 208:1274–1276, 1996.
13. Eddlestone S, Taboada J, Senior D, Paulsen DB: Renal haemangioma in a dog. *J Small Anim Pract* 40:132–135, 1999.
14. Lucke VM, Kelly DF: Renal carcinoma in the dog. *Vet Pathol* 13:264–276, 1976.
15. Arai C, Ono M, Une Y, et al: Canine renal carcinoma with extensive bone metastasis. *J Vet Med Sci* 53:495–497, 1991.
16. Madewell BR, Wilson DW, Hornof WJ, Gregory CR: Leukemoid blood response and bone infarcts in a dog with renal tubular adenocarcinoma. *JAVMA* 197:1623–1625, 1990.
17. Peeters D, Clercx C, Thiry A, et al: Resolution of paraneoplastic leukocytosis and hypertrophic osteopathy after resection of a renal transitional cell carcinoma producing granulocytemacrophage colony-stimulating factor in a young Bull Terrier. *J Vet Intern Med* 15:407–411, 2001.
18. Gorse MJ: Polycythemia associated with renal fibrosarcoma in a dog. *JAVMA* 192:793–794, 1998.
19. Crow SE, Allen DP, Murphy CJ, Culbertson R: Concurrent renal adenocarcinoma and polycythemia in a dog. *JAAHA* 31:29–33, 1995.
20. Ghosh AK, Bhattacharjee GC: Primary multicentric carcinomas of kidney. *J Indian Med Assoc* 90:69–70, 1992.
21. Bryan J, Jackson T, Henry CJ, et al: Canine renal neoplasms: a retrospective of 30 cases. *Proc 22nd Annu Conf Vet Cancer Soc* 26, 2002.
22. Khan KN, Stanfield KM, Trajkovic D, Knapp DW: Expression of cyclooxygenase-2 in canine renal cell carcinoma. *Vet Pathol* 38:116–119, 2001.
23. Llum B, Moe L: Hereditary multifocal renal cystadenocarcinomas and nodular dermatofibrosis in the German Shepherd dog: Macroscopic and histopathologic changes. *Vet Pathol* 22:447–455, 1985.
24. Moe L, Lium B: Hereditary multifocal renal cystadenocarcinomas and nodular dermatofibrosis in 51 German shepherd dogs. *J Small Anim Pract* 38:498–505, 1997.
25. Atlee BA, DeBoer DJ, Ihrke PJ, et al: Nodular dermatofibrosis in German Shepherd dogs as a marker for renal cystadenocarcinoma. *JAAHA* 27:481–487, 1991.
26. Perry W: Generalised nodular dermatofibrosis and renal cystadenoma in a series of 10 closely related German Shepherd dogs. *Aust Vet Practit* 25:90–93, 1995.
27. Jonasdottir TJ, Mellersh CS, Moe L, et al: Genetic mapping of a naturally occurring hereditary renal cancer syndrome in dogs. *Proc Natl Acad Sci* USA 97:4132–4137, 2000.
28. White SD, Rosychuk AW, Schultheiss P, Scott KV: Nodular dermatofibrosis and cystic renal disease in three mixed-breed dogs and a Boxer dog. *Vet Dermatol* 9:119–126, 1998.
29. Marks SL, Farman CA, Peaston A: Nodular dermatofibrosis and renal cystadenomas in a golden retriever. *Vet Dermatol* 4:133–137, 1994.
30. Vilafranca M, Fondevila D, Marlasca MJ, Ferrer L: Chromophilic-eosinophilic (oncocyte-like) renal cell carcinoma in a dog with nodular dermatofibrosis. *Vet Pathol* 31:713–716, 1994.
31. Moe L, Lium B: Computed tomography of hereditary multifocal renal cystadenocarcinomas in German shepherd dogs. *Vet Radiol Ultrasound* 38:335–343, 1997.
32. Moe L, Gamlem H, Jonasdottir TJ, Lingaas F: Renal microcystic tubular lesions in two 1year-old dogs—An early sign of hereditary renal cystadenocarcinoma? *J Comp Pathol* 123:218–221, 2000.
33. Cosenza SF, Seely JC: Generalized nodular dermatofibrosis and renal cystadenocarcinomas in a German Shepherd dog. *JAVMA* 189:1587–1590, 1986.
34. Jones TL: Embryonal nephroma in a dog. *Can J Comp Med* 164:153–154, 1952.
35. Savage A, Isa JM: Embryonal nephroma with metastasis in a dog. *JAVMA* 124:185–186, 1954.
36. Medway W, Nielsen SW: Canine renal disorders II. Embryonal

37. Coleman GL, Gralla EJ, Knirsch AK, Stebbons RB: Canine embryonal nephroma: a case report. *Am J Vet Res* 31:1315–1320, 1970.
38. Simpson RM, Gliatto JM, Caseey HW, Henk WG: The histologic, ultrastructural, and immunohistochemical features of a blastema-predominant canine nephroblastoma. *Vet Pathol* 26:281–282, 1989.
39. Takeda T, Makita T, Nakamura N, Horie H: Congenital mesoblastic nephroma in a dog: A benign variant of nephroblastoma. *Vet Pathol* 26:281–282, 1989.
40. Frimberger AE, Moore AS, Schelling SH: treatment of nephroblastoma in a juvenile dog. *JAVMA* 207:596–598, 1995.
41. Caywood DD, Osborne CA, Stevens JB, et al: Hypertrophic osteoarthropathy associated with an atypical nephroblastoma in a dog. *JAAHA* 16:855–865, 1980.
42. Abrahamsson K, Uhlhorn M, Lamb CR: What is your diagnosis? Embryonal nephroma. *J Small Anim Pract* 37:154–184, 1996.
43. Sagartz JW, Ayers KM, Cashell IG, Robinson FR: Malignant embryonal nephroma in an aged dog. *JAVMA* 161:1658–1660, 1972.
44. Nakayama H, Hayashi T, Takahashi R, Fujiwara K: Nephroblastoma with liver and lung metastases in an adult dog. *Japanese J Vet Science* 46:897–900, 1984.
45. Seaman RL, Patton CS: treatment of renal nephroblastoma in an adult dog. *JAAHA* 39:76–79, 2003.
46. Hartmann M, Steidel T: Sekundäre polyzythämie infolge neophroblastom bei einem beutschen schäferhund. *Kleintierpraxis* 42:577–588, 1997.
47. Gasser AM, Bush WW, Smith S, Walton R: Extradural spinal, bone marrow, and renal nephroblastoma. *JAAHA* 39:80–85, 2003.
48. Seibold HR, Hoerlein BF: Embryonal nephroma (nephroblastoma) in a dog. *JAVMA* 130:82–85, 1957.
49. Coleman GL, Gralla EJ, Knirsch AK, Stebbins RB: Mithramycin treatment of metastatic canine embryonal nephroma (Radiographic evidence of regression was associated with histopathologic changes). *Fed Proc* 28:686, 1969.
50. Reichle JK, Peterson RA, Mahaffey MB, et al: Ureteral fibroepithelial polyps in four dogs. *Vet Radiol Ultrasound* 44:433–437, 2003.
51. Mutsaers AJ, Widmer WR, Knapp DW: Canine transitional cell carcinoma. *J Vet Intern Med* 17:136–144, 2003.
52. Hayes HM Jr: Canine bladder cancer: Epidemiologic features. *Am J Epidemiol* 104:673–677, 1976.
53. Norris AM, Laing EJ, Valli VE, et al: Canine bladder and urethral tumors: A retrospective study of 115 cases (1980–1985). *J Vet Intern Med* 6:145–153, 1992.
54. Burnie AG, Weaver AD: Urinary bladder neoplasia in the dog; a review of seventy cases. *J Small Anim Pract* 24:129–143, 1983.
55. Osborne CA, Low DG, Perman V, Barnes DM: Neoplasms of the canine and feline urinary bladder: Incidence, etiologic factors, occurrence and pathologic features. *Am J Vet Res* 29:2041–2055, 1968.
56. Moroff SD, Brown BA, Matthiesen DT, Scott RC: Infiltrative urethral disease in female dogs: 41 cases (1980–1987). *JAVMA* 199:247–251, 1991.
57. Esplin DG: Urinary bladder fibromas in dogs: 51 cases (1981–1985). *JAVMA* 190:440–444, 1987.
58. Leav I, Schelling KH, Adams JY, et al: Role of canine basal cells in postnatal prostatic development, induction of hyperplasia, and sex hormone-stimulated growth; and the ductal origin of carcinoma. *Prostate* 48:210–224, 2001.
59. Sorenmo KU, Goldschmidt M, Shofer F, et al: Immunohistochemical characterization of canine prostatic carcinoma and correlation with castration status and castration time. *Vet & Comp Oncology* 1:48–56, 2003.
60. Kelly DF: Rhabdomyosarcoma of the urinary bladder in dogs. *Vet Pathol* 10:375–384, 1973.
61. Davies JV, Read HM: Urethral tumours in dogs. *J Small Anim Pract* 31:131–136, 1990.
62. Nikula KJ, Benjamin SA, Angleton GM, Lee AC: Transitional cell carcinomas of the urinary tract in a colony of beagle dogs. *Vet Pathol* 26:455–461, 1989.
63. Glickman LT, Schofer FS, McKee LJ, et al: Epidemiologic study of insecticide exposure, obesity, and risk of bladder cancer in household dogs. *J Toxicol Environ Health* 28:407–414, 1989.
64. Glickman LT, Raghavan M, Knapp DW, et al: Herbicide exposure and the risk of transitional cell carcinoma of the urinary bladder in Scottish terriers. *JAVMA* 224:1290–1297, 2004.
65. Hayes HM, Tarone RE, Cantor KP, et al: Case-control study of canine malignant lymphoma: positive association with dog owners use of 2, 4-dichlorophenoxyacetic acid herbicides. *J Natl Cancer Inst* 83:1226–1231, 1991
66. Raghavan M, Knapp DW, Dawson MH, et al: Topical flea and tick pesticides and the risk of transitional cell carcinoma of the urinary bladder in Scottish terriers. *JAVMA* 225: 389–394, 2004.
67. Macy DW, Withrow SJ, Hoopes J: Transitional cell carcinoma of the bladder associated with cyclophosphamide administration. *JAAHA* 19:965–969, 1983.
68. Samma S, Uemura H, Tabata S, et al: Rapid induction of carcinoma in situ in dog urinary bladder by sequential treatment with N-methyl-N'-nitrosourea and N-butyl-N-(4-hydroxybutyl)-nitrosamine. *Gann* 75:385–387, 1984.
69. Osborne CA, Low DG, Perman V: Neoplasms of the canine and feline urinary bladder: Clinical findings, diagnosis and treatment. *JAVMA* 152:247–259, 1968.
70. Fontaine J, Coignoul F, Moureau P, Penninck D: Un cas d'ostéoarthropathie hypertrophique. *Ann Med Vet* 128:545–554, 1984.
71. Knapp DW, Glickman NW, DeNicola DB, et al: Naturally occurring canine transitional cell carcinoma of the urinary bladder. A relevant model of human invasive bladder cancer. *Urologic Oncol* 5:47–59, 2000.
72. Rozengaurt N, Hyman WJ, Berry A, et al: Urinary cytology of a canine bladder carcinoma. *J Comp Path* 96:581–585, 1986.
73. Holt PE, Lucke VM, Brown PJ: Evaluation of a catheter biopsy technique as a diagnostic aid in lower urinary tract disease. *Vet Record* 118:681–684, 1986.
74. Gilson SD, Stone EA: Surgically induced tumor seeding in eight dogs and two cats. *JAVMA* 196:1811–1815, 1990.
75. Anderson WI, Dunham BM, King JM, Scott DW: Presumptive subcutaneous surgical transplantation of a urinary bladder transitional cell carcinoma in a dog. *Cornell Vet* 7989:263–266, 1989.
76. Magrie ML, Hoopes PJ, Kainer RA, et al: Urinary tract carcinomas involving the canine vagina and vestibule. *JAAHA* 21:767–772, 1985.
77. Hanson JA, Tidwell AS: Ultrasonographic appearance of urethral transitional cell carcinoma in ten dogs. *Vet Radiol Ultrasound* 37:293–299, 1996.
78. Nyland TG, Wallack ST, Wisner ER: Needle-tract implantation following US-guided fine-needle aspiration biopsy of transitional cell carcinoma of the bladder, urethra, and prostate. *Vet Radiol Ultrasound* 43:50–53, 2002.
79. Lamb CR, Trower ND, Gregory SP: Ultrasound-guided catheter biopsy of the lower urinary tract: technique and results in 12 dogs. *J Small Anim Pract* 37:413–416, 1996.
80. Allen DK, Waters DJ, Knapp DW, Kuczek T: High urine concentrations of basic fibroblast growth factor in dogs with bladder cancer. *J Vet Intern Med* 10:231–234, 1996.
81. Borjesson DL, Christopher MM, Ling GV: Detection of canine transitional cell carcinoma using a bladder tumor antigen urine dipstick test. *Vet Clin Pathol* 28:33–38, 1999.
82. Billet JP, Moore AH, Holt PE: Evaluation of a bladder tumor antigen test for the diagnosis of lower urinary tract malignancies in dogs. *Am J Vet Res* 63:370–373, 2002.
83. Valli VE, Norris A, Jacobs RM, et al: Pathology of canine bladder and urethral cancer and correlation with tumour progression and survival. *J Comp Pathol* 113:113–130, 1995.
84. Stone EA, George TF, Gilson SD, Page RL: Partial cystectomy for urinary bladder neoplasia: surgical technique and outcome in 11 dogs. *J Small Anim Pract* 37:480–485, 1996.
85. Walter PA, Haynes JS, Feeney DA, Johnston GR: Radiographic appearance of pulmonary metastases from transitional cell carcinoma of the bladder and urethra of the dog. *JAVMA* 185:411–418, 1984.
86. Weber KO, Willimzik HF: Mechanisches gliedmaßenödem durch eine lymphangiosis carcinomatosa infolge eines metastasierenden übergangszellkarzinoms der harnblase bein einem hund. *Kleintierpraxis* 44:35–41, 1999.
87. Clemo FA, DeNicola DB, Carlton WW, et al: Flow cytometric DNA ploidy analysis in canine transitional cell carcinoma of urinary bladders. *Vet Pathol* 31:207–215, 1994.
88. Clemo FA, DeNicola DB, Carlton WW, et al: Immunoreactivity of canine transitional cell carcinoma of the urinary bladder with monoclonal antibodies to tumor-associated glycoprotein 72. *Vet Pathol* 32:155–161, 1995.
89. Bove KC, Pass MA, Wardley R, et al: Trigonal-colonic anastomosis: A urinary diversion procedure in dogs. *JAVMA* 174: 184–191, 1979.
90. Montgomery RD, Hankes GH: Ureterocolonic anastomosis in a dog with transitional cell carcinoma of the urinary bladder. *JAVMA* 190:1427–1429, 1987.
91. Stone EA, Withrow SJ, Page RL, et al: Ureterocolonic anastomosis in ten dogs with transitional cell carcinoma. *Vet Surg* 17:147–153, 1988.
92. Kadosawa T, Takagi S, Osaki T, Fujinaga T: Total cystectomy and ureterourethral anastomosis in dogs 6 dogs with transitional cell carcinoma of bladder. *Proc 23rd Annu Conf Vet Cancer Soc*:18, 2003.
93. Josel JR, Pagor CA, Glickman NW, et al: The role of surgical debulkment in dogs with transitional cell carcinoma of the urinary bladder: a retrospective study of 122 dogs. *Proc 22nd Annu Conf Vet Cancer Soc*:5, 2002.
94. Liptak JM, Brutscher SP, Monnet E, et al: Transurethral resection

in the management of urethral and prostatic neoplasia in 6 dogs. *Vet Surg* 33:1–12, 2004.

95. Smith JD, Stone EA, Gilson SD: Placement of a permanent cystostomy catheter to relieve urine outflow obstruction in dogs with transitional cell carcinoma. *JAVMA* 206:496–499, 1995.

96. Stiffler KS, McCrackin Stevenson MA, Cornell KK, et al: Clinical use of low-profile cystostomy tubes in four dogs and a cat. *JAVMA* 223:325–10, 2003.

97. Walker M, Breider M: Intraoperative radiotherapy of canine bladder cancer. *Vet Radiol* 28:200–204, 1987.

98. Withrow SJ, Gillette EL, Hoopes PJ, McChesney SL: Intraoperative irradiation of 16 spontaneously occurring canine neoplasms. *Vet Surg* 18:7–11, 1989.

99. Anderson CR, McNiel EA, Gillette EL, et al: Late complications of pelvic irradiation in 16 dogs. *Vet Radiol Ultrasound* 43:187–192, 2002.

100. McCaw DL, Lattimer JC: Radiation and cisplatin for treatment of canine urinary bladder carcinoma: a report of two case histories. *Vet Radiol* 29:264–268, 1988.

101. Turner AI, Hahn KA, King GK, Carreras JK: Mitoxantrone, piroxicam and external beam radiation therapy in the treatment of canine bladder tumors, 15 cases (2001–2003). *Proc 23rd Annu Conf Vet Cancer Soc*:20, 2003.

102. Poirier VJ, Forrest LJ, Adams WM, Vail DM: Piroxicam, mitoxantrone, and coarse fraction radiotherapy for the treatment of transitional cell carcinoma of the bladder in 10 dogs: A pilot study. *JAAHA* 40:131–136, 2004.

103. Moore AS, Cardona A, Shapiro W, Madewell BR: Cisplatin (cisdiamminedichloroplatinum) for treatment of transitional cell carcinoma of the urinary bladder or urethra. A retrospective study of 15 dogs. *J Vet Intern Med* 4:148–152, 1990.

104. Chun R, Knapp DW, Widmer WR, et al: Cisplatin treatment of transitional cell carcinoma of the urinary bladder in dogs: 18 cases (1983–1993). *JAVMA* 209:1588–1591, 1996.

105. Chun R, Knapp DW, Widmer WR, et al: Phase II clinical trial of carboplatin in canine transitional cell carcinoma of the urinary bladder. *J Vet Intern Med* 11:279–283, 1997.

106. Knapp DW, Richardson RC, Bottoms GD, et al: Phase I trial of piroxicam in 62 dogs bearing naturally occurring tumors. *Cancer Chemother Pharmacol* 29:214–218, 1992.

107. Knapp DW, Richardson RC, Chan TC, et al: Piroxicam therapy in 34 dogs with transitional cell carcinoma of the urinary bladder. *J Vet Intern Med* 8:273–278, 1994.

108. Mohammed SI, Bennett PF, Craig BA, et al: Effects of the cyclooxygenase inhibitor, piroxicam, on tumor response, apoptosis, and angiogenesis in a canine model of human invasive urinary bladder cancer. *Cancer Res* 62:356–358, 2002.

109. Kahn KN, Knapp DW, DeNicola DB, Harris RK: Expression of cyclooxygenase-2 in transitional cell carcinoma of the urinary bladder in dogs. *Am J Vet Res* 61:478–481, 2000.

110. Boria PA, Biolsi SA, Greenberg CB, et al: Preliminary evaluation of deracoxib in canine transitional cell carcinoma of the urinary bladder. *Proc 23rd Annu Conf Vet Cancer Soc*:17, 2003.

111. Knapp DW, Glickman NW, Widmer WR, et al: Cisplatin versus cisplatin combined with piroxicam in a canine model of human invasive urinary bladder cancer. *Cancer Chemother Pharmacol* 46:221–226, 2000.

112. Greene SN, Lucroy MD, Greenberg CB, et al: Evaluation of cisplatin (40–50 mg/m^2) and piroxicam in dogs with transitional cell carcinoma of the urinary bladder. *Proc 24th Annu Conf Vet Cancer Soc*:9, 2004.

113. Boria PA, Mutsaers AJ, DiBernardi L, et al: Carboplatin and piroxicam therapy in 31 dogs with transitional cell carcinoma. *Proc 22nd Annu Conf Vet Cancer Soc*:25, 2002.

114. Ogilvie GK, Obradovich JE, Elmslie RE, et al: Efficacy of mitoxantrone against various neoplasms in dogs. *JAVMA* 198:1618–1621, 1991.

115. Henry CJ, McCaw DL, Turnquist SE, et al: Clinical evaluation of mitoxantrone and piroxicam in a canine model of human invasive urinary bladder carcinoma. *Clinical Cancer Research* 9:906–911, 2003.

116. Helfand SC, Hamilton TA, Hungerford L, et al: Comparison of three treatments for transitional cell carcinoma of the bladder in the dog. *JAAHA* 30:270–275, 1994.

117. Harrold MW, Edwards CN, Gravey FK: treatment of bladder tumors by direct instillation of 5-fluorouracil. Experimental observations in dogs. *Invest Urol* 15:47–51, 1964.

118. Lucroy MD, Ridgway TD, Peavy GM, et al: Preclinical evaluation of 5-aminolevulinic acid-based photodynamic therapy for canine transitional cell carcinoma. *Vet Comp Oncology* 1:76–85, 2003.

119. Fulkerson CM, Knapp DW. Management of transitional cell carcinoma of the urinary bladder in dogs: A review. *Vet J* pii: S1090-0233(15)00035-0, 2015.

120. Budreckis DM, Byrne BA, Pollard RE, et al: Bacterial urinary tract infections associated with tansitional cell carcinoma in dogs. *J Vet Intern Med* doi: 10.1111/jvim.12578, 2015.

121. Cerf DJ, Lindquist EC. Palliative ultrasound-guided endoscopic diode laser ablation of transitional cellcarcinomas of the lower urinary tract in dogs. *JAVMA* 240(1):51-60, 2012.

122. Allstadt SD, Rodriguez CO Jr, Boostrom B, et al: Randomized phase III trial of piroxicam in combination with mitoxantrone or carboplatin for first-line treatment of urogenital tract transitional cell carcinoma in dogs. *J Vet Intern Med* 29(1):261-267, 2015.

123. Saeki K, Fujita A, Fujita N, et al: Total cystectomy and subsequent urinary diversion to the prepuce or vagina in dogs withtransitional cell carcinoma of the trigone area: a report of 10 cases (2005-2011). *Can Vet J* 56(1):73-80, 2015.

124. Halliwell WH, Ackerman N: Botryoid rhabdomyosarcoma of the urinary bladder and hypertrophic osteoarthropathy in a young dog. *JAVMA* 165:911–913, 1974.

125. Takiguchi M, Watanabe T, Okada H, et al: Rhabdomyosarcoma (botryoid sarcoma) of the urinary bladder in a Maltese. *J Small Anim Pract* 43:269–271, 2002.

126. Roszel JF: Cytology of urine from dogs with botryoid sarcoma of the bladder. *Acta Cytol* 16:443–446, 1972.

127. Senior DF, Lawrence DT, Gunson C, et al: Successful treatment of botryoid rhabdomyosarcoma in the bladder of a dog. *JAAHA* 29:386–390, 1993.

128. Rassnick KM, Frimberger AE, Wood CA, et al: Evaluation of ifosfamide for treatment of various canine neoplasms. *J Vet Intern Med* 14:271–276, 2000.

Chapter 40

Canine tumors of bone

CANINE OSTEOSARCOMA OF THE APPENDICULAR SKELETON

Clinical presentation

- Common, especially in large to giant breed dogs.
- Painful as long as tumor is present.
- Lameness and pain at metaphyseal sites, particularly distal radius, proximal humerus, proximal tibia, and distal femur.
- Lytic and productive bone lesion on radiographs.
- Most commonly osteoblastic osteosarcoma.
- Affects large to giant-breed dogs with no sex predilection.
  - One study confirmed the hypothesis that dogs dying due to primary bone cancer would be larger measured by bodyweight and the circumference of the distal radius and ulna than those of the same breed that died of other causes.[1]
- Usually middle-aged to older dogs.

> **Key point**
> This painful tumor of long bones usually occurs at or near the metaphysis of large or giant breed dogs. The micrometastatic rate that is most often away from the elbow and around the knee is at or above 90%.

Staging and diagnosis

- Minimum data base (MDB): includes a CBC, biochemical profile, urinalysis, and three-view thoracic radiographs or computerized tomography of the chest. Note serum alkaline phosphatase (ALP) particularly (prognostic).
- Aspirate or bone biopsy can help confirm the diagnosis, and biopsy can confirm the grade of

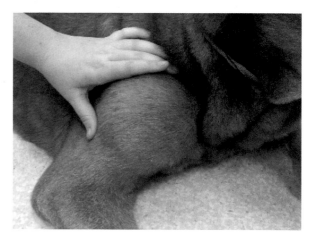

Figure 40-1: Dogs with appendicular osteosarcoma usually present for lameness. Most but not all dogs are larger in size. The tumors most commonly occur in the metaphysis of long bones. The long bones that are most commonly involved are away from the elbow and near the knee. This dog presented for chronic lameness and a mass over the proximal humerus. Statistics show that dogs with osteosarcoma of this location tend to have a worse prognosis than other appendicular osteosarcomas.

the tumor. Ultrasound-guided needle aspiration of aggressive bone lesions is a viable, cost effective and minimally invasive technique for identifying malignant mesenchymal cells and for diagnosing sarcomas of bone.[2]
- High-detail radiographs of lesion.
- Serum total or bone alkaline phosphatase (ALP) can be predictive of outcome.
- Metastasis occurs early but is usually not clinically evident.
- Scintigraphy may assist in identifying bone metastases.

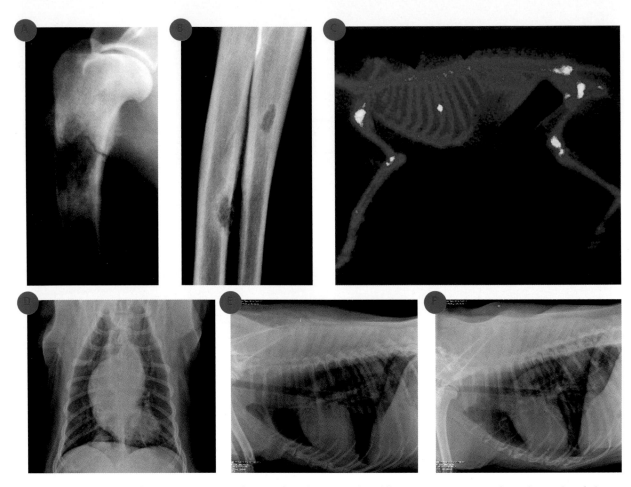

Figure 40-2: Dogs with osteosarcoma rarely present with tumor related fractures as seen in A. The radiographs of almost all dogs with this malignancy are used to confirm the presence of a lytic, proliferative pattern (A). Up to 90% of dogs with appendicular osteosarcoma do not present with detectable metastases yet most of them do spread to other parts of the body sometime in the course of the disease. The most common sites of metastases is bone (B and C) or chest (D-F). Staging each patient by obtaining blood work and chest radiographs is a good first step in the management of the disease. Imaging courtesy of Lenore Anderson Mohammadian, DVM, MSpVM, Diplomate ACVR.

Key point

An elevated alkaline phosphatase level in dogs with osteosarcoma, the presence of metastatic disease (most commonly of lung or bone), and the treatment pursued can be associated with a poor prognosis.

Prognostic factors

- Adjunctive chemotherapy improves survival markedly.
- Serum ALP above normal confers worse prognosis.
- Low-grade osteosarcoma confers better prognosis.
- Dogs with proximal humoral osteosarcoma have a worse prognosis.
- When chemotherapy is used, smaller dogs have better prognosis.
- Dogs with osteosarcoma that lived longer that one year after diagnosis had a median survival time beyond the initial year of approximately 8 months. In that study the development of a surgical-site infection in dogs undergoing a limb-sparing surgery significantly affected prognosis.[3]
- Small-breed dogs with appendicular osteosarcoma tend to do better than similarly affected and treated dogs. For example, when small dogs with appendicular osteosarcoma were treated without surgery, amputation alone, or amputation plus chemotherapy, the median survival times 112, 257, and 415 days.[4]

Treatment

This section is divided into three options:
- Comfort for those who want to improve quality of life.
- Comfort and control for those who want to improve quality of life while trying to provide some control of the tumor.

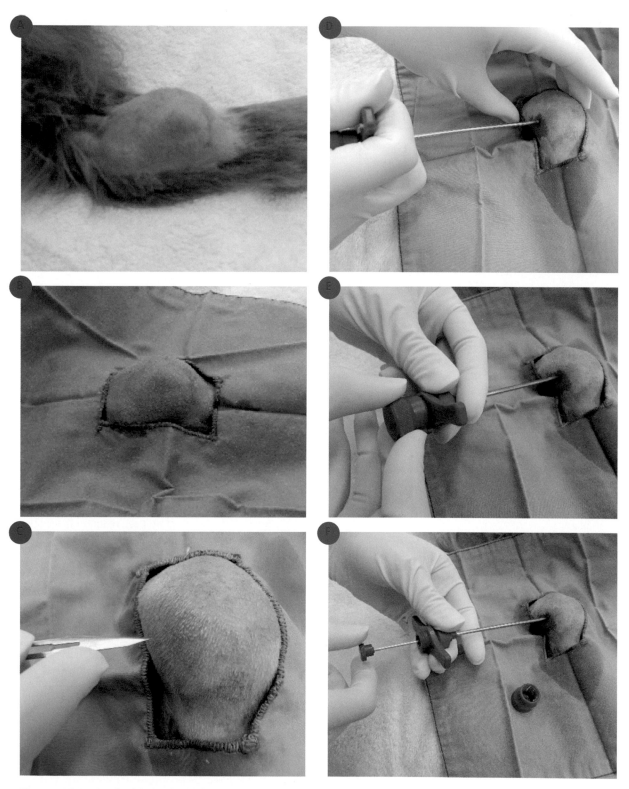

Figure 40-3: The "gold standard" for making a diagnosis of osteosarcoma is performing a bone biopsy on a patient that is anesthetized and given appropriate analgesics. The procedure is affordable, easy to perform and relatively safe. The extremity is clipped, draped and prepared for surgery (A and B). A number 11 or 15 surgical blade is used to make a stab incision through the skin (C) enabling the surgeon to place the bone biopsy needle through the skin and subcutaneous tissues to the level of the tumor whereupon the cap and then the inner trocar is removed from the inside of the needle (D-F).

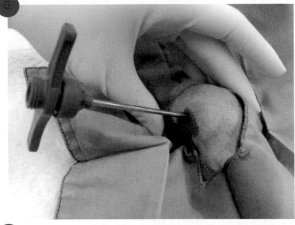

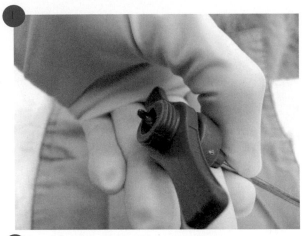

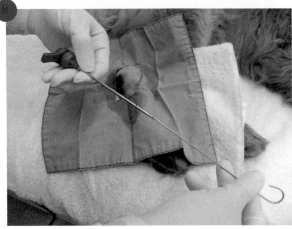

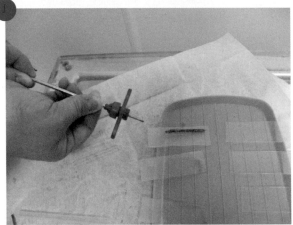

Figure 40-3 (*cont.*): The biopsy needle is then advanced through the center of the tumor (G) before the needle is removed. The biopsy sample is then advanced from the tip to the back of the biopsy instrument with the small wire provided (H-J). Impression smears can be made by rolling the sample onto the slides before submission of the biopsy to for review by a histopathologist.

Key point

Pain relief is an absolute requirement as long as the tumor is present. Radiation or surgical removal of the tumor can also relieve the tumor-associated discomfort, but chemotherapy is essential to extend the length of life by delaying or preventing metastases.

- Comfort and longer-term control for those who want to improve quality of life while trying to maximize the chance of controlling the tumor.

Comfort

- Therapy to enhance comfort and freedom from nausea, vomiting, diarrhea and lack of appetite. NSAIDs (e.g.: piroxicam) plus tramadol, plus gabapentin, plus docosahexaenoic acid may be helpful to reduce discomfort. Bisphosphonates are used by some for comfort, but they do not appear to have significant anticancer effects.

Comfort and control

Above mentioned therapy for comfort plus:
- Palliative radiation (e.g.: 2-5 dosages of radiation) to first enhance comfort, second, to reduce the rate of growth and third, occasionally to reduce the size of the tumor. Note that the body's attempt to heal damage to the bone may result in significant non neoplastic boney changes around the tumor that is often designated as reactive bone histologically. The benefit of palliative radiation may be enhanced with carboplatin chemotherapy.
  - In one study, the survival times of 50 dogs with primary bone tumors that were treated with palliative radiation therapy alone, and in combination with chemotherapy, pamidronate, or both was determined.[11] The median survival times were longest for dogs receiving radiation therapy and chemotherapy (307 days) and shortest in dogs receiving radiation and pamidronate (69 days).

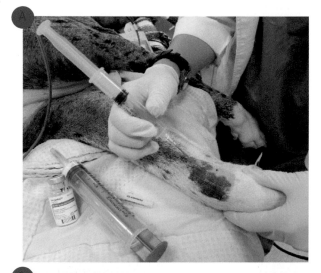

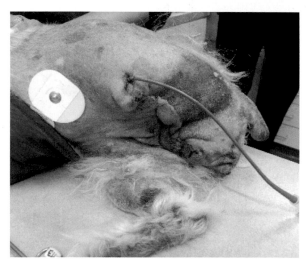

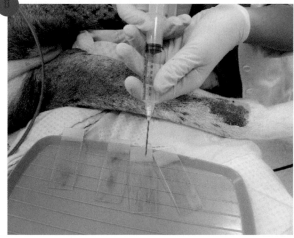

Figure 40-5: Many options exist to manage the primary appendicular osteosarcoma including palliative radiation, stereotactic radiosurgery and surgery. If an amputation is performed, systemic and local pain control is very important. One method of providing local analgesia is the placement of a soaker catheter in the surgical wound so that local analgesic agents lidocaine and prilocaine can be administered by constant rate infusion for the first 24-72 hours. The dog pictured here is 20 years old. He had had a right proximal femoral osteosarcoma that was treated with a hemipelvectomy followed by carboplatin. A red rubber catheter was placed along the length of the surgical wound before it exited a separate skin incision. The catheter had the tip sealed. The entire length inside the wound was perforated with a needle so that local anesthetic agents would drip out into the incision along the entire length of the wound. Commercially available soaker catheters do exist.

Figure 40-4: A simple procedure for making a diagnosis of a lytic bone lesion is done by performing a bone aspirate. This diagnostic test is done an anesthetized patient that was given appropriate analgesics. The bone aspirate is more affordable than a bone biopsy, easy to perform and relatively safe. The extremity is clipped, and prepared as if for surgery before the 14, 16 or 18 gage needle attached to a syringe filled with air is repeatedly advanced through the outer cortex of the bone into the center of the lesion (A). Radiographs or diagnostic ultrasound are used to direct or guide the needle into the center of the bone through defects the integrity of the cortical bone. Once the needle is removed from the middle of the tumor, the contents of the needle is expressed into slides and appropriate smears are made. (B). A slide is stained to confirm that the sample is adequate before the rest of the slides are submitted to a clinical pathologist.

- Another study affirmed in a randomized study design that when pamidronate is combined with standardized palliative therapy, it did not improve pain control and bone biologic effects in dogs with osteosarcoma.[12]

Comfort and longer-term control

Above mentioned therapy for comfort plus:
- Surgical resection of the tumor via amputation or limb sparing surgery if indicated with evaluation and biopsy of regional lymph nodes.
  - Neoadjuvant definitive radiation therapy has also been used preoperatively prior to limb sparing surgery (e.g.: 16-19 dosages of radiation).
  - With amputation alone, median survival is 162 days; 11% of dogs alive at 1 year[6]; limb sparing provides good limb function for distal radial tumors.
- Chemotherapy with cisplatin, carboplatin, doxorubicin with or without a biological response modifier, liposome encapsulated muramyl tripeptide (L-MTP-PE).
  - Despite dose intensification with standard chemotherapeutic agents, survival times for dogs diagnosed with high-grade osteosarcoma have not changed in the past 20 years. One study[15] assessed in 470 dogs with appendicular osteosarcoma the efficacy of amputation followed by 1 of 5 chemotherapy with carboplatin (300

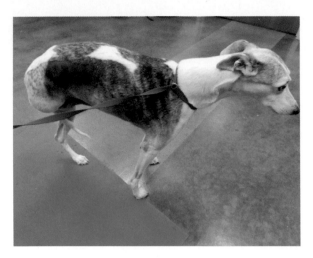

Figure 40-6: Most dogs that have an amputation for osteosarcoma do quite well. Dogs that get up and walk prior to surgery tend to adapt to being an amputee. This type of surgery is the most cost effective way of alleviating pain and suffering while controlling the tumor locally. The administration of adjuvant therapy (e.g.: carboplatin is very important to improve survival time by delaying or preventing metastases and tumor recurrence.

mg/m² IV q21d for 4 or 6 cycles), doxorubicin (30 mg/m² IV q14d or q21d for 5 cycles) or alternating carboplatin and doxorubicin (300 mg/m² IV and 30 mg/m², respectively, IV q21d for 3 cycles). The authors concluded that choice of protocol did not result in significant differences in disease-free interval or survival time, but the dogs treated with carboplatin alone had fewer adverse effects which contributed to a better quality of life.
- A separate study[13] showed that the median survival time and adverse effects in dogs with osteosarcoma that received a single subcutaneous infusion of carboplatin over a 3-, 5-, or 7-day period as adjunctive treatment following limb amputation or limb-sparing surgery were comparable to those of previously reported chemotherapy protocols requiring intravenous drug administration as noted below. Chemoimmunotherapy may help break this impasse.
- Other studies confirm the general efficacy of single agent chemotherapy is as follows[12,51-70]:
  - Cisplatin: median survival 10.5 months; 1 year survival 46%.
  - Doxorubicin: median survival 9.5 months; 1 year survival 40%.
  - Carboplatin: median survival 10.5 months; 1 year survival 35%.
- In one study, dogs with osteosarcoma that has metastasized to bone and those treated palliatively with radiation therapy and carboplatin chemotherapy had a significantly longer survival time (130 days) than dogs with other sites of metastases or those not treated, or those treated with surgery alone.
  - When dogs were randomized to receive either six doses of carboplatin or three doses each of carboplatin and doxorubicin on an alternating schedule, the dogs that received carboplatin alone (disease-free interval of 425 days) did better than those that received the alternating protocol (disease-free interval of 135 days).
- Stereotactic body radiation therapy (SBRT) or CyberKnife robotic radiosurgery (e.g.: 1-3 dosages) plus chemotherapy can be used for ultraprecise treatments to enhance tumor control while minimizing normal tissue injury in those tumors that have defined margins. Carboplatin is encouraged to delay or prevent recurrence or metastases.
- Standard course curative intent radiation therapy with or without carboplatin chemotherapy can be used to treat dogs with appendicular osteosarcoma.
  - In one study involving dogs with appendicular osteosarcoma, it was determined that full-course radiation therapy in conjunction with chemotherapy did not yield equivalent results to the standard of care options.[16]
- Toceranib has been reported to have some efficacy for the treatment of osteosarcoma, however this was not proven valuable in one study[17] that was done to test the hypothesis that the addition of toceranib to metronomic cyclophosphamide/piroxicam therapy would significantly improve disease-free interval and overall survival in dogs with appendicular osteosarcoma following amputation and carboplatin chemotherapy.

CANINE OSTEOSARCOMA OF THE AXIAL SKELETON

Clinical presentation

- Tumors of the appendicular skeleton are four times more common than axial tumors.
- Sometimes painful.
- Older dogs (except rib tumors, which often affect young dogs).
- No breed predilection; more females may be affected.

Key point

Dogs with osteosarcoma of the maxilla, mandible and calvarium generally have a better prognosis and a lower rate of metastases than dogs with appendicular osteosarcoma, especially if the tumor is completely excised.

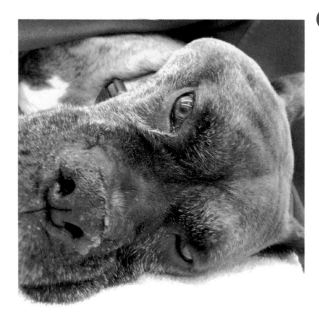

Figure 40-7: Dogs with osteosarcoma of the axial skeleton can present with a mass that is deviating the normal anatomy. These tumors can spread to lungs, lymph nodes and elsewhere, however they tend to have a less aggressive biological behavior then appendicular osteosarcoma. Chemotherapy is recommend to delay or prevent recurrence and metastases. This dog has a relatively uncommon malignancy called multilobular osteochondrosarcoma. This tumor type is invasive, relatively slow growing and the rate and pace of metastases is generally low. Radiation therapy and/or surgery can be helpful especially if followed with adjuvant chemotherapy.

> **Key point**
>
> Dogs with multilobular osteochondrosarcoma often have a long clinical course resulting in a mass-like lesion of the head that can progress over months or years.

Staging and diagnosis

- Minimum data base (MDB): includes a CBC, biochemical profile, urinalysis, and three-view thoracic radiographs or computerized tomography of the chest and site of the tumor.
- Ultrasound-guided aspirate or bone biopsy can help confirm the diagnosis and can be used to grade the tumor.
- High-detail radiographs of lesion.
- CT or MRI of lesion.
- Highly metastatic, but local recurrence usually occurs earlier.
  - Up to 18% of cases present with detectable metastatic disease.
- Mandibular osteosarcoma may have lower metastatic rate.

> **Key point**
>
> Metastases to lung, bone and lymph nodes may be seen, therefore radiographs, CT and aspirates of any enlarged lymph nodes are recommended.

Prognostic factors

- Complete excision confers longer survival.
- Smaller dogs may live longer than larger dogs.
- Mandibular osteosarcoma appears to confer better prognosis than any other site.

Treatment

This section is divided into three options:
- Comfort for those who want to improve quality of life.
- Comfort and control for those who want to improve quality of life while trying to provide some control of the tumor.
- Comfort and longer-term control for those who want to improve quality of life while trying to maximize the chance of controlling the tumor.

> **Key point**
>
> Wide surgical excision is the treatment of choice for dogs with axial osteosarcoma. Palliative or definitive radiation can also be quite helpful.

> **Key point**
>
> While complete excision of a multilobular osteochondrosarcoma is preferred, dogs that have their tumors incompletely excised and/or irradiated often have a long progression-free survival due to the slow growth rate of many of these tumors.

Comfort

- Therapy to enhance comfort and freedom from nausea, vomiting, diarrhea and lack of appetite. Pain control can be enhanced with NSAID plus tramadol plus gabapentin plus docosahexaenoic acid. Bisphosphonates are used by some to enhance comfort.

Comfort and control

Above mentioned therapy for comfort plus:
- Palliative radiation (e.g.: 2-5 dosages of radiation) to first enhance comfort, second, to reduce the rate of growth and third, occasionally to reduce the size of the tumor.

Comfort and longer-term control

Above mentioned therapy for comfort plus:

- Surgical resection of the tumor(s) with evaluation and biopsy of regional lymph nodes.
  - Tumors of maxilla, mandible and rib can be resected to resolve local tumors.
    - When dogs with osteosarcoma of the maxilla, mandible were treated with at least one of the following: surgery, radiation and chemotherapy for calvarium were evaluated, it was determined that the local recurrence or progression occurred in 51.3% of dogs, and 38.5% dogs developed distant metastases.[97] Median survival time for all dogs was 239 days and those dogs that underwent surgery had a median survival time of 329 days.
    - Median survival time for dogs with rib osteosarcoma that had a chest wall resection was 290 days.[98]
- Definitive radiation therapy may be helpful (e.g.: 16-19 dosages of radiation).
- Chemotherapy with cisplatin, carboplatin or doxorubicin seems appropriate given the relatively high rate of recurrence and metastases.
- Stereotactic body radiation therapy (SBRT) or CyberKnife robotic radiosurgery (e.g.: 1-3 dosages) can be used for ultraprecise treatments to enhance tumor control while minimizing normal tissue injury in those tumors that have defined margins.

CANINE NONOSTEOSARCOMA BONE TUMORS

Clinical presentation

- Relatively uncommon.
- May be painful.
- More often affect axial skeleton than appendicular skeleton.
- Usually chondrosarcoma, fibrosarcoma, and hemangiosarcoma.
- Older dogs, except oral fibrosarcoma, in which younger dogs predominate.
- Tumors that involve the digits can cause lameness and discomfort of the local site.

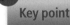

Key point

Chondrosarcoma, fibrosarcoma, and hemangiosarcoma are examples of these tumors that often appear acutely as lameness or discomfort.

Staging and diagnosis

- Minimum data base (MDB): includes a CBC, biochemical profile, urinalysis, biopsy and or fine needle aspiration cytology and three-view thoracic radiographs or computerized tomography of the chest.
- High-detail radiographs, CT or MRI of the lesion.

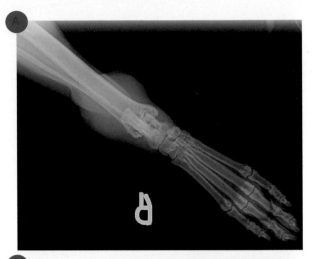

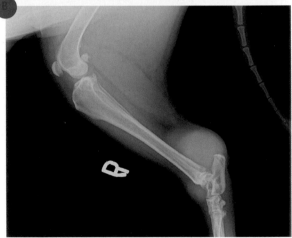

Figure 40-8: Dogs with tumors that originate at or around bones but that do not originate from bone are moderately common. This dog has a synovial cell sarcoma (A and B) that can spread to lungs and lymph nodes. These tumors seem to originate around joints. Amputation or radiation is used to help control the local disease. Imaging courtesy of Lenore Anderson Mohammadian, DVM, MSpVM, Diplomate ACVR.

- Metastases occur at a lower rate than osteosarcoma and may occur late in the course of the disease.
- Care required in interpreting incisional biopsy specimens, as small biopsies may miss the true histologic diagnosis.

Key point

Dogs with hemangiosarcoma of bone often have metastatic disease to lung, heart, spleen or liver, and therefore full staging is recommended.

Prognostic factors

- Complete excision confers longer survival.

- In one study,[152] the records of 428 dogs who had their digits amputated were reviewed to confirm that squamous cell carcinoma was the most commonly identified tumor (36.3%) and was associated with greater metastatic potential than that occurring elsewhere in the body. Other common diagnoses included melanoma (17.3%), soft-tissue sarcoma (9.7%), and mast cell tumor (6.7%). Melanomas were associated with poor prognoses, with a median survival time of 365 days.

Treatment

This section is divided into three options:
- Comfort for those who want to improve quality of life.
- Comfort and control for those who want to improve quality of life while trying to provide some control of the tumor.
- Comfort and longer-term control for those who want to improve quality of life while trying to maximize the chance of controlling the tumor.

> **Key point**
> Amputation or radiation is the treatment of choice along with appropriate analgesics.

Comfort

- Therapy to enhance comfort and freedom from nausea, vomiting, diarrhea and lack of appetite.

Comfort and control

Above mentioned therapy for comfort plus:
- Palliative radiation (e.g.: 2-5 dosages of radiation) to first enhance comfort, second, to reduce the rate of growth and third, occasionally to reduce the size of the tumor. Given the sensitivity of the paw, this may or may not be considered for tumors of the digit.

Comfort and longer-term control

Above mentioned therapy for comfort plus:
- Surgical resection of the tumor(s) with evaluation and biopsy of regional lymph nodes.
  - Fibrosarcoma of the mandible or maxilla that was treated surgically resulted in a median survival of 12 months.[112,143]
  - Dogs with appendicular chondrosarcomas have been reported to have a median survival time of up to 18 months.[140]
  - Dogs with rib resections for chondrosarcomas have been report to have a median survival time exceeding 3 years without adjuvant chemotherapy.[106,107,140]
  - Digital amputation of melanomas of the toe has

been associated with poor prognoses than other toe tumors, with a median survival time of 365 days.[152]
- Definitive radiation therapy may be helpful if margins are questionable (e.g.: 16-19 dosages of radiation).
- Doxorubicin or carboplatin chemotherapy may be wise due to the relatively high metastatic rate.
- Stereotactic body radiation therapy (SBRT) or CyberKnife robotic radiosurgery (e.g.: 1-3 dosages) can be used for ultraprecise treatments to enhance tumor control while minimizing normal tissue injury in those tumors that have defined margins.
  - Standard non SBRT or CyberKnife definitive radiation therapy of nasal chondrosarcomas resulted in a median survival of 500 days.[147]

References

1. Anfinsen KP, Grotmol T, Bruland OS, et al: Primary bone cancer in Leonbergers may be associated with a higher bodyweight during adolescence. *Prev Vet Med* 119(1-2):48-53, 2015.
2. Britt T, Clifford C, Barger A, et al: Diagnosing appendicular osteosarcoma with ultrasound-guided fine-needle aspiration: 36 cases. *J Small Anim Pract* 48(3):145-150, 2007.
3. Culp WT, Olea-Popelka F, Sefton J, et al: Evaluation of outcome and prognostic factors for dogs living greater than one year after diagnosis of osteosarcoma: 90 cases (1997-2008). *JAVMA* 245(10):1141-1146, 2014.
4. Amsellem PM, Selmic LE, Wypij JM, et al: Appendicular osteosarcoma in small-breed dogs: 51 cases (1986-2011). *JAVMA* 245(2):203-210, 2014.
5. Gellasch KL, Kalscheur VL, Clayton MK, Muir P: Fatigue microdamage in the radical predilection site for osteosarcoma in dogs. *Am J Vet Res* 63:896–899, 2002.
6. Spodnick GJ, Berg J, Rand W, et al: Prognosis for dogs with appendicular osteosarcoma treated by amputation alone: 162 cases (1978–1988). *JAVMA* 200:995–999, 1992.
7. Misdorp W, Hart AA: Some prognostic and epidemiologic factors in canine osteosarcoma. *J Natl Cancer Inst* 62:537–545, 1979.
8. Brodey RS, Riser WH: Canine osteosarcoma: A clinicopathy study of 194 cases. *Clin Orthop Rel Res* 62:54–64, 1969.
9. Cooley DM, Beranek BC, Schlittler DL, et al: Endogenous gonadal hormone exposure and bone sarcoma risk. *Cancer Epidemiol Biomarkers Prev* 11:1434–1440, 2002.
10. Sinibaldi KR, Pugh J, Rosen H, Liu SK: Osteomyelitis and neoplasia associated with use of the Jonas intramedullary splint in small animals. *JAVMA* 181:885–890, 1982.
11. Oblak ML, Boston SE, Higginson G, et al: The impact of pamidronate and chemotherapy on survival times in dogs with appendicular primary bone tumors treated with palliative radiation therapy. *Vet Surg* 41(3):430-435, 2012.
12. Fan TM, Charney SC, de Lorimier LP, et al: Double-blind placebo-controlled trial of adjuvant pamidronate with palliative radiotherapy and intravenous doxorubicin for canine appendicular osteosarcoma bone pain. *J Vet Intern Med* 23(1):152-160, 2009.
13. Simcock JO, Withers SS, Prpich CY, et al: Evaluation of a single subcutaneous infusion of carboplatin as adjuvant chemotherapy for dogs with osteosarcoma: 17 cases (2006-2010). *J Am Vet Med Assoc* 241(5):608-614, 2012.
14. Saam DE, Liptak JM, Stalker MJ, et al: Predictors of outcome in dogs treated with adjuvant carboplatin for appendicular osteosarcoma: 65 cases (1996-2006). *J Am Vet Med Assoc* 238(2):195-206, 2011.
15. Selmic LE, Burton JH, Thamm DH, et al: Comparison of carboplatin and doxorubicin-based chemotherapy protocols in 470 dogs after amputation for treatment of appendicular osteosarcoma. *J Vet Intern Med* 28(2):554-563, 2014.
16. Walter CU, Dernell WS, LaRue SM, et al: Curative-intent radiation therapy as a treatment modality for appendicular and axial osteosarcoma: a preliminary retrospective evaluation of 14 dogs with the disease. *JAVMA* 228(12):1905-1908, 2006.
17. London CA, Gardner HL, Mathie T, et al: Impact of toceranib/piroxicam/cyclophosphamide maintenance therapy on outcome of dogs with appendicular osteosarcoma following amputation and carboplatin chemotherapy: A multi-institutional study. *PLoS One* 10(4):e0124889, 2015.

18. Boston SE, Ehrhart NP, Dernell WS, et al: Evaluation of survival time in dogs with stage III osteosarcoma that undergo treatment: 90 cases (1985-2004). *JAVMA* 228(12):1905-1908, 2006.

19. Cooley DM, Waters DJ: Skeletal neoplasms of small dogs: A retrospective study and literature review. *JAAHA* 33:11–23, 1997.

20. Wallack ST, Wisner ER, Werner JA, et al: Accuracy of magnetic resonance imaging for estimating intramedullary osteosarcoma extent in pre-operative planning of canine limbsalvage procedures. *Vet Radiol Ultrasound* 43:432–441, 2002.

21. Davis GJ, Kapatkin AS, Craig LE, et al: Comparison of radiography, computed tomography, and magnetic resonance imaging for evaluation of appendicular osteosarcoma in dogs. *JAVMA* 220:1171–1176, 2002.

22. Lamb CR, Berg J, Bengston AE: Preoperative measurement of canine primary bone tumors, using radiography and bone scintigraphy. *JAVMA* 196:1474–1478, 1990.

23. Daniel GB, Avenell JS, Young K, et al: Scintigraphic detection of subcutaneous metastasis in a dog with appendicular osteosarcoma. *Vet Radiol Ultrasound* 37:146–149, 1996.

24. Berg J, Lamb CR, O'Callaghan MW: Bone scintigraphy in the initial evaluation of dogs with primary bone tumors. *JAVMA* 196:917–920, 1990.

25. Jankowski MK, Uhriteyn PF, Lana SE, et al: Nuclear scanning with 99mTc-HDP for the initial evaluation of osseous metastasis in canine osteosarcoma. *Vet Comp Oncol* 1:152–158, 2003.

26. Lang J, Wortman JA, Glickman LT, et al: Sensitivity of radiographic detection of lung metastases in the dog. *Vet Radiol* 27, 74–78, 1986.

27. Hillers KR, Lana SE, Lafferty MH, et al: A retrospective study: the incidence and significance of lymph node metastasis in canine osteosarcoma. *Proc 23rd Annu Conf Vet Cancer Soc*:13, 2003.

28. Samii VF, Nyland TG, Werner LL, Baker TW: Ultrasound-guided fine-needle aspiration biopsy of bone lesions: A preliminary report. *Vet Radiol Ultrasound* 40:82–86, 1999.

29. Wykes PM, Withrow SJ, Powers BE, Park RD: Closed biopsy for diagnosis of long bone tumors: Accuracy and results. *JAAHA* 21:489–494, 1985.

30. Kirpensteijn JK, Kik M, Rutteman GR, Teske E: Prognostic significance of a new histologic grading system for canine osteosarcoma. *Vet Pathol* 39, 240–246, 2002.

31. Ehrhart N, Dernell WS, Hoffmann WE, et al: Prognostic importance of alkaline phosphatase activity in serum from dogs with appendicular osteosarcoma: 75 cases (1990–1996). *JAVMA* 213:1002–1006, 1998.

32. Garzotto CK, Berg J, Hoffmann WE, Rand WM: Prognostic significance of serum alkaline phosphatase activity in canine appendicular osteosarcoma. *J Vet Intern Med* 14:587–592, 2000.

33. Kirpensteijn J, Teske E, Kik M, et al: Lobaplatin as an adjuvant chemotherapy to surgery in canine appendicular osteosarcoma: A phase II evaluation. *Anticancer Res* 22:2765–2770, 2002.

34. Vail DM, Kurzman ID, Glawe PC, et al: STEALTH liposome-encapsulated cisplatin (SPI-77) versus carboplatin as adjuvant therapy for spontaneously arising osteosarcoma (OSA) in the dog: A randomized multicenter clinical trial. *Cancer Chemother Pharmacol* 50:131–136, 2002.

35. Moore AS, Dernell WS, Ogilvie GK, et al: Doxorubicin for osteosarcoma treatment in dogs. *21st Ann ACVIM Forum Proc*:309–310, 2003.

36. Cooper S, Black AP, Smith BA, et al: Low-grade osteosarcoma in a dog. *Aust Vet Pract* 32:104, 2002.

37. Weinstein MJ, Berg J, Kusazaki K, et al: In vitro assays of nuclear uptake of doxorubicin hydrochloride in osteosarcoma cells of dogs. *Am J Vet Res* 52:1951–1955, 1991.

38. Powers BE, Withrow SJ, Thrall DE: Percent tumor necrosis as a predictor of treatment response in canine osteosarcoma. *Cancer* 67:126–134, 1991.

39. Kirpensteijn J, van Den Bos R, Endenburg N: Adaptation of dogs to the amputation of a limb and their owner's satisfaction with the procedure. *Vet Rec* 144:115–118, 1999.

40. Carberry CA, Harvey HJ: Owner satisfaction with limb amputation in dogs and cats. *JAAHA* 23:227–232, 1987.

41. Brodey RS: Results of surgical treatment in 65 dogs with osteosarcoma. *JAVMA* 168:1032–1035, 1993.

42. Straw RC, Withrow SJ: Limb-sparing surgery versus amputation for dogs with bone tumors. *Vet Clin North Am Small Anim Pract* 26:135–143, 1996.

43. O'Brien MG, Straw RC, Withrow SJ: Recent advances in the treatment of canine appendicular osteosarcoma. *Comp Contin Educ Pract Vet* 15:939–947, 1993.

44. Kuntz CA, Asselin TL, Dernell WS, et al: Limb salvage surgery for osteosarcoma of the proximal humerus: outcome in 17 dogs. *Vet Surg* 27:417–422, 1998.

45. Trout NJ, Pavletic MM, Kraus KH: Partial scapulectomy for management of sarcomas in three dogs and two cats. *JAVMA* 207:585–587, 1995.

46. LaRue SM, Withrow SJ, Power BE, et al: Limb-sparing treatment for osteosarcoma in dogs. *JAAHA* 195:1734–1744, 1989.

47. Morello E, Vasconi E, Martano M, et al: Pasteurized tumoral autograft and adjuvant chemotherapy for the treatment of canine distal radial osteosarcoma: 13 cases. *Vet Surg* 32:539–544, 2003.

48. Withrow SJ, Thrall DE, Straw RS: Intra-arterial cisplatin with or without radiation in limb sparing for canine osteosarcoma. *Cancer* 71:2484–2490, 1993.

49. Degna MT, Ehrhart N, Feretti A, Buracco P: Bone transport osteogenesis for limb salvage. *Vet Comp Orthop Traumatol* 13: 18–22, 2000.

50. Ehrhart N, Eurell JA, Tommasini M, et al: Effect of cisplatin on bone transport osteogenesis in dogs. *Am J Vet Res* 63:703–711, 2002.

51. Cotter SM, Parker LM: High-dose methotrexate and leucovorin rescue in dogs with osteogenic sarcoma. *Am J Vet Res* 39: 1943–1945, 1978.

52. Hernigou P, Thiery JP, Benoit J, et al: Methotrexate diffusion from acrylic cement. Local chemotherapy for bone tumours. *J Bone Joint Surg Br* 71:804–811, 1989.

53. Shapiro W, Fossum TW, Kitchell BE, et al: Use of cisplatin for treatment of appendicular osteosarcoma in dogs. *JAVMA* 192:507–511, 1988.

54. Straw RC, Withrow SJ, Richter SL, et al: Amputation and cisplatin for treatment of canine osteosarcoma. *J Vet Intern Med* 5:205–210, 1991.

55. Thompson JP, Feguent MJ: Evaluation of survival time after limb amputation, with and without subsequent administration of cisplatin, for treatment of appendicular osteosarcoma in dogs: 30 cases (1979–1990). *JAVMA* 200:531–533, 1992.

56. Kraegel SA, Madewell BR, Simonson E, Gregory CR: Osteogenic sarcoma and cisplatin chemotherapy in dogs: 16 cases (1986–1989). *JAVMA* 199:1057–1059, 1991.

57. Berg RJ, Weinstein MJ, Schelling SH, Rand MW: treatment of dogs with osteosarcoma by administration of cisplatin after amputation or limb-sparing surgery: 22 cases (1987–1990). *JAVMA* 200:2005–2008, 1992.

58. Withrow SJ, Straw RC, Brekke JH: Slow-release adjuvant cisplatin for the treatment of metastatic canine osteosarcoma. *Eur J Musculoskel Res* 4:110, 1995.

59. Liptak JM, Dernell WS, Straw RC, et al: Intercalary bone grafts for joint and limb preservation in 17 dogs with high-grade malignant tumors of the diaphysis. *Vet Surg* 33:457–467, 2004.

60. Dernell WS, Withrow SJ, Straw RC, Lafferty MH: Adjuvant chemotherapy using cisplatin by subcutaneous administration. *In Vivo* 11:345–350, 1997.

61. Hahn KA, Richardson RC, Blevins WE, et al: Intramedullary cisplatin chemotherapy: Experience in four dogs with osteosarcoma. *J Small Anim Pract* 37:187–192, 1996.

62. Madewell BR, Leighton RL, Theilen GH: Amputation and doxorubicin for treatment of canine and feline osteogenic sarcoma. *Eur J Cancer* 14:287–293, 1978.

63. Berg J, Weinstein MJ, Rand WM: Results of surgery and doxorubicin chemotherapy in dogs with osteosarcoma. *JAVMA* 206:1555–1560, 1995.

64. Bergman PJ, MacEwen EG, Kurzman ID, et al: Amputation and carboplatin for treatment of dogs with osteosarcoma: 48 cases (1991–1993). *J Vet Intern Med* 10:76–81, 1996.

65. Mauldin GN, Matus RE, Withrow SJ, Patnaik AK: Canine osteosarcoma. treatment by amputation versus amputation and adjuvant chemotherapy using doxorubicin and cisplatin. *J Vet Intern Med* 2:177–180, 1988.

66. Berg J, Gebhardt MC, Rand WM: Effect of timing of postoperative chemotherapy on survival of dogs with osteosarcoma. *Cancer* 79:1343–1350, 1997.

67. DeRegis CJ, Moore AS, Rand WM, Berg J: Cisplatin and doxorubicin toxicosis in dogs with osteosarcoma. *J Vet Intern Med* 17:668–673, 2003.

68. Chun R, Kurzman ID, Couto CG, et al: Cisplatin and doxorubicin combination chemotherapy for the treatment of canine osteosarcoma: A pilot study. *J Vet Intern Med* 14:495–498, 2000.

69. Bailey D, Erb H, Williams L, et al: Carboplatin and doxorubicin combination chemotherapy for the treatment of appendicular osteosarcoma in the dog. *J Vet Intern Med* 17: 199–205, 2003.

70. Kent MS, Strom A, London CA, Seguin B: Alternating carboplatin and doxorubicin as adjunctive chemotherapy to amputation or limb-sparing surgery in the treatment of appendicular osteosarcoma in dogs. *J Vet Intern Med* 18:540–544, 2004.

71. Bech-Nielsen S, Brodey RS, Fidler IJ, et al: The effect of BCG on in vitro immune reactivity and clinical course in dogs treated surgically for osteosarcoma. *Eur J Cancer* 13:33–41, 1977.

72. MacEwen EG, Kurzman TD, Rosenthal RC, et al: Therapy for osteosarcoma in dogs with intravenous injection of liposome encapsulated muramyl tripeptide. *J Natl Cancer Inst* 81:935–938, 1989.

73. Kurzman ID, MacEwan EG, Rosenthal RC, et al: Adjuvant therapy

for osteosarcoma in dogs: Results of randomized clinical trials using combined liposome-encapsulated muramyl tripeptide and cisplatin. *Clin Cancer Res* 1:1595–1601, 1995.

74. Visonneau S, Cesano A, Jeglum KA, Santoli D: Adjuvant treatment of canine osteosarcoma with the human cytotoxic T-cell line TALL-104. *Clin Cancer Res* 5:1868–1875, 1999.

75. Khanna C, Anderson PM, Hasz DE, et al: Interleukin-2 liposome inhalation therapy is safe and effective for dogs with spontaneous pulmonary metastases. *Cancer* 79:1409–1421, 1997.

76. Coomber BL, Denton J, Sylvestre A, Kruth S: Blood vessel density in canine osteosarcoma. *Can J Vet Res* 62:199–204, 1998.

77. Lana SE, Ogilvie GK, Hansen RA, et al: Identification of matrix metalloproteinases in canine neoplastic tissue. *Am J Vet Res* 61:111–114, 2000.

78. Cakir Y, Hahn KA: Direct action by doxycycline against canine osteosarcoma cell proliferation and collagenase (MMP-1) activity in vitro. *In Vivo* 13:327–332, 1999.

79. Mehl ML, Withrow SJ, Seguin B, et al: Spontaneous regression of osteosarcoma in four dogs. *JAVMA* 219:614–617, 2001.

80. Greenberg, C. B., Snyder, P. W., Khan, K. N, et al: Cyclooxygenase-2 expression in naturally-occurring canine osteosarcoma: A preliminary report. *Proc 23rd Annu Conf Vet Cancer Soc*:11, 2003.

81. Mullins MN, Ehrhart EJ, Lana SE, et al: Cyclooxygenase-2 expression in canine appendicular osteosarcomas. *Proc 23rd Annu Conf Vet Cancer Soc*:15, 2003.

82. Knapp DW, Richardson RC, Bonney PL, Hahn K: Cisplatin therapy in 41 dogs with malignant tumors. *J Vet Intern Med* 2:41–46, 1988.

83. Ogilvie GK, Straw RC, Jameson VJ: Evaluation of single agent chemotherapy for treatment of clinically evident osteosarcoma metastasis in dogs: 45 cases (1987–1991). *JAVMA* 202:304–306, 1993.

84. O'Brien MG, Straw RC, Withrow SJ: Resection of pulmonary metastases in canine osteosarcoma: Thirty-one cases (1983–1992). *Vet Surg* 22:105–109, 1993.

85. Boston, S., Ehrhart, N., Dernell, W., et al: Retrospective evaluation of survival time of dogs with stage III osteosarcoma that undergo treatment. *Proc 24th Annu Conf Vet Cancer Soc*:38, 2004.

86. McEntee MC, Page RL, Novotney CA, Thrall DE: Palliative radiotherapy for canine appendicular osteosarcoma. *Vet Radiol Ultrasound* 34:367–370, 1993.

87. Green EM, Adams WM, Forrest LJ: Four fraction palliative radiotherapy for osteosarcoma in 24 dogs. *JAAHA* 38:445–451, 2002.

88. Ramirez O, III, Dodge RK, Page RL, et al: Palliative radiotherapy of appendicular osteosarcoma in 95 dogs. *Vet Radiol Ultrasound* 40:517–522, 1999.

89. Farese JP, Milner R, Thompson M, et al: Stereotactic radiosurgery for the treatment of lower extremity canine appendicular osteosarcoma. *Proc 23rd Annu Conf Vet Cancer Soc*. 2003.

90. Lattimer JC, Corwin LA, Stapleton J, et al: Clinical and clinicopathologic response of canine bone tumor patients to treatment with samarium-153-EDTMP. *J Nucl Med* 31:1316–1325, 1990.

91. Milner RJ, Dormehl I, Louw WK, Croft S: Targeted radiotherapy with Sm-153-EDTMP in nine cases of canine primary bone tumours. *J S Afr Vet Assoc* 69:12–17, 1998.

92. Moe L, Boysen M, Aas M, et al: Maxillectomy and targeted radionuclide therapy with 153Sm-EDTMP in a recurrent canine osteosarcoma. *J Small Anim Pract* 37:241–246, 1996.

93. Tomlin JL, Sturgeon C, Pead MJ, Muir P: Use of the bisphosphonate drug alendronate for palliative management of osteosarcoma in two dogs. *Vet Rec* 147:129–132, 2000.

94. Mazzaferro EM, Hackett TB, Stein TP, et al: Metabolic alterations in dogs with osteosarcoma. *Am J Vet Res* 62:1234–1239, 2001.

95. Lucroy MD, Peck JN, Berry CR: Osteosarcoma of the patella with pulmonary metastases in a dog. *Vet Radiol Ultrasound* 42:218–220, 2001.

96. Maute AM, Grundmann S, Grest P, von Werthern CJ: Osteosarkom der patella beim hund. *Kleintierpraxis* 45:295–298, 2000.

97. Selmic LE, Lafferty MH, Kamstock DA, et al: Outcome and prognostic factors for osteosarcoma of the maxilla, mandible, or calvarium in dogs: 183 cases (1986-2012). *JAVMA* 245(8):930-938, 2014.

98. Liptak JM, Kamstock DA, Dernell WS, et al: Oncologic outcome after curative-intent treatment in 39 dogs with primary chest wall tumors (1992-2005). *Vet Surg* 37(5):488–496, 2008.

99. Straw RC, Withrow SJ, Powers: Primary osteosarcoma of the ulna in 12 dogs. *JAAHA* 27:323–326, 1991.

100. Heymann SJ, Diefender DL, Goldschmidt MH, Newton CD: Canine axial skeletal osteosarcoma. A retrospective study of 116 cases (1986 to 1989). *Vet Surg* 21:304–310, 1992.

101. Hammer AS, Weeren FR, Weisbrode SE, Padgett SL: Prognostic factors in dogs with osteosarcomas of the flat or irregular bones. *JAAHA* 31:321–326, 1995.

102. Dickerson, M. E., Page, R. L., LaDue, T. A., et al: Retrospective analysis of axial skeleton osteosarcoma in 22 largebreed dogs. *J Vet Intern Med* 15, 120–124. 2001.

103. Patnaik AK, Lieberman PH, Erlandson RA, Liu SK: Canine sinonasal skeletal neoplasms: chondrosarcomas and osteosarcomas. *Vet Pathol* 21:475–482, 1984.

104. Straw RC, Powers BE, Klausner J, Henderson RA, et al: Canine mandibular osteosarcoma: 51 cases (1980–1992). *JAAHA* 32:257–262, 1996.

105. Dernell WS, Van Vechten BJ, Straw RC, et al: Outcome following treatment of vertebral tumors in 20 dogs (1986–1995). *JAAHA* 36:245–251, 2000.

106. Pirkey-Ehrhart N, Withrow SJ, Straw RC, et al: Primary rib tumors in 54 dogs. *JAAHA* 31:65–69, 1995.

107. Baines SJ, Lewis S, White RA: Primary thoracic wall tumours of mesenchymal origin in dogs: A retrospective study of 46 cases. *Vet Rec* 150:335–339, 2002.

108. Feeney DA, Johnston GR, Grindem CB, et al: Malignant neoplasia of canine ribs: Clinical, radiographic, and pathologic findings. *JAVMA* 180:927–933, 1982.

109. Matthiesen DT, Clark GN, Orsher RJ, et al: Enbloc resection of primary rib tumors in 40 dogs. *Vet Surg* 21:201–204, 1992.

110. Moore GE, Mathey WS, Eggers JS, Estep JS: Osteosarcoma in adjacent lumbar vertebrae in a dog. *JAVMA* 217:1038–40, 1008, 2000.

111. Wallace J, Matthiesen DT, Patnaik AK: Hemimaxillectomy for the treatment of oral tumors in 69 dogs. *Vet Surg* 21:337–341, 1992.

112. White RA: Mandibulectomy and maxillectomy in the dog: long term survival in 100 cases. *J Small Anim Pract* 32:69–74, 1991.

113. Beck JA, Strizek AA: Full-thickness resection of the hard palate for treatment of osteosarcoma in a dog. *Aust Vet J* 77: 163–165, 1999.

114. Withrow SJ, Doige CE: Enbloc resection of a juxtacortical and three intraosseous osteosarcoma of the zygomatic arch in dogs. *JAAHA* 16:867–872, 1980.

115. Hendrix DV, Gelatt KN: Diagnosis, treatment and outcome of orbital neoplasia in dogs: A retrospective study of 44 cases. *J Small Anim Pract* 41:105–108, 2000.

116. Straw RC, Withrow SJ, Powers BE: Partial or total hemipelvectomy in the management of sarcomas in nine dogs and two cats. *Vet Surg* 21:183–188, 1992.

117. Doige CE: Multiple cartilaginous exostoses in dogs. *Vet Pathol* 24:276–278, 1987.

118. Green EM, Adams WM, Steinberg H: Malignant transformation of solitary spinal osteochondroma in two mature dogs. *Vet Radiol Ultrasound* 40:634–637, 1999.

119. Dernell WS, Straw RC, Cooper MF, et al: Multilobular osteochondrosarcoma in 39 dogs: 1979–1993. *JAAHA* 34: 11–18, 1998.

120. Hathcock JT, Newton JC: Computed tomographic characteristics of multilobular tumor of bone involving the cranium in 7 dogs and zygomatic arch in 2 dogs. *Vet Radiol Ultrasound* 41:214–217, 2000.

121. Lipsitz D, Levitski RE, Berry WL: Magnetic resonance imaging features of multilobular osteochondrosarcoma in 3 dogs. *Vet Radiol Ultrasound* 42:14–19, 2001.

122. Johnston TC: Osteosarcoma of the canine skull (a case report). *Vet Med Small Anim Clin* 71:629–631, 1976.

123. Straw RC, LeCouter RA, Power BE, Withrow SJ: Multilobular osteosarcoma of the canine skull: 16 cases (1978–1988). *JAVMA* 195:1764–1769, 1989.

124. Mclain DL, Hill JR, Pulley LT: Multilobular osteoma and chondroma (chondroma rodeus) with pulmonary metastasis in a dog. *JAAHA* 19:359–362, 1983.

125. Losco DL, Hill JR, Pulley LT: Canine multilobar osteosarcoma of the skull with metastasis. *J Comp Pathol* 94:621–624, 1984.

126. Bryant KJ, Steinberg H, McAnulty JF: Cranioplasty by means of molded polymethylmethacrylate prosthetic reconstruction after radical excision of neoplasms of the skull in two dogs. *JAVMA* 223:67–72, 59, 2003.

127. Pletcher JM, Koch SA, Stedham MA: Orbital chondroma rodens in a dog. *JAVMA* 175:187–190, 1979.

128. Banks WC: Parosteal osteosarcoma in a dog and a cat. *JAVMA* 158:1412–1415, 1971.

129. Brogdon JD, Brightman AH, Helper LC, et al: Parosteal osteosarcoma of the mandible in a dog. *JAVMA* 194:1079–1081, 1989.

130. Moores AP, Beck AL, Baker JF: High-grade surface osteosarcoma in a dog. *J Small Anim Pract* 44:218–220, 2003.

131. Thomas WB, Daniel GB, McGavin MD: Parosteal osteosarcoma of the cervical vertebra in a dog. *Vet Radiol Ultrasound* 38:120–123, 1997.

132. Cook JL, Huss BT, Johnson GC: Periosteal osteosarcoma in the long head of the triceps in a dog. *JAAHA* 31:317–320, 1995.

133. Langenbach A, Anderson MA, Dambach DM, et al: Extraskeletal osteosarcoma in dogs: A retrospective study of 169 cases (1986–1996). *JAAHA* 34:113–120, 1998.

134. Patnaik AK: Canine extraskeletal osteosarcoma and chondrosarcoma: A clinicopathologic study of 14 cases. *Vet Pathol* 27:46–55, 1990.

135. Weinstein MJ, Carpenter JL, Schunk CJ: Nonangiogenic and nonlymphomatous sarcomas of the canine spleen: 57 cases (1975–1987). *JAVMA* 195:784–788, 1989.

136. Kuntz CA, Dernell WS, Powers BE, Withrow S: Extraskeletal osteosarcoma in dogs: 14 cases. *JAAHA* 34:26–30, 1998.

137. Pardo AD, Adams WH, McCracken MD, Legendre AM: Primary jejunal osteosarcoma associated with a surgical sponge in a dog. *JAVMA* 196:935–938, 1990.

138. Bradley WA: Extraskeletal soft tissue compound osteosarcoma intimately associated with a retained surgical sponge. *Aust Vet Pract* 25:172–175, 1995.

139. Brodey RS, Misdorp W, Riser WH, van der Heul RO: Canine skeletal chondrosarcoma: A clinicopathological study of 35 cases. *JAVMA* 165:68–78, 1974.

140. Popovitch CA, Weinstein MJ, Goldschmidt MH, Shofer FS: Chondrosarcoma: A retrospective study of 97 dogs (1987–1990). *JAAHA* 30:81–85, 1994.

141. Gibbs C, Denny HR, Lucke VM: The radiological features of non osteogenic malignant tumors of bone in the appendicular skeleton of the dog. *J Small Anim Pract* 26:537–553, 1985.

142. Wesselhoeft-Albin L, Berg J, Schelling SH: Fibrosarcoma of the canine appendicular skeleton. *JAAHA* 27:303–309, 1991.

143. Salisbury SK, Lantz GC: Long-term results of partial mandibulectomy for treatment of oral tumors in 30 dogs. *JAAHA* 24:285–294, 1988.

144. Chauvet AE, Hogge GS, Sandin JA, Lipsitz D: Vertebrectomy, bone allograft fusion, and antitumor vaccination for the treatment of vertebral fibrosarcoma in a dog. *Vet Surg* 28:480–488, 1999.

145. Liu SK, Dorfman HD, Hurvitz AI, Patnaik AK: Primary and secondary bone tumors in the dog. *J Small Anim Pract* 18: 313–326, 1977.

146. Barnhart MD: Malignant transformation of an aneurismal bone cyst in a dog. *Vet Surg* 31:519–524, 2002.

147. Obradovich, J. E., Straw, R. C., Powers, B. E., Withrow, S. J. Canine chondrosarcoma: A clinicopathologic review of 55 cases. *Proc 10th Annu Conf Vet Cancer Soc:*29–30, 1990.

148. Boudrieau RJ, Schelling SH, Pisanelli ER: Chondrosarcoma of the radius with distant metastasis in a dog. *JAVMA* 205: 580–583, 1994.

149. The Veterinary Cooperative Oncology Group: Retrospective study of 26 primary tumors of the osseous thoracic wall in dogs. *JAAHA* 29:68–72, 1993.

150. Theon AP, Madewell BR, Harb MF, Dungworth DL: Megavoltage irradiation of neoplasms of the nasal and paranasal cavities in 77 dogs. *JAVMA* 202:1469–1475, 1993.

151. Rusbridge C, Wheeler SJ, Lamb CR, et al: Vertebral plasma cell tumors in 8 dogs. *J Vet Intern Med* 13:126–133, 1999.

152. Wobeser BK, Kidney BA, Powers BE, et al: Diagnoses and clinical outcomes associated with surgically amputated canine digits submitted to multiple veterinary diagnostic laboratories. *Vet Pathol* 44(3):355-361, 2007.

Chapter 41

Canine soft tissue sarcomas

Clinical presentation

- Very common.
- Often not painful.
- Highly locally invasive with most types of soft tissue sarcomas having a relatively low metastatic rate.
- Firm, often irregular mass that appears (but is not) encapsulated.
- Often subcutaneous.
- Ulceration may occur in larger tumors.
- Common histologic types include fibrosarcoma, hemangiopericytoma, nerve sheath tumor, rhabdomyosarcoma, leiomyosarcoma, myxosarcoma, liposarcoma, and histiocytic sarcoma. Histiocytic sarcomas are generally more aggressive with a higher metastatic rate and are thus in a separate class.

> **Key point**
>
> This common and highly invasive malignancy has a relatively low probability of distant metastases, yet it is generally not painful.

Staging and diagnosis

- Minimum data base: (MDB): includes a CBC, biochemical profile, urinalysis, biopsy and three-view thoracic radiographs and abdominal ultrasound, or computerized tomography of the chest.
- CT scan or MRI and biopsy before definitive treatment.
- Tumor grade and mitotic index.
- Lymph node cytology if lymphadenopathy.
- Metastasis relatively uncommon, usually to lungs.

> **Key point**
>
> The extent of the local disease is generally underestimated, therefore a CT scan of the tumor, regional lymph nodes and lungs is ideal, however radiographs of the chest and the tumor are more economical.

Prognostic factors

- Tumor grade is an important predictor of recurrence after surgery and development of metastases.
- AgNORs and possibly Ki-67 should be routinely evaluated with histologic grading for STSs in dogs as they can predict outcome.[3]

Treatment

This section is divided into three options:
- Comfort for those who want to improve quality of life.
- Comfort and control for those who want to improve quality of life while trying to provide some control of the tumor.
- Comfort and longer-term control for those who want to improve quality of life while trying to maximize the chance of controlling the tumor.

> **Key point**
>
> Definitive radiation and/or metronomic therapy (cyclophosphamide, piroxicam and docosahexaenoic acid) are important and effective adjuvant postoperative treatments to delay or prevent local regrowth of soft tissue sarcomas that may have been removed with limited or insufficient margins.

Comfort

- Therapy to enhance comfort and freedom from nausea, vomiting, diarrhea and lack of appetite.

Comfort and control

Above mentioned therapy for comfort plus:
- Palliative radiation (e.g.: 2-5 dosages of radiation) to first enhance comfort, second, to reduce the rate of growth and third, occasionally to reduce the size of the tumor.
  - In one study[5], 48 dogs with histologically confirmed incomplete or closely excised STSs were treated with a hypofractionated protocol

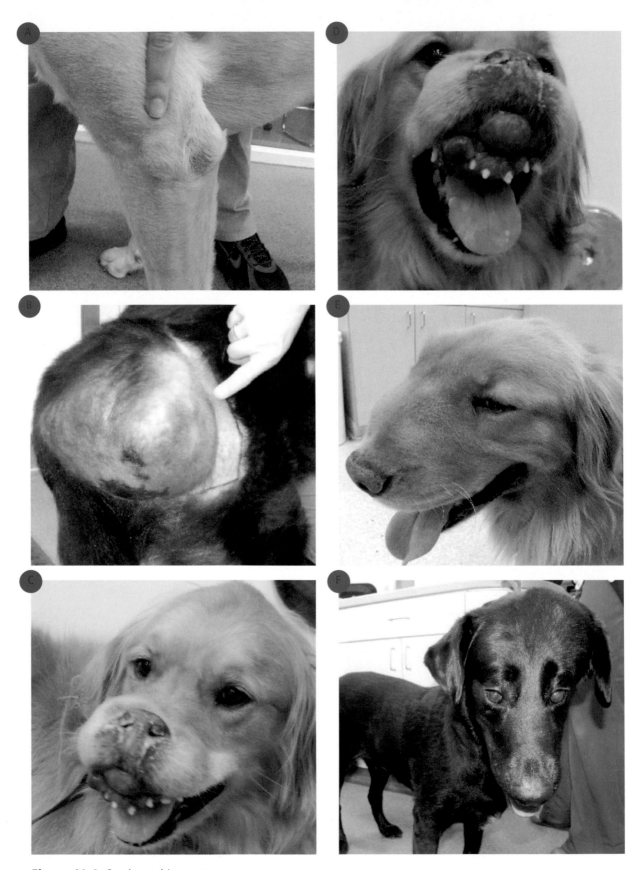

Figure 41-1: See legend in next page.

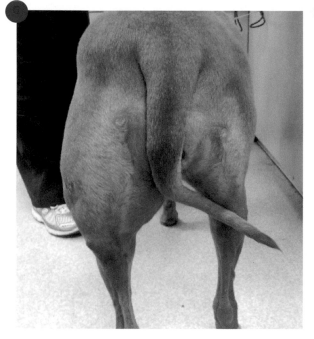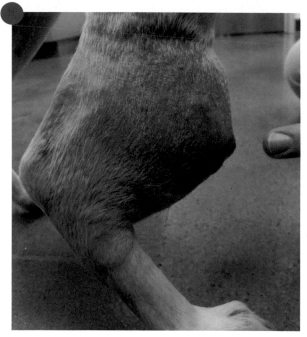

Figure 41-1 (*cont.*): Soft tissue sarcomas are a family of highly invasive tumors with a relatively low probability of distant metastases. Because their biological behavior is so similar, they are discussed as a group rather than as individuals based on their cell of origin. The grade of the tumor is predictive of outcome, but even high grade soft tissue sarcomas only have only a 20-30% chance of spread. The tumors imaged in figures A-H depict a few of the many clinical presentations. A unique subtype of soft tissue sarcomas seen most frequently on the head of golden retrievers looks fairly benign histologically, yet the tumor is highly invasive and relentless (C-E). Regardless of location, a chest radiograph and an assessment of regional lymph nodes is important. Distal extremity soft tissue sarcomas can be marginally excised but must be treated with definitive radiation and or piroxicam, metronomic cyclophosphamide and docosahexaenic acid to delay or prevent recurrence.

that is typically reserved for palliative radiation therapy (6-8 Gy/weekly fractions to a total dose of 24-32 Gy). In this group of dogs, 21% developed local recurrence and 23% developed metastasis. The median progression-free survival was 698 days; the local failure-free probability at 1 and 3 years was 81 and 73%; and the 1 and 3 years tumor-specific overall survival was 81 and 61%.

Comfort and longer-term control

Above mentioned therapy for comfort plus:
- Wide and deep (3 cm margins) surgical resection of the tumor(s) with evaluation and biopsy of regional lymph nodes.
  - A study was done that generally confirmed a good outcome for 350 dogs with soft tissue sarcoma treated with surgery in general practice.[6] Median survival time for all dogs was not reached with 70% proportional survival at 5 years and confirmed local recurrence in 20.8% of cases.
  - Another study involving 104 dogs with soft tissue sarcomas that were treated with surgery in general practice confirmed a median survival time of 1013 days and a local recurrence rate of 27.9%.[6]

- A publication confirmed that low-grade spindle cell sarcomas located at or distal to the elbow and stifle joints can be excised without need for wide or radical surgery with a mean disease-free and survival time of 697.8 and 703 days, respectively.[7]
- Definitive radiation therapy may be helpful if margins are not free of tumor (e.g.: 16-19 dosages of radiation).
  - Adjuvant external beam radiation therapy of >60 Gy gives control of 80%–90% at 4 years for grade 1-2 tumors.
  - Preoperative radiation may be used for tumors that are a challenge to remove with wide margins.
  - In one study involving 39 dogs had 40 soft-tissue sarcomas and received 51 Gy orthovoltage radiation in 17 daily 3 Gy fractions plus 10 mg/m(2) doxorubicin once a week administered intravenously one hour before the dose of radiation.[8] The median follow-up time was 910 days. The tumors recurred locally in seven of the dogs, in five of them within the radiation field; the median time to their recurrence was 213 days (range 63 to 555 days). Six of the dogs developed a distant metastasis after a median time of 276

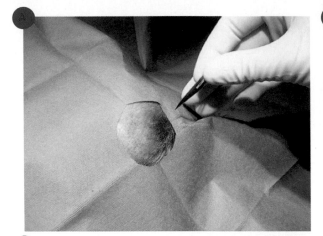

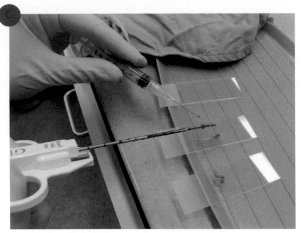

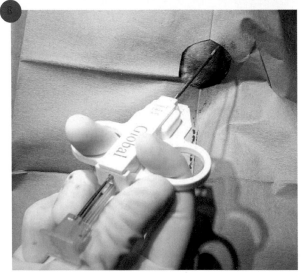

Figure 41-2: Soft tissue sarcomas can be diagnosed via cytology and histopathology. A simple, relatively inexpensive way of obtaining a biopsy of many tumors including soft tissue sarcomas is a needle core biopsy. The patient is given local and systemic analgesia with or without anesthesia. A surgical blade is used to penetrate the skin (A) to allow the cocked 12, 14, 16 or 18 gauge needle core biopsy instrument to be advanced through the skin and then up to the edge of the tumor (B). The inner cannula is advanced through the tumor by advancing it with a finger. Once the cannula is advanced, the spring-loaded mechanism fires automatically, which cuts a core of tumor tissue. The core of tissue is then re-cocked so that the inner cannula can be advanced to reveal the tumor. That tissue is then removed with a needle (C), placed into a cassette, put into formalin and submitted to obtain a histopathologic diagnosis.

days (range eight to 826 days). The one-year and two- to four-year tumor control rates were 84 and 81%, respectively, and the one-, two- and three- to four-year survival rates were 85, 79 and 72%, respectively.

- When the results of 31 dogs with oral fibrosarcomas that were treated with curative radiotherapy (median total dose: 52.5 Gy) or palliatively (3 x 8 Gy or 5 x 6 Gy), it was determined that the time-to-progression for the curatively-treated dogs was 333 days versus 180 days for the palliatively-treated dogs.[10] The overall survival was 331 days for the curative group and 310 days for the palliative group.

- Doxorubicin chemotherapy may be helpful, especially for grade III tumors, however data are limited affirming efficacy.

References

1. Williamson MM, Middleton DJ: Cutaneous soft tissue tumors in dogs: Classification, differentiation, and histogenesis. *Vet Dermatol* 9:43–48, 1998.
2. Vascellari M, Melchiotti E, Bozza MA, Mutinelli F: Fibrosarcomas at presumed sites of injection in dogs: Characteristics and comparison with non-vaccination site fibrosarcomas and feline post-vaccinal fibrosarcomas. *J Vet Med A Physiol Pathol Clin Med* 50:286–291, 2003.
3. Ettinger SN, Scase TJ, Oberthaler KT, et al: Association of argyrophilic nucleolar organizing regions, Ki-67, and proliferating cell nuclear antigen scores with histologic grade and survival in dogs with soft tissue sarcomas: 60 cases (1996-2002). *JAVMA* 228(7):1053-1062, 2006.
4. Kuntz CA, Dernell WS, Powers BE, et al: Prognostic factors for surgical treatment of soft-tissue sarcomas in dogs: 75 cases (1986–1996). *JAVMA* 211:1147–1151, 1997.
5. Kung MB, Poirier VJ, Dennis MM, et al: Hypofractionated radiation therapy for the treatment of microscopic canine soft tissue sarcoma. *Vet Comp Oncol* doi: 10.1111/vco.12121, 2014.
6. Bray JP, Polton GA, McSporran KD, et al: Canine soft tissue sarcoma managed in first opinion practice: outcome in 350 cases. *Vet Surg* 43(7):774-782, 2014.
7. Chase D, Bray J, Ide A, et al: Outcome following removal of canine spindle cell tumours in first opinion practice: 104 cases. *J Small Anim Pract* 50(11):568-574, 2009.
8. Stefanello D, Morello E, Roccabianca P, et al: Marginal excision of low-grade spindle cell sarcoma of canine extremities: 35 dogs (1996-2006). *Vet Surg* 37(5):461-465, 2008.
9. Simon D, Ruslander DM, Rassnick KM, et al: Orthovoltage radiation and weekly low dose of doxorubicin for the treatment of incompletely excised soft-tissue sarcomas in 39 dogs. *Vet Rec* 160(10):321-326, 2007.
10. Poirier VJ, Bley CR, Roos M, et al: Efficacy of radiation therapy for the treatment of macroscopic canine oral soft tissue sarcoma. *In Vivo* 20(3):415-419, 2006.
11. Seitz SE, Foley GL, Marretta SM: Evaluation of marking materials for cutaneous surgical margins. *Am J Vet Res* 56:826–833, 1995.
12. Banks TA, Straw RC, Withrow SJ, et al: Prospective study of canine soft tissue sarcoma treated by wide surgical excision:

quantitative evaluation of surgical margins. *Proc 23rd Annu Conf Vet Cancer Soc:*21, 2003.

13. Trout NJ, Pavletic MM, Kraus KH: Partial scapulectomy for management of sarcomas in three dogs and two cats. *JAVMA* 207:585–587, 1995.

14. Connery NA, Bellenger CR: Surgical management of haemangiopericytoma involving the biceps femoris muscle in four dogs. *J Small Anim Pract* 43:497–500, 2002.

15. Hilmas DE, Gillette EL: Radiotherapy of spontaneous fibrous connective-tissue sarcomas in animals. *J Natl Cancer Inst* 56: 365–368, 1976.

16. Brewer WG Jr, Turrel JM: Radiotherapy and hyperthermia in the treatment of fibrosarcomas in the dog. *JAVMA* 181:146–150, 1982.

17. Graves GM, Bjorling DE, Mahaffey E: Canine hemangiopericytoma: 23 cases (1967–1984). *JAVMA* 192:99–101, 1988.

18. McChesney SL, Withrow SJ, Gillette EL, et al: Radiotherapy of soft tissue sarcomas in dogs. *JAVMA* 194:60–63, 1989.

19. McChesney SL, Gillette EL, Dewhirst MW, Withrow SJ: Influence of WR 2721 on radiation response of canine soft tissue sarcomas. *Int J Radiat Oncol Biol Phys* 12:1957–1963, 1986.

20. Simon D, Ruslander DM, Rassnick KM, et al: Combination of orthovoltage radiation therapy and weekly low-dose doxorubicin for incompletely excised soft tissue sarcomas in 39 dogs. *Vet Comp Oncol* 2004.

21. McKnight JA, Mauldin GN, McEntee MC, et al: Radiation treatment for incompletely resected soft-tissue sarcomas in dogs. *JAVMA* 217:205–210, 2000.

22. Ogilvie GK, Reynolds HA, Richardson RC, et al: Phase II evaluation of doxorubicin for treatment of various canine neoplasms. *JAVMA* 195:1580–1583, 1989.

23. Schoster JV, Wyman M: Remission of orbital sarcoma in a dog, using doxorubicin therapy. *JAVMA* 172:1101–1103, 1978.

24. Ogilvie GK, Obradovich JE, Elmslie RE, et al: Efficacy of mitoxantrone against various neoplasms in dogs. *JAVMA* 198:1618–1621, 1991.

25. Rassnick KM, Frimberger AE, Wood CA, et al: Evaluation of ifosfamide for treatment of various canine neoplasms. *J Vet Intern Med* 14:271–276, 2000.

26. Payne SE, Rassnick KM, Northrup NC, et al: treatment of vascular and soft-tissue sarcomas in dogs using an alternating protocol of ifosfamide and doxorubicin. *Vet Comp Oncol* 1:171–179, 2003.

27. Hahn KA, Richardson RC: Use of cisplatin for control of metastatic malignant mesenchymoma and hypertrophic osteopathy in a dog. *JAVMA* 195:351–353, 1989.

28. Orenberg EK, Luck EE, Brown DM, Kitchell BE: Implant delivery system: Intralesional delivery of chemotherapeutic agents for treatment of spontaneous skin tumors in veterinary patients. *Clin Dermatol* 9:561–568, 1992.

29. Theon AP, Madewell BR, Ryu J, Castro J: Concurrent irradiation and intratumoral chemotherapy with cisplatin: A pilot study in dogs with spontaneous tumors. *Int J Radiat Oncol Biol Phys* 29:1027–1034, 1994.

30. London CA, Hannah AL, Zadovoskaya R, et al: Phase I dose-escalating study of SU11654, a small molecule receptor tyrosine kinase inhibitor, in dogs with spontaneous malignancies. *Clin Cancer Res* 9:2755–2768, 2003.

31. McCaw DL, Payne JT, Pope ER, et al: treatment of canine hemangiopericytomas with photodynamic therapy. Lasers Surg Med 29:23–26, 2001.

32. Goldschmidt MH, Shofer FS: Cutaneous fibrosarcoma. In Goldschmidt MH, Shofer FS (eds): *Skin Tumors of the Dog and Cat.* Tarrytown, NY, Pergamon Press, 1992, pp 158–167.

33. Goldschmidt MH, Shofer FS: Canine hemangiopericytoma. In Goldschmidt MH, Shofer FS (eds): *Skin Tumors of the Dog and Cat.* Tarrytown, NY, Pergamon Press, 1992, pp 168–174.

34. Perez J, Bautista MJ, Rollon E, et al: Immunohistochemical characterization of hemangiopericytomas and other spindle cell tumors in the dog. *Vet Pathol* 33:391–397, 1996.

35. Mazzei M, Millanta F, Citi S, et al: Haemangiopericytoma: Histological spectrum, immunohistochemical characterization and prognosis. *Vet Dermatol* 13:15–21, 2002.

36. Goldschmidt MH, Shofer FS: Cutaneous myxoma and myxosarcoma. In Goldschmidt MH, Shofer FS (eds): *Skin Tumors of the Dog and Cat.* Tarrytown, NY, Pergamon Press, 1992, pp 179–183.

37. Goldschmidt MH, Shofer FS: Uncommon skin tumors. In Goldschmidt MH, Shofer FS (eds): *Skin Tumors of the Dog and Cat.* Tarrytown, NY, Pergamon Press, 1992, pp 291–295.

38. Goldschmidt MH, Shofer FS: Cutaneous tumors of neural differentiation. In Goldschmidt MH, Shofer FS (eds): *Skin Tumors of the Dog and Cat.* Tarrytown, NY, Pergamon Press, 1992, pp 184–191.

39. Bradley RL, Withrow SJ, Shyder SP: Nerve sheath tumors in the dog. *JAAHA* 18:915–921, 1982.

40. Forterre F, Matiasek K, Schmahl W, Brunnberg L: Periphere nervenerkrankungen: Teil I Monoparese, -plegie bei hund und katze: Retrospective studie über 94 fälle. *Kleintierpraxis* 48:141–150, 2003.

41. Brehm DV, Vite CH, Steinberg HS, et al: A retrospective evaluation of 51 cases of peripheral nerve sheath tumors in the dog. *JAAHA* 31:349–359, 1995.

42. Rudich SR, Feeney DA, Anderson KL, Walter PA: Computed tomography of masses of the brachial plexus and contributing nerve roots in dogs. *Vet Radiol Ultrasound* 45:46–50, 2004.

43. Bagley RS, Wheeler SJ, Klopp L, et al: Clinical features of trigeminal nerve-sheath tumor in 10 dogs. *JAAHA* 34:19–25, 1998.

44. Simpson DJ, Beck JA, Allan GS, Culvenor JA: Diagnosis and excision of a brachial plexus nerve sheath tumour in a dog. *Aust Vet J* 77:222–224, 1999.

45. Liptak JM, Dernell WS, Ehrhart EJ, et al: Retroperitoneal sarcomas in dogs: 14 cases (1992–2002). *JAVMA* 224:1471–1477, 2004.

46. Robinson TM, Dubielzig RR, McAnulty JF: Malignant mesenchymoma associated with an unusual vasoinvasive metastasis in a dog. *JAAHA* 34:295–299, 1998.

47. Munday JS, Prahl A: Retroperitoneal extraskeletal mesenchymal chondrosarcoma in a dog. *J Vet Diagn Invest* 14:498–500, 2002.

48. Rhind SM, Welsh E: Mesenchymal chondrosarcoma in a young German shepherd dog. *J Small Anim Pract* 40:443–445, 1999.

49. McGlennon NJ, Houlton JEF, Gorman NT: Synovial sarcoma in the dog—A review. *J Small Anim Pract* 29:139–152, 1988.

50. Vail DM, Powers BE, Getzy DM, et al: Evaluation of prognostic factors for dogs with synovial sarcoma: 36 cases (1986–1991). *JAVMA* 205:1300–1307, 1994.

51. Fox DB, Cook JL, Kreeger JM, et al: Canine synovial sarcoma: a retrospective assessment of described prognostic criteria in 16 cases (1994–1999). *JAAHA* 38:347–355, 2002.

52. Whitelock RG, Dyce J, Houlton JE, Jefferies AR: A review of 30 tumours affecting joints. *Vet Comp Orthop Traumatol* 10:152, 1997.

53. Craig LE, Julian ME, Ferracone JD: The diagnosis and prognosis of synovial tumors in dogs: 35 cases. *Vet Pathol* 39:66–73, 2002.

54. Madewell BR, Pool R: Neoplasms of joints and related structures. *Vet Clin North Am* 8:511–521, 1978.

55. Kramer M, Stengel H, Gerwing M, et al: Sonography of the canine stifle. *Vet Radiol Ultrasound* 40:282–293, 1999.

56. Berrocal A, Millan Y, Ordas J, de las Mulas JM: A joint myxoma in a dog. *J Comp Pathol* 124:223–226, 2001.

57. Lipowitz AJ, Fetter AW, Walker MA: Synovial sarcoma of the dog. *JAVMA* 174:76–81, 1979.

58. Tilmant LL, Gorman NT, Ackerman N, et al: Chemotherapy of synovial cell sarcoma in a dog. *JAVMA* 188:530–532, 1986.

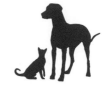

Chapter 42

Canine tumors of the body cavities

CANINE MESOTHELIOMA

Clinical presentation

- Relatively uncommon.
- Not usually uncomfortable however effusions may cause discomfort.
- Effusion of body cavities causing abdominal discomfort, tachypnea, and respiratory distress.
- In decreasing order of incidence, affects pleural, peritoneal, or pericardial cavities
- Epithelial-type mesothelioma is most common.
- Occurs in older dogs.
- Exposure to asbestos and pesticide powders may be associated with development of mesothelioma.

Key point

Dogs with mesotheliomas often present for dyspnea due to pleural effusion.

Staging and diagnosis

- Minimum data base (MDB): includes a CBC, biochemical profile, urinalysis, biopsy and three-view thoracic radiographs or computerized tomography of the chest.
- Thoracic and abdominal ultrasonography.
- Metastasis uncommon.

Key point

The diagnosis of mesothelioma is best made with a biopsy of involved tissue, however occasionally malignant cells can be identified in the pleural effusion, especially if it is concentrated.

Prognostic factors

- None identified.

Treatment

This section is divided into two options:
- Comfort for those who want to improve quality of life.
- Comfort and control for those who want to improve quality of life while trying to provide some control of the tumor.

Key point

Intracavitary chemotherapy is often used with some success at controlling mesotheliomas and the effusion that results from it.

Comfort

- Therapy to enhance comfort and freedom from nausea, vomiting, diarrhea and lack of appetite. Thoracic or abdominal cavity evacuation may be needed.

Comfort and control

Above mentioned therapy for comfort plus:
- Surgery is rarely if ever curative, but in some cases, it may be palliative.
- Intracavitary cisplatin, carboplatin or mitoxantrone chemotherapy may be palliative.
  - One set of investigators confirmed efficacy when dogs with mesotheliomas were treated with four cycles of intracavitary cisplatin at the dose of 50 mg/m^2 every three weeks with a diuresis coupled with daily administration of piroxicam at the dose of 0.3 mg/kg.[2] Effusion was reduced or eliminated for variable periods of time.
  - When dogs with carcinomatosis, sarcomatosis, or mesothelioma, with or without malignant effusions were treated with intracavitary (IC) carboplatin and mitoxantrone in dogs and

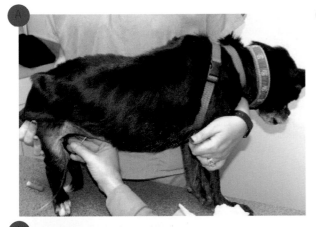

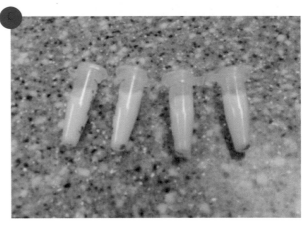

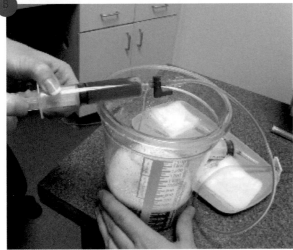

Figure 42-1: Dogs with mesothelioma are often thin and cachectic (A). The neoplastic cells often induce fluid production in the chest and abdomen. Unless effective therapy (e.g.: Intracavitary chemotherapy at 180 mg/m² body surface area), the fluid buildup impairs bodily function such as respiration. Abdominocentesis and or thoracocentesis temporarily relieves clinical signs. Fluid may be accumulated, spun down to acquire a pellet of cells to be evaluated for a specific diagnosis (B and C).

compared to those that were not treated, the median survival time for untreated dogs was 25 days, whereas the treated dogs was 332 days.[3]

CANINE THYMOMA

Clinical presentation

- Relatively uncommon.
- Not painful.
- In one study it was determined that at the time of initial diagnosis, 34% dogs with thymoma had hypercalcemia, 7% dogs had a concurrent immune-mediated disease and 27% had another tumor. Fourteen percent of dogs developed a second nonthymic tumor at a later date.[37]
- Labrador and Golden retrievers may be over represented.
- Cough may be seen, dyspnea, regurgitation and lethargy; rarely PU/PD from hypercalcemia.
- May have aspiration pneumonia secondary to myasthenia gravis and megaesophagus.
  - Dogs with megaesophagus may regurgitate and have weight loss.
  - If myasthenia gravis is present, generalized weakness predominates.

- Epithelial malignant component associated with mature lymphocytes and mast cells.
- Older dogs and females dogs possibly predisposed.
- Usually large, invasive, slow-growing tumors with low metastatic rate.
- Paraneoplastic syndromes are common. Myasthenia gravis is most common; polymyositis, hypercalcemia, and second malignancies may occur.

Key point

Thymomas often present exactly like dogs with mediastinal lymphoma, including the presence of the thoracic mass, weight loss, lethargy, anorexia and, occasionally, hypercalcemia of malignancy.

Staging and diagnosis

- Minimum data base (MDB): includes a CBC, biochemical profile, urinalysis, biopsy and three-view thoracic radiographs, abdominal ultrasound or computerized tomography of the chest and abdomen if indicated.
- Metastasis uncommon.

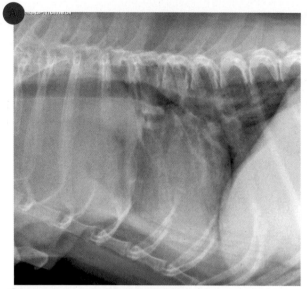

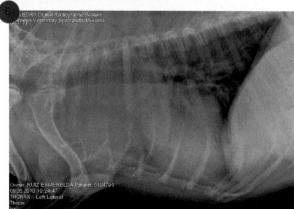

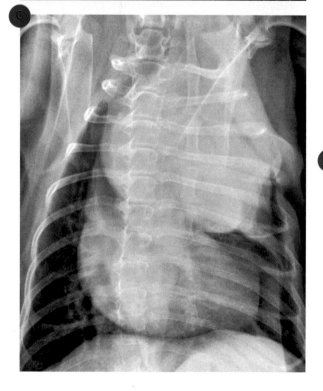

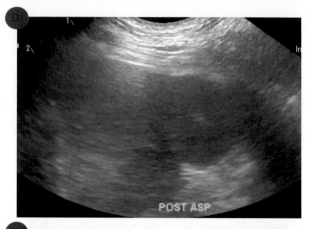

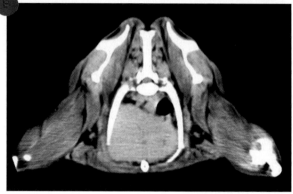

Figure 42-2: Thymomas in the dog are often large and sometimes invasive when they are discovered. They must be differentiated from mediastinal lymphoma, heart based tumor, ectopic thyroid neoplasia, cysts and granulomas with imaging and a biopsy. Imaging via chest radiographs (A-C) and ultrasound (D) is very helpful for identifying an anterior mediastinal mass. Ultrasound guided aspirates and needle core biopsies help confirm the diagnosis. Because some thymomas are very invasive, computerized tomography (E) is often very helpful for determining the extent and invasiveness of the disease before proceeding with radiation and or surgery. Some thymomas, especially those that are lymphocytic rich can have a partial resoponse to chemotherapy. Imaging courtesy of Lenore Anderson Mohammadian, DVM, MSpVM, Diplomate ACVR.

Key point

While cytology may suggest the presence of a thymoma, a tissue biopsy and histopathology is often required to confirm the diagnosis.

Prognostic factors

• Dogs with megaesophagus may have very poor prognosis if aspiration pneumonia occurs.

Treatment

This section is divided into three options:

- Comfort for those who want to improve quality of life.
- Comfort and control for those who want to improve quality of life while trying to provide some control of the tumor.
- Comfort and longer-term control for those who want to improve quality of life while trying to maximize the chance of controlling the tumor.

> **Key point**
>
> Surgery or radiation are the most commonly used treatments for the treatment of canine thymoma. The surgeon may be faced with an invasive mass that may result in an incomplete resection which may be subsequently benefitted with radiation therapy.

Comfort

Therapy to enhance comfort and freedom from nausea, vomiting, diarrhea and lack of appetite. Corticosteroids and possibly anticholinesterase therapy (pyridostigmine) if needed to reduce myasthenia gravis and resolve megaesophagus. Antibiotics to reduce risk of aspiration pneumonia.

Comfort and control

Above mentioned therapy for comfort plus:
- Palliative radiation (e.g.: 2-5 dosages of radiation) to first enhance comfort, second, to reduce the rate of growth and third, occasionally to reduce the size of the tumor.

Comfort and longer-term control

Above mentioned therapy for comfort plus:
- Surgical resection of well-defined thymoma, keeping in mind that may be invasive. Small tumors may be cured. Dogs with megaesophagus need to be monitored for aspiration pneumonia. Preoperative or postoperative definitive radiation therapy may be helpful (e.g.: 16-19 dosages of radiation).
  - In one study, tumor excision was performed for 84 dogs with thymomas, after which 17% had tumor recurrence; prognosis was good for dogs undergoing a second surgery. Median survival time with and without surgical treatment was 635 and 76 days, respectively.[37]
  - Another study confirmed a median overall survival time for 11 dogs that had their thymomas removed was 790 days, with a 1-year survival rate of 64% and a 3-year survival rate of 42%.[38]
  - A retrospective study was performed of 17 dogs with various stages of thymoma treated with radiation alone or as an adjunctive therapy. Analysis revealed an overall response rate of 75% with a median survival time of 248 days.[39]

- Prednisone and platinum agents may be most active. Lymphocyte-rich thymomas can respond to drugs used to treat lymphoma.

CANINE HISTIOCYTIC DISEASES

Clinical presentation

- Benign cutaneous histiocytoma form single or multiple masses with following diagnoses:
  - Reactive histiocytic diseases.
  - Cutaneous histiocytosis.
  - Systemic histiocytosis.
  - Splenic histiocytic nodules and splenic histiocytosis.
- Malignant histiocytic diseases are invasive and often have a high metastatic rate and may be one of the following diagnoses:
  - Disseminated histiocytic sarcoma (malignant histiocytosis).
    - Often involves multi-organs including lungs, abdomen, brain periarticular bones, vertebrae, proximal humerus, rib and bone marrow.
  - Localized histiocytic sarcoma.
- These diseases form a spectrum of signs and outcomes.

> **Key point**
>
> Benign cutaneous histiocytomas are localized benign tumors, whereas malignant histiocytosis is an aggressive disease that is highly metastatic.

Staging and diagnosis

- Minimum data base (MDB): includes a CBC, biochemical profile, urinalysis, biopsy and three-view thoracic radiographs, abdominal ultrasound or computerized tomography of the chest and abdomen if indicated.
- Immunohistochemistry to differentiate malignant forms from other neoplasms (CD-18 positive).

> **Key point**
>
> Malignant histiocytosis is a disease that can and often does metastasize to multiple sites, requiring a full evaluation of lungs, abdomen, brain, periarticular bones, vertebrae, proximal humerus, rib and bone marrow.

Prognostic factors

- Thrombocytopenia and hypoalbuminemia are predictors of poor prognosis for malignant forms.
- Metastatic disease suggests a poor prognosis for malignant forms.

- Dogs with periarticular histiocytic sarcoma, even with metastatic disease, may have a more favorable prognosis than those with the same tumor of other locations.[74]

Treatment

This section is divided into three options:
- Comfort for those who want to improve quality of life.
- Comfort and control for those who want to improve quality of life while trying to provide some control of the tumor.
- Comfort and longer-term control for those who want to improve quality of life while trying to maximize the chance of controlling the tumor.

> **Key point**
>
> Benign histiocytomas often spontaneously regress, although they can be excised with good results.

> **Key point**
>
> Dogs with malignant histiocytosis can be treated with surgery, although many patients require chemotherapy. CCNU and doxorubicin have been reported to be effective.

Comfort

- Therapy to enhance comfort and freedom from nausea, vomiting, diarrhea and lack of appetite.

Comfort and control

Above mentioned therapy for comfort plus:
- Palliative radiation (e.g.: 2-5 dosages of radiation) to first enhance comfort, second, to reduce the rate of growth and third, occasionally to reduce the size of the tumor.

Comfort and longer-term control

Above mentioned therapy for comfort plus:
- Surgical resection of the tumor(s) with evaluation and biopsy of regional lymph nodes.
  - Benign cutaneous histiocytoma.
    - Initial surgery should be curative. Even multiple tumors regress spontaneously.
  - Reactive histiocytic diseases.
    - Some regress spontaneously.
    - Immunosuppressive therapy has been suggested by some as helpful (corticosteroids, cyclosporine, and leflunomide).
- Definitive radiation therapy may be helpful at controlling local disease (e.g.: 16-19 dosages of radiation).
- Doxorubicin and CCNU based chemotherapy has

been suggested to be helpful for malignant forms of the disease.
- Treatment with CCNU at 60 to 90 mg/m^2 resulted in an overall response rate of 46% in the 56 dogs with gross measurable histiocytic sarcoma.[75] The dogs with minimal residual disease experienced tumor relapse but lived 433 days or more after starting CCNU, whereas the median survival of all dogs was 106 days.
- Dogs with histiocytic sarcoma treated with lomustine and doxorubicin (± cyclophosphamide) alternating every 2 weeks had an overall response rate of 58%, with a median time to tumor progression of 185 days for responders and an overall median survival time was 185 days.[76]
- In one study, dogs with periarticular histiocytic sarcoma had an overall median survival times of 391, whereas those dogs with histiocytic sarcoma of other sites had a median survival time of 128 days, despite the presence of suspected metastasis at diagnosis in those dogs with the periarticular malignancy.[77] Dogs with periarticular histiocytic sarcoma without evidence of metastasis at diagnosis had a median survival times of 980 days, whereas those with evidence of metastasis had a median survival time of 253 days. Interestingly enough, the administration of prednisone in dogs with periarticular histiocytic sarcoma was associated with a significantly shorter time to tumor progression and increased risk of tumor progression and death.

References

1. Glickman LT, Domanski LM, MacGuire TG, et al: Mesothelioma in pet dogs associated with exposure of their owners to asbestos. *Environ Res* 32:305–313, 1983.
2. Spugnini EP, Crispi S, Scarabello A, et al: Piroxicam and intracavitary platinum-based chemotherapy for the treatment of advancedmesothelioma in pets: preliminary observations. *J Exp Clin Cancer Res* doi: 10.1186/1756-9966-27-6, 2008.
3. Charney SC, Bergman PJ, McKnight JA, et al: Evaluation of intracavitary mitoxantrone and carboplatin for treatment of carcinomatosis, sarcomatosis and mesothelioma, with or without malignant effusions: A retrospective analysis of 12 cases (1997-2002). *Vet Comp Oncol* 3(4):171-181, 2005.
4. Ikede BO, Zubaidy A, Gill CW: Pericardial mesothelioma with cardiac tamponade in a dog. *Vet Pathol* 17:496–501, 1980.
5. Thrall DE, Goldschmidt MH: Mesothelioma in the dog: Six case reports. *J Am Vet Radiol Soc* 19:107–115, 1978.
6. Smith DA, Hill FW: Metastatic malignant mesothelioma in a dog. *J Comp Path* 100:97–101, 1989.
7. Cihak RW, Roen DR, Klaassen J: Malignant mesothelioma of the tunica vaginalis in a dog. *J Comp Path* 96:459–462, 1986.
8. DiPinto MN, Dunstan RW, Lee C: Cystic, peritoneal mesothelioma in a dog. *JAAHA* 31:385–389, 1995.
9. Kim JH, Choi YK, Yoon HY, et al: Juvenile malignant mesothelioma in a dog. *J Vet Med Sci* 64:269–271, 2002.
10. Breeze RG, Lauder IM: Pleural mesothelioma in a dog. *Vet Record* 96:243–246, 1975.T
11. Morrison WB, Trigo FJ: Clinical characterization of pleural mesothelioma in seven dogs. *Comp Contin Educ Pract Vet* 6:342–348, 1984.
12. Stepien RL, Whitley NT, Dubielzig RR: Idiopathic or mesothelioma-related pericardial effusion: Clinical findings and survival in 17 dogs studied retrospectively. *J Small Anim Pract* 41:342–347, 2000.
13. Girard C, Helie P, Odin M: Intrapericardial neoplasia in dogs. *J Vet Diagn Invest* 11, 73–78. 1999.
14. Kovak JR, Ludwig LL, Bergman PJ, et al: Use of thoracoscopy to

determine the etiology of pleural effusion in dogs and cats: 18 cases (1998–2001). *JAVMA* 221:990–994, 2002.

15. Jackson J, Richter KP, Launer DP: Thoracoscopic partial pericardiectomy in 13 dogs. *J Vet Intern Med* 13:529–533, 1999.

16. Moore AS, Kirk C, Cardona A: Intracavitary cisplatin chemotherapy experience with six dogs. *J Vet Intern Med* 5:227–231, 1991.

17. Geninet C, Bernex F, Rakotovao F et al: Sclerosing peritoneal mesothelioma in a dog: A case report. *J Vet Med A Physiol Pathol Clin Med* 50:402–405, 2003.

18. Fine DM, Tobias AH, Jacob KA: Use of pericardial fluid pH to distinguish between idiopathic and neoplastic effusions. *J Vet Intern Med* 17:525–529, 2003.

19. Peters M, Tenhundfeld J, Stephan I, Hewicker-Trautwein M: Embolized mesothelial cells within mediastinal lymph nodes of three dogs with idiopathic haemorrhagic pericardial effusion. *J Comp Pathol* 128:107–112, 2003.

20. Liu KX, Bird AE, Lenz SD, et al: Antigen expression in normal and neoplastic canine tissues defined by a monoclonal antibody generated against canine mesothelioma cells. *Vet Pathol* 31:663–673, 1994.

21. Gallagher LA, Birchard SJ, Weisbrode SE. Effects of tetracycline hydrochloride on pleurae in dogs with induced pleural effusion. *Am J Vet Res* 51:1682–1687, 1990.

22. Birchard SJ, Gallagher L: Use of pleurodesis in treating selected pleural diseases. *Comp Contin Educ Pract Vet* 10:826–832, 1988.

23. Dunning D, Monnet E, Orton EC, Salman MD: Analysis of prognostic indicators for dogs with pericardial effusion: 46 cases (1985–1996). *JAVMA* 212:1276–1280, 1998.

24. Ogilvie GK, Obradovich JE, Elmslie RE, et al: Efficacy of mitoxantrone against various neoplasms in dogs. *JAVMA* 198:1618–1621, 1991.

25. Ogilvie GK, Reynolds HA, Richardson RC, et al: Phase II evaluation of doxorubicin for treatment of various canine neoplasms. *JAVMA* 195:1580–1583, 1989.

26. Balli A, Lachat M, Gerber B, et al: [Cardiac tamponade due to pericardial mesothelioma in an 11-year-old dog: diagnosis, medical and interventional treatments]. *Schweiz Arch Tierheilkd* 145:82–87, 2003.

27. Closa JM, Font A, Mascort J: Pericardial mesothelioma in a dog: Long-term survival after pericardiectomy in combination with chemotherapy. *J Small Anim Pract* 40:383–386, 1999.

28. Atwater SW, Powers BE, Park RD, et al: Thymoma in dogs: 23 cases (1980–1991). *JAVMA* 205:1007–1013, 1994.

29. Aronsohn MG, Schunk KL, Carpenter JL, King NW: Clinical and pathologic features of thymoma in 15 dogs. *JAVMA* 184:1355–1362, 1984.

30. Bellah JR, Stiff ME, Russsell RG: Thymoma in the dog: Two case reports and review of 20 additional cases. *JAVMA* 183: 306–311, 1983.

31. Hitt ME, Shaw DP, Hogan PM, et al: Radiation treatment for thymoma in a dog. *JAVMA* 190:1187–1190, 1987.

32. Hunt GB, Churcher RK, Church DB, Mahoney P: Excision of a locally invasive thymoma causing cranial vena caval syndrome in a dog. *JAVMA* 210:1628–1630, 1997.

33. Lainesse MF, Taylor SM, Myers SL, et al: Focal myasthenia gravis as a paraneoplastic syndrome of canine thymoma: improvement following thymectomy. *JAAHA* 32:111–117, 1996.

34. Dewey CW, Bailey CS, Shelton GD, et al: Clinical forms of acquired myasthenia gravis in dogs: 25 cases (1988–1995). *J Vet Intern Med* 11:50–57, 1997.

35. Stenner VJ, Parry BW, Holloway SA: Acquired myasthenia gravis associated with a non-invasive thymic carcinoma in a dog. *Aust Vet J* 81:543–546, 2003.

36. Shelton GD, Skeie GO, Kass PH, Aarli JA: Titin and ryanodine receptor autoantibodies in dogs with thymoma and late-onset myasthenia gravis. *Vet Immunol Immunopathol* 78:97–105, 2001.

37. Robat CS, Cesario L, Gaeta R, et al: Clinical features, treatment options, and outcome in dogs with thymoma: 116 cases (1999-2010). *JAVMA* 243(10):1448-1454. 2013.

38. Zitz JC, Birchard SJ, Couto GC, et al: Results of excision of thymoma in cats and dogs: 20 cases (1984-2005). *JAVMA* 232(8):1186-1192, 2008.

39. Smith AN, Wright JC, Brawner WR Jr, et al: Radiation therapy in the treatment of canine and feline thymomas: A retrospective study (1985–1999). *JAAHA* 37:489–496, 2001.

40. Rusbridge C, White RN, Elwood CM, Wheeler SJ: treatment of acquired myasthenia gravis associated with thymoma in two dogs. *J Small Anim Pract* 37:376–380, 1996.

41. Dewey CW, Coates JR, Ducoté JM, et al: Azathioprine therapy for acquired myasthenia gravis in five dogs. *JAAHA* 35: 396–402, 1999.

42. Goldschmidt MH, Shofer FS: Canine cutaneous histiocytoma. In Goldschmidt MH, Shofer FS (eds): *Skin Tumors of the Dog and Cat*, ed 1. Tarrytown NY, Pergamon Press, 1992, pp 222–230.

43. Morris JS, Bostock DE, McInnes EF, et al: Histopathological survey of neoplasms in flat-coated retrievers, 1990 to 1998. *Vet Rec* 147:291–295, 2000.

44. Morris JS, McInnes EF, Bostock DE, et al: Immunohistochemical and histopathologic features of 14 malignant fibrous histiocytomas from flat-coated retrievers. *Vet Pathol* 39:473–479, 2002.

45. Cockerell GL, Slauson DO: Patterns of lymphoid infiltrate in the canine cutaneous histiocytoma. *J Comp Pathol* 89:193–203, 1979.

46. Kipar A, Baumgartner W, Kremmer E, et al: Expression of major histocompatibility complex class II antigen in neoplastic cells of canine cutaneous histiocytoma. *Vet Immunol Immunopathol* 62:1–13, 1998.

47. Bender WM, Muller GH: Multiple, resolving, cutaneous histiocytoma in a dog. *JAVMA* 194:535–537, 1989.

48. Linek M, Mecklenburg L: Multiple kutane histiozytome bei einem flat-coated retriever. *Kleintierpraxis* 46:507–511, 2001.

49. Affolter VK, Moore PF: Canine cutaneous and systemic histiocytosis: Reactive histiocytosis of dermal dendritic cells. *Am J Dermatopathol* 22:40–48, 2000.

50. Carpenter JL, Thornton GW, Moore FM, King NW Jr: Idiopathic periadnexal multinodular granulomatous dermatitis in twenty-two dogs. *Vet Pathol* 24:5–10, 1987.

51. Paterson S, Boydell P, Pike R: Systemic histiocytosis in the Bernese mountain dog. *J Small Anim Pract* 36:233–236, 1995.

52. Calderwood-Mays M, Bergeron JA: Cutaneous histiocytosis in dogs. *JAVMA* 188:377–381, 1986.

53. Baines SJ, McCormick D, McInnes E, et al: Cutaneous T-cell lymphoma mimicking cutaneous histiocytosis: Differentiation by flow cytometry. *Vet Rec* 147:11–16, 2000.

54. Gregory CR: Immunosuppressive agents. In Bonagura JD (ed): *Kirk's Current Veterinary Therapy*, ed. XIII. Philadelphia, WB Saunders, 2000, pp 509–513.

55. Moriello KA, MacEwen G, Schultz KT: PEG-L-asparaginase in the treatment of canine epitheliotropic lymphoma and histiocytic proliferative dermatitis. In Ihrke, PJ, Mason, IS, White SD (eds): *Advances in Vet Dermatology*, vol 2. Tarrytown, NY, Pergamon Press, 1992.

56. Moore PF: Utilization of cytoplasmic lysozyme immunoreactivity as a histiocytic marker in canine histiocytic disorders. *Vet Pathol* 23:757–762, 1986.

57. Weiss DJ: Flow cytometric evaluation of hemophagocytic disorders in canine. *Vet Clin Pathol* 31:36–41, 2002.

58. Visonneau S, Cesano A, Tran T, et al: Successful treatment of canine malignant histiocytosis with the human major histocompatibility complex nonrestricted cytotoxic T-cell line TALL-104. *Clin Cancer Res* 3:1789–1797, 1997.

59. Spangler WL, Kass PH: Splenic myeloid metaplasia, histiocytosis, and hypersplenism in the dog (65 cases). *Vet Pathol* 36:583–593, 1999.

60. Spangler WL, Kass PH: Pathologic and prognostic characteristics of splenomegaly in dogs due to fibrohistiocytic nodules: 98 cases. *Vet Pathol* 35:488–498, 1998.

61. Ramsey IK, McKay JS, Rudorf H, Dobson JM: Malignant histiocytosis in three Bernese mountain dogs. *Vet Rec* 138:440–444, 1996.

62. Padgett GA, Madewell BR, Keller ET, et al: Inheritance of histiocytosis in Bernese mountain dogs. *J Small Anim Pract* 36:93–98, 1995.

63. Moore PF, Rosin A: Malignant histiocytosis of Bernese mountain dogs. *Vet Pathol* 23:1–10, 1986.

64. Shimizu Y, Nakamura S, Harada T, Takahashi K: Malignant histiocytosis of a Bernese mountain dog. *J Vet Med (Tokyo)* 52:370–374, 1999.

65. Schmidt ML, Rutteman G, Wolvekamp P: Canine malignant histiocytosis (MH): Clinical and radiographic findings. *Tijdschr Diergeneeskd* 117(suppl 1):43–44, 1992.

66. Affolter VK, Moore PF: Localized and disseminated histiocytic sarcoma of dendritic cell origin in dogs. *Vet Pathol* 39:74– 83, 2002.

67. Goldschmidt MH, Shofer FS: Uncommon skin tumors. In Goldschmidt MH, Shofer FS (eds): *Skin Tumors of the Dog and Cat*, ed 1. Tarrytown NY, Pergamon Press, 1992, pp 291–295.

68. Ramirez S, Douglass JP, Robertson ID: Ultrasonographic features of canine abdominal malignant histiocytosis. *Vet Radiol Ultrasound* 43:167–170, 2002.

69. Uchida K, Morozumi M, Yamaguchi R, Tateyama S: Diffuse leptomeningeal malignant histiocytosis in the brain and spinal cord of a Tibetan Terrier. *Vet Pathol* 38:219–222, 2001.

70. Chandra AM, Ginn PE: Primary malignant histiocytosis of the brain in a dog. *J Comp Pathol* 121:77–82, 1999.

71. Uchida K, Morozumi M, Yamaguchi R, Tateyama S: Diffuse leptomeningeal malignant histiocytosis in the brain and spinal cord of a Tibetan Terrier. *Vet Pathol* 38:219–222, 2001.

72. Suzuki M, Uchida K, Morozumi M, et al: A comparative pathological study on granulomatous

meningoencephalomyelitis and central malignant histiocytosis in dogs. *J Vet Med Sci* 65:1319–1324, 2003.

73. Klahn SL, Kitchell BE, Dervisis NG. Evaluation and comparison of outcomes in dogs with periarticular and nonperiarticular histiocytic sarcoma. *JAVMA* 239(1):90-96, 2011.

74. Skorupski KA, Clifford CA, Paoloni MC, et al: CCNU for the treatment of dogs with histiocytic sarcoma. *J Vet Intern Med* 21(1):121-126, 2007.

75. Cannon C, Borgatti A, Henson M, et al: Evaluation of a combination chemotherapy protocol including lomustine and doxorubicin in canine histiocytic sarcoma. *J Small Anim Pract* doi: 10.1111/jsap.12354, 2015.

76. Weiss DJ, Evanson OA, Sykes J: A retrospective study of canine pancytopenia. *Vet Clin Pathol* 28:83–88, 1999.

77. Hugnet C, Hugnet-Bruchon C, Degorie-Rubiales F, Poujadee A: Histiocytose maligne associee a une hypercalcemie paraneoplasique. *Pract Med Chirurgicale* 36:23–27, 2001.

78. Brown DE, Thrall MA, Getzy DM, et al: Cytology of canine malignant histiocytosis. *Vet Clin Pathol* 23:118–123, 1994.

79. Skorupski KA, Clifford CA, Paoloni MC, et al: CCNU for the treatment of dogs with metastatic or disseminated histiocytic sarcoma. *Proc 23rd Annu Conf Vet Cancer Soc*:36, 2003.

80. Poirier VJ, Hershey AE, Burgess KE, et al: Efficacy and toxicity of paclitaxel (Taxol) for the treatment of canine malignant tumors. *J Vet Intern Med* 18:219–222, 2004.

81. Kerlin RL, Hendrick MJ: Malignant fibrous histiocytoma and malignant histiocytosis in the dog: Convergent or divergent phenotypic differentiation? *Vet Pathol* 33:713–716, 1996.

82. Pires MA: Malignant fibrous histiocytoma in a puppy. *Vet Rec* 140:234–235, 1997.

83. Craig LE, Julian ME, Ferracone JD: The diagnosis and prognosis of synovial tumors in dogs: 35 cases. *Vet Pathol* 39:66–73, 2002.

84. Hendrick MJ, Brooks JJ, Bruce EH: Six cases of malignant fibrous histiocytoma of the canine spleen. *Vet Pathol* 29:351–354, 1992.

85. Booth MJ, Bastianello SS, Jiminez M, van Heerden A: Malignant fibrous histiocytoma of the deep peri-articular tissue of the stifle in a dog. *J S Afr Vet Assoc* 69:163–168, 1998.

Chapter 43

Canine tumors of the skin and surrounding structures

CANINE CUTANEOUS SQUAMOUS CELL CARCINOMA

Clinical presentation

- Skin tumors common in dogs with non-pigmented skin and in those that have thin, short hair coat.
- May be painful.
- Ulcerated cutaneous lesions.
- Most often on the trunk (induced by sunlight; actinic).
- Most cutaneous squamous cell carcinomas are well differentiated and rarely metastasize.
- Digital (subungual) lesions are more likely to metastasize.
- Large, black-breed dogs are prone to subungual tumors.
- Light-skinned dogs are prone to actinically induced tumors.

> **Key point**
>
> Solar-induced squamous cell carcinoma is often found on the ventrum in regions of sparse hair coat and pink skin. They are often multiple, but they rarely metastasize.

> **Key point**
>
> Digital squamous cell carcinomas may metastasize to regional lymph nodes or lungs, and they may also be seen in larger black dogs.

Staging and diagnosis

- Minimum data base (MDB): includes a CBC, biochemical profile, urinalysis, biopsy and three-view thoracic radiographs, abdominal ultrasound or computerized tomography of the chest and abdomen if indicated.
- Careful examination of regional nodes for subungual.
- CT or MRI if involves nasal planum.

> **Key point**
>
> Chest radiographs and evaluation of all regional lymph nodes is important, especially in dogs with digital squamous cell carcinoma.

Prognostic factors

- Higher grade tumors are more likely to be invasive and, therefore, more difficult to excise; they are also more likely to metastasize.

Treatment

This section is divided into three options:
- Comfort for those who want to improve quality of life.
- Comfort and control for those who want to improve quality of life while trying to provide some control of the tumor.
- Comfort and longer-term control for those who want to improve quality of life while trying to maximize the chance of controlling the tumor.

> **Key point**
>
> Wide excision of the tumor is always ideal. Cryotherapy is optimal for small (<2 cm) cutaneous lesions. Radiation may be of value if other therapy is not appropriate or effective.

Comfort

- Therapy to enhance comfort and freedom from nausea, vomiting, diarrhea and lack of appetite.

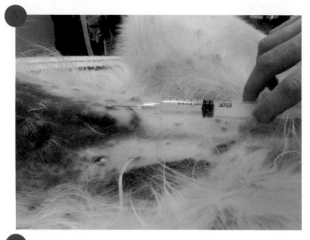

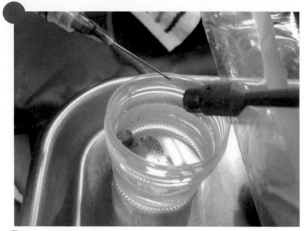

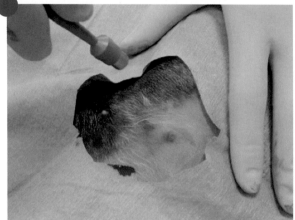

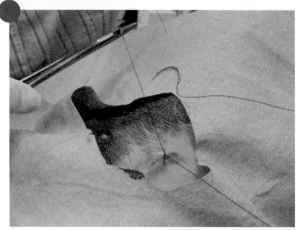

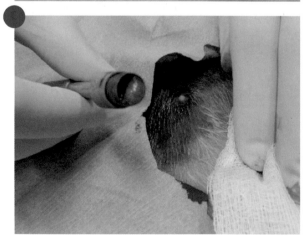

Figure 43-1: Obtaining a skin biopsy via a skin biopsy punch allows the surgeon to secure a histopathologic diagnosis, but it can in some cases actually remove small cutaneous lesions. The patient should be given local and systemic analgesics (A) after the local site is prepared for surgery. A biopsy punch of appropriate size is selected and placed in the skin (B). The biopsy punch is then rotated in one direction until a full thickness sample of the skin is secured (C) and the tissue is placed into formalin (D) prior to submission for a histopathologic diagnosis. A suture is placed for closure of the biopsy wound (E).

Piroxicam, docosahexaenoic acid, retinoids and sun avoidance and/or sunscreen may be helpful.

Comfort and control

Above mentioned therapy for comfort plus:
- Early cutaneous lesions are best treated with complete surgical excision, retinoids, topical 5-FU or BCNU ointments, and cryotherapy if lesions are <1 cm.
- Digital tumors are best treated with removal of the entire digit at least one joint above any evidence of the tumor.
- Nasal planum tumors may be best treated with removal of the tumor with an appropriate margin. This may involve removing the rostral maxilla as well.

Comfort and longer-term control

Above mentioned therapy for comfort plus:
- Surgical resection of the tumor(s) with evaluation and biopsy of regional lymph nodes followed by

definitive radiation therapy may be helpful (e.g.: 16-19 dosages of radiation).

- Cisplatin or mitoxantrone chemotherapy may be helpful to delay or prevent recurrence or metastases.

CANINE CUTANEOUS AND EXTRAMEDULLARY PLASMACYTOMAS

Clinical presentation

- Common.
- Generally not painful.
- Usually do not metastasize.
- Often multiple.
- Solitary cutaneous mass in trunk or limbs.
- May affect oral cavity, ears, and head; less commonly, may occur in multiple sites.
- Older dogs; cutaneous tumors are usually benign.

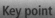

Key point

May present as cutaneous "wart-like" lesions around the head, mouth, ears and legs.

Staging and diagnosis

- Minimum data base (MDB): includes a CBC, biochemical profile, urinalysis, biopsy and three-view thoracic radiographs, abdominal ultrasound.

Prognostic factors

- Tumors with amyloid may be more likely to recur.

Treatment

This section is divided into two options:
- Comfort for those who want to improve quality of life.
- Comfort and control for those who want to improve quality of life while trying to provide some control of the tumor.
- Comfort and longer-term control for those who want to improve quality of life while trying to maximize the chance of controlling the tumor.

Key point

Surgery is the treatment of choice for extramedullary plasmacytomas of the skin.

Comfort

- Therapy to enhance comfort and freedom from nausea, vomiting, diarrhea and lack of appetite.

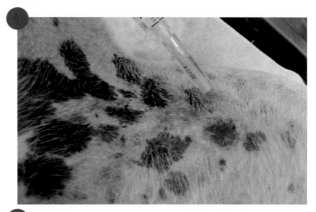

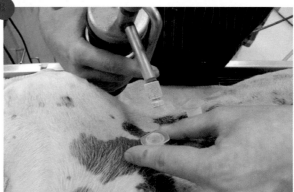

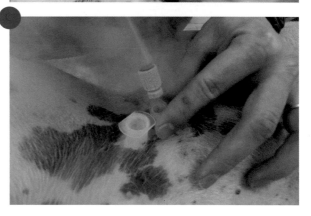

Figure 43-2: Solar induced squamous cell carcinoma is quite common in light skinned, poorly haired dogs (A). Excluding dogs at high risk of these tumors from sunlight is important. These tumors don't usually spread to lungs and lymph nodes but it is appropriate to stage them before proceeding with any therapeutics such as cryotherapy or surgery. In this patient, multiple small tumors were identified and treated first with systemic and local analgesia, and second with cryotherapy. A liquid nitrogen spray device is used. A 3 cc syringe barrel is cut in half and used to minimize the breadth of tissue to be frozen (B and C). Three quick freezes followed by slow, complete thaws is often quite effective. Additional lesions are often seen and if treated when they are small can be kept under control. Retinoids and NSAIDs have been used with some success to minimize progression and recurrence.

Comfort and control

Above mentioned therapy for comfort plus:
- Surgical resection of each tumor should be curative.
  - In one study, 11 dogs with extramedullary plasmacytomas died with a median survival time of 474 days.[11] The dogs without complete surgical removal of the EMP and no adjuvant therapy had a median survival time of 138 days.
- Chemotherapy with melphalan, prednisone, and doxorubicin have all caused tumor responses.

CANINE CUTANEOUS LYMPHOMA

Clinical presentation

- Common.
- May be uncomfortable locally.
- May be localized and treated that way, or multifocal requiring systemic therapy.
- Dogs with cutaneous epitheliotropic T-cell lymphoma have been reported to present with diffuse erythema (86.6%) with scaling (60%) and focal hypopigmentation (50%). The skin is often uniformly involved but muco-cutaneous junctions or mucosae were affected in 50% of cases.[117]
- T-cell variant is usually epitheliotropic and called mycosis fungoides.

Key point
The cutaneous lesions may present as a single lesion and are most commonly found around the mucocutaneous regions of the body, but most patients have multiple lesions that can result in crusty, scaly skin or large "mushroom-like" lesions that are red and inflamed.

Staging and diagnosis

- Minimum data base (MDB): includes a CBC, biochemical profile, urinalysis, biopsy bone marrow aspirate, three-view thoracic radiographs and abdominal ultrasound or computerized tomography of the chest and abdomen if indicated.
- Often systemic involvement is not seen until later stages.

Prognostic factors

- Dogs with cutaneous epitheliotropic T-cell lymphoma have a median survival of 6 months.

Treatment

This section is divided into three options:
- Comfort for those who want to improve quality of life.

- Comfort and control for those who want to improve quality of life while trying to provide some control of the tumor.
- Comfort and longer-term control for those who want to improve quality of life while trying to maximize the chance of controlling the tumor.

Key point
Surgery or radiation may be quite effective for localized lesions, however the more commonly noted multiple skin tumors are often best treated with CCNU-based chemotherapy protocols with retinoids such as isotretinoin.

Comfort

- Therapy to enhance comfort and freedom from nausea, vomiting, diarrhea and lack of appetite. Retinoids (e.g.: isotretinoin) may induce transient remissions in some patients with mycosis fungoides.

Comfort and control (see lymphoma)

Above mentioned therapy for comfort plus:
- Wide surgical resection of localized tumor(s) with evaluation and biopsy of regional lymph nodes if indicated.
- Definitive radiation therapy may be helpful alone for localized disease or in areas where surgical margins are inadequate (e.g.: 16-19 dosages of radiation).
- Chemotherapy with CCNU alone or with CCNU-enriched protocols is often quite helpful.

References

1. Goldschmidt MH, Shofer FS: Introduction. In Goldschmidt MH, Shofer FS (eds): *Skin Tumors of the Dog and Cat*, ed 1. Tarrytown NY, Pergamon Press, 1992, pp 1–10.
2. Pulley LT, Stannard AA: Tumors of the skin and soft tissues. In Moulton JE (ed): *Tumors in Domestic Animals*, ed 3. Berkeley, CA, University of California Press, 1990, pp 23–87.
3. Hahn KA, Lantz GC, Salisbury SK, et al: Comparison of survey radiography with ultrasonography and x-ray computed tomography for clinical staging of subcutaneous neoplasms in dogs. *JAVMA* 196:1795–1798, 1990.
4. Aitken ML, Patnaik AK: Comparison of needle-core (Tru-cut) biopsy and surgical biopsy for the diagnosis of cutaneous and subcutaneous masses: A prospective study of 51 cases (November 1997–August 1998). *JAAHA* 36:153–157, 2000.
5. Er JC, Sutton RH: A survey of skin neoplasms in dogs from the Brisbane region. *Aust Vet J* 66:225–227, 1989.
6. Rothwell TL, Howlett CR, Middleton DJ, et al: Skin neoplasms of dogs in Sydney. *Aust Vet J* 64:161–164, 1987.
7. Goldschmidt MH, Shofer FS: Cutaneous papillomas. In Goldschmidt MH, Shofer FS (eds): *Skin Tumors of the Dog and Cat*, ed 1. Tarrytown NY, Pergamon Press, 1992, pp 11–15.
8. Nicholls PK, Stanley MA: Canine papillomavirus: A centenary review. *J Comp Pathol* 120:219–233, 1999.
9. Wright ZM, Rogers KS, Mansell J. Survival data for canine oral extramedullary plasmacytomas: a retrospective analysis (1996-2006). *J Am Anim Hosp Assoc* 44(2):75-81, 2008.
10. Bregman CL, Hirth RS, Sundberg JP, Christensen EF: Cutaneous neoplasms in dogs associated with canine oral papillomavirus vaccine. *Vet Pathol* 24:477–487, 1987.
11. Goldschmidt MH, Shofer FS: Basal cell tumors and Basosquamous carcinomas. In Goldschmidt MH, Shofer FS (eds): *Skin Tumors of the Dog and Cat*, ed 1. Tarrytown NY, Pergamon Press, 1992, pp 16–36.

12. Stockhaus C, Teske E, Rudolph R, Werner HG: Assessment of cytological criteria for diagnosing basal cell tumours in the dog and cat. *J Small Anim Pract* 42:582–586, 2001.

13. Nikula KJ, Benjamin SA, Angleton GM, Saunders WJ, Lee AC: Ultraviolet radiation, solar dermatosis, and cutaneous neoplasia in beagle dogs. *Radiat Res* 129:11–18, 1992.

14. Goldschmidt MH, Shofer FS: Squamous cell carcinoma. In Goldschmidt MH, Shofer FS (eds): *Skin Tumors of the Dog and Cat*, ed 1. Tarrytown NY, Pergamon Press, 1992, pp 37–49.

15. Scott DW, Teixeira EAC: Multiple squamous cell carcinomas arising from multiple cutaneous follicular cysts in a dog. *Vet Dermatol* 6:27–31, 1995.

16. Scott DW, Miller WH Jr: Squamous cell carcinoma arising in chronic discoid lupus erythematosus nasal lesions in two German Shepherd dogs. *Vet Dermatol* 6:99–104, 1995.

17. Madewell BR, Conroy JD, Hodgkins EM: Sunlight-skin cancer association in the dog: A report of three cases. *J Cutan Pathol* 8:434–443, 1981.

18. Marks SL, Song MD, Stannard AA, Power HT: Clinical evaluation of etretinate for the treatment of canine solar-induced squamous cell carcinoma and preneoplastic lesions. *J Am Acad Dermatol* 27:11–16, 1992.

19. Pestili de Almeida EM, Piché C, Sirois J, Doré M: Expression of cyclo-oxygenase-2 in naturally occurring squamous cell carcinomas in dogs. *J Histochem Cytochem* 49:867–875, 2001.

20. Schmidt BR, Glickman NW, DeNicola DB, et al: Evaluation of piroxicam for the treatment of oral squamous cell carcinoma in dogs. *JAVMA* 218:1783–1786, 2001.

21. Gross TL, Brimacomb BH: Multifocal intraepidermal carcinoma in a dog histologically resembling Bowen's disease. *Am J Dermatopathol* 8:509–515, 1986.

22. Kitchell BE, Orenberg EK, Brown DM, et al: Intralesional sustained-release chemotherapy with therapeutic implants for treatment of canine sun-induced squamous cell carcinoma. *Eur J Cancer* 31(suppl A):2093–2098, 1995.

23. Orenberg EK, Luck EE, Brown DM, Kitchell BE: Implant delivery system: Intralesional delivery of chemotherapeutic agents for treatment of spontaneous skin tumors in veterinary patients. *Clin Dermatol* 9:561–568, 1992.

24. McCaw DL, Pope ER, Payne JT, et al: treatment of canine oral squamous cell carcinomas with photodynamic therapy. *Br J Cancer* 82:1297–1299, 2000.

25. Frimberger AE, Moore AS, Cincotta L, et al: Photodynamic therapy of naturally occurring tumors in animals using a novel benzophenothiazine photosensitizer. *Clin Cancer Res* 4:2207–2218, 1998.

26. Himsel CA, Richardson RC, Craig JA: Cisplatin chemotherapy for metastatic squamous cell carcinoma in two dogs. *JAVMA* 189:1575–1578, 1986.

27. Buhles WC, Theilen GH: Preliminary evaluation of bleomycin in feline and canine squamous cell carcinoma. *Am J Vet Res* 34:289–291, 1973.

28. Ogilvie GK, Obradovich JE, Elmslie RE, et al: Efficacy of mitoxantrone against various neoplasms in dogs. *JAVMA* 198:1618–1621, 1991.

29. Paradis M, Scott DW, Breton L: Squamous cell carcinoma of the nail bed in three related giant schnauzers. *Vet Rec* 125: 322–324, 1989.

30. Madewell BR, Pool RR, Theilen GH, Brewer WG: Multiple subungual squamous cell carcinomas in five dogs. *JAVMA* 180:731–734, 1982.

31. Guerin SR, Jones BR, Alley MR, Broome C: Multiple digital tumours in a rottweiler. *J Small Anim Pract* 39:200–202, 1998.

32. O'Brien MG, Berg J, Engler SJ: treatment by digital amputation of subungual squamous cell carcinoma in dogs: 21 cases (1987–1988). *JAVMA* 201:759–761, 1992.

33. Liu S-K, Hohn RB: Squamous cell carcinoma of the digit of the dog. *JAVMA* 153:411–424, 1968.

34. Brewer WG Jr, Mitley E, Ogilvie GK, et al: Canine digital tumors: retrospective review of 63 cases (1980–1990): A VCOG cooperative study—Preliminary results. *Vet Cancer Soc News* 2003.

35. Marino DJ, Matthiesen DT, Stefanacci JD, Moroff SD: Evaluation of dogs with digit masses: 117 cases (1981–1991). *JAVMA* 207:726–728, 1995.

36. Maiolino P, De Vico G, Restucci B: Expression of vascular endothelial growth factor in basal cell tumours and in squamous cell carcinomas of canine skin. *J Comp Pathol* 123:141–145, 2000.

37. Shapiro W, Kitchell BE, Fossum TW, et al: Cisplatin for treatment of transitional cell and squamous cell carcinomas in dogs. *JAVMA* 193:1530–1533, 1988.

38. Rogers KS, Helman RG, Walker MA: Squamous cell carcinoma of the canine nasal planum: eight cases (1988–1994). *JAAHA* 31:373–378, 1995.

39. Lascelles BDX, Parry AT, Stidworthy MF, Dobson JM, White RAS: Squamous cell carcinoma of the nasal planum in 17 dogs. *Vet Rec* 473–476, 2000.

40. Thrall DE, Adams WM: Radiotherapy of squamous cell carcinomas of the canine nasal plane. *Vet Radiol* 23:193–196, 1982.

41. Peters J, Scott DW, Erb HN, Miller WH: Hereditary nasal parakeratosis in Labrador retrievers: 11 new cases and a retrospective study on the presence of accumulations of serum ("serum lakes") in the epidermis of parakeratotic dermatoses and inflamed nasal plana of dogs. *Vet Dermatol* 14:197–203, 2003.

42. Theon AP, Madewell BR, Moore AS, et al: Localized thermocisplatin therapy: A pilot study in spontaneous canine and feline tumors. *Int J Hypertherm* 7:881–892, 1991.

43. Holt D, Prymak C, Evans S: Excision of tumors in the nasal vestibule of two dogs. *Vet Surg* 19:418–423, 1990.

44. Withrow SJ, Straw RC: Resection of the nasal planum in nine cats and five dogs. *JAAHA* 26:219–222, 1990.

45. Kirpensteijn J, Withrow SJ, Straw RC: Combined resection of the nasal planum and premaxilla in three dogs. *Vet Surg* 23:341–346, 1994.

46. Goldschmidt MH, Shofer FS: Sebaceous tumors. In Goldschmidt MH, Shofer FS (eds): *Skin Tumors of the Dog and Cat*, ed 1. Tarrytown NY, Pergamon Press, 1992, pp 50–65.

47. White SD, Rosychuk RA, Scott KV, et al: Sebaceous adenitis in dogs and results of treatment with isotretinoin and etretinate: 30 cases (1990–1994). *JAVMA* 207:197–200, 1995.

48. Kalaher KM, Anderson WI, Scott DW: Neoplasms of the apocrine sweat glands in 44 dogs and 10 cats. *Vet Record* 127:400–403, 1990.

49. Goldschmidt MH, Shofer FS: Apocrine gland tumors. In Goldschmidt MH, Shofer FS (eds): *Skin Tumors of the Dog and Cat*, ed 1. Tarrytown NY, Pergamon Press, 1992, pp 80–95.

50. Simko E, Wilcock BP, Yager JA: A retrospective study of 44 canine apocrine sweat gland adenocarcinomas. *Can Vet J* 44:38–42, 2003.

51. Kusters AH, Peperkamp KH, Hazewinkel HA: Atrichial sweat gland adenocarcinoma in the dog. *Vet Dermatol* 10:51–54, 1999.

52. Ogilvie GK, Reynolds HA, Richardson RC, et al: Phase II evaluation of doxorubicin for treatment of various canine neoplasms. *JAVMA* 195:1580–1583, 1989.

53. Goldschmidt MH, Shofer FS: Intracutaneous cornifying epithelioma. In Goldschmidt MH, Shofer FS (eds): *Skin Tumors of the Dog and Cat*, ed 1. Tarrytown NY, Pergamon Press, 1992, pp 109–114.

54. White SD, Rosychuk RA, Scott KV, et al: Use of isotretinoin and etretinate for the treatment of benign cutaneous neoplasia and cutaneous lymphoma in dogs. *JAVMA* 202:387–391, 1993.

55. Goldschmidt MH, Shofer FS: Trichoepithelioma. In Goldschmidt MH, Shofer FS (eds): *Skin Tumors of the Dog and Cat*, ed 1. Tarrytown NY, Pergamon Press, 1992, pp 115–124.

56. Goldschmidt MH, Shofer FS: Pilomatrixoma. In Goldschmidt MH, Shofer FS (eds): *Skin Tumors of the Dog and Cat*, ed 1. Tarrytown NY, Pergamon Press, 1992, pp 125–130.

57. Goldschmidt MH, Thrall DE, Jeglum KA, et al: Malignant pilomatricoma in a dog. *J Cutan Pathol* 8:375–381, 1981.

58. Rodriguez F, Herraez P, Rodriguez E, et al: Metastatic pilomatrixoma associated with neurological signs in a dog. *Vet Rec* 137:247–248, 1995.

59. Sells DM, Conroy JD: Malignant epithelial neoplasia with hair follicle differentiation in dogs. Malignant pilomatrixoma. *J Comp Pathol* 86:121–129, 1976.

60. Rodriguez F, Herráez P, Rodriguez E, et al: Metastatic pilomatrixoma associated with neurological signs in a dog. *Vet Rec* 137:247–248, 1995.

61. Lüttgenau H, Flaig K, Kirchhoff A: Malignes pilomatrixom bei einem hund. *Kleintierpraxis* 46:653–660, 2001.

62. Vascellari M, Mutinelli F, Cossettini R, Altinier E: Liposarcoma at the site of an implanted microchip in a dog. *Vet J* 168:188–190, 2004.

63. Goldschmidt MH, Shofer FS: Cutaneous lipoma and liposarcoma. In Goldschmidt MH, Shofer FS (eds): *Skin Tumors of the Dog and Cat*, ed 1. Tarrytown NY, Pergamon Press, 1992, pp 192–203.

64. Reimann N, Nolte I, Bonk U, et al: Cytogenetic investigation of canine lipomas. *Cancer Genet Cytogenet* 111:172–174, 1999.

65. Liggett AD, Frazier KS, Styer EL: Angiolipomatous tumors in dogs and cats. *Vet Pathol* 39:286–289, 2002.

66. Albers GW, Theilen GH: Calcium chloride for treatment of subcutaneous lipomas in dogs *JAVMA* 186:492–494, 1985.

67. Mayhew PD, Brockman DJ: Body cavity lipomas in six dogs. *J Small Anim Pract* 43:177–181, 2002.

68. Brown PJ, Lucke VM, Sozmen M, et al: Lipomatous infiltration of the canine salivary gland. *J Small Anim Pract* 38:234–236, 1997.

69. Bergman PJ, Withrow SJ, Straw RC, Powers BE: Infiltrative lipoma in dogs: 16 cases (1981–1992). *JAVMA* 205:322–324, 1994.

70. Saik JE, Diters RW, Wortman JA: Metastasis of a well-differentiated liposarcoma in a dog and a note on nomenclature of fatty tumours. *J Comp Pathol* 97:369–373, 1987.

71. McEntee MC, Thrall DE: Computed tomographic imaging of infiltration lipoma in 22 dogs. *Vet Radiol Ultrasound* 42:221–225, 2001.

72. McChesney AE, Stephens LC, Lebel J, et al: Infiltrative lipoma in dogs. *Vet Pathol* 17:316–322, 1980.

73. Kramek BA, Spackman CJA, Hayden DW: Infiltrative lipoma in three dogs. *JAVMA* 186:81–82, 1985.

74. Thomson MJ, Withrow SJ, Dernell WS, Powers BE: Intermuscular lipomas of the thigh region in dogs: 11 cases. *JAAHA* 35:165–167, 1999.

75. McEntee MC, Page RL, Mauldin GN, Thrall DE: Results of irradiation of infiltrative lipoma in 13 dogs. *Vet Radiol Ultrasound* 41:554–556, 2000.

76. McCarthy PE, Hedlund CS, Veazy RS, et al: Liposarcoma associated with a glass foreign body in a dog. *JAVMA* 209:612–614, 1996.

77. Strafuss AC, Bozarth AJ: Liposarcoma in dogs. *JAAHA* 9: 183–187, 1973.

78. Baez JL, Hendrick MJ, Shofer FS, et al: Liposarcomas in dogs: 56 cases (1989–2000). *JAVMA* 224:887–891, 2004.

79. Bozarth AJ, Strafuss AC: Metastatic liposarcoma in a dog. *JAVMA* 162:1043–1044, 1973.

80. Zwicker GM: Liposarcoma in a dog. *Pathol Vet* 7:145–147, 1970.

81. Davis PE, Dixon RT, Johnson JA, Paris R: Multiple liposarcoma of bone marrow origin in a Greyhound. *J Small Anim Pract* 15:445–456, 1974.

82. Meierhenry EF: Metastatic liposarcoma with extensive osteolysis in the dog. *JAAHA* 10:478–481, 1974.

83. Konno A, Nagata M, Nanko H: Immunohistochemical diagnosis of a merkel cell tumor in a dog. *Vet Pathol* 35:538–540, 1998.

84. Duncan JR, Prasse KW: Cytology of canine cutaneous round cell tumors. Mast cell tumor, histiocytoma, lymphosarcoma and transmissible venereal tumor. *Vet Pathol* 16:673–679, 1979.

85. Sandusky GE, Carlton WW, Wightman KA: Diagnostic immunohistochemistry of canine round cell tumors. *Vet Pathol* 24:495–499, 1987.

86. Lucke VM: Primary cutaneous plasmacytomas in the dog and cat. *J Small Anim Pract* 28:49–55, 1987.

87. Clark GN, Berg J, Engler SJ, Bronson RT: Extramedullary plasmacytomas in dogs: results of surgical excision in 131 cases. *JAAHA* 28:105–111, 1992.

88. Rakich PM, Latimer KS, Weiss R, Steffans WL: Mucocutaneous plasmacytomas in dogs: 75 cases (1980–1987). *JAVMA* 194:803–810, 1989.

89. Baer KE, Patnaik AK, Gilbertson SR, Hurvitz AI: Cutaneous plasmacytomas in dogs: A morphologic and immunohistochemical study. *Vet Pathol* 26:216–221, 1989.

90. Rowland PH, Valentine BA, Stebbons KE, Smith CA: Cutaneous plasmacytomas with amyloid in six dogs. *Vet Pathol* 28:125–130, 1991.

91. Walton GS, Gopinath C: Multiple myeloma in a dog with some unusual features. *J Small Anim Pract* 13:703–708, 1972.

92. Goldschmidt MH, Shofer FS: Cutaneous plasmacytoma. In Goldschmidt MH, Shofer FS (eds): *Skin Tumors of the Dog and Cat*, ed 1. Tarrytown NY, Pergamon Press, 1992, pp 265–270.

93. Brener W, Colbatzky F, Platz S, Hermanns W: Immunoglobulin-producing tumours in dogs and cats. *J Comp Pathol* 109:203–216, 1993.

94. Trigo FJ, Hargis AM: Canine cutaneous plasmacytoma with regional lymph node metastasis. *Vet Med Small Anim Clin* 78:1749–1751, 1983.

95. Platz SJ, Breuer W, Pfleghaar S, et al: Prognostic value of histopathological grading in canine extramedullary plasmacytomas. *Vet Pathol* 36:23–27, 1999.

96. Morton LD, Barton CL, Ellissalde GS, Wilson SR: Oral extramedullary plasmacytoma in two dogs. *Vet Pathol* 26: 637–639, 1986.

97. Brunnert SR, Dee LA, Herron AJ, Altman NH: Gastric extramedullary plasmacytoma in a dog *JAVMA* 200:1501–1502, 1992.

98. Goldschmidt MH, Shofer FS: Cutaneous lymphosarcoma. In Goldschmidt MH, Shofer FS (eds): *Skin Tumors of the Dog and Cat*, ed 1. Tarrytown NY, Pergamon Press, 1992, pp 252–264.

99. Day MJ: Immunophenotypic characterization of cutaneous lymphoid neoplasia in the dog and cat. *J Comp Pathol* 112: 79–96, 1995.

100. Kleiter M, Wagner R, Day MJ: Eine generalisierte demodikose in verbindung mit einem kutanen B-zell lymphosarkom beim adulten hund. *Kleintierpraxis* 43:537–548, 1998.

101. Ridyard AE, Rhind SM, French AT, et al: Myasthenia gravis associated with cutaneous lymphoma in a dog. *J Small Anim Pract* 41:348–351, 2000.

102. O'Brown NO, Nesbitt GH, Patnaik AK, MacEwen EG: Cutaneous lymphosarcoma in the dog: A disease with variable clinical and histologic manifestations. *JAAHA* 16:565–572, 1980.

103. Graham JC, Myers RK: Pilot study of the use of lomustine (CCNU) for the treatment of cutaneous lymphoma in dogs. *J Vet Intern Med* 13, 257. 1999.

104. Foster AP, Evans E, Kerlin RL, Vail DM: Cutaneous T-cell lymphoma with Sezary syndrome in a dog. *Vet Clin Pathol* 26: 188–192, 1997.

105. Thrall MA, Macy DW, Snyder SP, Hall RL: Cutaneous lymphosarcoma and leukemia in a dog resembling Sezary syndrome in man. *Vet Pathol* 21:182–186, 1984.

106. DeBoer DJ, Turrel JM, Moore PF: Mycosis fungoides in a dog: Demonstration of T-cell specificity and response to radiotherapy. *JAAHA* 26:566–572, 1990.

107. Donaldson D, Day MJ: Epitheliotropic lymphoma (mycosis fungoides) presenting as blepharoconjunctivitis in an Irish setter. *J Small Anim Pract* 41:317–320, 2000.

108. Czasch S, Risse K, Baumgartner W: Central nervous system metastasis of a cutaneous epitheliotropic lymphosarcoma in a dog. *J Comp Pathol* 123:59–63, 2000.

109. Brain PH, Howlett CR: Two cases of epidermotropic lymphoma in dogs. *Aust Vet J* 68:247–248, 1991.

110. McKeever PJ, Grindem CB, Stevens JB, Osborne CA: Canine cutaneous lymphoma. *JAVMA* 180:531–536, 1982.

111. Iwamoto KS, Bennett LR, Norman A, et al: Linoleate produces remission in canine mycosis fungoides. *Cancer Lett* 64:17–22, 1992.

112. Williams LE, Rassnick KM, Power H, et al:. CCNU (Lomustine) for the treatment of canine epitheliotropic lymphoma. *J Vet Intern Med* 2006, in press.

113. Risbon R, Burgess K, Skorupski K, et al: Response of epitheliotropic lymphoma to CCNU. *Proc 24th Annu Conf Vet Cancer Soc* 2004.

114. Lemarié SL, Eddlestone SM: treatment of cutaneous T-cell lymphoma with dacarbazine in a dog. *Vet Dermatol* 8:41–46, 1997

115. Moriello KA, MacEwen G, Schultz KT: PEG-L-asparaginase in the treatment of canine epitheliotropic lymphoma and histiocytic proliferative dermatitis. In Ihrke, PJ, Mason, IS, White SD (eds): *Advances in Vet Dermatology*, vol 2. Tarrytown, NY, Pergamon Press, 1992.

116. Prescott DM, Gordon J: Total skin electron beam irradiation for generalized cutaneous lymphoma. *Proc 24th Annu Conf Vet Cancer Soc* 2004.

117. Fontaine J, Heimann M, Day MJ. Canine cutaneous epitheliotropic T-cell lymphoma: a review of 30 cases. *Vet Dermatol* 21(3):267-275, 2010.

Chapter 44

Canine mast cell tumors

Clinical presentation

- Very common.
- Generally not painful, but can be itchy due to release of histamines.
- Raised or ulcerated intracutaneous mass. May be hairless or haired, single or multiple.
- Mast cell tumors can look and feel like anything!
- Most do not metastasize.
- Most patients are cured with appropriate therapy (surgery and/or radiation).
- Bulldog-derived breeds (Boxers, Boston terriers) and golden retrievers are predisposed, but MCTs can occur in any breed and at any age.

> **Key point**
>
> Mast cell tumors may be single or multiple, and they are often noted to increase and decrease in size.

Staging and diagnosis

- Metastasis similar to other hematopoietic tumors: to regional lymph nodes as well as to liver, spleen, and bone marrow.
- Minimum data base (MDB): includes a CBC, biochemical profile, urinalysis, biopsy and three-view thoracic radiographs or computerized tomography of the chest.
- Ultrasonography with aspirates of liver, spleen, enlarged lymph nodes and bone marrow. Liver and spleen aspirates should be secured regardless of the ultrasound findings. Bone marrow aspirates are recommended regardless of the results of the hemogram.

> **Key point**
>
> High grade mast cell tumors can and do metastasize to the liver, spleen, lymph nodes and bone marrow. Blood work, abdominal ultrasound and aspiration of the regional or enlarged lymph nodes, liver, spleen and bone marrow may be indicated.

Prognostic factors

- Tumors on limbs have better prognosis than trunk.
- Slow growth and long duration of presence may be favorable.
- Complete surgical margins are associated with long control.
- The most important prognostic factor is histologic grade.
  - The three-tier (grade I-III) Patnaik grading system is commonly used and has been shown to be predictive of survival, although it is subjective.
  - To improve concordance among pathologists and to provide better prognostic significance, a two-tier histologic grading system was devised. High-grade mast cell tumors are associated with shorter time to metastasis or new tumor development, and with shorter survival time (4 months) vs. low-grade tumors (>2 years).
- Intestinal location is associated with high a metastatic rate and poor prognosis.

Treatment

There are many options for the treatment of mast cell tumors. The general overview of the optimal approach is as follows:

- Patnaik grade I/II tumors (low-grade tumors on the two tier grading system)[69]: Wide surgical excision.
- Patnaik grade II tumors (the more well differentiated of which are low-grade tumors on the two tier grading system): Wide surgical excision; adjunctive radiation therapy if incompletely excised (86% achieve 5-year control); chemotherapy only with incompletely excised, disseminated or metastatic disease: vinblastine, lomustine (CCNU), paclitaxel, chlorambucil and prednisone appear to be most active agents.
- Patnaik grade II/III tumors (high-grade tumors on the two tier grading system): Surgery with or without radiation therapy to the regional lymph node may provide local control; chemotherapy is strongly encouraged.

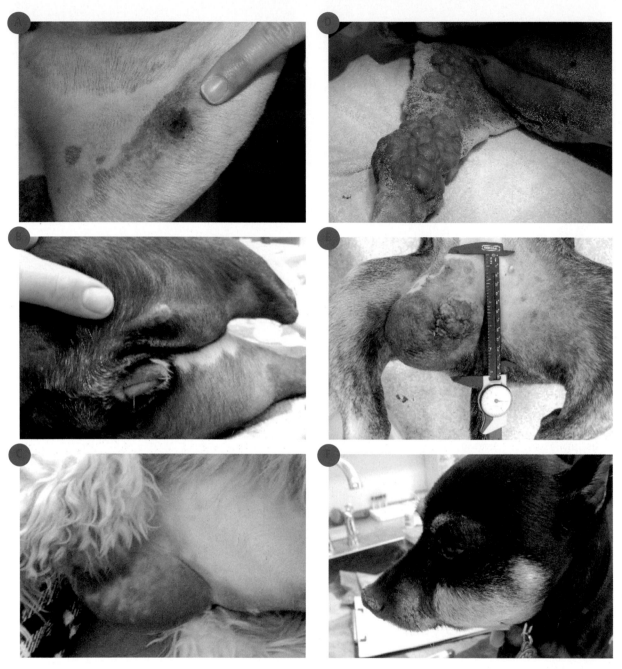

Figure 44-1: Mast cell tumors are often called the great imposters because they can look like anything (A-F). This tumor type is very common but it is different than almost any other tumor in the dog because it may cause bruising, bleeding, swelling, inflammation and stomach ulcers. The dog depicted in figure F has a tiny mast cell tumor yet his head is completely swollen due to the consequences of the tiny mast cell tumor. There are two grading schemes use to predict outcome. The more recent two tiered grading system separates the tumors into those that are relatively well behaved (grade 1) vs those that are more aggressive grade II) with a higher risk of metastases, recurrence and a shorter survival time. Mast cell tumors may spread to liver, spleen, lymph node and bone marrow. This is one tumor that has a characteristic cell type with metachromatic granules (B-D) A normal abdominal ultrasound (A) and complete blood count does not provide assurance that the tumor has not spread to liver, spleen lymph node or bone marrow. Only an aspirate of these tissues can enhance confidence that the disease has not metastasized to these sites. Essentially, the clinician must decide if the disease is localized or if it is systemic. If localized, then the primary tumor type can be controlled with wide and deep surgery, radiation therapy or medical management (e.g.: tyrosine kinase receptor antagonists, vinblastine and/or CCNU). Regardless, supportive care should be considered by giving docosahexaenoic acid, famotidine, prednisone, and if needed, diphenhydramine. Ultimately, it should be remembered that with appropriate therapy, most mast cell tumors can be cured or controlled long term.

The remainder of this section is divided into three options:

- Comfort for those who want to improve quality of life.
- Comfort and control for those who want to improve quality of life while trying to provide some control of the tumor.
- Comfort and longer-term control for those who want to improve quality of life while trying to maximize the chance of controlling the tumor.

> **Key point**
>
> Most mast cell tumors are cured with wide and deep surgical excision, however those that are not completely resectable can respond quite well to medical therapy (tyrosine kinase inhibitors and/or vinblastine) and/or radiation therapy.

Comfort

- Therapy to enhance comfort and freedom from nausea, vomiting, diarrhea and lack of appetite. Pepcid and H2 receptor antagonists or proton pump inhibitors may be helpful.

Comfort and control

Above mentioned therapy for comfort plus:
- Tyrosine cinase inhibitors (TKI):
  - Toceranib (Palladia®) (2.5-2.8 mg/kg PO Monday, Wednesday and Friday).
  - Masitinib (Masivet®, Kinavet®) 12.5 mg/kg PO q 24 h.
  - Imatinib (Gleevec®) 5 to 10 mg/kg PO q 24 h.

Comfort and longer-term control

Above mentioned therapy for comfort plus:
- Surgical resection of the tumor(s) with evaluation and biopsy of regional lymph nodes.
  - The outcomes of dogs with mast cell tumors that had incomplete or close surgical resection were evaluated after additional local therapy (primary re-excision or radiation therapy) or no additional local therapy.[69] Median survival times for the dogs that a re-excision of the tumor (2930 days) or radiation therapy (2194 days) were significantly longer than those that did not have surgery or radiation (710 days).
  - The outcome of 21 dogs with grade II mast cell tumors with regional lymph node metastases treated with adequate local therapy and adjuvant systemic chemotherapy (prednisone, vinblastine and CCNU) were assessed to find that the median survival and disease-free interval for all dogs was 1359 and 2120 days, respectively.[70] Dogs treated with surgery and chemotherapy had shorter survival (median, 1103 days) than those that underwent surgery, radiation therapy and

chemotherapy as part of their treatment (median, 2056 days).
- Definitive radiation therapy may be helpful if excision is incomplete or questionable (e.g.: 16-19 dosages of radiation).
  - Tyrosine kinase inhibitors or chemotherapy can be included for high-grade tumors, if radiation therapy is not desired or if there is confirmed metastatic disease.
- Chemotherapy.
  - Prednisone and vinblastine.
    - Prednisone: 2 mg/kg PO q 24 h.
    - Vinblastine: 2 mg/m² IV q weekly for 5 weeks, followed by 5 treatments every 2 weeks.
    - Continue vinblastine 2 mg/m² IV q 2 weeks for as long as appears to have an objective response. Taper and discontinue prednisone over 12–26 weeks.
    - Prednisone and vinblastine chemotherapy was shown to be well tolerated with good outcomes following surgery in dogs with mast cell tumors at high risk for metastasis.[71] The disease-free interval was 1305 days, and the overall survival time was not reached, with 65% alive at 3 years. The overall survival time for dogs with grade III mast cell tumors was 1374 days.
    - The survival outcome of 94 dogs with high metastatic risk mast cell tumors treated with a cytotoxic chemotherapy protocol or the tyrosine kinase inhibitor masitinib, in the presence of gross disease or as an adjunct to surgical resection of the primary tumor was assessed.[72] Dogs with metastatic disease that has the primary tumor surgically removed followed with adjunctive therapy with any chemotherapy incurred a significant survival advantage (median survival time: 278 days) compared to patients receiving chemotherapy without surgical excision of the primary tumor (median survival time: 91 days). Those dogs with surgically excised Patnaik grade II tumor and high Ki-67 in the absence of metastatic disease treated with vinblastine and prednisolone showed a significantly longer survival (median survival time: 1946 days) than those treated with masitinib (median survival time: 369 days).
    - In another study, 26 dogs with non resectable and metastatic mast cell tumors were treated with masitinib.[72,73] The overall response rate to masitinib was 50%. The median survival time for dogs that responded to masitinib was 630 days versus 137 days for dogs that did not respond.
    - Dogs with measurable mast cell tumors amenable to radiation therapy were treated.[74] The combination of toceranib, prednisone,

and hypofractionated radiation treatment was well tolerated and efficacious with an overall response rate was 76.4%, with 58.8% of dogs achieving a complete response. The median progression-free interval was 316 days and the overall median survival time was not reached with a median follow-up of 374 days.

- CCNU (lomustine): 60–80 mg/m² PO q 21 days.
- Vinblastine and CCNU (lomustine).
  - Vinblastine: 2 mg/m² IV week 1, then every 4 weeks.
  - CCNU (lomustine): 60 mg/m² PO week 3, then every 4 weeks.
- CVP: CCNU, vinblastine, prednisone.
  - Vinblastine: 2 mg/m² IV week 1, then every 4 weeks.
  - CCNU (lomustine): 60-70 mg/m² PO week 3, then every 4 weeks.
  - Prednisone: 0.5 mg/kg PO q 48 hours.
- Cremophor-free formulation of paclitaxel (Paccal Vet®): 145 mg/m² IV once every 21 days for three cycles.
- Chlorambucil and prednisone.
  - Chlorambucil: 6 mg/m² PO daily.
  - Prednisone: 0.5-1 mg/kg PO q 24 hours.

References

1. Macy DW: Canine and feline mast cell tumors: biologic behavior, diagnosis, and therapy. *Semin Vet Med Surg (Small Anim)* 1:72–83, 1986.
2. Goldschmidt MH, Shofer FS: Mast cell tumors. In Goldschmidt MH, Shofer FS (eds): *Skin Tumors of the Dog and Cat*, ed 1. Tarrytown NY, Pergamon Press, 1992, 1992, pp 231–251.
3. Miller DM: The occurrence of mast cell tumors in young Shar-Peis. *J Vet Diagn Invest* 7:360–363, 1995.
4. London CA, Kisseberth WC, Galli SJ, G, et al: Expression of stem cell factor receptor (c-kit) by the malignant mast cells from spontaneous canine mast cell tumours. *J Comp Pathol* 115:399–414, 1996.
5. Zemke D, Yamini B, Yuzbasiyan-Gurkan V: Mutations in the juxtamembrane domain of c-KIT are associated with higher grade mast cell tumors in dogs. *Vet Pathol* 39:529–535, 2002.
6. Downing S, Chien MB, Kass PH, et al: Prevalence and importance of internal tandem duplications in exons 11 and 12 of ckit in mast cell tumors of dogs. *Am J Vet Res* 63:1718–1723, 2002.
7. Zemke D, Yamini B, Yuzbasiyan-Gurkan V: Characterization of an undifferentiated malignancy as a mast cell tumor using mutation analysis in the proto-oncogene c-KIT. *J Vet Diagn Invest* 13:341–345, 2001.
8. Sato AF, Solano M: Ultrasonographic findings in abdominal mast cell disease: A retrospective study of 19 patients. *Vet Radiol Ultrasound* 45:51–57, 2004.
9. Bookbinder PF, Butt MT, Harvey HJ: Determination of the number of mast cells in lymph node, bone marrow, and buffy coat cytologic specimens from dogs. *JAVMA* 200:1648–1650, 1992.
10. O'Keefe DA, Couto CG, Burke-Schwartz C, Jacobs RM: Systemic mastocytosis in 16 dogs. *J Vet Intern Med* 1:75–80, 1987.
11. Endicott MM, Charney SC, McKnight JA, Bergman PJ: Incidence of bone marrow infiltration and hematologic abnormalities in canine cutaneous mast cell tumors: 157 cases (1999–2002). *Proc 23rd Annu Conf Vet Cancer Soc:*22, 2003.
12. Howard EB, Sawa TR, Nielsen SW, Kenyon AJ: Mastocytoma and gastroduodenal ulceration. Gastric and duodenal ulcers in dogs with mastocytoma. *Pathol Vet* 6:146–158, 1969.
13. McManus PM: Frequency and severity of mastocytemia in dogs with and without mast cell tumors: 120 cases (1995–1997). *JAVMA* 215:355–357, 1999.
14. Gerritsen RJ, Teske E, Kraus JS, Rutteman GR: Multi-agent chemotherapy for mast cell tumours in the dog. *Vet Quart* 20:28–31, 1998.
15. Sfiligoi G, Rassnick KM, Scarlett JM, et al: Outcome of dogs with mast cell tumors in the inguinal or perineal region versus other cutaneous locations: 124 cases (1990–2001). *JAVMA* 226:1368–1374, 2005.
16. Bostock DE: The prognosis following surgical removal of mastocytomas in dogs. *J Small Anim Pract* 14:27–41, 1973.
17. Strefezzi RF, Xavier JG, Catao-Dias JL: Morphometry of canine cutaneous mast cell tumors. *Vet Pathol* 40:268–275, 2003.
18. Hottendorf, GH, Nielsen SW: Pathologic study of 300 extirpated canine mastocytomas. *Zbl Vet Med* A14, 272–281, 1967.
19. Patnaik AK, Ehler WJ, MacEwen EG: Canine cutaneous mast cell tumor: morphologic grading and survival time in 83 dogs. *Vet Pathol* 21:469–474, 1984.
20. Gieger TL, Theon AP, Werner JA, et al: Biologic behavior and prognostic factors for mast cell tumors of the canine muzzle: 24 cases (1990–2001). *J Vet Intern Med* 17:687–692, 2003.
21. Baker-Gabb M, Hunt GB, France MP: Soft tissue sarcomas and mast cell tumours in dogs; clinical behaviour and response to surgery. *Aust Vet J* 81:732–738, 2003.
22. Murphy S, Sparkes AH, Smith KC, et al: Relationships between the histological grade of cutaneous mast cell tumours in dogs, their survival and the efficacy of surgical resection. *Vet Rec* 154:743–746, 2004.
23. Northrup NC, Howerth EW, Harmon BG, et al: Variation among pathologists in histopathologic grading of canine cutaneous mast cell tumors. *Proc 23rd Annu Conf Vet Cancer Soc:*73, 2003.
24. Séguin B, Leibman NF, Bregazzi VS, et al: Clinical outcome of dogs with grade-II mast cell tumors treated with surgery alone: 55 cases (1996–1999). *JAVMA* 218:1120–1123, 2001.
25. Davies DR, Wyatt KM, Jardine JE, et al: Vinblastine and prednisolone as adjunctive therapy for canine cutaneous mast cell tumors. *JAAHA* 40:124–130, 2004.
26. Michels GM, Knapp DW, DeNicola DB, et al: Prognosis following surgical excision of canine cutaneous mast cell tumors with histopathologically tumor-free versus nontumor-free margins: A retrospective study of 31 cases. *JAAHA* 38:458–466, 2002.
27. Turrel JM, Kitchell BE, Miller LM, Theon A: Prognostic factors for radiation treatment of mast cell tumor in 85 dogs. *JAVMA* 193:936–940, 1988.
28. Weisse C, Shofer FS, Sorenmo K: Recurrence rates and sites for grade II canine cutaneous mast cell tumors following complete surgical excision. *JAAHA* 38:71–73, 2002.
29. Cahalane AK, Payne S, Barber LG, et al: Prognostic factors for survival of dogs with inguinal and perineal mast cell tumors treated with surgery with or without adjunctive treatment. 68 cases. *JAVMA* 225:401–408, 2004.
30. Murphy S, Sparkes AH, Blunden AS, et al: Canine cutaneous mast cell tumours: Do dogs with multiple tumours have a poorer prognosis? *Vet Rec* 2006, in press.
31. Mullins M, Dernell W, Ehrhart E, et al: Multiple cutaneous canine mast cell tumors: A retrospective analysis. *Proc 24th Annu Conf Vet Cancer Soc:*13, 2004.
32. Bostock DE, Crocker J, Harris K, Smith P: Nucleolar organizer regions as indicators of post-surgical prognosis in canine spontaneous mast cell tumours. *Br J Cancer* 59:915–918, 1989.
33. Kravis LD, Vail DM, Kisseberth WC, et al: Frequency of argyrophilic nucleolar organizer regions in fine-needle aspirates and biopsy specimens from mast cell tumors in dogs. *JAVMA* 209:1418–1420, 1996.
34. Simoes JPC, Schoning P, Butine M: Prognosis of canine mast cell tumors: A comparison of three methods. *Vet Pathol* 31:637–647, 1994.
35. Abadie JJ, Amardeilh MA, Delverdier ME: Immunohistochemical detection of proliferating cell nuclear antigen and Ki-67 in mast cell tumors from dogs. *JAVMA* 15:1629–1634, 1999
36. Sakai H, Noda A, Shirai N, et al: Proliferative activity of canine mast cell tumours evaluated by bromodeoxyuridine incorporation and Ki-67 expression. *J Comp Pathol* 127:233–238, 2002.
37. Ayl RD, Couto CG, Hammer AS, Weisbrode S, Ericson JG, Mathes L: Correlation of DNA ploidy to tumor histologic grade, clinical variables, and survival in dogs with mast cell tumors. *Vet Pathol* 29:386–390, 1992.
38. Kiupel M, Webster JD, Kaneene JB, et al: The use of KIT and tryptase expression patterns as prognostic tools for canine cutaneous mast cell tumors. *Vet Pathol* 41:371–377, 2004.
39. Leibman NF, Lana SE, Hansen RA, et al: Identification of matrix metalloproteinases in canine cutaneous mast cell tumors. *J Vet Intern Med* 14:583–586, 2000.
40. Ginn PE, Fox LE, Brower JC, et al: Immunohistochemical detection of p53 tumor-suppressor protein is a poor indicator of prognosis for canine cutaneous mast cell tumors. *Vet Pathol* 37:33–39, 2000.
41. Jaffe MH, Hosgood G: Immunohistochemical and clinical evaluation of p53 in canine cutaneous mast cell tumors. *Vet Pathol* 37:40–46, 2000.
42. Davis BJ, Page R, Sannes PL, Meuten DJ: Cutaneous mastocytosis in a dog. *Vet Pathol* 29:363–365, 1992.

43. Simpson AM, Ludwig LL, Newman SJ, et al: Evaluation of surgical margins required for complete excision of cutaneous mast cell tumors in dogs. *JAVMA* 224:236–240, 2004.
44. Slusher R, Roengik WJ, Wilson GP: Effect of x-irradiation on mastocytoma in dogs. *JAVMA* 151:1049–1054, 1967.
45. LaDue T, Price S, Dodge R, et al: Radiation therapy for incompletely resected canine mast cell tumors. *Vet Radiol Ultrasound* 39:57–62, 1998.
46. Al Sarraf R, Mauldin GN, Patnaik AK, Meleo KA: A prospective study of radiation therapy for the treatment of grade 2 mast cell tumors in 32 dogs. *J Vet Intern Med* 10:376–378, 1996.
47. Frimberger AE, Moore AS, LaRue SM, et al: Radiotherapy of incompletely resected, moderately differentiated mast cell tumors in the dog: 37 cases (1989–1993). *JAAHA* 33:320–324, 1997.
48. Northrup NC, Roberts RE, Harrell TW, et al: Iridium-192 interstitial brachytherapy as adjunctive treatment for canine cutaneous mast cell tumors. *JAAHA* 40:309–315, 2004.
49. Chaffin K, Thrall DE: Results of radiation therapy in 19 dogs with cutaneous mast cell tumor and regional lymph node metastasis. *Vet Radiol Ultrasound* 43:392–395, 2002.
50. Hahn KA, King GK, Carreras JK: Efficacy of radiation therapy for incompletely resected grade-III mast cell tumors in dogs: 31 cases (1987–1998). *JAVMA* 224:79–82, 2004.
51. Dobson J, Cohen S, Gould S: treatment of canine mast cell tumours with prednisolone and radiotherapy. *Vet Compar Oncol* 2:132–141, 2004.
52. Grier RL, Di Guardo G, Schaffer CB, et al: Mast cell tumor destruction by deionized water. *Am J Vet Res* 51:1116–1120, 1990.
53. Grier RL, DiGuardo G, Myers R, Merkley DF: Mast cell tumour destruction in dogs by hypotonic solution. *J Small Anim Pract* 36:385–388, 1995.
54. Jaffe MH, Hosgood G, Kerwin SC, et al Deionised water as an adjunct to surgery for the treatment of canine cutaneous mast cell tumours. *J Small Anim Pract* 41:7–11, 2000.
55. Takahashi T, Kadosawa T, Nagase M, et al: Inhibitory effects of glucocorticoids on proliferation of canine mast cell tumor. *J Vet Med Sci* 59:995–1001, 1997.
56. McCaw DL, Miller MA, Ogilvie GK, et al: Response of canine mast cell tumors to treatment with oral prednisone. *J Vet Intern Med* 8:406–408, 1994.
57. Miyoshi N, Tojo E, Oishi A, et al: Immunohistochemical detection of P-glycoprotein (PGP) and multidrug resistance-associated protein (MRP) in canine cutaneous mast cell tumors. *J Vet Med Sci* 64:531–533, 2002.
58. Thamm DH, Mauldin EA, Vail DM: Prednisone and vinblastine chemotherapy for canine mast cell tumor: 41 cases (1992–1997). *J Vet Intern Med* 13:491–497, 1999.
59. Santoro SK, Chun R, Garret, LD: Vinblastine and prednisone for the treatment of grade 2 mast cell tumors in dogs. *Proc 24th Annu Conf Vet Cancer Soc.*10, 2004.

60. Elmslie RE: Combination chemotherapy with and without surgery for dogs with high-grade mast cell tumors with regional lymph node metastases. *Vet Cancer Soc Newsletter* 20:6–7, 1997.
61. Rassnick KM, Moore AS, Williams LE, et al: treatment of canine mast cell tumors with CCNU (lomustine). *J Vet Intern Med* 13:601–605, 1999.
62. McCaw DL, Miller MA, Bergman PJ, et al: Vincristine therapy for mast cell tumors in dogs. *J Vet Intern Med* 11:375–378, 1997.
63. Hardy WD Jr, Old LJ: L-asparaginase in the treatment of neoplastic diseases of the dog, cat and cow. *Cancer Res* 33:131–139, 1970.
64. Legrand J-J, Carlier B, Parodi A-L: Apport de la cytologie au diagnostic, au pronostic et au suivi thérapeuticque du mastocytome chez le chien. *Bull Acad Vet* 60:269–278, 1987.
65. Hershey AE, Jones PD, Klein MK: Evaluation of combination vinblastine, lomustine and prednisone for the treatment of canine mast cell tumors. *Proc 23rd Annu Conf Vet Cancer Soc.*71, 2003.
66. Bennett P, Langova V: Response of mast cell tumours to combination therapy with lomustine and vinblastine. *Proc 24th Annu Conf Vet Cancer Soc.*76, 2004.
67. Owen LN, Lewis JC, Morgan DR, Gorman NT: The effects of *Corynebacterium parvum* in dogs and a study of its distribution following intravenous injection. *Eur J Cancer* 16:999–1005, 1980.
68. Tinsley PE Jr, Taylor DO: Immunotherapy for multicentric malignant mastocytoma in a dog. *Mod Vet Pract* 225–228, 1987.
69. Kry KL, Boston SE. Additional local therapy with primary re-excision or radiation therapy improves survival and local control after incomplete or close surgical excision of mast cell tumors in dogs. *Vet Surg* 43(2):182-189, 2014.
70. Lejeune A, Skorupski K, Frazier S, et al: Aggressive local therapy combined with systemic chemotherapy provides long-term control in grade II stage 2 canine mast cell tumour: 21 cases (1999-2012). *Vet Comp Oncol* doi: 10.1111/vco.12042, 2013.
71. Miller RL, Van Lelyveld S, Warland J, et al: A retrospective review of treatment and response of high-risk mast cell tumours in dogs. *Vet Comp Oncol.* doi: 10.1111/vco.12116, 2014.
72. Smrkovski OA, Essick L, Rohrbach BW, et al: Masitinib mesylate for metastatic and non-resectable canine cutaneous mast cell tumours. *Vet Comp Oncol.* doi: 10.1111/vco.12053, 2013.
73. Hahn KA, Ogilvie G, Rusk T, et al: Masitinib is safe and effective for the treatment of canine mast cell tumors. *J Vet Intern Med* 22(6):1301-1309, 2008.
74. Carlsten KS, London CA, Haney S, et al: Multicenter prospective trial of hypofractionated radiation treatment, toceranib, and prednisone for measurable canine mast cell tumors. *J Vet Intern Med* 26(1):135-141, 2012.
75. Taylor F, Gear R, Hoather T, Dobson J. Chlorambucil and prednisolone chemotherapy for dogs with inoperable mast celltumours: 21 cases. *J Small Anim Pract* 50(6):284-289, 2009.

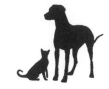

Chapter 45

Feline lymphoma

Clinical presentation

- Moderately common.
- May be uncomfortable.
- Weight loss, anorexia and lethargy are common.
- Clinical presentation often relates to anatomic location of the disease.

> **Key point**
>
> GI lymphoma generally occurs in older, FeLV-negative cats, whereas mediastinal lymphoma is seen more commonly in FeLV-positive cats, often of Siamese/Oriental breed.

Alimentary lymphoma

- Most common type; usually affects older, FeLV-negative cats.
- Vomiting, diarrhea, weakness, cachexia seen with lymphoma of the gastrointestinal tract.
- May be large cell (best treated with modified CHOP protocol) or small cell lymphoma (best treated with chlorambucil and prednisolone).

Mediastinal lymphoma

- Usually affects young, FeLV-positive cats, often of Siamese/Oriental breed.
- Respiratory difficulty, cyanosis, and tachypnea may be seen with mediastinal lymphoma.

Spinal lymphoma

- Usually affects FeLV-positive cats. Demographics may be changing as FeLV infection is becoming less common.
- Weakness, ataxia, cranial nerve abnormalities and conscious proprioception deficits seen with lymphoma of the central nervous system.

Renal lymphoma

- Cats may be FeLV-positive.
- Large kidneys, uremic breath, and cachexia seen with renal lymphoma.

Nasal lymphoma

- Chronic nasal discharge that may be transiently responsive to antibiotics due to secondary bacterial infection.
- Must be differentiated from cryptococcus, herpes and calici-induced upper respiratory infections.

Hodgkin's-like lymphoma

- Cervical lymphadenopathy may be seen with Hodgkin's-like lymphoma.
- Pale mucous membranes, weakness, petechial and ecchymosis with bone marrow involvement.

Lymphoma of large granular cell lymphocytes

- Enlarged lymph nodes at or around the gastrointestinal tract that stain intensely with intra-cytoplasmic granules.
- Weight loss, vomiting and diarrhea are common with LGL lymphoma

Staging and diagnosis

> **Key point**
>
> Small cell lymphoma of the gastrointestinal tract causes loss of layering of the intestine, whereas large cell lymphoma is more commonly associated with masses of the bowel wall, sometimes with marked lymph node enlargement. A biopsy is needed to definitively determine the difference between the two.

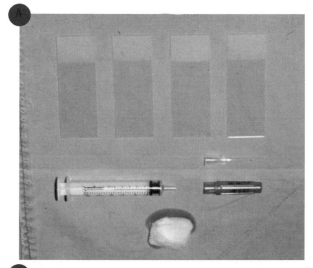

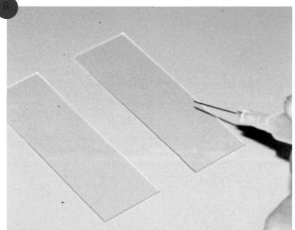

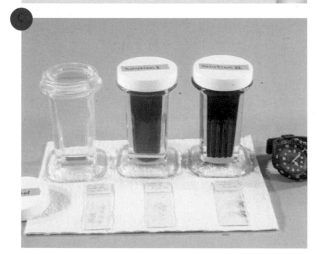

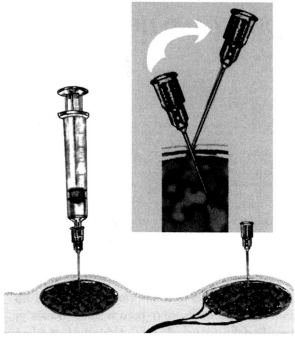

Figure 45-2: Directing the needle into the tissue with the needle attached to the syringe may be less effective than repeatedly directing only the needle into the tissue. Aspirating may cause rupture of cells and dilute out the sample by drawing in blood and other fluids. Once the needle is filled with tissue, it is attached to a syringe filled with air to forcibly eject the contents onto a slide for further preparation. Reprinted with permission from: Ogilvie GK, Moore AS. *Feline Oncology: A Comprehensive Guide for Compassionate Care.* Trenton NJ, Veterinary Learning Systems. 2002

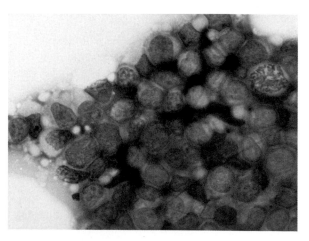

Figure 45-1: Fine needle aspirate cytology is a commonly used diagnostic tool for the diagnosis of feline lymphoma. Slides and 20-22 gauge needles (A) and a microscope are all that is needed. Once the needle is placed through the tissue, it is forcibly blown out of the needle and on to the slide (B) and stained appropriately such as with Diff Quick Stain (C).

Figure 45-3: Large or intermediate cell lymphoma is common in the cat and is characterized by very large immature lymphocytes. These malignant lymphocytes have scanty cytoplasm and an open, non-condensed chromatin that may also contain nucleoli. These tumors are most effectively treated with multiagent chemotherapy protocols such as the CHOP protocol.

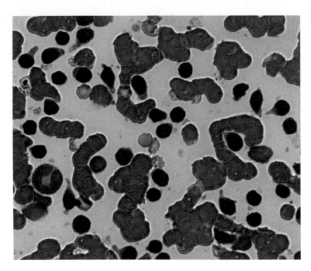

Figure 45-4: Small cell lymphoma is composed of small lymphocytes that are most often smaller than neutrophils. They often have dense nuclei and cannot be distinguished from normal circulating lymphocytes. This disease may have a prolonged asymptomatic period. Once clinical signs are noted, treatment with chlorambucil and prednisolone is usually quite effective for enhancing and improving quality of life.

Key point

Whenever cats are biopsied to confirm the presence of nasal lymphoma, the biopsy instrument (curette, cup biopsy instrument, etc.) is best passed up the nostril to secure a sample of the tissue in question. The instrument should never be passed further caudal than the medial canthus of the eye.

- Minimum data base (MDB): includes a CBC, biochemical profile, urinalysis, FIV/FeLV serology, T4 testing, biopsy, three-view thoracic radiographs or computerized tomography of the chest, ultrasound or CT of the abdomen.
- Aspirate or biopsy considered essential.
- Unique diagnostic tests depend on anatomic location of the disease:

Alimentary lymphoma

- Large or intermediate cell lymphoma is almost always associated with enlarged lymph nodes and thickening of the gastrointestinal tract. Ultrasound-guided aspirates or biopsies, upper or lower GI endoscopy, or surgical biopsies may be indicated.
- Small cell lymphoma may be associated with infiltration of the pancreas, liver and intestinal tract, but it is not commonly associated with significant intra-abdominal lymphadenopathy. Surgical or gastrointestinal endoscopic biopsies or ultrasound-guided biopsies or aspirates may be diagnostic.

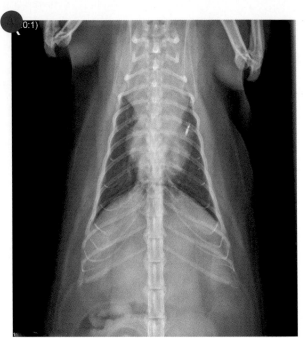

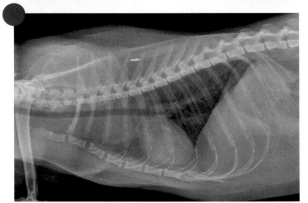

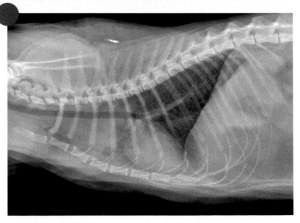

Figure 45-5: Lymphoma of the gastrointestinal tract is now more common than mediastinal lymphoma. The latter is associated with a non-compressible chest and a mass noted in the cranial mediastinum that can be seen on radiographs (A-C). Imaging courtesy of Lenore Anderson Mohammadian, DVM, MSpVM, Diplomate ACVR.

- Cats with low grade lymphoma almost never have a palpable or ultrasonographically evident abdominal mass. Those with intermediate or high grade gastrointestinal lymphoma have a mass almost half the time.

Mediastinal lymphoma

- Important to differentiate from thymomas, heart based tumors and primary lung tumors and cystic structures.
- Aspirates or biopsies obtained via ultrasound or computerized tomographic imaging.

Spinal lymphoma

- Often extradural and in FeLV-positive cats that also have lymphoma in the bone marrow. Therefore, testing for FeLV and performing a bone marrow aspirate is reasonable.
- Magnetic resonance or computerized tomographic imaging of the spinal cord is logical. If unavailable, then consider a myelogram with or without obtaining cerebrospinal fluid. Securing cells or a biopsy from the abnormal region is important.

Renal lymphoma

- Lymphoma is almost always bilateral. Occasionally there are lymph nodes that are involved.
- Aspirate or biopsy of one or both enlarged kidneys and associated enlarged lymph nodes can be diagnostic.

Nasal lymphoma

- Computerized tomography or nasal radiographs plus a biopsy of abnormal tissue visualized on imaging may help determine the extent of the disease.
- Rhinoscopy and biopsy may be helpful in some cases.

Hodgkin's-like lymphoma

- Cervical lymph nodes are often enlarged. Aspirates may be misleading, therefore a Tru-Cut, incisional or excisional biopsy of an enlarged lymph node is often necessary to make a definitive diagnosis.

Lymphoma of large granular cell lymphocytes

- Obtaining aspirates or a biopsy with ultrasound-guidance or during an abdominal exploratory may be needed.
- Stage of disease, as defined by Mooney,[55] was significantly related to response in one study,[56] in which cats with stage I lymphoma had higher response rates (93%) than those with stage IV to V disease (40% to 60%); in addition, cats with stage I and II lymphoma had longer survival times (7.6 months versus 3 months).

- A positive response to therapy is favorable prognostic indicator.
- Cats that are relatively healthy, FeLV-negative, and those that are treated with a doxorubicin-containing protocol generally do well.

Treatment

This section is divided into three options:
- Comfort for those who want to improve quality of life.
- Comfort and control for those who want to improve quality of life while trying to provide some control of the tumor.
- Comfort and longer-term control for those who want to improve quality of life while trying to maximize the chance of controlling the tumor.

> **Key point**
> Cats with nasal lymphoma have been reported to respond to combination chemotherapy and/or radiation therapy. Survival times exceeding a year are common.

> **Key point**
> Cats with small cell lymphoma usually respond quite well when treated with chlorambucil and prednisolone, whereas those cats with intermediate and large cell lymphoma generally respond favorably to combination chemotherapy.

Comfort

- Therapy to provide some benefit for the lymphoma by prescribing prednisolone plus therapy to enhance comfort and freedom from nausea, vomiting (e.g.: maropitant and/or metoclopramide), diarrhea (e.g.: metronidazole) and lack of appetite (e.g.: mirtazapine, cyproheptadine).

Comfort and control (first remission)

Above mentioned therapy for comfort plus:
CCNU (lomustine) at 60 mg/m² body surface area PO q3 weeks for 5 treatments. Note that treatment delays may be required due to neutropenia or thrombocytopenia.
- CCNU was used in one study as a rescue agent for 39 cases of resistant feline lymphoma. The overall median progression-free interval (MPFI) was 39 days (range 7-708 days). The MPFI for large versus small and intermediate cell lymphomas was 21 versus 169 days, respectively. The MPFI for gastrointestinal versus non-gastrointestinal lymphomas was 180 versus 25.5 days, respectively.[64]
- COP protocol (cyclophosphamide, vincristine and prednisolone) has been shown to be helpful for cats with lymphoma.

Table 45-1. COP Protocol for treatment of lymphoma[66,106]

Agent	Week						
	1	2	3	6	9	12	15[a]
Vincristine (0.7 mg/m^2 IV)	•	•	•	•	•	•	• →
Cyclophosphamide (250 mg/m^2 IV or PO [to nearest 25 mg])	•			•	•	•	•
Prednisolone (10 mg PO daily throughout the protocol)	•	→					

[a]After week-15, administer protocol every 3 weeks to 1 year, then stop therapy.

- In one study, 61 cats with lymphoma were treated with a COP chemotherapy protocol (cyclophosphamide, vincristine, and prednisolone) in the Netherlands. Complete remission (CR) was achieved in 46 of the 61 cats (75.4%). The estimated 1- and 2-year disease-free periods in the 46 cats with CR were 51.4 and 37.8%, respectively, whereas the median duration of remission was 251 days. The overall estimated 1-year survival rate in all cats was 48.7%, and the 2-year survival rate was 39.9%, with a median survival of 266 days. While these numbers are impressive, most believe that a doxorubicin containing combination protocol is likely preferable.[66]
- Palliative radiation, especially for those with localized or extranodal lymphoma, may be quite helpful (e.g.: 2-5 dosages of radiation) to first enhance comfort, second, to reduce the rate of growth and third, to occasionally to reduce the size of the tumor.
  - A study was performed to evaluate the efficacy of hypofractionated radiation for the treatment of 65 cats with nasal lymphoma. The median overall survival time and progression-free interval in 65 cats was 432 days and 229 days, respectively.[19]

Comfort and longer-term control (first remission)

Above mentioned therapy for comfort plus:
- CHOP chemotherapy to include cyclophosphamide, vincristine, prednisolone, doxorubicin and in some cases, L-asparaginase.
  - A study was completed to describe the outcome of 119 cats with intermediate- to high-grade lymphoma that were prescribed a modified 25-week University of Wisconsin-Madison (UW-25) chemotherapy protocol. The Kaplan-Meier median progression-free interval (PFI) and survival time (MST) were 56 and 97 (range

Table 45-2. Modified CHOP protocol for the treatment of lymphoma[69,160]

Week 1	Vincristine 0.5 mg/m^2 IV L-asparaginase 400 IU/kg or 10,000 IU/m^2 IM Prednisolone 2 mg/kg PO once daily
Week 2	Cyclophosphamide 250 mg/m^2 IV L-asparaginase 400 IU/kg or 10,000 IU/m^2 IM Prednisolone 1.5 mg/kg PO once daily
Week 3	Vincristine 0.5 mg/m^2 IV Prednisolone, 1.0 mg/kg PO once daily
Week 4	Doxorubicin 25 mg/m^2 or 1 mg/kg IV Prednisolone 0.5 mg/kg PO once daily
Week 6	Vincristine 0.5 mg/m^2 IV
Week 7	Cyclophosphamide 250 mg/m^2 IV
Week 8	Vincristine 0.5 mg/m^2 IV
Week 9	Doxorubicin 25 mg/m^2 or 1 mg/kg IV
Week 11	Vincristine 0.5 mg/m^2 IV
Week 13	Cyclophosphamide 250 mg/m^2 IV
Week 15	Vincristine 0.5 mg/m^2 IV
Week 17	Doxorubicin 25 mg/m^2 or 1 mg/kg IV
Week 19	Vincristine 0.5 mg/m^2 IV
Week 21	Cyclophosphamide 250 mg/m^2 IV
Week 23	Vincristine 0.5 mg/m^2 IV
Week 25	Doxorubicin 25 mg/m^2 or 1 mg/kg IV

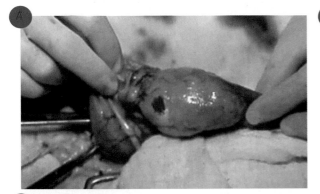

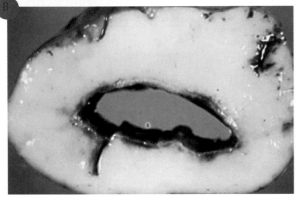

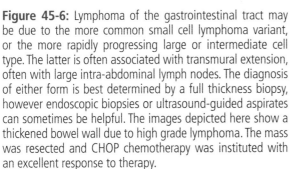

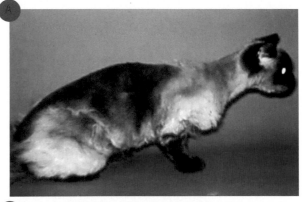

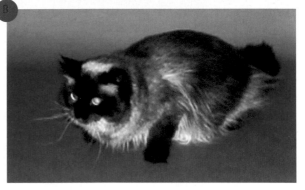

Figure 45-6: Lymphoma of the gastrointestinal tract may be due to the more common small cell lymphoma variant, or the more rapidly progressing large or intermediate cell type. The latter is often associated with transmural extension, often with large intra-abdominal lymph nodes. The diagnosis of either form is best determined by a full thickness biopsy, however endoscopic biopsies or ultrasound-guided aspirates can sometimes be helpful. The images depicted here show a thickened bowel wall due to high grade lymphoma. The mass was resected and CHOP chemotherapy was instituted with an excellent response to therapy.

Figure 45-7: Cats may present with posterior paresis due to lymphoma. The cats, as the one pictured above, may drag or scuff their hind limbs during ambulation. These cats generally have excellent femoral pulses with an extradural compressive lesion that may be evident on MRI. These cats are often FeLV-positive and may have lymphoma in the bone marrow. Radiation to the compressive site and/or multiagent chemotherapy has the best chance for restoring function.

2-2019) days, respectively. Cats assessed as having a complete response (CR) to therapy had significantly longer PFI and MST than those with partial or no response (PFI 205 versus 54 versus 21 days, respectively, and MST 318 versus 85 versus 27 days, respectively [69]).

- Another study was done to assess the efficacy and toxicity of a short-term, maintenance-free 12-week chemotherapy protocol in 26 cats with high and intermediate-grade lymphoma. These cats were treated with a 12-week protocol consisting of cyclic administration of L-asparaginase, vincristine, cyclophosphamide, doxorubicin and prednisolone. Complete (CR) and partial remission (PR) rates were 46 and 27%, respectively. Median duration of first complete remission was 394 days, compared with a median partial remission duration of 41 days. Median survival in those cats that developed a complete remission was 454 days.

The cats that had a partial remission had a median survival of 82 days. Toxicities were mainly low grade with anorexia seen most frequently.[70]

- Sixty cats with lymphoma were treated with a CHOP protocol using L-asparaginase, vincristine, cyclophosphamide, doxorubicin, methotrexate and prednisolone. The median survival time for these 60 cats was 116 days. Of the 60 cats, 48 rapidly went into complete remission (complete remission rate 80%) and these cats had a median survival of 187 days. Twenty cats were classed as 'long-term survivors' based on survival time in excess of one year. Long-term survivors were more likely to be less than 4-years and to have tumors of the T-cell phenotype. Eighty-five percent of clients expressed complete satisfaction with their decision to pursue chemotherapy, and 70% believed their cat's health status improved during the first two weeks of treatment. Methotrexate, while used in this study, is generally not used by others as it is thought to be minimally effective.[71]

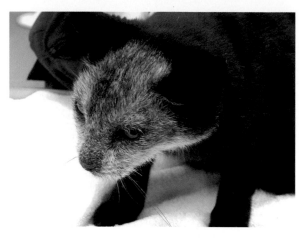

Figure 45-8: Nasal lymphoma often responds extraordinarily well to either localized radiation or to systemic multiagent chemotherapy. Long-term remissions often occur with either. If radiation is used, there may be hair color changes as noted in this patient.

Specific comments on the different anatomic types of lymphoma include:

Alimentary lymphoma

- High or intermediate grade lymphoma should be treated with at least CCNU, if not a CCNU-enriched combination protocol or a CHOP protocol.
- Small cell lymphoma should be treated with chlorambucil (6 mg/m² PO daily compounded or 2 mg 2-3 times per week) and prednisolone (1-2 mg/kg/day).

Mediastinal lymphoma

- Combination chemotherapy with or without radiation to the mediastinum is ideal.

Spinal lymphoma

- Combination chemotherapy with or without radiation to the site of involvement of the central nervous system is ideal.

Renal lymphoma

- This extranodal lymphoma generally responds quite well to combination CHOP chemotherapy protocols. Some advocate including cytosine arabinoside or CCNU, as the cats with longer-term remissions may have involvement of the central nervous system.

Nasal lymphoma

- Combination chemotherapy or radiation therapy have been shown to be quite effective for inducing durable remissions.
- The survival times of 97 cats with nasal lymphoma treated with radiation therapy (RT) alone,

chemotherapy alone, or RT + chemotherapy were assessed to identify potential prognostic variables that affected survival. The median survival time, regardless of therapy modality, was 536 days.[72]
- One hundred and forty-nine cats with extranodal lymphoma were treated and assessed. Sixty-six cats received cyclophosphamide, vincristine, and prednisolone (COP); 25 cats received the Wisconsin-Madison doxorubicin-containing multiagent protocol; 10 prednisolone alone, and nine other combinations. The response rate for the 110 treated cats was 85.5%. Of cyclophosphamide, vincristine, prednisolone treated cats, 72.7% achieved complete remission, with a median survival of 239 days. Sixty-four percent of Wisconsin-Madison treated cats achieved complete remission, with a median survival time of 563 days. Cats with nasal lymphoma achieving complete remission had the longest survival (749 days), and cats with central nervous system lymphoma the shortest (70 days).[73]

Hodgkin's-Like lymphoma

- Chemotherapy with regional radiation therapy has been advocated for this unusual lymphoma.

Lymphoma of large granular cell lymphocytes

- Combination chemotherapy is preferred for this type of lymphoma.

Rescue Protocols

The treatment protocols listed above are also used to attain second and third, and occasionally fourth remissions. The choice of rescue protocols depends on the response to the prior protocol. If, for example, the patient has a long, durable remission to a modified CHOP protocol, then that protocol can be repeated. If the patient has a poor response to the modified CHOP protocol, then it would be important to choose a protocol or a single agent that does not contain the previously used protocol. For example, a modification of the CHOP protocol where vinblastine is used instead of vincristine, mitoxantrone instead of doxorubicin, lomustine (CCNU) instead of cyclophosphamide, and dexamethasone instead of prednisolone. Alternatively, CCNU can be used as a single agent. In general, the duration of remission for a rescue protocol is half the duration of the previous remission. Options include, but are not limited to:
- Single agents —Lomustine, DTIC, mitoxantrone, Actinomycin-D and doxorubicin.
- MOPP—Mechlorethamine, vincristine, procarbazine and prednisolone.

References

1. Nielsen SW, Holzworth J: Visceral lymphosarcoma of the cat. *JAVMA* 122:189–197, 1953.
2. Takahashi R, Goto N, Ishii H, et al: Pathological observations

of natural cases of feline lymphosarcomatosis. *Jap J Vet Sci* 36:163–173, 1974.

3. Carpenter JL, Andrews LK, Holzworth J: Tumors and tumor-like lesions. In Holzworth J (ed): *Diseases of the Cat Medicine and Surgery*. Philadelphia, WB Saunders Co, 1987, pp 407–596.

4. Nielsen SW: Spontaneous hematopoietic neoplasms of the domestic cat [monograph]. *Natl Cancer Inst* 32:73–94, 1969.

5. Cotter SM: Feline viral neoplasia. In Greene CE (ed): *Infectious Diseases of the Dog and Cat*, ed 3. Philadelphia, WB Saunders, 1998, pp 71–83.

6. Anderson WI, Miller DM, Davis JM: Multicentric lymphosarcoma in a kitten. *Modern Vet Pract* 66:206, 1985.

7. Meincke JE, Hobbie Jr WV, Hardy Jr WD: Lymphoreticular malignancies in the cat: Clinical findings. *JAVMA* 160:1093–1099, 1972.

8. Slayter MV, Farver TB, Schneider R: Feline malignant lymphoma: Log-linear multiway frequency analysis of a population involving the factors of sex and age of animal and tumor cell type and location. *Am J Vet Res* 45:2178–2181, 1984.

9. Hardy Jr WD: Hematopoietic tumors of cats. *JAAHA* 17:921–940, 1981.

10. Crighton GW: Clinical aspects of lymphosarcoma in the cat. *Vet Rec* 83:122–126, 1968.

11. Sabine M, Wright RG, Love DN: Studies on feline lymphosarcoma in the Sydney area. *Aust J Exp Biol Med Sci* 52:331–340, 1974.

12. Holzworth J: Leukemia and related neoplasms in the cat: I. Lymphoid malignancies *JAVMA* 136:47–69, 1960.

13. Court EA, Watson ADJ, Peaston AE: Retrospective study of 60 cases of feline lymphosarcoma. *Aust Vet J* 75:424–427, 1997.

14. Gabor LJ, Malik R, Canfield PJ: Clinical and anatomical features of lymphosarcoma in 118 cats. *Aust Vet J* 76:725–732, 1998.

15. Vail DM, Moore AS, Ogilvie GK, Volk LM: Feline lymphoma (145 cases): Proliferation indices, cluster of differentiation 3 immunoreactivity, and their association with prognosis in 90 cats. *J Vet Intern Med* 12:349–354, 1998.

16. Dorn CR, Taylor DON, Schneider R, et al: Survey of animal neoplasms in Alameda and Contra Costa Counties, California: II Cancer morbidity in dogs and cats from Alameda County. *J Natl Cancer Inst* 40:307–318, 1968.

17. Jarrett WFH, Crawford EM, Martin WB, Davie F: Leukemia in the cat. *Nature* 202:566–568, 1964.

18. Schneider R, Frye FL, Taylor DON, Dorn CR: A household cluster of feline malignant lymphoma. *Cancer Res* 27:1316–1322, 1967.

19. Schneider R: Feline malignant lymphoma: Environmental factors and the occurrence of this viral cancer in cats. *Int J Cancer* 10:345–350, 1972.

20. Theilen GH, Dungworth DL, Kawakami TG, et al: Experimental induction of lymphosarcoma in the cat with "C"-type virus. *Cancer Res* 30:401–408, 1970.

21. Cotter SM, Hardy Jr WD, Essex M: Association of feline leukemia virus with lymphosarcoma and other disorders in the cat. *JAVMA* 166:449–454, 1975.

22. Hardy Jr WD, Zuckerman EE, MacEwen EG, et al: A feline leukemia and sarcoma virus-induced tumor-specific antigen. *Nature (Lond)* 270:249–251, 1977.

23. Snyder Jr HW, Singhal MC, Zuckerman EE, et al: The feline oncornavirus-associated cell membrane antigen (FOCMA) is related to, but distinguishable from, FeLV-C gp70. *Virology* 131:315–327, 1983.

24. Reinacher M, Theilen GH: Frequency and significance of feline leukemia virus infection in necropsied cats. *Am J Vet Res* 48:939–945, 1987.

25. Reinacher M: Diseases associated with spontaneous feline leukemia virus (FeLV) infection in cats. *Vet Immun Immunopath* 21:85–95, 1989.

26. Francis DP, Cotter SM, Hardy Jr WD, Essex M: Comparison of virus positive and virus negative cases of feline leukemia and lymphoma. *Cancer Res* 39:3866–3870, 1979.

27. Rezanka LJ, Rojko JL, Neil JC: Feline leukemia virus: Pathogenesis of neoplastic disease. *Cancer Invest* 10:371–389, 1992.

28. Miura T, Tsujimoto H, Fukasawa M, et al: Structural abnormality and over-expression of the *myc* gene in feline leukemias. *Int J Cancer* 40:564–569, 1987.

29. Pantginis J, Beaty RM, Levy LS, Lenz J: The feline leukemia virus long terminal repeat contains a potent genetic determinant of T-cell lymphomagenicity. *J Virology* 71:9786–9791, 1997.

30. Pandey R, Bechtel MK, Su Y, et al: Feline leukemia virus variants in experimentally induced thymic lymphosarcomas. *Virology* 214:584–592, 1995.

31. Athas GB, Choi B, Prabhu S, et al: Genetic determinants of feline leukemia virus-induced multicentric lymphomas. *Virology* 214:431–438, 1995.

32. Okuda M, Umeda A, Sakai T, et al: Cloning of the feline p53 tumor-suppressor gene and its aberration in hematopoietic tumors. *Int J Cancer* 58:602–607, 1994.

33. Casey JW, Roach A, Mullins JE, et al: The U3 portion of feline leukemia virus DNA identifies horizontally acquired proviruses in leukemia cats. *Proc Natl Acad Sci USA* 78:7778–7782, 1981.

34. Sheets RL, Pandey R, Jen W-C, Roy-Burman P: Recombinant feline leukemia virus genes detected in naturally occurring feline lymphosarcomas. *J Virology* 67:3118–3125, 1993.

35. Jackson ML, Haines DM, Meric SM, Misra V: Feline leukemia virus detection by immunohistochemistry and polymerase chain reaction in formalin-fixed, paraffin-embedded tumor tissue from cats with lymphosarcoma. *Can J Vet Res* 57:269–276, 1993.

36. Gregory CR, Madewell BR, Griffey S, Torten M: Feline leukemia virus-associated lymphosarcoma following renal *transplantation* in a cat. Transplantation 1097–1099, 1991.

37. Gabor LJ, Jackson ML, Trask B, et al: Feline leukemia virus status of Australian cats with lymphosarcoma. *Aust Vet J* 79(7):476-81, 2001.

38. Jackson ML, Wood SL, Misra V, Haines DM: Immunohistochemical identification of B and T lymphocytes in formalin-fixed, paraffin-embedded feline lymphosarcomas: Relation to feline leukemia virus status, tumor site, and patient age. *Can J Vet Res* 60:199–204, 1996.

39. Shelton GH, Grant CK, Cotter SM, et al: Feline immunodeficiency virus and feline leukemia virus infections and their relationships to lymphoid malignancies in cats: A retrospective study (1968–1988). *J Acquir Immune Defic Syndr* 3:623–630, 1990.

40. Hutson CA, Rideout BA, Pedersen NC: Neoplasia associated with feline immunodeficiency virus infection in cats of Southern California. *JAVMA* 199:1357–1362, 1991.

41. Callanan JJ, Jones BA, Irvine J, et al: Histologic classification and immunophenotype of lymphosarcomas in cats with naturally and experimentally acquired feline immunodeficiency virus infections. *Vet Pathol* 33:264–272, 1996.

42. Poli A, Abramo F, Baldinotti F, et al: Malignant lymphoma associated with experimentally induced feline immunodeficiency virus infection. *J Comp Pathol* 110:319–328, 1994.

43. Alexander R, Robinson WF, Mills JN, et al: Isolation of feline immunodeficiency virus from three cats with lymphoma. *Aust Vet Practit* 19:93–97, 1989.

44. Jarrett O, Edney ATB, Toth S, Hay D: Feline leukaemia virus-free lymphosarcoma in a specific pathogen free cat. Vet Rec 115:249–250, 1984.

45. Gulino SE: Chromosome abnormalities and oncogenesis in cat leukemias. *Cancer Genet Cytogenet* 64:149–157, 1992.

46. Holmberg CA, Manning JS, Osburn BI: Feline malignant lymphomas: Comparison of morphologic and immunologic characteristics. *Am J Vet Res* 37:1455–1460, 1976.

47. Wellman ML, Kociba GJ, Rojko JL: Guinea pig erythrocyte rosette formation as a non-specific cell surface receptor assay in the cat. *Am J Vet Res* 47:433–437, 1986.

48. Rojko JL, Kociba GJ, Abkowitz JL, et al: Feline lymphomas: Immunological and cytochemical characterization. *Cancer Res* 49:345–351, 1989.

49. Darbès J, Majzoub M, Hermanns W: Evaluation of the cross-reactivity between human and feline or canine leucocyte antigens using commercially available antibodies. *J Vet Diagn Invest* 9:94–97, 1997.

50. Monteith CE, Chelack BJ, Davis WC, Haines DM: Identification of monoclonal antibodies for immunohistochemical staining of feline B lymphocytes in frozen and formalin-fixed paraffin-embedded tissues. *Can J Vet Res* 60:193–198, 1996.

51. Shimojima M, Pecoraro MR, Maeda K, et al: Characterization of anti-feline CD8 monoclonal antibodies. *Vet Immun Immunopath* 61:17–23, 1998.

52. Gabor LJ, Canfield PJ, Malik R: Immunophenotypic and histological characterization of 109 cases of feline lymphosarcoma. *Aust Vet J* 77:436–441, 1999.

53. Moore AS: treatment of feline lymphoma. *Feline Pract* 24:17–20, 1996.

54. Mooney SC, Hayes AA, Matus R, MacEwen EG: Renal lymphoma in cats: 28 cases (1977–1984). *JAVMA* 191:1473–1477, 1987.

55. Mooney SC, Hayes AA: Lymphoma in the cat: An approach to diagnosis and management. *Semin Vet Med Surg Small Anim* 1:51–57, 1986.

56. Mooney SC, Hayes AA, MacEwen EG, et al: treatment and in lymphoma in cats: 103 cases (1977–1981). *JAVMA* 194:696–699, 1989.

57. Pennick DG, Moore AS, Tidwell AS, et al: Ultrasonography of alimentary lymphosarcoma in the cat. *Vet Radiol* 35:299–304, 1994.

58. Penninck DG, Crystal MA, Matz ME, Pearson SH: The technique of percutaneous ultrasound guided fine-needle aspiration biopsy and automated microcore biopsy in small animal gastrointestinal diseases. *Vet Radiol Ultrasound* 34:433–436, 1993.

59. Lamb CR, Hartzband LE, Tidwell AS, Pearson SH: Ultrasonographic findings in hepatic and splenic lymphosarcoma in dogs and cats. *Vet Radiol* 32:117–120, 1991.

60. Gabor LJ, Canfield PJ, Malik R: Haematological and biomedical findings in cats in Australia with lymphosarcoma. *Aust Vet J* 78:456–461, 2000.

61. Fritz D, Saignes C-F, Hopfner C: Usefulness of bone marrow biopsy for the diagnosis of deep-seated lymphomas in cat: One case. *Revue Méd Vét* 147:681–686, 1996.

62. Spodnick GJ, Berg J, Moore FMCSM: Spinal lymphoma in cats: 21 cases (1976—1989). *JAVMA* 200:373–376, 1992.

63. Todorovic D, Gafner F, Knezevic M, Kovacevic S: Lymphosarcoma in cats. *Acta Veterinarian (Beograd)* 40:341–344, 1990.

64. Dutelle AL, Bulman-Fleming JC, Lewis CA, et al: Evaluation of lomustine as a rescue agent for cats with resistant lymphoma. J Feline Med Surg. (10):694-700. 2012.

65. Teske E, van Straten G, van Noort R, et al. Chemotherapy with cyclophosphamide, vincristine, and prednisolone (COP) in cats with malignant lymphoma: new results with an old protocol. J Vet Intern Med. 16(2):179-186, 2002.

66. Walton RM, Hendrick MJ: Feline Hodgkin's-like lymphosarcoma: 20 cases (1992–1998) [abstract 64]. *Vet Pathol* 36:496, 1999.

67. Day MJ, Kyaw-Tanner M, Silkstone MA, et al: T-cell-rich B-cell lymphoma in the cat. *J Comp Pathol* 120:155–167, 1999.

68. Valli VE, Jacobs RM, Norris A, et al: The histological classification of 602 cases of feline lymphoproliferative disease using the national cancer institute working formulation. *J Vet Diagn Invest* 12:295–306, 2000.

69. Collette SA, Allstadt SD, Chon EM, et al: treatment of feline intermediate- to high-grade lymphoma with a modified university of Wisconsin-Madison protocol: 119 cases (2004-2012). Vet Comp Oncol. doi: 10.1111/vco.12158, 2015.

70. Limmer S, Eberle N, Nerschbach V, et al: treatment of feline lymphoma using a 12-week, maintenance-free combination chemotherapy protocol in 26 cats. Vet Comp Oncol. doi: 10.1111/vco.12082, 2014.

71. Malik R, Gabor LJ, Foster SF, et al: Therapy for Australian cats with lymphosarcoma. Aust Vet J. 79(12):808-817, 2001.

72. Haney SM, Beaver L, Turrel J, et al: Survival analysis of 97 cats with nasal lymphoma: a multi-institutional retrospective study (1986-2006). J Vet Intern Med. 23(2):287-294, 2009.

73. Taylor SS, Goodfellow MR, Browne WJ, et al: Feline extranodal lymphoma: response to chemotherapy and survival in 110 cats. J Small Anim Pract. 50(11):584-592, 2009.

74. Qureshi SR, Olander HJ: Feline lymphosarcoma with heterotopic bone. *JAAHA* 13:616–618, 1977.

75. Thilsted JP, Bolton RG: Thymic lymphosarcoma with bony metaplasia in a cat. *Vet Pathol* 22:424–425, 1985.

76. Provencher-Bollinger A, Graham PA, Refsal KR, et al: Detection of parathyroid hormone related peptide (PTHrP) in serum of cats with hypercalcemia of malignancy [abstract 12]. *Am Soc Vet Clin Path Vet Pathol* 36:483, 1999.

77. Kehoe JM, Hurvitsz AI, Capra JD: Characterization of three feline paraproteins. *J Immunol* 109:511–516, 1972.

78. Glick AD, Horn RG, Holscher M: Characterization of feline glomerulonephritis associated with viral-induced hematopoietic neoplasms. *Am J Pathol* 92:321–327, 1978.

79. Jeraj KP, Hardy R, O'Leary TP, et al: Immune complex glomerulonephritis in a cat with renal lymphosarcoma. *Vet Pathol* 22:287–290, 1985.

80. Anderson LJ, Jarrett WFH: Membranous glomerulonephritis associated with leukaemia in cats. *Res Vet Sci* 12:179–180, 1971.

81. Ashley PF, Bowman LA: Symmetric cutaneous necrosis of the hind feet and multicentric follicular lymphoma in a cat. *JAVMA* 214:211–214, 1999.

82. Daniels-McQueen SM, Directo AC, Palomo HA: Chorea in a cat with malignant lymphoma. *Vet Med Small Anim Clin*: 413–415, 1974.

83. Parnell NK, Powell LL, Hohenhaus AE, et al: Hypoadrenocortism as the primary manifestation of lymphoma in two cats. *JAVMA* 8:1208–1211, 1999.

84. Farrelly J, Hohenhaus AE, Peterson ME, et al: Evaluation of pituitary-adrenal function in cats with lymphoma. *Proc Vet Cancer Soc.* 19th Annual Conf: 33, 1999.

85. Madewell BR, Holmberg CA, Ackerman N: Lymphosarcoma and cryptococcosis in a cat. *JAVMA* 175:65–68, 1979.

86. Edwards JF, Ficken MD, Luttgen PJ, Frey MS: Disseminated sarcocystosis in a cat with lymphosarcoma. *JAVMA* 193:831–832, 1988.

87. Aronson E, Bendickson JC, Miles KG, et al: Disseminated histoplasmosis with osseous lesions in a cat with feline lymphosarcoma. *Vet Radiol* 27:50–53, 1986.

88. Lent SF, Burkhardt JE, Bolka D: Coincident enteric cryptosporidiosis and lymphosarcoma in a cat with diarrhea. *JAAHA* 29:492–496, 1993.

89. Hohenhaus AE, Rosenberg MP, Moroff SD: Concurrent lymphoma and salmonellosis in a cat. *Can Vet J* 31:38–40, 1990.

90. Järplid B, Feldman BF: Large granular lymphoma with toxoplasmosis in a cat. *Comp Haematol Int* 3:241–243, 1993.

91. Zwahlen CH, Lucroy MD, Kraegel SA, Madewell BR: Results of chemotherapy for cats with alimentary malignant lymphoma: 21 cases (1993–1997). *JAVMA* 213:1144–1149, 1998.

92. Head KW, Else RW: Neoplasia and allied conditions of the canine and feline intestine. *Small Anim Intest Neoplasia* 190–208, 1981.

93. Mahony O, Moore AS, Cotter SM: Alimentary lymphoma in cats: 28 cases (1988–1993). *JAVMA* 207:1593–1598, 1995.

94. Brodey RS: Alimentary tract neoplasms in the cat: A clinicopathologic survey of 46 cases. *Am J Vet Res* 27:74–80, 1966.

95. Groothers AM, Biller DS, Ward H, et al: Ultrasonographic appearance of feline alimentary lymphoma. *Vet Radiol Ultrasound* 35:468–472, 1994.

96. Patterson DF, Meier H: Surgical intervention in intestinal lymphosarcoma in two cats. *JAVMA* 127:495–498, 1955.

97. Jeglum KA, Whereat A, Young K: Chemotherapy of lymphoma in 75 cats. *JAVMA* 190:174–178, 1987.

98. Wieser JR: What is your diagnosis? *JAVMA* 205:685–686, 1994.

99. Weller RE, Hornof WJ: Gastric malignant lymphoma in two cats. *Modern Vet Pract* 60:701–704, 1979.

100. Slawienski MJ, Mauldin GE, Mauldin GN, Patnaik AK: Malignant colonic neoplasia in cats: 46 cases (1990–1996). *JAVMA* 211:878–881, 1997.

101. Loupal G, Pfeil C: Tumoren im darmtrakt der katze unter besonderer Berücksightung der nicht-hämatopoetischen Geschwiilste. *Berl Münch Teirärztl Wschr* 97:208–213, 1984.

102. Strand RD: treatment of recurrent feline intestinal lymphoma. *Mod Vet Pract* 67:823–824, 1986.

103. Münster M: Effizienz der endoskopie bei magen-darm-erkrankungen von hund und katze. *Der Praktische Tierarzt* 4:309–312, 1993.

104. Wasmer ML, Willard MD, Helman RG, Edwards JF: Food intolerance mimicking alimentary lymphosarcoma. *JAAHA* 31:463–466, 1995.

105. Gores BR, Berg J, Carpenter JL, Ullman SL: Chylous ascites in cats: Nine cases (1978–1993). *JAVMA* 205:1161–1164, 1994.

106. Cotter SM: treatment of lymphoma and leukemia with cyclophosphamide, vincristine, and prednisone: II. treatment of cats. *JAAHA* 19:166–172, 1983.

107. Moore AS, Cotter SM, Frimberger AE, et al: A comparison of doxorubicin and COP for maintenance of remission in cats with lymphoma. *J Vet Intern Med* 10:372–375, 1996.

108. Franks PT, Harvey JW, Calderwood Mays M, et al: Feline large granular lymphoma. *Vet Pathol* 23:200–202, 1986.

109. Honor DJ, DeNicola DB, Turek JJ, et al: A neoplasm of globule leukocytes in a cat. *Vet Pathol* 23:287–292, 1986.

110. Konno A, Hashimoto Y, Kon Y, Sugimura M: Perforin-like immunoreactivity in feline globule leukocytes and their distribution. *J Vet Med Sci* 56:1101–1105, 1994.

111. Goitsuka R, Tsuji M, Matsumoto Y, et al: A case of feline large granular lymphoma. *Jpn J Vet Sci* 50:593–595, 1988.

112. Kariya K, Konno A, Ishida T, et al: Globule leukocyte neoplasm in a cat. *Jpn J Vet Sci* 52:403–405, 1990.

113. Darbés J, Majzoub M, Breuer W, Hermanns W: Large granular lymphocyte leukemia/lymphoma in six cats. *Vet Pathol* 35:370–379, 1988.

114. Finn JP, Schwartz LW: A neoplasm of globule leucocytes in the intestine of a cat. *J Comp Pathol* 82:323–326, 1972.

115. Moore FM, Kaufman J: What is your diagnosis? *Vet Clin Pathol* 18:37–38, 2000.

116. Cheney CM, Rojko JL, Kociba GJ, et al: A feline large granular lymphoma and its derived cell line. *In Vitro Cell Dev Biol* 26:455–463, 1990.

117. Buracco P, Guglielmino R, Abate O, et al: Large granular lymphoma in an FIV-positive and FeLV-negative cat. *J Small Anim Pract* 33:279–284, 1992.

118. Wellman ML, Hammer AS, DiBartola SP, et al: Lymphoma involving large granular lymphocytes in cats: 11 cases (1982–1991). *JAVMA* 201:1265–1269, 1992.

119. McEntee MF, Horton S, Blue J, Meuten DJ: Granulated round cell tumor of cats. *Vet Pathol* 30:195–203, 1993.

120. Drobatz KJ, Fred R, Waddle J: Globule leukocyte tumor in six cats. *JAAHA* 29:391–396, 1993.

121. McPherron MA, Chavkin MJ, Powers BE, Seim III HB: Globule leukocyte tumor involving the small intestine in a cat. *JAVMA* 204:241–245, 1994.

122. von Beust BR, Guscetti F, Kohn B: Neoplasien ausgehend von großen granulierten lymphzyten bei hund und katze. *Tierarztl Prax* 23:70–74, 1995.

123. Goitsuka R, Ohno K, Matsumoto Y, et al: Establishment and characterization of a feline large granular lymphoma cell line expressing interleukin 2 receptor a-chain. *J Vet Med Sci* 55:863–865, 1993.

124. Tobey JC, Houston DM, Breur GJ, et al: Cutaneous T-cell lymphoma in a cat. *JAVMA* 204:606–609, 1994.

125. Gruffydd-Jones TJ, Gaskell CJ, Gibbs C: Clinical and radiological features of anterior mediastinal lymphosarcoma in the cat: A review of 30 cases. *Vet Rec* 104:304–307, 1979.

126. Mauldin GE, Mooney SC, Meleo KA, et al: Chemotherapy in 132 cats with lymphoma (1988–1994). *Proc 15th Vet Cancer Soc*: 35–36, 1995.

127. Shimoda T: Clinicopathological findings in 12 cases of feline thymic lymphoma. *J Jpn Vet Med Assoc* 46:227–230, 1993.

128. Day MJ: Review of thymic pathology in 30 cats and 36 dogs. *J Small Anim Pract* 38:393–403, 1997.

129. Forrester SD, Fossum TW, Rogers KS: Diagnosis and treatment of chylothorax associated with lymphoblastic lymphosarcoma in four cats. *JAVMA* 198:291–294, 1991.

130. Fossum TW, Dru Forrester S, Swenson CL, et al: Chylothorax in cats: 37 cases (1969–1989). *JAVMA* 198:672–678, 1991.

131. Murphy MG: Thymic lymphosarcoma in a cat. *Irish Vet J* 41:332–334, 1987.

132. Sottiaux J, Franck M: Cranial vena caval thrombosis secondary to invasive mediastinal lymphosarcoma in a cat. *J Small Anim Pract* 39:352–355, 1998.

133. Hinko PJ, Rickards DA, Morse Jr EM: Malignant lymphoma of thymus gland. *Feline Pract* 2:17–18, 1972.

134. Cotter SM, Essex M, McLane MF, et al: Chemotherapy and passive immunotherapy in naturally occurring feline mediastinal lymphoma. In Hardy Jr WD, Essex M, McClelland AJ (eds): *Feline Leukemia Virus.* New York, Elselvier North Holland, Inc, 1980, pp 219–225.

135. Gruffydd-Jones TJ, Flecknell PA: The prognosis and treatment related to the gross appearance and laboratory characteristics of pathological thoracic fluids in the cat. *J Small Anim Pract* 19:315–328, 1978.

136. Mackey L, Jarrett W, Jarrett O, Wilson L: B and T cells in a cat with thymic lymphosarcoma. *J Natl Cancer Inst* 54:1483–1485, 1975.

137. Freitag WA, Norsworthy GD: Lymphosarcoma treatment. *Feline Pract* 6:11–14, 1976.

138. Zaki FA, Hurvitz AI: Spontaneous neoplasms of the central nervous system of the cat. *J Small Anim Pract* 17:773–782, 1976.

139. Lane SB, Kornegay JN, Duncan Jr, Oliver Jr JE: Feline spinal lymphosarcoma: A retrospective evaluation of 23 cats. *J Vet Intern Med* 8:99–104, 1994.

140. Noonan M, Kline KL, Meleo K: Lymphoma of the central nervous system: A retrospective study of 18 cats. *Compen Contin Educ Pract Vet* 19:497–504, 1997.

141. LeCouteur RA, Fike JR, Cann CE, et al: X-ray computed tomography of brain tumors in cats. *JAVMA* 183:301–305, 1983.

142. Lapointe J-M, Higgins RJ, Kortz GD, et al: Intravascular malignant T-cell lymphoma (malignant angioendotheliomatosis) in a cat. *Vet Pathol* 34:247–250, 1997.

143. Fondevila D, Vilafranca M, Pumarola M: Primary central nervous system T-cell lymphoma in a cat. *Vet Pathol* 35:550–553, 1998.

144. Allen JG, Amis T: Lymphosarcoma involving cranial nerves in a cat. *Aust Vet J* 51:155–158, 1975.

145. Northington JW, Juliana MM: Extradural lymphosarcoma in six cats. *J Small Anim Pract* 19:409–416, 1978.

146. Schappert HR, Geib LW: Reticuloendothelial neoplasms involving the spinal canal in cats. *JAVMA* 150:753–757, 1967.

147. Fox JG, Gutnick MJ: Horner's syndrome and brachial paralysis due to lymphosarcoma in a cat. *JAVMA* 160:977–980, 1972.

148. Rowe WS, Bradford TS, Martin P: Posterior paralysis due to lymphosarcoma. *Feline Pract* 7:34–36, 1977.

149. Heavner JE: Neural lymphomatosis in cats. *Mod Vet Pract* 59:122–124, 1978.

150. Mitchell M: Feline spinal lymphosarcoma—A case report. *Southwest Vet* 33:72–75, 1980.

151. Ogilvie GK: Extradural lymphoma in a cat. *Vet Med Report* 1:57–61, 1988.

152. Suess Jr RP, Martin RA, Shell LG, et al: Vertebral lymphosarcoma in a cat. *JAVMA* 197:101–103, 1990.

153. Parker AJ, Park RD: Myelographic diagnosis of a spinal cord tumor in a cat. *Feline Pract* 4:28–33, 1974.

154. Chrisman CL: Electromyography in the localization of spinal cord and nerve root neoplasia in dogs and cats. *JAVMA* 166:1074–1079, 1975.

155. Barr MC, Butt MT, Anderson KL, et al: Spinal lymphosarcoma and disseminated mastocytoma associated with feline immunodeficiency virus infection in a cat. *JAVMA* 202:1978–1980, 1993.

156. Swaim SF, Shields RP: Paraplegia in the cat. *Vet Med Small Anim Clin* 66:787–798, 1971.

157. Weller RE, Stann SE: Renal lymphosarcoma in the cat. *JAAHA* 19:363–367, 1983.

158. Podell M, DiBartola SP, Rosol TJ: Polycystic kidney disease and renal lymphoma in a cat. *JAVMA* 201:906–909, 1992.

159. Osborne CA, Johnson KH, Kurtz HJ, Hanlon GF: Renal lymphoma in the dog and cat. *JAVMA* 158:2058–2070, 1971.

160. Moore FM, Emerson WE, Cotter SM, Delellis RA: Distinctive peripheral lymph node hyperplasia of young cats. *Vet Pathol* 23:386–391, 1986.

161. Brown PJ, Hopper CD, Harbour DA: Pathological features of lymphoid tissues in cats with natural feline immunodeficiency virus infection. *J Comp Pathol* 104:345–355, 1991.

162. Lucke VM, Davies JD, Wood CA, Whitbread TJ: Plexiform vascularization of lymph nodes: An unusual but distinctive lymphadenopathy in cat. *J Comp Pathol* 97:109–119, 1987.

163. Mooney SC, Patnaik AK, Hayes AA, MacEwen EG: Generalized lymphadenopathy resembling lymphoma in cats: Six cases (1972–1976). *J Comp Pathol* 190:897–900, 1987.

164. Steele KE, Saunders GK, Coleman GD: T cell-rich B-cell lymphoma in a cat. *Vet Pathol* 34:47–49, 1997.

165. Day MJ, Kyaw-Tanner M, Silkstone MA, et al: T-cell rich B-cell lymphoma in the cat. *J Comp Pathol* 120:155–167, 1999.

166. Carlton WW: Intraocular lymphosarcoma: Two cases in Siamese cats. *JAAHA* 12:83–87, 1976.

167. Peiffer Jr RL, Wilcock BP: Histopathologic study of uveitis in cats: 139 cases (1978–1988). *JAVMA* 198:135–138, 1991.

168. Corcoran KA, Peiffer Jr RL, Koch SA: Histopathologic features of feline ocular lymphosarcoma: 49 cases (1978–1992). *Vet Comp Ophthalmology* 5:35–41, 1995.

169. Hittmair K, Walzer C: Generalisierte lymphidezellige infiltration des fettgewebes und exophthalmus bei einer leukosekranken katze. *Wien Tierärztl Mschr* 79:81–86, 1992.

170. Meincke JE: Reticuloendothelial malignancies, with intraocular involvement in the cat. *JAVMA* 148:157–161, 1966.

171. Saunders LZ, Barron CN: Intraocular tumors in animals. *Br Vet J* 120:25–35, 1964.

172. Barclay SM: Lymphosarcoma in tarsi of a cat. *JAVMA* 175:582–583, 1979.

173. Wilson JW: Reticulum cell sarcoma of long bone terminating as respiratory distress. *Vet Med Small Anim Clin* 68:1393–1401, 1973.

174. Elmslie RE, Ogilvie GK, Gillette EL, McChesney-Gillette S: Radiotherapy with and without chemotherapy for localized lymphoma in 10 cats. *Vet Radiol* 32:277–280, 1991.

175. Squire RA: Feline lymphoma: A comparison with the Burkitt tumor of children. *Cancer* 19:447–453, 1966.

176. Ladiges WC, Zeidner NS: An overview of feline cancer therapy. *Feline Pract* 10:38–43, 1980.

177. Brick JO, Roenigk WJ, Wilson GP: Chemotherapy of malignant lymphoma in dogs and cats. *JAVMA* 153:47–52, 1968.

178. Carpenter JL, Holzworth J: treatment of leukemia in the cat. *JAVMA* 158:1130–1131, 1971.

179. Squires RA, Bush M: The therapy of canine and feline lymphosarcoma, in: *Unifying Concepts of Leukemia.* Basel, Switzerland, Bibl Haemat Karger, 1973,: pp 189-197.

180. McClelland RB: Chemotherapy in reticulum-cell sarcoma in five dogs and a cat and in mast cell leukemia in a cat. *Cornell Vet* 61:477–481, 1971.

181. Ogilvie GK, Moore AS, Obradovich JE, et al: Toxicoses and efficacy associated with the administration of mitoxantrone to cats with malignant tumors. *JAVMA* 202:1839–1844, 1993.

182. Hahn KA, Fletcher CM, Legendre AM: Marked neutropenia in five tumor-bearing cats one week following single agent vincristine sulfate chemotherapy. *Vet Clin Pathol* 25:121–123, 1996.

183. Peaston AE, Maddison JE: Efficacy of doxorubicin as an induction agent for cats with lymphosarcoma. *Aust Vet J* 77:442–444, 1999.

184. Kristal O, Lana SE, Moore AS, et al: Single agent chemotherapy with doxorubicin for feline lymphoma. *Proc 18th Vet Cancer Soc*:25, 1998.

185. Matus RE: Chemotherapy of lymphoma and leukemia. In Kirk RW (ed): *Current Veterinary Therapy X. Small Animal Practice.* Philadelphia, WB Saunders, 1989, pp 482–488.

186. Marks SL, Cook AK, Griffey S, et al: Dietary modulation of methotrexate-induced enteritis in cats. *Am J Vet Res* 58:989–996, 1997.
187. Rassnick KM, Geiger TL, Williams LE, et al: Phase I evaluation of CCNU (lomustine) in tumor-bearing cats. *J Vet Internal Med* 15:196–199, 2001.
188. Mauldin GE, Mooney SC, Mauldin GN: MOPP chemotherapy for cats with refractory lymphoma. *Proc 17th Vet Cancer Soc*: 98, 1997.
189. Klein MK, Powers BE, Johnson CS, et al: Feline nasal lymphoma: A retrospective analysis. *Veterinary Cancer Society*, Tucson, 1995.
190. Calia CM, Hohenhaus AE, Fox PR, Meleo KA: Acute tumor lysis syndrome in a cat with lymphoma. *J Vet Intern Med* 10:409–411, 1996.
191. Hardy Jr WD, Hess PW, MacEwan EG, Hayes AA, Kassel RL, Day NK, Old LJ: treatment of feline lymphosarcoma with feline blood constituents, in: *Comparative Leukemia Research. Bibliotheca Haematologica*. Basel, Switzerland, Karger, 1976;43:518-521.
192. Kassel RL, Old LJ, Day NK, et al: Plasma mediated leukemic cell destruction: Current status. *Blood Cells* 3:605–621, 1977.
193. Snyder Jr HW, Jones FR, Day NK, Hardy Jr WD: Isolation and characterization of circulating feline leukemia virus-immune complexes from plasma of persistently infected pet cats removed by ex vivo immunosorption. *J Immunol* 128:2726–2730, 1982.
194. MacEwan EG: Current concepts in cancer therapy: Biologic therapy and chemotherapy. *Semin Vet Med & Surg (Small Anim)* 1:5–16, 1986.
195. Engelman RW, Good RA, Day NK: Clearance of retroviremia and regression of malignancy in cats with leukemia-lymphoma during treatment with staphylococcal protein A. *Cancer Detect Prevent* 10:435–444, 1987.
196. Harper HD, Sjöquist J, Hardy Jr WD, Jones FR: Antitumor activity of protein A administered intravenously to pet cats with leukemia or lymphosarcoma. *Cancer* 55:1863–1867, 1985.
197. Snyder Jr HW, Singhal MC, Hardy Jr WD, Jones FR: Clearance of feline leukemia virus from persistently infected pet cats treated by extracorporeal immunoadsorption is correlated with an enhanced antibody response to FeLV gp 70. *J Immunol* 132:1538–1543, 1984.
198. Jones FR, Grant CK, Snyder Jr HW: Lymphosarcoma and persistent feline leukemia virus infection of pet cats: A system to study responses during extracorporeal treatments. *J Biol Resp Modif* 3:286–292, 1984.
199. Gordon BR, Matus RE, Hurvitz AI, et al: Perfusion of plasma over *Staphylococcus aureus*: Release of bacterial product is related to regression of tumor. *J Biol Resp Modif* 3:266–270, 1984.
200. Sheets MA, Unger BA, Giggleman GF Jr, Tizard IR: Studies of the effect of acemannan on retrovirus infections: Clinical stabilization of feline leukemia virus-infected cats. *Mol Biother* 3:41–45, 1991.

Chapter 46

Feline bone marrow neoplasias

FELINE MYELODYSPLASIA (PRELEUKEMIA)

Clinical presentation

- Moderately common and sometimes associated with infection with FeLV.
- Usually not painful.
- Myelodysplasia or preleukemia may progress to a true neoplastic process or leukemia.
- Clinically, it is often important to distinguish chronic leukemias and myeloproliferative diseases from acute leukemias and to differentiate between acute lymphoblastic leukemia (ALL) and acute nonlymphoid leukemia (ANLL).
- Myelodysplasia is distinguished from the acute leukemias by the presence of less than 30% abnormal blast cells and abnormal cellular maturation in the bone marrow aspirate in the former.

Key point

Clinical signs secondary to this disease are often related to the anemia, which results in fatigue, anorexia, lethargy and chronic weight loss.

Staging and diagnosis

- Minimum data base (MDB): includes a CBC, biochemical profile, urinalysis, FIV/FeLV serology, T4 testing, biopsy and three-view thoracic radiographs.
- Bone marrow aspiration and cytology is essential to make a definitive diagnosis.

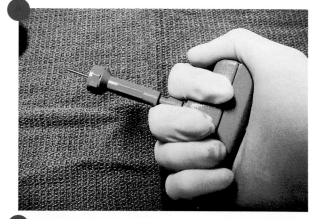

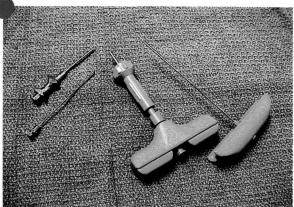

Figure 46-1: Bone marrow aspirates can be done safely, easily and with little training or expertise. There are several types of bone marrow needles that are commercially available including Illiniois bone marrow needles and disposable plastic-handled marrow needles. When doing a bone marrow in a cat, a 20 gauge bone marrow needle is preferred.

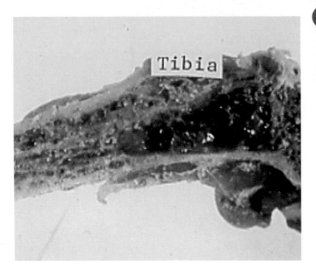

Figure 46-2: The marrow in this bone is almost completely replaced by neoplastic cells. Obtaining a sample from this site may be the only way of making a diagnosis of bone marrow neoplasia. Reprinted with permission from: Ogilvie GK, Moore AS. *Feline Oncology: A Comprehensive Guide for Compassionate Care.* Trenton NJ, Veterinary Learning Systems. 2002.

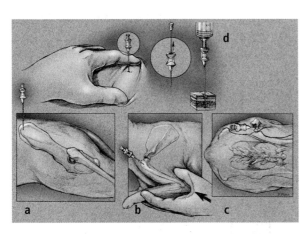

Figure 46-3: A bone marrow aspirate can be done in many bony locations in an anesthetized cat that has been given appropriate analgesia. The area to be sampled is clipped and prepared for anesthesia. A lidocaine block is administered for local analgesia. The bone marrow needle is placed through the skin and directed toward the iliac crest (a), proximal humerus (b) or femoral fossa (c) as depicted above. Once the needle is secured into bone, the stylette is removed and the syringe is attached (d). The marrow is immediately aspirated and slides are quickly prepared to ensure the marrow is smeared into a thin film. Most acute and chronic leukemias cannot be accurately diagnosed without a bone marrow aspirate and review by an accomplished pathologist. Reprinted with permission from: Ogilvie GK, Moore AS. *Feline Oncology: A Comprehensive Guide for Compassionate Care.* Trenton NJ, Veterinary Learning Systems. 2002.

Key point

Impossible to diagnose or to differentiate from other lymphoproliferative diseases without an analysis of the cytology obtained from a bone marrow aspirate or histopathology from a bone marrow core biopsy.

Treatment

This section is divided into two options:
- Comfort for those who want to improve quality of life.
- Comfort and control for those who want to improve quality of life while trying to provide some control of the tumor.

Comfort

- Therapy to enhance comfort and freedom from nausea, vomiting (e.g.: maropitant and/or metoclopramide), diarrhea (e.g.: metronidazole) and lack of appetite (e.g.: mirtazapine or cyproheptadine). Transfusions, erythropoietin therapy and steroids may be helpful in some cats.

Comfort and control

Above mentioned therapy for comfort plus:
- Bone marrow transplantation, however this is experimental.
- Cytosine arabinoside or synthetic retinoids have been used as differentiating agents.

FELINE ACUTE NON-LYMPHOID LEUKEMIA

Clinical presentation

- Relatively uncommon.
- This type of leukemia may develop from myelodysplastic syndrome.
- May be uncomfortable or associated with pain, especially at end stages of the disease.
- Young cats seem to predominate.
- FeLV antigenemia is common.
- Rapidly progressive and often associated with anorexia, lethargy and weakness.
- Cytopenias, hepatosplenomegaly common.

Key point

Lethargy, anorexia and weight loss.

Staging and diagnosis

- Minimum data base (MDB): includes a CBC, biochemical profile, urinalysis, FIV/FeLV serology,

T4 testing, biopsy, three-view thoracic radiographs or, if available, computerized tomography of the chest.
- Bone marrow aspirate and cytology.
- Anemia and an increased number of nucleated red blood cells are commonly seen on the complete blood count.
- Hypercalcemia of malignancy is occasionally seen.

Treatment

This section is divided into two options:
- Comfort for those who want to improve quality of life.
- Comfort and control for those who want to improve quality of life while trying to provide some control of the tumor.

Comfort

- Therapy to enhance comfort (e.g.: NSAID, tramadol, buprenorphine) and freedom from nausea, vomiting (e.g.: maropitant and/or metoclopramide), diarrhea (e.g.: metronidazole) and lack of appetite (e.g.: mirtazapine or cyproheptadine).
- Transfusions or blood product therapy and/or erythropoietin may be very helpful to treat anemia or thrombocytopenia.
- Neutropenia may be associated with the development of infections that may respond to antibiotics.
- Thrombocytopenia may result in bleeding that may respond to Yunnan Baiyao.

Comfort and control

Above mentioned therapy for comfort plus:
- Bone marrow transplantation, however this is experimental.
- Cytosine arabinoside or synthetic retinoids have been used as differentiating agents.

FELINE ACUTE LYMPHOID LEUKEMIA

Clinical presentation

- Moderately common, but less common than lymphoma.
- May be painful.
- Young cats (median age, 5 years); no breed or gender predilection.
- Most cats are FeLV antigenemic.
- Rapid onset of anorexia and weight loss; lymphadenopathy is common, which may make differentiating acute lymphoid leukemia from lymphoma difficult.

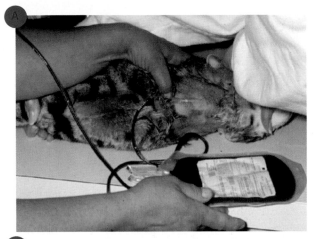

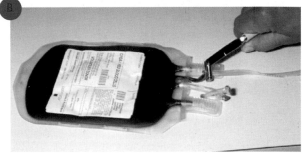

Figure 46-4: All leukemias can cause pancytopenia requiring whole blood transfusion support. Blood can be harvested from a larger healthy adult cat and given to the recipient to ensure that the patient has the best chance to respond well to therapy. All cells degrade with time, especially white blood cells and platelets. Therefore fresh whole blood is preferred to treat pancytopenic cats.

> **Key point**
> Clinical signs for cats with acute lymphoid leukemia are often nonspecific and include anorexia, weight loss and lethargy.

Staging and diagnosis

- Minimum data base (MDB): includes a CBC, biochemical profile, urinalysis, FIV/FeLV serology, T4 testing, biopsy, three-view thoracic radiographs or computerized tomography of the chest.
- Ultrasonography and/or radiographs are practical and cost effective, however computerized tomography or magnetic resonance imaging of the tumor may be preferable.
- Bone marrow aspirate and cytology.
- Blast cells may be found in the circulation in most cats, or in the bone marrow aspirates, but they may be difficult to identify definitively on morphologic criteria alone. Therefore immunocytochemical staining, flow cytometry or PPAR of peripheral blood or bone marrow is indicated.

> **Key point**
> Some cats with acute lymphoid leukemia have only hematologic changes noted on CBC (anemia, thrombocytopenia, leukemia? or leukopenia) and bone marrow aspirate cytology, whereas others may also have intra-abdominal lymphadenopathy as well as involvement of the liver and spleen.

Treatment

This section is divided into three options:
- Comfort for those who want to improve quality of life.
- Comfort and control for those who want to improve quality of life while trying to provide some control of the tumor.
- Comfort and longer-term control for those who want to improve quality of life while trying to maximize the chance of controlling the tumor.

Comfort

- Therapy to enhance comfort (e.g.: tramadol, buprenorphine) and freedom from nausea, vomiting (e.g.: maropitant and/or metoclopramide), diarrhea (e.g.: metronidazole) and lack of appetite (e.g.: mirtazapine or cyproheptadine).
- Transfusions or blood product therapy and/or erythropoietin may be very helpful to treat anemia or thrombocytopenia.
- Neutropenia may be associated with the development of infections that may respond to antibiotics.
- Thrombocytopenia may result in bleeding that may respond to Yunnan Baiyao.

Comfort and control

Above mentioned therapy for comfort plus:
- COP protocol (vincristine, 0.75 mg/m^2 IV; cyclophosphamide, 300 mg/m^2 PO every 3 weeks; and prednisolone, 40 mg/m^2 PO daily) with a median remission of 7 months.[51]

Comfort and longer-term control

Above mentioned therapy for comfort plus:
- CHOP protocol.

FELINE CHRONIC LYMPHOCYTIC LEUKEMIA

Clinical presentation

- Relatively uncommon.
- Usually not painful.
- Patients may be asymptomatic, however anemia is commonly seen with this disease, therefore weakness, lethargy, weight loss and anorexia is occasionally seen.

> **Key point**
> Most cats with CLL have a long, clinically silent period that is followed by vague clinical signs of weakness, lethargy, anorexia and infections.

Staging and diagnosis

- Minimum data base (MDB): includes a CBC, biochemical profile, urinalysis, FIV/FeLV serology, T4 testing, biopsy, three-view thoracic radiographs or computerized tomography of the chest.
- Determining the causes of lymphocytosis should include evaluation of signalment, concurrent disease conditions, lymphocyte morphology, lymphocyte distribution in bone marrow, and immunophenotype by PPAR or flow cytometry.
- Cats with chronic lymphocytic leukemia tend to be older, and lymphocytes are often T-cells, slightly larger than expected and have cleaved or lobulated nuclei.
- Cats with a B-cell immunophenotype that are often described as a reactive lymphocytosis are usually associated with immune-mediated anemias and inflammatory diseases.
- Bone marrow aspirate and cytology.
- Infiltration of the bone marrow with more than 15% mature lymphocytes confirms the diagnosis of CLL in cats. Unlike dogs, normal cats may have lymphocytes accounting for as much as 5% of their bone marrow.
- Mature lymphocytes may have infiltrated other organs.

Treatment

This section is divided into two options:
- Comfort for those who want to improve quality of life.
- Comfort and control for those who want to improve quality of life while trying to provide some control of the tumor.

> **Key point**
> Most cats with CLL positively respond to chlorambucil and prednisolone therapy, however complete remissions may take months to occur.

Comfort

- Therapy to enhance comfort (e.g.: NSAID, tramadol, buprenorphine) and freedom from nausea, vomiting (e.g.: maropitant and/or metoclopramide), diarrhea (e.g.: metronidazole) and lack of appetite (e.g.: mirtazapine or cyproheptadine).

Comfort and control

Above mentioned therapy for comfort plus:

- Chlorambucil and prednisolone.
  - In one study of cats treated with chlorambucil and prednisolone or a CHOP protocol, complete and partial remissions were confirmed in 88% of cats, with a median overall remission duration of 15.7 months and a median overall survival of 14.4 months. The authors concluded that CLL affects older-aged cats and responds favorably to treatment with oral chlorambucil and prednisolone.[49]

FELINE HYPEREOSINOPHILIC DISEASE

Clinical presentation

- Relatively uncommon.
- May be associated with discomfort.
- Adult cats (median age, 8 years).
- Females may be predisposed.
- May have widespread organ infiltration.
- Chronic history of vomiting, diarrhea and weight loss is relatively common.
- Differential diagnoses include allergies, eosinophilic granuloma complex, and parasitic disease.
- Physical examination may reveal thickened loops of bowel, abdominal masses, pyrexia, pruritus, and hepatosplenomegaly.

Staging and diagnosis

- Minimum data base (MDB): includes a CBC, biochemical profile, urinalysis, FIV/FeLV serology, T4 testing, biopsy, three-view thoracic radiographs or computerized tomography of the chest.
- Abdominal ultrasound.
- Bone marrow aspirate.

Treatment

This section is divided into two options:

- Comfort for those who want to improve quality of life.
- Comfort and control for those who want to improve quality of life while trying to provide some control of the tumor.

Comfort

- Therapy to enhance comfort (e.g.: NSAID, tramadol, buprenorphine) and freedom from nausea, vomiting (e.g.: maropitant and/or metoclopramide), diarrhea (e.g.: metronidazole) and lack of appetite (e.g.: mirtazapine or cyproheptadine).

Comfort and control

Above mentioned therapy for comfort plus:

- Palliative radiation, especially for those with extension into surrounding structures or regional metastases (e.g.: 2-5 dosages of radiation), to first enhance comfort, second, to reduce the rate of growth and third, occasionally to reduce the size of the tumor.

FELINE PRIMARY ERYTHROCYTOSIS (POLYCYTHEMIA VERA)

Clinical presentation

- Uncommon.
- May be uncomfortable.
- Polycythemia (increase in PCV, hemoglobin and number of red blood cells) may be primary (polycythemia vera) or secondary (disorders due to an increase in erythropoietin).
- Polycythemia vera is an abnormal clonal expansion of the red blood cell line independent of erythropoietin.
- Secondary polycythemia may be caused by systemic hypoxia from cardiorespiratory disease, high altitude, altered hemoglobin or erythropoietin producing tumors, most commonly renal tumors.
- Middle-age (median 6 years old) male cats may predominate.
- Hyperviscosity syndrome causes signs of neurologic disturbances (e.g., seizures and ataxia) and dark mucous membranes.

> **Key point**
>
> Cats with feline primary erythrocytosis may occur secondary increased amounts of endogenous erythropoietin or secondary to a malignancy of red blood cell precursors that causes an increased number of red blood cells.

Staging and diagnosis

- Minimum data base (MDB): includes a CBC, biochemical profile, urinalysis, FIV/FeLV serology, T4 testing, biopsy, three-view thoracic radiographs or computerized tomography or magnetic resonance imaging of the chest and abdomen.
- Bone marrow aspiration.
- Eliminate secondary causes with cardiac ultrasound, aspiration of any masses, echocardiography, serum erythropoietin concentration, as well as pulse oximetry or blood gas determination at rest and exercise.

27. Groulade P, Guilhon JC: Syndrome érythrémique chez le chat. *Bull Acad Vt France* 39:127–131, 1966.
28. Watson ADJ, Huxtable CRR, Hoskins LP: Erythremic myelosis in two cats. *Aust Vet J* 50:29–33, 1974.
29. Zawidzka ZZ, Janzen E, Grice HC: Erythremic myelosis in a cat. A case resembling Di Guglielmo's syndrome in man. *Pathol Vet* 1:530–541, 1964.
30. Saar C: Erythrämie und erythroleukämie bei der katze bericht über je einen fall. *Berl Münch Teirärztl Wschr* 21:423–426, 1968.
31. Cotter SM, Holzworth J: Disorders of the hematopoietic system. In Holzworth J (ed): *Diseases of the cat. Medicine and Surgery.* Philadelphia, WB Saunders Co, 1987, pp 755–807.
32. Case MT: A case of myelogenous leukemia in a cat. *Zentralbl Veterinärmed A* 17:273–277, 1970.
33. Eyestone WH: Myelogenous leukemia in the cat. *J Natl Cancer Inst* 1951;12:599–613.
34. Gilbride AP: Myelogenous leukemia in a cat complicated by otitis media. *Can J Comp Med* 28:207–211, 1964.
35. Henness AM, Crow SE: treatment of feline myelogenous leukemia. Four case reports. *JAVMA* 171:263–266, 1977.
36. Meier H, Patterson DF: Myelogenous leukemia in a cat. *JAVMA* 128:211–214, 1956.
37. Reid JA, Marcus LC: Granulocytic leukemia in a cat. *J Small Anim Pract* 7:421–425, 1966.
38. Fraser CJ, Joiner GN, Jardine JH, Gleiser CA: Acute granulocytic leukemia in cats. *JAVMA* 165:355–359, 1974.
39. Henness AM, Crow SE, Anderson BC: Monocytic leukemia in three cats. *JAVMA* 170:1325–1328, 1977.
40. Saar C, Reichel C: Einige besondere leukoseformen bei der katze. *Praktische Tierarzt* 5:443–450, 1983.
41. Holscher MA, Collins RD, Cousar JB, et al: Megakaryocytic leukemia in a cat. *Feline Pract* 13:8–12, 1983.
42. Michel RL, O'Handley P, Dade AW: Megakaryocytic myelosis in a cat. *JAVMA* 168:1021–1025, 1976.
43. Sutton RH, McKellow AM, Bottrill MB: Myeloproliferative disease in the cat: A granulocytic and megakaryocytic disorder. *NZ Vet J* 26:273–279, 1978.
44. Miyamoto T, Takeda T, Kuwamura M, et al: An unusual feline case of suspected myelomonocytic leukemia with severe leukopenia. *Feline Pract* 27:15–17, 1999.
45. Loeb WF, Rininger B: Myelomonocytic leukemia in a cat. *Vet Pathol* 12:464–467, 1975.
46. Stann SE: Myelomonocytic leukemia in a cat. *JAVMA* 174:722–725, 1979.
47. Engleman RW, Tyler RD, Mosier DA: Changing manifestations of a chronic feline haematopoietic proliferative disease during immunotherapy with staphylococcal protein A. *J Comp Pathol* 96:177–188, 1986.
48. Crow SE, Madewell BR, Henness AM: Feline reticuloendotheliosis: a report of four cases. *JAVMA* 170:1329–1332, 1977.
49. Campbell MW, Hess PR, Williams LE. Chronic lymphocytic leukaemia in the cat: 18 cases (2000-2010). *Vet Comp Oncol* 11(4):256-264, 2013.
50. Moore AS, Ruslander D, Cotter SM, et al: Efficacy of, and toxicoses associated with, oral idarubicin administration in cats with neoplasia. *JAVMA* 206:1550–1554, 1995.
51. Cotter SM: treatment of lymphoma and leukemia with cyclophosphamide, vincristine, and prednisone: II. treatment of cats. *JAAHA* 19:166–172, 1983.
52. Cotter SM, Holzworth J: Disorders of the hematopoetic system. In Holzworth J (ed): *Diseases of the Cat. Medicine and Surgery.* Philadelphia, WB Saunders, 1987, pp 755–807.
53. Thrall MA: Lymphoproliferative disorders: Lymphocytic leukemia and plasma cell myeloma. *Vet Clin North Am Small Anim Clin* 11:321–347, 1981.
54. Center SA, Randolph JF, Erb HN, Reiter S: Eosinophilia in the cat: A retrospective study of 312 cases (1975 to 1986). *JAAHA* 26:349–358, 1990.
55. Neer TM: Hypereosinophilic syndrome in cats. *Compend Contin Educ Pract Vet* 13:549–555, 1991.
56. Simon N, Holzworth J: Eosinophilic leukemia in a cat. *Cornell Vet* 7:579–597, 1967.
57. Silverman J: Eosinophilic leukemia in a cat. *JAVMA* 158:199, 1971
58. Harvey RG: Feline hypereosinophilia with cutaneous lesions. *J Small Anim Pract* 31:453–456, 1990.
59. Scott DW, Randolph JF, Walsh KM: Hypereosinophilic syndrome in a cat. *Feline Pract* 15:22–30, 1985.
60. Watson ADJ, Moore AS, Helfand SC: Primary erythrocytosis in the cat: treatment with hydroxyurea. *J Small Anim Pract* 35:320–325, 1994.
61. Reed C, Ling GV, Gould D, Kaneko JJ: Polycythemia vera in a cat. *JAVMA* 157:85–91, 1970.
62. Duff BC, Allan GS, Howlett CR: A presumptive case of polycythemia vera in a cat. *Aust Vet Pract* 3:78–79, 1973.
63. Foster ES, Lothrop Jr CD: Polycythemia vera in a cat with cardiac hypertrophy. *JAVMA* 192:1736–1738, 1988.
64. Mellor PJ, Haugland S, Murphy S, et al: Myeloma-related disorders in cats commonly present as extramedullary neoplasms in contrast to myeloma in human patients: 24 cases with clinical follow-up. *J Vet Intern Med* 20(6):1376-1383, 2006.
65. Patel RT, Caceres A, French AF, et al: Multiple myeloma in 16 cats: a retrospective study. *Vet Clin Pathol.* 34(4):341-352, 2005.
66. Jacobs T: Multiple myeloma in a cat with paraparesis. *Feline Pract* 22:28–32, 1994.
67. Holzworth J, Meier H: Reticulum cell myeloma in a cat. *Cornell Vet* 47:302–316, 1957.
68. Mills JN, Eger CE, Robinson WF, et al: A case of multiple myeloma in a cat. *JAAHA* 18:79–82, 1982.
69. Ward DA, McEntee MF, Weddle DL: Orbital plasmacytoma in a cat. *J Small Anim Pract* 38:576–578, 1997.
70. Drazner FH: Multiple myeloma in the cat. *Compend Contin Educ Pract Vet* 4:206–216, 1982.
71. MacEwen EG, Huruitz AI: Diagnosis and management of monoclonal gammopathies. *Vet Clin North Am Small Anim Clin* 7:119–132, 1977.
72. Williams DA, Goldschmidt MH: Hyperviscosity syndrome with IgM monoclonal gammopathy and hepatic plasmacytoid lymphosarcoma in a cat. *J Small Anim Pract* 23:311–323, 1982.
73. Saar C, Saar U, Opitz M, Burow H, Teichert G: Paraproteinämische retikulosen bei der katze. *Berl Münch Teirärztl Wschr* 86:11–15, 1973.
74. Mandel NS, Esplin DG: A retroperitoneal extramedullary plasmacytoma in a cat with a monoclonal gammopathy. *JAAHA* 30:603–608, 1994.
75. Weber NA, Tebeau CS: An unusual presentation of multiple myeloma in two cats. *JAAHA* 34:477–483, 1998.
76. Hay LE: Multiple myeloma in a cat. *Aust Vet Pract* 8:45–48, 1978.
77. Hribernik TN, Barta O, Gaunt SD, Boudreaux MK: Serum hyperviscosity syndrome associated with IgG myeloma in a cat. *JAVMA* 181:169–170, 1982.
78. Forrester SD, Greco DS, Relford RL: Serum hyperviscosity syndrome associated with multiple myeloma in two cats. *JAVMA* 200:79–82, 1992.
79. Forrester SD, Fossum TW, Rogers KS: Diagnosis and treatment of chylothorax associated with lymphoblastic lymphosarcoma in four cats. *JAVMA* 198:291–294, 1991.
80. Farrow BRH, Penny R: Multiple myeloma in a cat. *JAVMA* 158:606–611, 1971.
81. Bertoy RW, Brightman AH, Regan K: Intraocular melanoma with multiple metastases in a cat. *JAVMA* 192:87–89, 1988.
82. Kehoe JM, Hurvitsz AI, Capra JD: Characterization of three feline paraproteins. *J Immunol* 109:511–516, 1972.
83. Rowland PH, Linke RP: Immunohistochemical characterization of lambda light-chain-derived amyloid in one feline and five canine plasma cell tumors. *Vet Pathol* 31:390–393, 1994.
84. Port CD, Maschgan ER, Pond J, Scarpelli DG: Multiple neoplasia in a jaguar *(Panthera onca). J Comp Pathol* 91:115–122, 1981.

Chapter 47

Feline tumors of bone

FELINE OSTEOSARCOMA

Clinical presentation

- Moderately common.
- May be painful.
- Appendicular and axial skeleton equally affected.
- As in dogs and humans, fractures or repair thereof has been associated with tumor formation, although this is quite rare.
- Hind limb and skull most common sites.
- Extraosseous osteosarcoma may be associated with injections (i.e.: injection site sarcomas).
- Metastases are uncommon.
- Pathologic fracture at the site of an appendicular osteosarcoma is common in cats.
- Hypertrophic osteopathy may occur with pulmonary metastases.

> **Key point**
>
> Lameness and/or change in the structure of the bone is common in cats with osteosarcoma.

Staging and diagnosis

- Minimum data base (MDB): includes a CBC, biochemical profile, urinalysis, FIV/FeLV serology, T4 testing, biopsy, three-view thoracic radiographs or computerized tomography of the chest.
- Ultrasonography and/or radiographs are practical and cost effective, however computerized tomography or magnetic resonance imaging of the tumor may be preferable in some cases.
- While metastases are uncommon, regional lymph nodes and the thoracic cavity should be carefully assessed for metastases.
- Taking a sample with a 16 or 18 gauge needle through the center of the lesion may allow a

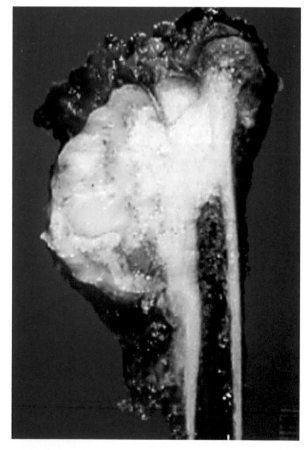

Figure 47-1: Cats with appendicular osteosarcoma may have a history of lameness of one limb or another. If osteosarcoma is the cause, a mass or thickening of the metaphysis of long bones or elsewhere is commonly found, as depicted in this image. Fortunately, osteosarcoma in the cat rarely metastasizes. Differentials that must be considered in these types of cases include infectious, inflammatory, degenerative or neoplastic conditions.

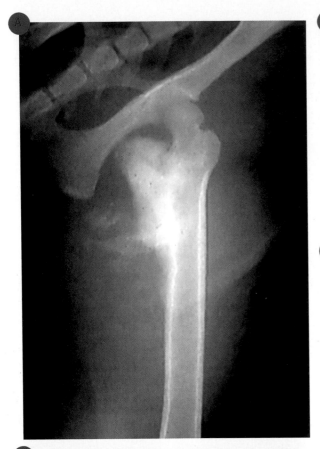

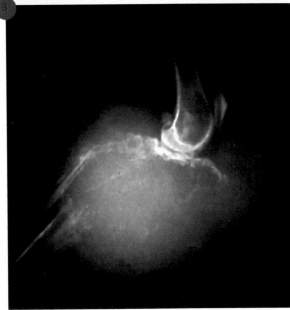

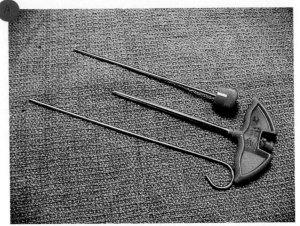

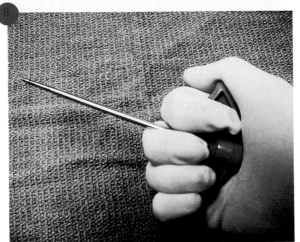

Figure 47-3: Once a bony lesion is identified on physical examination, radiographs or CT, a sample of that bone must be acquired to determine the diagnosis. The "gold standard" is a bone biopsy that can be secured with a bone marrow biopsy needle. This biopsy system comes complete with a biopsy needle, a stylettte within the needle, and a wire to push the biopsy from the tip of the biopsy needle out the "back" of the biopsy apparatus (47e). The assembled biopsy needle with the stylette within the needle is prepared for the actual biopsy (47f). A comfortable handle allows for the clinician to begin the biopsy system.

Figure 47-2: Radiographs, CT or MRI of the bony lesions often confirm a lytic, proliferative lesion. An aspirate or biopsy of the lesion confirms the diagnosis. Note the lysis of the metaphyseal region of the tibia (A) and proximal femur (B). Removal of the entire tumor and surrounding tissue often results in long-term control. Imaging courtesy of Lenore Anderson Mohammadian, DVM, MSpVM, Diplomate ACVR.

clinical pathologist to confirm that the lesion in question is likely due to a malignancy. This can be an inexpensive way of confirming a diagnosis of a malignancy. The specific type of malignancy may require either an excisional or incisional biopsy.

- Biopsies, either needle core, Jamshidi, wedge or
- excisional may be helpful. If removal of the tumor is attempted, the entire specimen should be submitted for a definitive diagnosis and to evaluate margins for completeness of excision.
- The presence of metastases is a poor prognostic indicator, although this is rare.

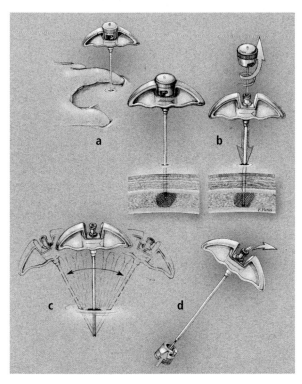

Figure 47-4: Cytology from the lytic boney lesion may allow the clinician to confirm malignancy of a bony lesion, however histopathology is considered the gold standard. The bone biopsy needle is used to secure a biopsy sample. The biopsy needle is advanced through the skin and underlying structures, up to the level of the bone to be biopsied (a). The objective is to secure at least one core of the lesion going through the center of the bony growth. Once the needle is resting on top of the bony lesion, the cap is removed (b) and the needle is then advanced through the center of the bone by rotating the handle back and forth while applying direct downward pressure. Once the needle has been advanced to the appropriate depth, the needle is then rotated laterally to the left and to the right several times (c). The bone biopsy needle is removed from the patient and the wire is used to push the biopsy core from the tip of the needle out the back end at the handle (d). Reprinted with permission from: Ogilvie GK, Moore AS. *Feline Oncology: A Comprehensive Guide for Compassionate Care.* Trenton NJ, Veterinary Learning Systems. 2002.

Key point

A histopathologic biopsy or fine needle aspirate cytology of osteosarcoma is ideal to make the diagnosis, however the sample should be taken within the center of the bony change.

Treatment

This section is divided into three options:
- Comfort for those who want to improve quality of life.

- Comfort and control for those who want to improve quality of life while trying to provide some control of the tumor.
- Comfort and longer-term control for those who want to improve quality of life while trying to maximize the chance of controlling the tumor.

Key point

Analgesics, radiation and/or surgical removal of the involved lesion often results in long-term progression-free survival in cats with osteosarcoma.

Comfort

- Therapy to enhance comfort (e.g.: NSAID, tramadol, buprenorphine) and freedom from nausea, vomiting (e.g.: maropitant and/or metoclopramide), diarrhea (e.g.: metronidazole) and lack of appetite (e.g.: mirtazapine or cyproheptadine).

Comfort and control

Above mentioned therapy for comfort plus:
- Palliative radiation, especially for those with extension into surrounding structures or regional metastases (e.g.: 2-5 dosages of radiation), to first enhance comfort, second, to reduce the rate of growth and third, occasionally to reduce the size of the tumor.

Comfort and longer-term control

Above mentioned therapy for comfort plus:
- Surgery such as amputation for tumors of the extremity, or mass removal with wide and deep margins for tumors of soft tissues. Tumors of the skull and flat bones may require CT-guided surgical excision.
  - Survival times for cats with axial osteosarcoma may be greater than 1 year, even with incomplete resection.
- Definitive radiation if there is evidence of tumor extending beyond the surgical margins (e.g.: 16-19 dosages of radiation).
- Stereotactic radiosurgery (e.g.: IMRT, CyberKnife or Trilogy based) may be helpful in certain situations as an alternative to surgery.
- Carboplatin is used by some, however there is little evidence that it may help improve progression-free survival.

FELINE GIANT CELL TUMORS OF BONE

Clinical presentation

- Uncommon.
- May be painful, especially if it involves an extremity.

- May be a variant of osteosarcoma or synovial sarcoma; appendicular more common than axial.
- Metastases, while apparently rare, may be found in regional lymph nodes or lungs.

Staging and diagnosis

- Minimum data base (MDB): includes a CBC, biochemical profile, urinalysis, FIV/FeLV serology, T4 testing, biopsy, three-view thoracic radiographs or computerized tomography of the chest.
- Computerized tomography or magnetic resonance imaging of the tumor may be quite helpful to guide the surgeon to a successful excision.
- Biopsies, either needle core, Jamshidi, wedge or excisional may be helpful. If removal of the tumor is attempted, the entire specimen should be submitted for a definitive diagnosis and to evaluate margins for completeness of excision.

Treatment

This section is divided into three options:
- Comfort for those who want to improve quality of life.
- Comfort and control for those who want to improve quality of life while trying to provide some control of the tumor.
- Comfort and longer-term control for those who want to improve quality of life while trying to maximize the chance of controlling the tumor.

Comfort

- Therapy to enhance comfort (e.g.: NSAID, tramadol, buprenorphine) and freedom from nausea, vomiting (e.g.: maropitant and/or metoclopramide), diarrhea (e.g.: metronidazole) and lack of appetite (e.g.: mirtazapine or cyproheptadine).

Comfort and control

Above mentioned therapy for comfort plus:
- Palliative radiation, especially for those with extension into surrounding structures or that have regional metastases (e.g.: 2-5 dosages of radiation), to first enhance comfort, second, to reduce the rate of growth and third, occasionally to reduce the size of the tumor.

Comfort and longer-term control

Above mentioned therapy for comfort plus:
- Surgery such as amputation for giant cell tumors of the extremity, or mass removal with wide and deep margins for tumors of soft tissues. Tumors of the skull and flat bones may require CT-guided surgical excision.
- Definitive radiation if there is evidence of tumor extending beyond the surgical margins (e.g.: 16-19 dosages of radiation).

- Stereotactic radiosurgery (e.g.: IMRT, CyberKnife or Trilogy based) may be helpful in certain situations as an alternative to surgery.

FELINE OSTEOMA
Clinical presentation

- Moderately common.
- May be painful.
- May be seen throughout the body, including and especially where osteosarcomas occur.

Staging and diagnosis

- Minimum data base (MDB): includes a CBC, biochemical profile, urinalysis, FIV/FeLV serology, T4 testing, biopsy, three-view thoracic radiographs or computerized tomography of the chest.
- Computerized tomography or magnetic resonance imaging of the tumor may be quite helpful to guide the surgeon to a successful excision.
- Biopsies, either needle core, Jamshidi, wedge or excisional may be helpful. If removal of the tumor is attempted, the entire specimen should be submitted for a definitive diagnosis and to evaluate margins for completeness of excision.

Treatment

This section is divided into three options:
- Comfort for those who want to improve quality of life.
- Comfort and control for those who want to improve quality of life while trying to provide some control of the tumor.
- Comfort and longer-term control for those who want to improve quality of life while trying to maximize the chance of controlling the tumor.

Comfort

- Therapy to enhance comfort (e.g.: NSAID, tramadol, buprenorphine) and freedom from nausea, vomiting (e.g.: maropitant and/or metoclopramide), diarrhea (e.g.: metronidazole) and lack of appetite (e.g.: mirtazapine or cyproheptadine).

Comfort and control

Above mentioned therapy for comfort plus:
- Palliative radiation, especially for those with extension into surrounding structures or regional metastases (e.g.: 2-5 dosages of radiation), to first enhance comfort, second, to reduce the rate of growth and third, occasionally to reduce the size of the tumor.

Comfort and longer-term control

Above mentioned therapy for comfort plus:
- Surgery such as amputation for tumors of the

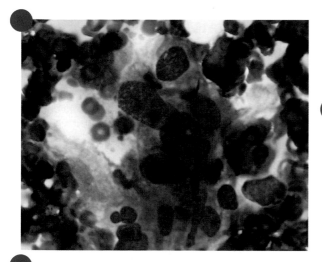

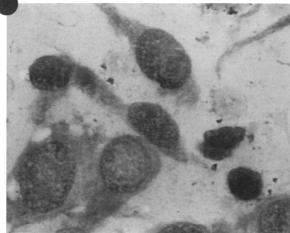

Figure 47-5: Cytology obtained by advancing an 18 gauge needle through the center of the bony lesion may allow the clinician to confirm malignancy of a bony lesion. Notice the elongated, streaming cells that have variable sized nuclei, often with nucleoli. A histopathological biopsy may be needed to distinguish the specific diagnosis.

extremity, or mass removal with wide and deep margins for tumors of soft tissues. Tumors of the skull and flat bones may require CT-guided surgical excision.
- Definitive radiation if there is evidence of tumor extending beyond the surgical margins (e.g.: 16-19 dosages of radiation).

FELINE CHONDROSARCOMA

Clinical presentation

- Moderately common.
- May be painful.
- Symptoms related to the location of the tumor.
- Rarely metastasizes, but if it does, it can spread to lungs and lymph nodes.

- Second most common tumor of bone after osteosarcoma.
- Slow growing malignancy that involves the axial skeleton more commonly than the appendicular skeleton.

Key point
Generally a slowly growing malignancy that may cause discomfort and functional abnormalities associated with clinical signs relating to the location of the tumor.

Staging and diagnosis

- Minimum data base (MDB): includes a CBC, biochemical profile, urinalysis, FIV/FeLV serology, T4 testing, biopsy, three-view thoracic radiographs or computerized tomography of the chest.
- Ultrasonography and/or radiographs are practical and cost effective, however computerized tomography or magnetic resonance imaging of the tumor may be preferable in some cases.
- Biopsies, either needle core, Jamshidi, wedge or excisional may be helpful. If removal of the tumor is attempted, the entire specimen should be submitted for a definitive diagnosis and to evaluate margins for completeness of excision.

Key point
While cytology may be suggestive of a chondrosarcoma, a biopsy is often required to accurately diagnose this malignancy.

Treatment

This section is divided into three options:
- Comfort for those who want to improve quality of life.
- Comfort and control for those who want to improve quality of life while trying to provide some control of the tumor.
- Comfort and longer-term control for those who want to improve quality of life while trying to maximize the chance of controlling the tumor.

Key point
Analgesia, radiation or complete removal of the tumor can be quite helpful for the treatment of chondrosarcoma.

Comfort

- Therapy to enhance comfort (e.g.: NSAID, tramadol, buprenorphine) and freedom from nausea, vomiting (e.g.: maropitant and/or metoclopramide), diarrhea

8. Madewell BR, Leighton RL, Theilen GH: Amputation and doxorubicin for treatment of canine and feline osteogenic sarcoma. *Europ J Cancer* 14:287–293, 1978.
9. Turrel JM, Pool RR: Primary bone tumors in the cat: A retrospective study of 15 cats and literature review. *Vet Radiol* 23:152–166, 1982.
10. Liu S-K, Dorfman HD, Patnaik AK: Primary and secondary bone tumours in the cat. *J Small Anim Pract* 15:141–156, 1974.
11. Kessler M, Tassani-Prell M, von Bomhard D, Matis U: Das osteosarkom der katze: epidemiologische, klinische und röntgenologische befunde bei 78 tieren (1990–1995). Tierärztl Prax 25:275–283, 1997.
12. Heldman E, Anderson MA, Wagner-Mann C: Feline osteosarcoma: 145 cases (1990–1995). *JAAHA* 36:518–521, 2000.
13. Berman E, Wright JF: What is your diagnosis. *JAVMA* 162:1065–1066, 1973.
14. Fry PD, Jukes HF: Fracture associated sarcoma in the cat. *J Small Anim Pract* 36:124–126, 1995.
15. Stubbs EL: Osteogenic chondrosarcoma in a cat. *JAVMA* 79:644–646, 1931.
16. Popp JA, Simpson CF: Feline malignant giant cell tumor of bone associated with C-type virus particles. *Cornell Vet* 66:528–535, 1976.
17. Howard EB, Kenyon AJ: Malignant osteoclastoma (giant cell tumor) in the cat with associated mast-cell response. *Cornell Vet* 57:398–409, 1967.
18. McClelland RB: A giant-cell tumor of the tibia in a cat. *Cornell Vet* 31:86–87, 1941.
19. Thornburg LP: Giant cell tumor of bone in a cat. *Vet Pathol* 16:255–257, 1979.
20. Bennett D, Campbell JR, Brown P: Osteosarcoma associated with healed fractures. *J Small Anim Pract* 20:13–18, 1979.
21. Thrasher JP, Riser WH: What is your diagnosis. *JAVMA* 141:1501–1502, 1962.
22. Goncalves M, Baptista R: Sarcoma osteogenico em felino. *Rep Trab* 14:63–66, 1982.
23. Quigley PJ, Leedale AH: Tumors involving bone in the domestic cat: A review of fifty-eight cases. *Vet Pathol* 20:670–686, 1983.
24. Purdy JG: Osteogeneic sarcoma in a cat. *Can Vet J* 2:156, 1961.
25. Thamm DH, MacEwen EG, Chun R, et al: Phase I clinical trial of Doxil, a stealth liposome encapsulated doxorubicin, in cats with malignant tumors. *Proc 17th Vet Cancer Soc*, 1997, p 38
26. Trout NJ, Pavletic MM, Kraus KH: Partial scapulectomy for management of sarcomas in three dogs and two cats. *JAVMA* 207:585–587, 1995.
27. Lord PF, Kapp DS, Schwartz A, Morrow DT: Osteogenic sarcoma of the nasal cavity in a cat: postoperative control with high dose-per-fraction radiation therapy and metronidazole. *Vet Radiol* 23:23–26, 1982.
28. Wolvekamp WThC, Boor-vd Putten IME, Gruys E: Wat is uw diagnose? *Tijdschr Diergeneesk* 101:1393–1397, 1976.
29. O'Brien D, Parker AJ, Tarvin G: Osteosarcoma of the vertebra causing compression of the thoracic spinal cord in a cat. *JAAHA* 16:497–499, 1980.
30. Levy MS, Mauldin G, Kapatkin AS, Patnaik AK: Nonlymphoid vertebral canal tumors in cats: 11 cases (1987–1995). *JAVMA* 5:663–664, 1997.
31. Griffith JW, Dubielzig RR, Riser WH, Jezyk P: Parosteal osteosarcoma with pulmonary metastases in a cat. *Vet Pathol* 21:123–125, 1984.
32. Banks WC: Parosteal osteosarcoma in a dog and a cat. *JAVMA* 158:1412–1415, 1971.
33. Pool RR: Tumors of bone and cartilage. In Moulton JE (ed):
Tumors in Domestic Animals. Berkley, University of California, 1990, pp 157–230.
34. Nielsen SW: Extraskeletal giant cell tumor in a cat. *Cornell Vet* 42:304–311, 1952.
35. Alexander JW, Riis RC, Dueland R: Extraskeletal giant cell tumor in a cat. *Vet Med Small Anim Clin* 1161–1166, 1975.
36. Whitehead JE: Neoplasia in the cat. *Vet Med Small Anim Clin* 357–358, 1967.
37. Knecht CD, Greene JA: Osteoma of the zygomatic arch in a cat. *JAVMA* 171:1077–1078, 1977.
38. Jabara AG, Paton JS: Extraskeletal osteoma in a cat. *Aust Vet J* 61:405–407, 1984.
39. Shell L, Sponenberg P: Chondrosarcoma in a cat presenting with forelimb monoparalysis. *Comp Small Anim* 9:391–398, 1987.
40. Hinko PJ, Burt JK, Fetter AW: Chondrosarcoma in the femur of a cat. *JAAHA* 15:737–739, 1979.
41. Brown NO, Patnaik AK, Mooney SC, et al: Soft tissue sarcomas in the cat. *JAVMA* 173:744–779, 1978.
42. Alden CL, Helzer LL: Humeral chondrosarcoma in a cat. *Modern Vet Pract* 214–216, 1981.
43. Morton D: Chondrosarcoma arising in a multilobular chondroma in a cat. *JAVMA* 186:804–806, 1985.
44. Herron ML: The musculoskeletal system. In Catcott EJ (ed): *Feline Medicine and Surgery*, ed 2. Santa Barbara, CA, American Veterinary Publications, 1975.
45. Butler R, Wrigley RH, Horsey R, Reuter R: Chondrosarcoma in a Sumatran tiger *(Panthera tigris sumatrae)*. *J Zoo Anim Med* 12:80–84, 1981.
46. Brown RJ, Trevethan WP, Henry VL: Multiple osteochondroma in a Siamese cat. *JAVMA* 160:433–435, 1972.
47. Riddle WE, Leighton RL: Osteochondromatosis in a cat. *JAVMA* 156:1428–1430, 1970.
48. Doige CE: Multiple osteochondromas with evidence of malignant transformation in a cat. *Vet Pathol* 24:457–459, 1987.
49. Pool RR, Harris JM: Feline osteochondromatosis. *Feline Pract* 5:24–30, 1975.
50. Pool RR, Carrig CB: Multiple cartilaginous exostoses in a cat. *Vet Pathol* 9:350–359, 1972.
51. Witt C: What is your diagnosis. *JAVMA* 185:451–452, 1984.
52. Cook JL, Turk JR, Tomlinson JL, et al: Fibrosarcoma in the distal radius and carpus of a four-year-old Persian. *JAAHA* 34:31–33, 1998.
53. Tischler SA, Owens JM: Ulnar fibrosarcoma in a cat. *Modern Vet Pract* 67:39,1986.
54. Sinibaldi KR, Pugh J, Rosen H, Liu S-K: Osteomyelitis and neoplasia associated with use of the Jonas intramedullary splint in small animals. *JAVMA* 181:885–890, 1982.
55. Madewell BR, Ackerman N, Sesline DH: Invasive carcinoma radiographically mimicking primary bone *cancer* in the mandibles of two cats. *Cancer* 17:213–215, 1976.
56. Bornstein N, Fayolle P, Moissonnier P: What is your diagnosis? *J Small Anim Pract* 40:205–207, 1999.
57. Silva-Krott IU, Tucker RL, Meeks JC: Synovial sarcoma in a cat. *JAVMA* 203:1430–1431, 1993.
58. Davies JD, Little NRF: Synovioma in a cat. *J Small Anim Pract* 13:127–133, 1972.
59. Hulse EV: A benign giant-cell synovioma in a cat. *J Pathol Bact* 91:269–271, 1966.
60. Thoday KL, Evans JG: Letters to the editor. *J Small Anim Pract* 13:399–402, 1972.

Chapter 48

Feline tumors of the nervous system

FELINE MENINGIOMA

Clinical presentation

- Meningiomas are the most common brain tumor in cats, with most occurring in the cerebral meninges above the temporal, frontal, parietal, or occipital regions of the brain.
- Rarely painful.
- Usually solitary.
- Multiple tumors seen in up to 20% of cats.
- Most common in older male cats.
- Slow growing, but changes in behavior, weakness, circling, or blindness may appear acutely.
- Paresis, usually tetraparesis, occurs in 60% to 80% of cats.[12,13]
- Seizures are not common.

> **Key point**
> While subtle neurologic signs including behavioral changes do occur in cats with meningiomas, most present with paresis and seizures.

Staging and diagnosis

- Minimum data base (MDB): includes a CBC, biochemical profile, urinalysis, FIV/FeLV serology, T4 testing, biopsy, three-view thoracic radiographs or computerized tomography of chest.
- Metastases are rare but they have been reported in the lungs.
- Radiographs of skull rarely helpful, however in some cats, hyperostotic, sclerotic or lytic lesions may be seen.
- Computerized tomography or magnetic resonance imaging of the tumor is important.

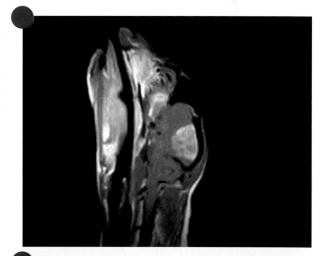
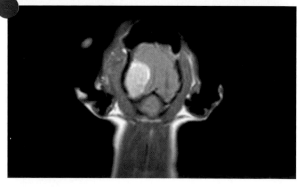

Figure 48-1: This MRI defines a large mass in the brain that is broad based and associated with the meninges. This is most consistent with a meningioma that is a common tumor in the brain of a cat. Surgery or radiation is generally quite effective at controlling most patients with this slowly growing tumor. Imaging courtesy of Lenore Anderson Mohammadian, DVM, MSpVM, Diplomate ACVR.

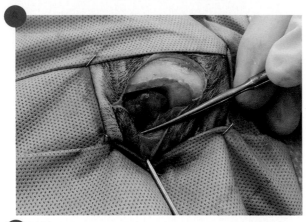

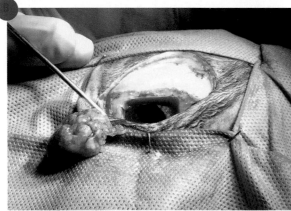

Figure 48-2: Surgery is often quite effective for removing meningiomas as imaged in A and B. Tumors can often be removed and the incision closed simply with no implants or replacement of bone. Survival time is generally excellent.

> **Key point**
> CT or MRI is important to make the diagnosis and to direct therapy in cats with meningioma.

Treatment

This section is divided into three options:
- Comfort for those who want to improve quality of life.
- Comfort and control for those who want to improve quality of life while trying to provide some control of the tumor.
- Comfort and longer-term control for those who want to improve quality of life while trying to maximize the chance of controlling the tumor.

> **Key point**
> Surgery or radiation can result in long-term improvement in cats with meningioma.

Comfort

- Therapy to enhance comfort and freedom from nausea, vomiting (e.g.: maropitant and/or metoclopramide), diarrhea (e.g.: metronidazole) and lack of appetite (e.g.: mirtazapine or cyproheptadine). Prednisolone and/or mannitol can be quite helpful for reducing edema of the central nervous system. Phenobarbital or levetiracetam may be helpful if seizures are a clinical concern.

Comfort and control

Above mentioned therapy for comfort plus:
- Palliative radiation, especially for those with extension into surrounding structures or regional metastases (e.g.: 2-5 dosages of radiation), to first enhance comfort, second, to reduce the rate of growth and third, occasionally to reduce the size of the tumor.

Comfort and longer-term control

Above mentioned therapy for comfort plus:
- Craniotomy to remove the involved bone and dura may be quite helpful and may be repeated if the tumor recurs. Some meningiomas may be seen on standard radiographs due to the presence of the lysis or thickening of bone.
  - Intraoperatively, hyperventilation (16 to 18 breaths/minute) decreases carbon dioxide concentration, thereby reducing cerebral blood flow, which in turn can help to reduce CNS edema and resultant postoperative complications.[16]
  - Prednisolone sodium succinate (25-50 mg/kg IV) may reduce postoperative inflammation associated with a craniotomy.
  - The incidence of herniation in studies is 10% to 20%.[12,16,17]
    - Survival beyond 1 year is common.[8,16,17,19,20,28] In one study, the median survival for cats that were released from the hospital was 22 months, with 66% of the cats alive 1 year and 50% 2 years after surgery.[12]
  - Incomplete excision may be treated with postoperative definitive radiation.
- An alternative to surgery is stereotactic radiosurgery via IMRT, Trilogy or CyberKnife therapy.

OTHER FELINE BRAIN TUMORS: EPENDYMOMA, OLIGODENDROGLIOMA, ASTROCYTOMA AND LYMPHOMA

Clinical presentation

- Uncommon.
- May be painful.

- Ependymomas arise from the wall of the ventricles.
  - Growth can be rapid, thus resulting in rapid onset or change in clinical signs, especially vestibular signs.
  - Interference with CSF distribution can lead to hydrocephalus, blindness, disorientation, and incoordination or tetraparesis with normal spinal reflexes.[30,34,35]
- Gliomas (oligodendrogliomas) are uncommon in the cat but they do cause many of the clinical signs typical for intracranial masses, including hemiparesis, head tilt, circling and ataxia, aggressive behavior and seizures.[8,37,39]
- Astrocytomas are uncommonly diagnosed tumors that have been shown to affect the frontal and parietal lobes of the cerebrum, the ventricular wall and the thalamus, resulting in abnormal behavior, facial deformity, blindness, and hemiparesis.[41]
- Lymphoma uncommonly involves the brain but it does cause compression of the spinal cord, usually via an extradural lesion. Clinical signs of brain involvement are not specific and are as noted with the other brain tumor types.

Staging and diagnosis

- Minimum data base (MDB): includes a CBC, biochemical profile, urinalysis, FIV/FeLV serology, T4 testing, biopsy, three-view thoracic radiographs or computerized tomography of the chest.
- Computerized tomography or magnetic resonance imaging of the brain is important.

Treatment

This section is divided into three options:
- Comfort for those who want to improve quality of life.
- Comfort and control for those who want to improve quality of life while trying to provide some control of the tumor.
- Comfort and longer-term control for those who want to improve quality of life while trying to maximize the chance of controlling the tumor.

Comfort

- Therapy to enhance comfort and freedom from nausea, vomiting (e.g.: maropitant and/or metoclopramide), diarrhea (e.g.: metronidazole) and lack of appetite (e.g.: mirtazapine or cyproheptadine). Prednisolone and mannitol may be quite helpful in managing clinical signs in the short term.

Comfort and control

Above mentioned therapy for comfort plus:
- Palliative radiation, especially for those with extension into surrounding structures or regional metastases (e.g.: 2-5 dosages of radiation), to first enhance comfort, second, to reduce the rate of growth and third, occasionally to reduce the size of the brain tumor. The most marked responses are seen with lymphoma.
- CCNU penetrates through the blood brain-barrier, and therefore this drug may be beneficial in some patients.

Comfort and longer-term control

Above mentioned therapy for comfort plus:
- Surgery for tumors other than lymphoma.
- Definitive radiation if there is evidence of tumor extending beyond the surgical margins (e.g.: 16-19 dosages of radiation).
- Stereotactic radiosurgery may be quite helpful in select patients via Trilogy or CyberKnife therapy.

FELINE SPINAL CORD TUMORS

Clinical presentation

- Relatively uncommon.
- May be painful.
- Lymphoma is most common; meningioma, ependymoma, astrocytoma, and sarcomas are less commonly diagnosed.
- Paresis, paralysis, gait abnormalities, diminished spinal cord reflexes and back pain are observed, regardless of the tumor type involved.
- Cats with lymphoma may be FeLV-positive and can have involvement of the bone marrow and other sites.

Staging and diagnosis

- Minimum data base (MDB): includes a CBC, biochemical profile, urinalysis, FIV/FeLV serology, T4 testing, biopsy, three-view thoracic radiographs or computerized tomography of the chest.
- A myelogram, or preferably contrast enhanced computerized tomography or magnetic resonance imaging of the spinal cord, is needed to localize the lesion beyond a physical examination.

Treatment

This section is divided into three options:
- Comfort for those who want to improve quality of life.
- Comfort and control for those who want to improve quality of life while trying to provide some control of the tumor.
- Comfort and longer-term control for those who want to improve quality of life while trying to maximize the chance of controlling the tumor.

Key point

Surgical decompression and/or radiation may improve clinical signs after the spinal cord lesion is localized and imaged via CT, MRI or myelogram.

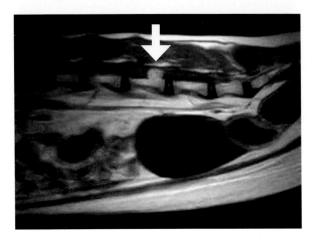

Figure 48-3: This MRI image confirms the presence of an intradural, extramedullary tumor in a cat with posterior paresis. The tumor was removed surgically and the cat recovered uneventfully. The histologic diagnosis was a meningioma. Imaging courtesy of Lenore Anderson Mohammadian, DVM, MSpVM, Diplomate ACVR.

Comfort

• Therapy to enhance comfort and freedom from nausea, vomiting (e.g.: maropitant and/or metoclopramide), diarrhea (e.g.: metronidazole) and lack of appetite (e.g.: mirtazapine or cyproheptadine). Prednisolone or other steroids may be ideal to reduce cord compression.

Comfort and control

Above mentioned therapy for comfort plus:
• Palliative radiation (e.g.: 2-5 dosages of radiation) to first enhance comfort, second, to reduce the rate of growth and third, occasionally to reduce the size of the spinal cord tumor.

Comfort and longer-term control

Above mentioned therapy for comfort plus:
• Surgical decompression of the cord compression.
• Definitive radiation (e.g.: 16-19 dosages of radiation).

References

1. Moore MP, Bagley RS, Harrington ML, Gavin PR: Intracranial tumors. *Vet Clin North Am Small Anim Pract* 26:759–777, 1996.
2. Kraus KH, McDonnell J: Identification and management of brain tumors. *Semin Vet Med Surg (Small Anim)* 11:218–224, 1996.
3. Gavin PR, Fike JR, Hoopes PJ: Central nervous system tumors. *Semin Vet Med Surg (Small Anim)* 10:180–189, 1995
4. Kornegay JN: Central nervous system neoplasia. In Kornegay JN (ed): *Neurologic Disorders. Contemporary Issues in Small Animal Practice.* New York, Churchill Livingston, 1986, pp 79–108.
5. Kornegay JN: Imaging brain neoplasms. Computed tomography and magnetic resonance imaging. *Vet Med Report* 2:372–390, 1990.
6. Dykes NL, Warnick LD, Summers BA, Wallace RJ, Kallfelz FA: Retrospective analysis of brain scintigraphy in 116 dogs and cats. *Vet Radiol Ultrasound* 35:59–65, 1994.
7. Gevel V, Machus B: Diagnosing brain tumors with a CSF sedimentation technique. *Vet Med Report* 2:403–408, 1990.
8. LeCouteur RA, Fike JR, Cann CE, et al: X-ray computed tomography of brain tumors in cats. *JAVMA* 183:301–305, 1983.
9. Smith MO, Turrell JM, Bailey CS, Cain GR: Neurological abnormalities as the predominant signs of neoplasia of the nasal cavity in dogs and cats: Seven cases (1973–1986). *JAVMA* 195:242–245, 1989.
10. Carpenter JL, Andrews LK, Holzworth J: Tumors and tumor-like lesions. In Holzworth J (ed): *Diseases of the Cat. Medicine and Surgery.* Philadelphia, WB Saunders, 1987, pp 407–596.
11. LeCouter RA: Brain tumors of dogs and cats: diagnosis and management. *Vet Med Report* 2:332–342, 1990.
12. Gordon LE, Thacher C, Matthiesen DT, Joseph RJ: Results of craniotomy for the treatment of cerebral meningioma in 42 cats. *Vet Surg* 23:94–100, 1994.
13. Nafe LA: Meningiomas in cats: A retrospective study of 36 cases. *JAVMA* 174:1224–1227, 1979.
14. Luginbuhl H: Studies on meningiomas in cats. *Am J Vet Res* 22:1030–1040, 1961.
15. Haskins ME, McGrath JT: Meningiomas in young cats with mucopolysaccharidosis. *J Neuropathol Exp Neurol* 42:664–670, 1983.
16. Gallagher JG, Berg J, Knowles KE, et al: Prognosis after surgical excision of cerebral meningiomas in cats: 17 cases (1986–1992). *JAVMA* 203:1437–1440, 1993.
17. Lawson DC, Burk RL, Prata RG: Cerebral meningioma in the cat: diagnosis and surgical treatment of ten cases. *JAAHA* 20:333–342, 1984.
18. Smit JD: The lesions found at autopsy in dogs and cats which manifest clinical signs referable to the central nervous system. *J S Afr Vet Med Assoc* 32:47–55, 1961.
19. Fingeroth JM, Hansen B, Myer CW: Diagnosis and successful removal of a brain tumor in a cat. *Comp Anim Pract* 2:6–15, 1988.
20. Shell L, Colter SB, Blass CE, Ingram JT: Surgical removal of a meningioma in a cat after detection by computerized axial tomography. *JAAHA* 21:439–442, 1985.
21. Gonzalez OG, Purpura DP: Epileptogenic effects of an auditory cortex meningioma in a cat. *Cornell Vet* 49:374–379, 1959.
22. Grahn BH, Stewart WA, Towner RA, Noseworthy MD: Magnetic resonance imaging of the canine and feline eye, orbit, and optic nerves and its clinical application. *Can Vet J* 34:418–424, 1993.
23. Ertürk E, Urman HK, Imren HY: Kedide meningioma olayi. *Yazi Dergi Yazi Kuruluna* 27:387–392, 1971.
24. Zaki FA, Hurvitz AI: Spontaneous neoplasms of the central nervous system of the cat. *J Small Anim Pract* 17:773–782, 1976.
25. Graham JP, Newell SM, Voges AK, et al: The dural tail sign in the diagnosis of meningiomas. *Vet Radiol Ultrasound* 39:297–302, 1998.
26. Dahme E: Meningome bei fleischfressern. *Berl Münch Teirärztl Wschr* 70:32–34, 1957.
27. Fusco JV, Hohenhaus AE, Aiken SW, et al: Autologous blood collection and transfusion in cats undergoing partial craniectomy. *JAVMA* 216:1584–1588, 2000.
28. Niebauer GW, Dayrell-Hart BL, Speciale J: Evaluation of craniotomy in dogs and cats. *JAVMA* 198:89–95, 1991.
29. Munson L, Nesbit JW, Meltzer DGA, et al: Diseases in captive cheetahs (*Acinonyx jubatus jubatus*) in South Africa: A 20-year retrospective survey. *J Zoo Wildl Med* 30:342–347, 1999.
30. Berry WL, Higgins RJ, LeCouteur RA, et al: Papillary ependymomas and hydrocephalus in three cats. *J Vet Intern Med* 12:243, 1998.
31. McKay JS, Targett MP, Jeffery ND: Histological characterization of an ependymoma in the fourth ventricle of a cat. *J Comp Pathol* 120:105–113, 1999.
32. Ingwersen W, Groom S, Parent J: Vestibular syndrome associated with an ependymoma in a cat. *JAVMA* 195:98–100, 1989.
33. Fox JG, Snyder SB, Reed C, Campbell LH: Malignant ependymoma in a cat. *J Small Anim Pract* 14:23–26, 1973.
34. Simpson DJ, Hunt GB, Tisdall PLC, et al: Surgical removal of an ependymoma from the third ventricle of a cat. *Aust Vet J* 77:645–648, 1999.
35. Tremblay C, Girard C, Quesnel A, et al: Ventricular ependymoma in a cat. *Can Vet J* 39:719–720, 1998.
36. Hayes Jr. HM, Priester WA, Pendergrass TW: Occurrence of nervous-tissue tumors in cattle, horses, cats and dogs. *Int J Cancer* 15:39–47, 1975.
37. Smith DA, Honhold N: Clinical and pathological features of a cerebellar oligodendroglioma in a cat. *J Small Anim Pract* 29:269–274 1988.
38. Cooper ERA, Howarth I: Some pathological changes in the cat brain. *J Comp Pathol* 66:35–38, 1956.
39. Knowlton FP: A case of tumor of the floor of the fourth ventricle with cerebellar symptoms, in a cat. *Am J Physiol* 13:20–21, 1905.
40. Dickinson PJ, Higgins RJ, Keel MK, et al: Diagnostic and

pathological features of caudal fossa oligodendrogliomas in two cats [abstract 197]. *J Vet Intern Med* 13:275, 1999.

41. Duniho S, Schulman FY, Morrison A, et al: A subependymal giant cell astrocytoma in a cat. *Vet Pathol* 37:275–278, 2000.

42. Chénier S, Quesnel A, Girard C: Intracranial teratoma and dermoid cyst in a kitten. *J Vet Diagn Invest* 10:381–384, 1998.

43. Ross J, Wyburn RS: A report on the clinical investigation of a paraplegic cat. *N Z Vet J* 17:251–253, 1969.

44. Jones BR: Spinal meningioma in a cat. *Aust Vet J* 50:229–231, 1974.

45. McGrath JT: Meningiomas in animals. *J Neuropathol Exp Neurol* 21:327–328, 1962.

46. Levy MS, Mauldin G, Kapatkin AS, Patnaik AK: Nonlymphoid vertebral canal tumors in cats: 11 cases (1987–1995). *JAVMA* 5:663–664, 1997.

47. Asperio RM, Marzola P, Zibellini E, et al: Use of magnetic resonance imaging for diagnosis of a spinal tumor in a cat. *Vet Radiol Ultrasound* 40:267–270, 1999.

48. Haynes JS, Leininger JR: A glioma in the spinal cord of a cat. *Vet Pathol* 19:713–715, 1982.

49. Milks HJ, Olafson P: Primary brain tumors in small animals. *Cornell Vet* 26:159–170, 1936.

50. Ruben JMS: Neurofibrosarcoma in a 19-year-old cat. *Vet Rec* 113:135, 1983.

51. Luttgen PJ, Braund Jr WR, Vandevelde M: A retrospective study of twenty-nine spinal tumors in the dog and cat. *J Vet Intern Med* 21:207–215, 1980.

52. Paul-Murphy J, Lloyd K, Turrel JM, et al: Management of a Schwannoma in the larynx of a lion. *JAVMA* 189:1202–1203, 1986.

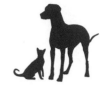

Chapter 49

Feline tumors of eyes and ears

FELINE TUMORS OF THE EAR AND EAR CANAL

Clinical presentation

- Moderately common and may be bilateral.
- May be uncomfortable.
- Tumors of the pinna are covered elsewhere, but squamous cell carcinoma, basal cell tumors and mast cell tumors are common.
- Ceruminous adenocarcinomas are most common.
- One-third of all tumors (and 40% of all malignant tumors) of the ear canal in a large survey.[3]
- Neurologic signs such as facial nerve paralysis, head tilt, circling, anisocoria (Horner's syndrome), and ataxia occur in 25% to 35% of cats.[3,6]
- In one study,[1] 28 of 56 malignant ear canal tumors appeared invasive. Nine of the tumors invaded the subcutis, while 19 invaded cartilage of the ear and canal.
- Vestibular signs may signal invasion of the middle ear.
- Metastasis most commonly to deep parotid, retropharyngeal, and prescapular lymph nodes.
- Adenomas and other carcinomas are less common.
- In a large study that included 56 cats with malignant tumors of the ear canal, 20 tumors were squamous cell carcinoma and 13 were undifferentiated carcinoma.
- Cats with SCC or undifferentiated carcinoma usually have evidence of bulla involvement on radiographs or CT scan.[1,8,10–14]

Key point

Squamous cell carcinoma of the pinna commonly causes a crusty, ulcerative condition, most commonly in white-haired cats with pink skin.

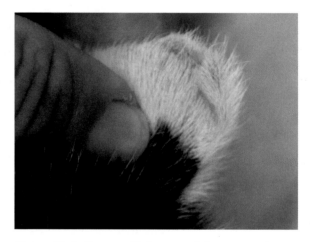

Figure 49-1: The most likely tumor of the pinna in this cat with white hair is the solar induced squamous cell carcinoma. A biopsy, either incisional or excisional is required to specifically diagnose the problem, however a partial or total pinnectomy is often required to resolve the disease.

Key point

Malignant ear canal tumors are almost always invasive and frequently cause clinical signs referable to an unresponsive otitis externa.

Staging and diagnosis

- Minimum data base (MDB): includes a CBC, biochemical profile, urinalysis, FeLV/FIV serology, T4testing, culture and cytology of the ear contents, biopsy and three-view thoracic radiographs or computerized tomography of the chest.
- Radiographs, computerized tomography, or magnetic resonance imaging is important to determine the local extent of the disease and to determine if it has metastasized.

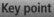

Key point

A CT of the skull in cats with ear canal tumors often increases cure rates and often decreases the overall cost of patient management.

Treatment

This section is divided into three options:
- Comfort for those who want to improve quality of life.
- Comfort and control for those who want to improve quality of life while trying to provide some control of the tumor.
- Comfort and longer-term control for those who want to improve quality of life while trying to maximize the chance of controlling the tumor.

Comfort

- Therapy to enhance comfort and freedom from nausea and vomiting that may be seen secondary to involvement of the middle and inner ear (e.g.: maropitant and/or metoclopramide), diarrhea that may be seen with stress or secondary to other medication (e.g.: metronidazole) and lack of appetite (e.g.: mirtazapine or cyproheptadine). Special attention should be directed toward ensuring that the patient is free from localized infection and discomfort.

Comfort and control

Above mentioned therapy for comfort plus:
- Palliative radiation, especially for those with extension into surrounding structures or regional metastases (e.g.: 2-5 dosages of radiation), to first enhance comfort, second, to reduce the rate of growth and third, occasionally to reduce the size of the tumor.

Comfort and longer-term control

Above mentioned therapy for comfort plus:
- Surgery. Localized surgery +/- cryotherapy for benign tumors may be effective. Most tumors invade into surrounding tissues, requiring an ear canal ablation and bulla osteotomy for tumor control.
  - Surgical resection of the ear canal in cats with ceruminous gland adenocarcinoma may be sufficient in cats with a tumor that affects only the vertical ear canal and has no bulla involvement.
    - One study involving 6 cats that were treated in this way showed a median disease-free period of 10 months (range, 1 to 14 months).[6]
  - Cats that have more invasive ceruminous gland adenocarcinomas require an ear canal ablation and lateral bulla osteotomy.
    - In one study[6] involving 16 cats, the median disease-free period treated in this manner was 42 months (range, 4 to 60 months).
  - Cats with squamous cell carcinoma or undifferentiated carcinoma do not do as well, with one study[8] confirming a median survival of 3.8 months for 20 cats with squamous cell carcinoma of the ear canal and 5.7 months for 13 cats with undifferentiated carcinoma.
- Definitive radiation if there is evidence of tumor extending beyond the surgical margins (e.g.: 16-19 dosages of radiation).
  - The median survival for cats with ceruminous gland carcinoma was longer than 49 months.[3]

FELINE OCULAR MELANOMA

Clinical presentation

- Moderately common.
- May be painful, especially if glaucoma occurs.
- Uveal melanoma is more common than limbal.
  - Most often unilateral and associated with chronic uveitis, pigment change, buphthalmos, cloudy eye, and glaucoma.
    - Pigment change may precede more serious changes by months[21,27] to years.[18,22,28]
    - In one study of 128 cats with glaucoma, 38 had uveal melanoma causing obliteration of the trabecular meshwork.[29]
    - Metastases may be widespread and have been reported in brain, lungs and liver, as well as the mediastinum, pericardium, pleura, diaphragm, adrenals, peritoneum, spleen, stomach, intestine, tonsils, and regional and distant lymph nodes.
    - Differentials for uveal melanomas include iris freckles (iris not thickened, indistinct margins) and iridial cysts (often at pupillary margin with smooth margins).
  - Patients with limbal melanomas often present for an ocular mass or swollen eyelid.
    - Widespread metastases may be seen with this form of the disease, especially to regional lymph nodes. Aspiration cytology of regional lymph nodes (mandibular, retropharyngeal, and parotid) should be performed.[18,39,41]

Staging and diagnosis

- Minimum data base (MDB): includes a CBC, biochemical profile, urinalysis, FIV/FeLV serology, T4 testing, biopsy via enucleation and three-view thoracic radiographs or computerized tomography of the chest.
- Ultrasonography and/or radiographs are practical and cost effective, however computerized tomography or magnetic resonance imaging of the tumor can be done but is most helpful for determining the presence of distant metastases.
  - In one study, survival appeared to be longer in cats with tumors limited to the iris and ciliary body.[18]

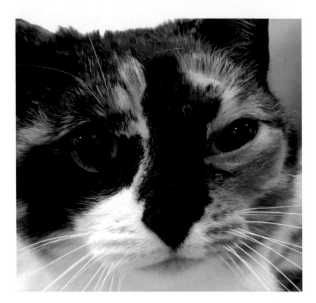

Figure 49-2: Uveal melanomas as in this cat with a left ocular tumor with invasion into surrounding structures can cause glaucoma, pain, mydriasis and blindness. Analgesia and supportive care are always indicated, while determining the extent of the disease and the presence of metastases with either radiographs, ultrasound, computerized tomography or magnetic resonance imaging. Removal of the eye and/or the entire orbit may be required for local tumor control.

- The number of mitotic figures on histopathologic sectioning has been shown to correlate with increasing tumor invasion of the surrounding sclera in one study.[35]

Key point

Widespread metastases may be present in cats with ocular melanoma, therefore evaluation of chest radiographs, blood work and aspirates of regional lymph nodes is often required.

Treatment

This section is divided into three options:
- Comfort for those who want to improve quality of life.
- Comfort and control for those who want to improve quality of life while trying to provide some control of the tumor.
- Comfort and longer-term control for those who want to improve quality of life while trying to maximize the chance of controlling the tumor.

Comfort

Therapy to enhance comfort by specifically addressing local discomfort and by resolving the presence of glaucoma. Similarly freedom from nausea, vomiting (e.g.: maropitant and/or metoclopramide), diarrhea (e.g.: metronidazole) and lack of appetite (e.g.: mirtazapine or cyproheptadine) must always be done.

Comfort and control

Above mentioned therapy for comfort plus:
- Palliative or course fractionated radiation, especially for those with extension into surrounding structures or regional metastases (e.g.: 2-5 dosages of radiation), to first enhance comfort, second, to reduce the rate of growth and third, occasionally to reduce the size of the tumor.

Comfort and longer-term control

Above mentioned therapy for comfort plus:
- Enucleation, including invasion into surrounding tissues.
  - One study found that cats with tumors involving only the iris and ciliary body had a median survival of 383 days, compared with 122 days for cats with tumors invading beyond these structures, and 14 days for those with tumors involving the whole eye.[18]
  - Lamellar sclerokeratectomy alone or followed by cryosurgery for limbal melanomas has been reported to be associated with long-term survival (>30 months).[38,42]
- Definitive radiation if there is evidence of tumor extending beyond the surgical margins (e.g.: 16-19 dosages of radiation).
- Carboplatin or the Merial DNA xenogeneic melanoma vaccine may be considered for systemic effects.

FELINE OCULAR SARCOMA

Clinical presentation

- Moderately common.
- May be painful.
- May occur after ocular trauma and/or inflammation.
- Biological behavior similar, regardless if the tumor is a fibrosarcoma, osteosarcoma, or undifferentiated sarcoma.
  - Clinical signs include increasing size of the globe, displacement or discoloration of the iris, presence of glaucoma, and a highly invasive mass. Metastases to regional lymph nodes or lungs may be noted.

Staging and diagnosis

- Minimum data base (MDB): includes a CBC, biochemical profile, urinalysis, FIV/FeLV serology, T4 testing, biopsy of the tumor via enucleation or a preoperative biopsy, and three-view thoracic radiographs or computerized tomography of the chest.
- Computerized tomography or magnetic resonance imaging of the head and tumor is optimal.

• Degree of local invasion of the primary tumor and presence of metastases are important.

Treatment

This section is divided into three options:
• Comfort for those who want to improve quality of life.
• Comfort and control for those who want to improve quality of life while trying to provide some control of the tumor.
• Comfort and longer-term control for those who want to improve quality of life while trying to maximize the chance of controlling the tumor.

Comfort

• Therapy to enhance comfort via local and systemic analgesics and freedom from nausea, vomiting (e.g.: maropitant and/or metoclopramide), diarrhea (e.g.: metronidazole) and lack of appetite (e.g.: mirtazapine or cyproheptadine). Medical treatment of uveitis or glaucoma.

Comfort and control

Above mentioned therapy for comfort plus:
• Palliative radiation, especially for those with extension into surrounding structures or regional metastases (e.g.: 2-5 dosages of radiation), to first enhance comfort, second, to reduce the rate of growth and third, occasionally to reduce the size of the tumor.

Comfort and longer-term control

Above mentioned therapy for comfort plus:
• Enucleation via removal of the tumor and a margin of surrounding tissue.
  • Follow-up information after enucleation was available for 21 cats.[43, 44, 46–48] Nineteen cats were dead within 8 months of surgery, and two cats lived more than a year after surgery.[44,48] Metastasis with or without tumor recurrence was seen in 8 cats 2-17 months after surgery, and extension to involve the CNS was seen in 8 cats.[43,44,48]
• Definitive radiation if there is evidence of tumor extending beyond the surgical margins (e.g.: 16-19 dosages of radiation).

FELINE ORBITAL/ RETROBULBAR TUMORS

Clinical presentation

• SCC is most common, usually as an extension of a maxillary or nasal tumor. Other tumors include fibrosarcoma, plasma cell tumor, and lymphoma. Exophthalmos and anterolateral globe deviation are commonly seen.
• Moderately common.

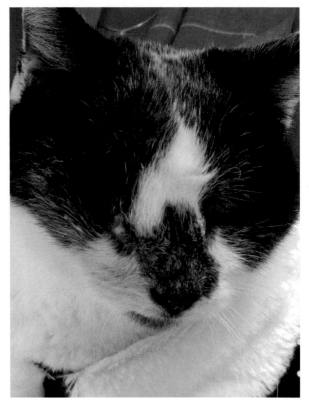

Figure 49-3: This cat had an orbitectomy for a sarcoma of the eye and surrounding structures followed by definitive radiation therapy five years ago. Soft tissue sarcomas are highly invasive but are unlikely to spread to distant sites.

• Often painful.
• Often associated with facial deformity, epiphora, nasal obstruction, exophthalmos, glaucoma, etc.

Staging and diagnosis

• Minimum data base (MDB): includes a CBC, biochemical profile, urinalysis, FIV/FeLV serology, T4 testing, biopsy, three-view thoracic radiographs or computerized tomography of the chest.
• Ultrasonography and/or radiographs are practical and cost effective, however computerized tomography or magnetic resonance imaging of the tumor may be preferable in some cases.
• An aspirate or biopsy is essential.

Treatment

This section is divided into three options:
• Comfort for those who want to improve quality of life.
• Comfort and control for those who want to improve quality of life while trying to provide some control of the tumor.
• Comfort and longer-term control for those who want to improve quality of life while trying to maximize the chance of controlling the tumor.

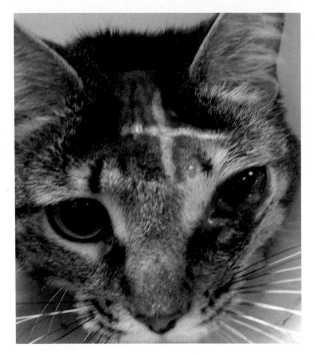

Figure 49-4: Cat prepared to start radiation therapy for a nasal tumor that has invaded the left orbit and caused some significant changes to the globe. The radiation resulted in substantial improvement in comfort and vision.

Comfort

• Therapy to enhance comfort (e.g.: NSAID, tramadol, gabapentin and/or opiates) and freedom from nausea, vomiting (e.g.: maropitant and/or metoclopramide), diarrhea (e.g.: metronidazole) and lack of appetite (e.g.: mirtazapine or cyproheptadine).

Comfort and control

Above mentioned therapy for comfort plus:

• Palliative radiation, especially for those with extension into surrounding structures or regional metastases (e.g.: 2-5 dosages of radiation), to first enhance comfort, second, to reduce the rate of growth and third, occasionally to reduce the size of the tumor.

Comfort and longer-term control

Above mentioned therapy for comfort plus:

• Orbitectomy with or without definitive radiation if there is evidence of tumor extending beyond the surgical margins (e.g.: 16-19 dosages of radiation).

References

1. Carpenter JL, Andrews LK, Holzworth J: Tumors and tumor-like lesions. In Holzworth J (ed): *Diseases of the Cat. Medicine and Surgery.* Philadelphia, WB Saunders 1987, pp 407–596.
2. Goldschmidt MH, Shofer FS: *Skin Tumors of the Dog and Cat.* New York, Pergamon Press, 1992.
3. London CA, Dubilzeig RR, Vail DM, et al: Evaluation of dogs and cats with tumors of the ear canal: 145 cases (1978–1992). *JAVMA* 208:1413–1418, 1996.
4. Cotchin E: Skin tumours of cats. *Res Vet Sci* 2:353–361, 1961.
5. Holzworth J: The ear. In Holzworth J (ed): *Diseases of the Cat. Medicine and Surgery.* Philadelphia, WB Saunders 1987, pp 724–738.
6. Marino DJ, MacDonald JM, Matthiesen DT, Patnaik AK: Results of surgery in cats with ceruminous gland adenocarcinoma. *JAAHA* 30:54–58, 1994.
7. Theon AP, Barthez PY, Madewell BR, Griffey SM: Radiation therapy of ceruminous gland carcinomas in dogs and cats. *JAVMA* 205:566–569, 1994.
8. Williams JM, White RAS: Total ear canal ablation combined with lateral bulla osteotomy in the cat. *J Small Anim Pract* 33:225–227, 1992.
9. Miller MA, Nelson SL, Turk JR, et al: Cutaneous neoplasia in 340 cats. *Vet Pathol* 28:389–395, 1991.
10. Stone EA, Goldschmidt MH, Littman MP: Squamous cell carcinoma of the middle ear in a cat. *J Small Anim Pract* 24:647–651, 1983.
11. Fiorito DA: Oral and peripheral vestibular signs in a cat with squamous cell carcinoma. *JAVMA* 188:71–72, 1986.
12. Trevor PB, Martin RA: Tympanic bulla osteotomy for treatment of middle-ear disease in cats: 19 cases (1984–1991). *JAVMA* 202:123–128, 1993.
13. Indrieri RJ, Taylor RF: Vestibular dysfunction caused by squamous cell carcinoma involving the middle and inner ear in two cats. *JAVMA* 184:471–473, 1984.
14. Pentlarge VW: Peripheral vestibular disease in a cat with middle and inner ear squamous cell carcinoma. *Compend Contin Educ Pract Vet* 6:731–736, 1984.
15. Peiffer Jr RL, Wilcock BP: Histopathologic study of uveitis in cats: 139 cases (1978–1988). *JAVMA* 198:135–138, 1991.
16. Schäffer EH, Funke K: Das primär-intraokulare maligne melanom bei hund and katze. *Tierärztl Prax* 13:343–359, 1985.
17. Peiffer Jr RL: The differential diagnosis of pigmented ocular lesions in the dog and cat. *California Vet* 5:14–18, 1981.
18. Patnaik AK, Mooney S: Feline melanoma: A comparative study of ocular, oral, and dermal neoplasms. *Vet Pathol* 25:105–112, 1988.
19. Souri E: Intraocular melanoma in a cat. *Feline Pract* 8:43–45, 1978.
20. Schulze Schleithoff N, Opitz M: Intraokuläres, metastasierendes, pigment armes melanom bei einer hauskatze. *Kleintierpraxis* 28:215–218, 1982.
21. Schwink K, Betts DM: Malignant melanoma of the iris in a cat. *Comp Anim Pract* 2:35–41, 1988.
22. Acland GM, McLean IW, Aquirre GD, Trucksa R: Diffuse iris melanoma in cats. *JAVMA* 176:52–56, 1980.
23. Schiller I, Spiess B, Pospischil A: Maligne melanome bei zwei katzen. *Schweiz Arch Tierheilk* 137:50–53, 1995.
24. Bellhorn RW, Henkind P: Intraocular malignant melanoma in domestic cats. *J Small Anim Pract* 10:631–637, 1970.
25. Shadduck JA, Albert DM, Niederkorn JY: Feline uveal melanomas induced with feline sarcoma virus: potential model of the human counterpart. *JNCI* 67:619–627, 1981.
26. Albert DM, Shadduck JA, Craft JL, Niederkorn JY: Feline uveal melanoma model induced with feline sarcoma virus. *Invest Ophthalmol Vis Sci* 20:606–624, 1981.
27. Bertoy RW, Brightman AH, Regan K: Intraocular melanoma with multiple metastases in a cat. *JAVMA* 192:87–89, 1988.
28. Wolfer J, Grahn B: Diagnostic ophthalmology. *Can Vet J* 32:440, 1991.
29. Wilcock BP, Peiffer Jr RJ, Davidson MG: The causes of glaucoma in cats. *Vet Pathol* 1990;27:35–40.
30. Cardy RH: Primary intraocular malignant melanoma in a Siamese cat. *Vet Pathol* 14:648–649, 1977.
31. Grahn B, Wolfer J: Diagnostic ophthalmology. *Can Vet J* 23:683, 1992.
32. Bjerkas E, Arnesen K, Peiffer Jr RL: Diffuse amelanotic iris melanoma in a cat. *Vet Comp Ophthalmol* 7:190–191, 1997.
33. Peiffer Jr RL, Seymour WG, Williams LW: Malignant melanoma of the iris and ciliary body in a cat. *Mod Vet Pract* 58:854–856, 1977.
34. Grahn BH, Stewart WA, Towner RA, Noseworthy MD: Magnetic resonance imaging of the canine and feline eye, orbit, and optic nerves and its clinical application. *Can Vet J* 34:418–424, 1993.
35. Day MJ, Lucke VM: Melanocytic neoplasia in the cat. *J Small Anim Pract* 36:207–213, 1995.
36. Schäffer EH, Pfleghaar S, Gordon S, Knödlseder M: Maligne nickhauttumoren bei hund und katze. *Tierärztl Prax* 22:382–391, 1994.

37. McLaughlin SA, Whitley RD, Gilger BC, et al: Eyelid neoplasms in cats: A review of demographic data (1979–1989). *JAAHA* 29:63–67, 1993.

38. Harling DE, Peiffer RL, Cook CS, Belkin PV: Feline limbal melanoma: Four cases. *JAAHA* 22:795–802, 1986.

39. Neumann W, Juchem R: Epibulbäres melanom bei einer katze. *Tierärztl Prax* 16:65–68, 1988.

40. Sullivan TC, Nasisse MP, Davidson MG, Glover TL: Photocoagulation of limbal melanoma in dogs and cats: 15 cases (1989–1993). *JAVMA* 208:891–894, 1996.

41. Cook CS, Rosenkrantz W, Peiffer RL, MacMillan A: Malignant melanoma of the conjunctiva in a cat. *JAVMA* 186:505–506, 1985.

42. Betton A, Healy LN, English RV, Bunch SE: Atypical limbal melanoma in a cat. *J Vet Intern Med* 13:379–381, 1999.

43. Peiffer RL, Monticello T, Bouldin TW: Primary ocular sarcomas in the cat. *J Small Anim Pract* 29:105–116, 1988.

44. Hakanson N, Shively JN, Reed RE, Merideth RE: Intraocular spindle cell sarcoma following ocular trauma in a cat: case report and literature review. *JAAHA* 26:63–66, 1990.

45. Barrett PM, Merideth RE, Alarcon FL: Central amaurosis induced by an intraocular, posttraumatic fibrosarcoma in a cat. *JAAHA* 31:242–245, 1995.

46. Miller WW, Boosinger TR: Intraocular osteosarcoma in a cat. *JAAHA* 23:317–320, 1987.

47. Woog J, Albert DM, Gonder JR, Carpenter JJ: Osteosarcoma in a phthisical feline eye. *Vet Pathol* 20:209–214, 1983.

48. Dubielzig RR, Everitt J, Shadduck JA, Albert DM: Clinical and morphologic features of post-traumatic ocular sarcomas in cats. *Vet Pathol* 27:62–65, 1990.

49. Peiffer Jr RL, Wilcock BP, Yin H: The pathogenesis and significance of pre-iridial fibrovascular membrane in domestic animals. *Vet Pathol* 27:41–45, 1990.

50. Bellhorn RW: Secondary ocular adenocarcinoma in three dogs and a cat. *JAVMA* 160:302–307, 1972.

51. O'Rouke MD, Geib LW: Endometrial adenocarcinoma in a cat. *Cornell Vet* 60:598–604, 1970.

52. Calia CM, Kirschner SE, Baer KE: The use of computed tomography scan for the evaluation of orbital disease in cats and dogs. *Vet Comp Ophthalmol* 4:24–30, 1998.

53. Gilger BC, McLaughlin SA, Whitley RD, Wright JC: Orbital neoplasms in cats: 21 cases (1974–1990). *JAVMA* 201:1083–1086, 1992.

54. Murphy CJ, Koblik P, Bellhorn RW, et al: Squamous cell carcinoma causing blindness and ophthalmoplegia in a cat. *JAVMA* 195:965–968, 1989.

55. Hayden DW: Squamous cell carcinoma in a cat with intraocular and orbital metastases. *Vet Pathol* 13:332–336, 1976.

56. Brown NO, Hayes AA, Mooney S, et al: Combined modality therapy in the treatment of solid tumors in cats. *JAAHA* 16:719–722, 1980.

57. Ward DA, McEntee MF, Weddle DL: Orbital plasmacytoma in a cat. *J Small Anim Pract* 38:576–578, 1997.

58. Chaitman J, van der Woerdt A, Bartick TE: Multiple eyelid cysts resembling apocrine hidrocystomas in three Persian cats and one Himalayan cat. *Vet Pathol* 36:474–476, 1999.

59. Komaromy AM, Ramsey DT, Render JA, Clark P: Primary adenocarcinoma of the gland of the nictitating membrane in a cat. *JAAHA* 33:333–336, 1997.

60. Roels S, Ducatelle R: Malignant melanoma of the nictitating membrane in a cat (Felis vulgaris). *J Comp Path* 119:189–193, 1998.

61. O'Brien MG, Withrow SJ, Straw RC, et al: Total and partial orbitectomy for the treatment of periorbital tumors in 24 dogs and 6 cats: A retrospective study. *Vet Surg* 25:471–479, 1996.

62. Neumann SM: Palpebral squamous cell carcinoma in a cat. *Modern Vet Pract* 63:547–549, 1982.

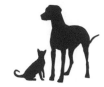

Chapter 50

Feline tumors of the gastrointestinal tract

FELINE ORAL SQUAMOUS CELL CARCINOMA

Clinical presentation

- Squamous cell carcinoma represents 60-80% of all oral tumors in cats.
- Passive smoking may increase risk of developing squamous cell carcinoma.
- Often seen in older cats.
- Squamous cell carcinoma often involves the tongue. Occasionally invades mandible or maxilla.
- Dysphagia and ptyalism are common.
- Often painful.
- Weight loss due to reduced intake of food is common and is best resolved with an esophagostomy tube early in the management of this disease.

Key point

Exposure to cigarette smoke may increase the risk of cats developing oral squamous cell carcinoma.

Staging and diagnosis

- Minimum data base (MDB): includes a CBC, biochemical profile, urinalysis, FIV/FeLV serology, T4 testing, biopsy, three-view thoracic radiographs or computerized tomography of the chest.
- Ultrasonography and/or radiographs are practical and cost effective, however computerized tomography or magnetic resonance imaging of the oral cavity that contains the tumor.
- Bone involvement and appropriate therapy are positive.

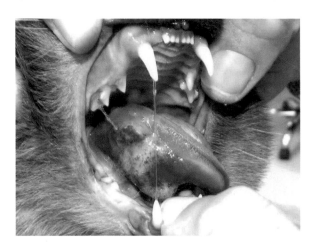

Figure 50-1: Sublingual squamous cell carcinoma results in weight loss, ptyalism, dysphagia, lethargy and debilitation. This tumor is almost always incurable. The single greatest thing that can be done for these cats is to place a feeding tube and to manage their pain. Many therapies have been tried, including radiation, surgery, chemotherapy and targeted therapy with drugs such as toceranib, with limited results.

Treatment

This section is divided into three options:
- Comfort for those who want to improve quality of life.
- Comfort and control for those who want to improve quality of life while trying to provide some control of the tumor.
- Comfort and longer-term control for those who want to improve quality of life while trying to maximize the chance of controlling the tumor.

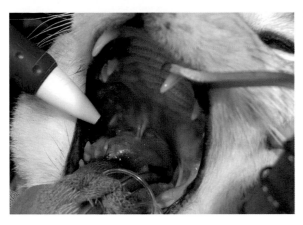

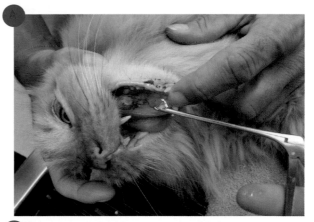

Figure 50-2: This cat presented for anorexia and dysphagia due to a tonsillar squamous cell carcinoma. A feeding tube was placed and the region treated with radiation therapy with supportive care.

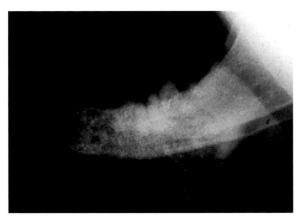

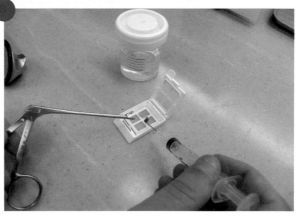

Figure 50-4: Tumors of the tongue, tonsils, lips, pharynx and surrounding structures can be biopsied a number of ways, including with cup biopsy instrument (A). Once the sample is obtained, it can be placed into a cassette and then into formalin for fixation (B).

Figure 50-3: Mandibular squamous cell carcinomas can be quite invasive into surrounding bone. A mandibulectomy and radiation for tumors that are confined just to that region may be helpful. Nutritional support via an esophagostomy tube is often indicated.

Comfort and control

Above mentioned therapy for comfort plus:

- Palliative radiation may provide transient benefit (e.g.: 2-5 dosages of radiation) to first enhance comfort, second, to reduce the rate of growth and third, occasionally to reduce the size of the tumor.
- A retrospective study was conducted[5] to describe outcomes for cats with oral squamous cell carcinoma that were treated with palliative radiation therapy with or without chemotherapy. Forty-nine patients had an overall mean and median survival times of 127 and 92 days. Mean and median survival times of cats receiving palliative radiation therapy alone were 157 and 113 days. Mean and median survival times of patients receiving both radiation therapy and chemotherapy were 116 and 80 days, although it could be argued that these cats tended to have more advanced disease. The median survival time for cats with sublingual tumors was 135 days versus 80 days for those with mandibular

Key point

Cats with sublingual squamous cell carcinoma generally respond poorly to therapy, whereas tumors that involve bone without lingual tissues generally respond well to surgery and/or radiation therapy.

Comfort

- Therapy to enhance comfort (e.g.: NSAID, tramadol, buprenorphine) and freedom from nausea, vomiting (e.g.: maropitant and/or metoclopramide), diarrhea (e.g.: metronidazole) and lack of appetite (e.g.: mirtazapine or cyproheptadine).

tumors. Sixty-five percent of clients stated their cat had a subjectively improved quality of life.
- In another study, 31 cats were treated twice daily for 14 fractions of 3.5 Gy given within a 9-day period with the addition of carboplatin given at 90-100 mg/m² on day 1 and day 4.5.[6] The median survival time was 135 days. Cats with tumors of tonsillar origin or cheek responded best to therapy and were long-term survivors with a mean survival of 724 days, and the median had not been reached.
- Clinician scientists did a study and concluded that their accelerated hypofractionated radiation therapy protocol (10, 4.8 Gy once-daily fractions given Monday through Friday) was well tolerated in cats with oral SCC, with manageable adverse events.[7] The median progression-free survival was 105 days (1 year PFS of 23%), median local progression-free survival was 219 days (1 year LPFS of 41%), and median overall survival was 174 days (1 year overall survival of 29%).

Comfort and longer-term control

Above mentioned therapy for comfort plus:
- Cures are obtained only in a small subset of cats whose tumors are amenable to complete resection, or where resection with microscopic residual disease is followed by definitive radiation therapy (e.g.: 16-19 dosages of radiation).

FELINE ORAL FIBROSARCOMA

Clinical presentation

- Moderately common.
- May be painful.
- Fibrosarcomas represent 10-20% of oral tumors.
- Often results in ptyalism, dysphagia, weight loss, anorexia, facial deformity, and exophthalmos.

Staging and diagnosis

- Minimum data base (MDB): includes a CBC, biochemical profile, urinalysis, FIV/FeLV serology, T4 testing, biopsy, three-view thoracic radiographs or computerized tomography of the chest.
- Radiographs, computerized tomography, or magnetic resonance imaging of the head.

Treatment

This section is divided into three options:
- Comfort for those who want to improve quality of life.
- Comfort and control for those who want to improve quality of life while trying to provide some control of the tumor.
- Comfort and longer-term control for those who want to improve quality of life while trying to maximize the chance of controlling the tumor.

> **Key point**
> Wide surgical removal of oral fibrosarcoma can result in long-term control of the disease.

Comfort

- Therapy to enhance comfort (e.g.: NSAID, tramadol, buprenorphine) and freedom from nausea, vomiting (e.g.: maropitant and/or metoclopramide), diarrhea (e.g.: metronidazole) and lack of appetite (e.g.: mirtazapine or cyproheptadine).

Comfort and control

Above mentioned therapy for comfort plus:
- Palliative radiation, especially for those with extension into surrounding structures or regional metastases (e.g.: 2-5 dosages of radiation), to first enhance comfort, second, to reduce the rate of growth and third, occasionally to reduce the size of the tumor.

Comfort and longer-term control

Above mentioned therapy for comfort plus:
- Surgery with or without definitive radiation if there is evidence of tumor extending beyond the surgical margins (e.g.: 16-19 dosages of radiation).
  - Surgical excision possible with wide excision that includes bone.
    - Maxillectomy needs to be aggressive in order to assure adequate surgical margins. Tumor recurrence was noted in one study 3.5 months after maxillectomy in one cat with a lesion centered around the upper canine,[26] whereas another cat had no evidence of tumor 24 months after a unilateral premaxillectomy.[32]
    - Medical records of 42 cats treated with mandibulectomy for oral neoplasia, including fibrosarcoma, were reviewed.[33] The progression-free and survival rates at 1 and 2 years were 56% and 49%, and 60% and 57%, respectively. Cats with fibrosarcoma or osteosarcoma had a longer survival time than cats with squamous cell carcinoma. Despite acute morbidity including dysphagia and anorexia, 83% of the owners providing information were satisfied with the outcome of mandibulectomy.
- Carboplatin, doxorubicin, and vincristine have shown efficacy and could be considered if radiation is not available.

FELINE ORAL MELANOMA

Clinical presentation

- Uncommon. In three surveys totaling 146 oral tumors in cats, only 4 were melanomas.[3-5]
- May be painful.

- There is a moderate chance of metastases, primarily to regional lymph nodes or lung.

Staging and diagnosis

- Minimum data base (MDB): includes a CBC, biochemical profile, urinalysis, FIV/FeLV serology, T4 testing, biopsy, three-view thoracic radiographs or computerized tomography of the chest.
- Ultrasonography and/or radiographs are practical and cost effective, however computerized tomography or magnetic resonance imaging of the tumor may be preferable in some cases.

Treatment

This section is divided into three options:
- Comfort for those who want to improve quality of life.
- Comfort and control for those who want to improve quality of life while trying to provide some control of the tumor.
- Comfort and longer-term control for those who want to improve quality of life while trying to maximize the chance of controlling the tumor.

Comfort

- Therapy to enhance comfort (e.g.: NSAID, tramadol, buprenorphine) and freedom from nausea, vomiting (e.g.: maropitant and/or metoclopramide), diarrhea (e.g.: metronidazole) and lack of appetite (e.g.: mirtazapine or cyproheptadine).

Comfort and control

Above mentioned therapy for comfort plus:
- Palliative or coarse fractionated radiation, especially for those with extension into surrounding structures or regional metastases (e.g.: 2-5 dosages of radiation), to first enhance comfort, second, to reduce the rate of growth and third, occasionally to reduce the size of the tumor.
  - In one study involving 5 cats with melanoma of the oral cavity that were treated with hypofractionated radiation therapy (three fractions of 8.0 Gray for a total dose of 24 Gy), 3 cats had a response to radiation, including one complete response and two partial responses, with a median survival time of 146 days (range 66-224 days) from the start of radiation.[44]

Comfort and longer-term control

Above mentioned therapy for comfort plus:
- Surgery.
- Definitive radiation if there is evidence of tumor extending beyond the surgical margins (e.g.: 16-19 dosages of radiation).

FELINE ODONTOGENIC TUMORS
Clinical presentation

- Moderately common.
- Non-neoplastic lesions in the mouth, such as eosinophilic granuloma or inflammatory polyps, may mimic malignant lesions. Always do a biopsy.
- May be painful.
- Inductive fibroameloblastoma are more commonly seen in cats less than 18 months of age; calcifying epithelial odontogenic tumor and epulides in older cats.
- Epulides are much less common in cats than in dogs, accounting for 3 of 89 oral neoplasms in one study[9] and 29 of 371[2] in a second study.

Staging and diagnosis

- Minimum data base (MDB): includes a CBC, biochemical profile, urinalysis, FIV/FeLV serology, T4 testing, biopsy, three-view thoracic radiographs or computerized tomography of the chest.
- Ultrasonography and/or radiographs are practical and cost effective, however computerized tomography or magnetic resonance imaging of the tumor may be preferable in some cases.

Treatment

This section is divided into three options:
- Comfort for those who want to improve quality of life.
- Comfort and control for those who want to improve quality of life while trying to provide some control of the tumor.
- Comfort and longer-term control for those who want to improve quality of life while trying to maximize the chance of controlling the tumor.

Comfort

- Therapy to enhance comfort (e.g.: NSAID, tramadol, buprenorphine) and freedom from nausea, vomiting (e.g.: maropitant and/or metoclopramide), diarrhea (e.g.: metronidazole) and lack of appetite (e.g.: mirtazapine or cyproheptadine).

Comfort and control

Above mentioned therapy for comfort plus:
- Palliative radiation, especially for those with extension into surrounding structures or regional metastases (e.g.: 2-5 dosages of radiation), to first enhance comfort, second, to reduce the rate of growth and third, occasionally to reduce the size of the tumor.

Comfort and longer-term control

Above mentioned therapy for comfort plus:

- Surgery with complete margins is likely curative.
  - Surgery is the treatment of choice, particularly for small inductive fibroameloblastomas. Localized excision may not be successful because of the high probability of bony invasion.
    - In 5 of 10 cats treated surgically, there was no recurrence 6 to 36 months after surgery.[52,54,56,57] Local recurrence was seen within 2 to 6 weeks of surgery in 3 of the remaining cats[56,57] and at 42 months after surgery in a fourth.[52].
  - Surgery should be curative for an epulis. Wide excision is essential as these tumors arise from the periodontal ligament, and thus the tooth with its socket must be removed to prevent recurrence.
- Definitive radiation alone or if there is evidence of tumor extending beyond the surgical margins (e.g.: 16-19 dosages of radiation).
  - Three cats with incompletely resected odontogenic tumors were treated with orthovoltage radiation therapy to a total radiation dose of 48-52 Gy over a period of 26-29 days.[56] Acute toxicities were mild and all cats had long-term (>35 months) control of their tumor.

FELINE TUMORS OF THE SALIVARY GLAND

Clinical presentation

- Moderately common.
- Most salivary gland tumors are adenocarcinomas, accounting for 89 of 106 tumors.[70,71]
- Carcinomas of other types are less common.
- Adenomas comprise approximately 5% of salivary tumors.[9,70-72]
- Mixed tumors (carcinosarcomas) are rare[73,74] and may occasionally be benign.[71]
- Some carcinomas appear to arise from the salivary duct rather than the glandular tissue.[75]
- Ulceration of the overlying skin is common, which may be exacerbated by secondary otitis externa from parotid tumors; deeper invasion may result in facial nerve damage[9] or vestibular signs.[72]
- Signs of hypersalivation, dysphagia, and weight loss are common, as is the case with other oral tumors such as SCC. Tumors can be very large, reaching more than 8 cm in diameter.[9,73,74]
- May be painful.
- Surgical excision curative if adenoma.
- Carcinomas are invasive and thus are rarely completely removed.

Staging and diagnosis

- Minimum data base (MDB): includes a CBC, biochemical profile, urinalysis, FIV/FeLV serology, T4 testing, biopsy, three-view thoracic radiographs or computerized tomography of the chest.
- Ultrasonography and/or radiographs are practical

and cost effective, however computerized tomography or magnetic resonance imaging of the tumor may be preferable in some cases.

Treatment

This section is divided into three options:
- Comfort for those who want to improve quality of life.
- Comfort and control for those who want to improve quality of life while trying to provide some control of the tumor.
- Comfort and longer-term control for those who want to improve quality of life while trying to maximize the chance of controlling the tumor.

> **Key point**
>
> Treatment of cats with salivary gland adenocarcinoma with surgery, radiation and chemotherapy has been shown to result in survival times that exceed a year.

Comfort

- Therapy to enhance comfort (e.g.: NSAID, tramadol, buprenorphine) and freedom from nausea, vomiting (e.g.: maropitant and/or metoclopramide), diarrhea (e.g.: metronidazole) and lack of appetite (e.g.: mirtazapine or cyproheptadine).

Comfort and control

Above mentioned therapy for comfort plus:
- Palliative radiation, especially for those with extension into surrounding structures or regional metastases (e.g.: 2-5 dosages of radiation), to first enhance comfort, second, to reduce the rate of growth and third, occasionally to reduce the size of the tumor.

Comfort and longer-term control

Above mentioned therapy for comfort plus:
- Surgery.
- Definitive radiation if there is evidence of tumor extending beyond the surgical margins (e.g.: 16-19 dosages of radiation).
- Doxorubicin chemotherapy resulted in greater than 50% reduction in the size of a salivary adenocarcinoma for 9 months.[37]
  - Combination therapy using surgery, radiation therapy, and chemotherapy with doxorubicin (or possibly carboplatin) is most likely to be successful in cats with salivary adenocarcinomas. A median survival of 516 days was achieved in 31 cats treated with any combination of these modalities.[78]

FELINE ESOPHAGEAL TUMORS

Clinical presentation

- Epithelial tumors of the esophagus are more common than mesenchymal tumors but are still considered very rare.
- Common locations are thoracic inlet or intrathoracic, but tumors can be anywhere in the esophagus.
- Regurgitation, ptyalism, gagging and weight loss are very common.
- May be painful.

Staging and diagnosis

- Minimum data base (MDB): includes a CBC, biochemical profile, urinalysis, FIV/FeLV serology, T4 testing, biopsy, three-view thoracic radiographs or computerized tomography of the chest.
- Endoscopy and biopsy are often key for making a diagnosis.
- Ultrasonography and/or radiographs are practical and cost effective, however computerized tomography or magnetic resonance imaging of the tumor may be preferable in some cases.

Treatment

This section is divided into three options:
- Comfort for those who want to improve quality of life.
- Comfort and control for those who want to improve quality of life while trying to provide some control of the tumor.
- Comfort and longer-term control for those who want to improve quality of life while trying to maximize the chance of controlling the tumor.

Comfort

- Therapy to enhance comfort (e.g.: NSAID, tramadol, buprenorphine) and freedom from nausea, vomiting (e.g.: maropitant and/or metoclopramide), diarrhea (e.g.: metronidazole) and lack of appetite (e.g.: mirtazapine or cyproheptadine).

Comfort and control

Above mentioned therapy for comfort plus:
- Palliative radiation, especially for those with extension into surrounding structures or regional metastases (e.g.: 2-5 dosages of radiation), to first enhance comfort, second, to reduce the rate of growth and third, occasionally to reduce the size of the tumor.

Comfort and longer-term control

Above mentioned therapy for comfort plus:
- Surgery.
- Definitive radiation if there is evidence of tumor extending beyond the surgical margins (e.g.: 16-19 dosages of radiation).

FELINE GASTRIC TUMORS

Clinical presentation

- Lymphoma is most common gastric tumor.
- Carcinomas and adenomas are uncommon. Other tumors are also seen.
- Vomiting and weight loss are common with all tumor types.
- May be painful.

> **Key point**
> Cats with gastric tumors often lose weight and may vomit.

Staging and diagnosis

- Minimum data base (MDB): includes a CBC, biochemical profile, urinalysis, FIV/FeLV serology, T4 testing, biopsy, three-view thoracic radiographs or computerized tomography of the chest.
- Endoscopic or ultrasound-guided biopsy.
- Ultrasonography and/or radiographs are practical and cost effective, however computerized tomography or magnetic resonance imaging of the tumor may be preferable in some cases.

> **Key point**
> Cats with lymphoma of the stomach often have lymphoma of the intra-abdominal lymph nodes and small intestine, all of which should be assessed by abdominal ultrasound or CT imaging.

Treatment

This section is divided into three options:
- Comfort for those who want to improve quality of life.
- Comfort and control for those who want to improve quality of life while trying to provide some control of the tumor.
- Comfort and longer-term control for those who want to improve quality of life while trying to maximize the chance of controlling the tumor.

> **Key point**
> Lymphoma of the gastrointestinal tract may respond well to combination chemotherapy.

Comfort

- Therapy to enhance comfort (e.g.: NSAID, tramadol, buprenorphine) and freedom from nausea, vomiting (e.g.: maropitant and/or metoclopramide), diarrhea (e.g.: metronidazole) and lack of appetite (e.g.: mirtazapine or cyproheptadine).

Treatment

This section is divided into two options:
- Comfort for those who want to improve quality of life.
- Comfort and longer-term control for those who want to improve quality of life while trying to maximize the chance of controlling the tumor.

> **Key point**
>
> Resection of intestinal adenocarcinoma with or without lymph node metastases has been shown to result in long-term (>1 year) control of the disease, even if there is lymph node metastases.

Comfort

- Therapy to enhance comfort (e.g.: NSAID, tramadol, buprenorphine) and freedom from nausea, vomiting (e.g.: maropitant and/or metoclopramide), diarrhea (e.g.: metronidazole) and lack of appetite (e.g.: mirtazapine or cyproheptadine).

Comfort and longer-term control

Above mentioned therapy for comfort plus:
- Surgical excision of a small intestinal carcinoma is best accomplished by resecting a minimum of 5 cm of normal-appearing bowel on either side of the lesion. Removal of possible metastatic lesions may be helpful. Rectal "pull-through" may be quite helpful for colonic tumors.
  - Cats with intestinal adenocarcinoma that survive the postoperative period have been reported with no evidence of tumor 6 to 54 months after surgery.[9,59,88,90]
  - Median survival of cats with intestinal adenocarcinoma that underwent surgical excision was 365 days and 22 days for those with suspected adenocarcinoma that did not undergo surgery.[108] Median survival of cats was 843 days for those without evidence of metastatic disease at the time of surgery and 358 days for those that had metastases.
- Doxorubicin or carboplatin may be beneficial to delay or prevent metastases or tumor growth.

FELINE INTESTINAL MAST CELL TUMORS

Clinical presentation

- The third most common tumor of the intestine.
  - Most mast cell tumors are in the small intestine.
- Clinical signs include vomiting, diarrhea, inappetence and weight loss.
- Most tumors are palpable.
- May be painful.

Staging and diagnosis

- Minimum data base (MDB): includes a CBC, biochemical profile, urinalysis, FIV/FeLV serology, T4 testing, tumor aspirate or biopsy and three-view thoracic radiographs or computerized tomography of the chest.
- Abdominal ultrasonography and/or radiographs are practical and cost effective, however computerized tomography or magnetic resonance imaging of the tumor may be preferable in some cases. Bone marrow aspirate.
  - More than half of cats with GI mast cell tumors have metastases to sites such as mesenteric lymph nodes, spleen, liver, bone marrow and, less commonly, the lung.

Treatment

This section is divided into three options:
- Comfort for those who want to improve quality of life.
- Comfort and control for those who want to improve quality of life while trying to provide some control of the tumor.
- Comfort and longer-term control for those who want to improve quality of life while trying to maximize the chance of controlling the tumor.

Comfort

- Therapy to enhance comfort (e.g.: NSAID, tramadol, buprenorphine) and freedom from nausea, vomiting (e.g.: maropitant and/or metoclopramide), diarrhea (e.g.: metronidazole) and lack of appetite (e.g.: mirtazapine or cyproheptadine).

Comfort and control

Above mentioned therapy for comfort plus:
- CCNU or vinblastine therapy with or without treatment with a tyrosine kinase inhibitor such as toceranib or masitinib may be helpful.

Comfort and longer-term control

Above mentioned therapy for comfort plus:
- Surgical resection of the involved bowel with 5-10 cm margins on either side followed by CCNU or vinblastine therapy with or without treatment with a tyrosine kinase inhibitor, such as toceranib or masitinib, may be helpful.[123] If metastases can be surgically concurrently downsized, that would be ideal.

References

1. Vos JH, van der Gaag I: Canine and feline oral-pharyngeal tumours. *J Vet Med A* 34:420–427, 1987.
2. Stebbins KE, Morse CE, Goldschmidt MH: Feline oral neoplasia: A ten year survey. *Vet Pathol* 26:121–128, 1989.
3. Cotter SM: Oral pharyngeal neoplasms in the cat. *JAAHA* 17:917–920, 1981.
4. Dorn CR, Priester WA: Epidemiologic analysis of oral and pharyngeal cancer in dogs, cats, horses and cattle. *JAVMA* 169:1202–1206, 1976.
5. Sabhlok A, Ayl R. Palliative radiation therapy outcomes for cats

with oral squamous cell carcinoma (1999-2005). *Vet Radiol Ultrasound* 55(5):565-570, 2014.

6. Fidel J, Lyons J, Tripp C, et al: treatment of oral squamous cell carcinoma with accelerated radiation therapy and concomitant carboplatin in cats. *J Vet Intern Med* 25(3):504-510, 2011.

7. Poirier VJ, Kaser-Hotz B, Vail DM, Straw RC. Efficacy and toxicity of an accelerated hypofractionated radiation therapy protocol in cats with oral squamous cell carcinoma. *Vet Radiol Ultrasound* 54(1):81-88, 2013.

8. Dorn CR, Taylor DON, Schneider R: Sunlight exposure and risk of developing cutaneous and oral squamous cell carcinomas in white cats. *J Natl Cancer Inst* 46:1073–1078, 1971.

9. Carpenter JL, Andrews LK, Holzworth J: Tumors and tumor-like lesions. In Holzworth J (ed): *Diseases of the Cat. Medicine and Surgery*. Philadelphia, WB Saunders, 1987, pp 407–596.

10. Miller AS, McCrea MW, Rhodes WH: Mandibular epidermoid carcinoma with reactive bone proliferation in a cat. *Am J Vet Res* 30:1465–1468, 1969.

11. Bradley RL, MacEwen EG, Loar AS: Mandibular resection for removal of oral tumors in 30 dogs and 6 cats. *JAVMA* 184:460–463, 1984.

12. Bond E, Dorfman HD: Squamous cell carcinoma of the tongue in cats. *JAVMA* 154:786–789, 1969.

13. Postorino Reeves NC, Turrel JM, Withrow SJ: Oral squamous cell carcinoma in the cat. *JAAHA* 29:438–441, 1993.

14. Quigley PJ, Leedale A, Dawson IMP: Carcinoma of mandible of cat and dog simulating osteosarcoma. *J Comp Pathol* 82:15–20, 1972.

15. Moisan PG, Lorenz MD, Stromberg PC, Simmons HA: Concurrent trichinosis and oral squamous cell carcinoma in a cat. *J Vet Diagn Invest* 10:199–202, 1998.

16. Young PL: Squamous cell carcinoma of the tongue of the cat. *Aust Vet J* 54:133–134, 1978.

17. Effron M, Griner L, Benirschke K: Nature and rate of neoplasia found in captive wild mammals, birds and reptiles at necropsy. *J Natl Cancer Inst* 59:185–198, 1977.

18. Martin HE: The zoologic distribution of intra-oral cancer. *Scientific Monthly* 262–266, 1998.

19. Madewell BR, Ackerman N, Sesline DH: Invasive carcinoma radiographically mimicking primary bone *cancer* in the mandibles of two cats. *Cancer* 17:213–215, 1976.

20. Liu S-K, Dorfman HD, Patnaik AK: Primary and secondary bone tumours in the cat. *J Small Anim Pract* 15:141–156, 1974.

21. Cotchin E: Further examples of spontaneous neoplasms in the domestic cat. *Br Vet J* 112:263–272, 1956.

22. Hutson CA, Willauer CC, Walder EJ, et al: treatment of mandibular squamous cell carcinoma in cats by use of mandibulectomy and radiotherapy: Seven cases (1987–1989). *JAVMA* 201:777–781, 1992.

23. Bostock DE: The prognosis in cats bearing squamous cell carcinoma. *J Small Anim Pract* 13:119–125, 1972.

24. Evans SM, LaCreta F, Helfand S, et al: Technique, pharmacokinetics, toxicity, and efficacy of intratumoral etanidazole and radiotherapy for treatment of spontaneous feline oral squamous cell carcinoma. *Int J Radiat Oncol* 20:703–708, 1991.

25. Quigley PJ, Leedale AH: Tumors involving bone in the domestic cat: A review of fifty-eight cases. *Vet Pathol* 20:670–686, 1983.

26. Emms SG, Harvey CE: Preliminary results of maxillectomy in the dog and cat. *J Small Anim Pract* 27:291–306, 1986.

27. Verstraete FJM, Kass PH, Terpak CH: Diagnostic value of full-mouth radiography in cats. *Am J Vet Res* 59:692–695, 1998.

28. Solano M, Penninck DG: Ultrasonography of the canine, feline and equine tongue: normal findings and case history reports. *Vet Radiol Ultrasound* 37:206–213, 1996.

29. Klausner JS, Bell FW, Hayden DW, et al: Hypercalcemia in two cats with squamous cell carcinomas. *JAVMA* 196:103–105, 1990.

30. Plotnick A, Brunt JE, Reitz BL: What is your diagnosis? *JAVMA* 202:991–994, 1993.

31. Penwick RC, Nunamaker DM: Rostral mandibulectomy: A treatment for oral neoplasia in the dog and cat. *JAAHA* 23:19–25, 1987.

32. Salisbury SK, Richardson DC, Lantz GC: Partial maxillectomy and premaxillectomy in the treatment of oral neoplasia in the dog and cat. *Vet Surg* 15:16–26, 1986.

33. Northrup NC Selting KA, Rassnick KM, et al: Outcomes of cats with oral tumors treated with mandibulectomy: 42 cases. *J Am Anim Hosp Assoc* 42(5):350-360, 2006.

34. Dewhirst MW, Sim DA, Wilson S, et al: Correlation between initial and long-term responses of spontaneous pet animal tumors to heat and radiation or radiation alone. *Cancer Res* 43:5735–5741, 1983.

35. Fox LE, Levine PB, King RR, et al: Use of cis-bis-neodocanoato-trans-R,R-1,2-diaminocyclohexane platinum (II), a liposomal cisplatin analogue, in cats with oral squamous cell carcinoma. *Am J Vet Res* 61:791–795, 2000.

36. Knapp DW, Richardson RC, BeNicola DB, et al: Cisplatin toxicity in cats. *J Vet Intern Med* 1:29–35, 1987.

37. Mauldin GN, Matus RE, Patnaik AK, et al: Efficacy and toxicity of doxorubicin and cyclophosphamide used in the treatment of selected malignant tumors in 23 cats. *J Vet Intern Med* 2:60–65, 1988.

38. Ogilvie GK, Moore AS, Obradovich JE, et al: Toxicoses and efficacy associated with the administration of mitoxantrone to cats with malignant tumors. *JAVMA* 202:1839–1844, 1993.

39. LaRue SM, Vail DM, Ogilvie GK, et al: Shrinking-field radiation therapy plus mitoxantrone for the treatment of oral squamous cell carcinoma in the cat. *Vet Cancer Soc Newsl* 15:4–7, 1991.

40. Wood CA, Moore AS, Frimberger AE, et al: Phase I evaluation of carboplatin in tumor bearing cats. *Proc Vet Cancer Soc 16th Annu .Conf*:39–40, 1996.

41. Frimberger AE, Moore AS, Cincotta L, et al: Photodynamic therapy of naturally occurring tumors in animals using a novel benzophenothiazine photosensitizer. *Clin Cancer Res* 4:2207–2218, 1998.

42. MacEwen EG: Anti-tumor evaluation of benzaldehyde in the dog and cat. *Am J Vet Res* 47:451–452, 1986.

43. Bradley RL, Sponenberg DP, Martin RA: Oral neoplasia in 15 dogs and 4 cats. *Semin Vet Med Surg Small Anim* 1:33–42, 1986.

44. Farrelly J, Denman DL, Hohenhaus AE et al: Hypofractionated radiation therapy of oral melanoma in five cats. *Vet Radiol Ultrasound* 45(1):91-93, 2004.

45. Wilson RB, Holscher MA, Casey TT, Berry KK: Tonsillar granular cell tumour in a cat. *J Comp Pathol* 101:109–112, 1989.

46. Patnaik AK: Histologic and immunohistochemical studies of granular cell tumors in seven dogs, three cats, one horse, and one bird. *Vet Pathol* 30:176–185, 1993.

47. Hahn KA: Vincristine sulfate as single-agent chemotherapy in a dog and a cat with malignant neoplasms. *JAVMA* 197:796–798, 1990.

48. Scott DW: Lentigo simplex in orange cats. *Compan Anim Pract* 23–25, 1987.

49. Patnaik AK, Mooney S: Feline melanoma: A comparative study of ocular, oral, and dermal neoplasms. *Vet Pathol* 25:105–112, 1988.

50. Sundberg JP, Van Ranst M, Montali R., et al: Feline papillomas and papillomaviruses. *Vet Pathol* 37:1–10, 2000.

51. Gardner DG: An orderly approach to the study of odontogenic tumours in animals. *J Comp Pathol* 107:427–438, 1992.

52. Poulet FM, Valentine BA, Summers BA: A survey of epithelial odontogenic tumors and cysts in dogs and cats. *Vet Pathol* 29:369–380, 1992.

53. Hawkins CD, Jones BR: Adamantinoma in a cat. *Aust Vet J* 59:54–55, 1982.

54. Dernell WS, Hullinger GH: Surgical management of ameloblastic fibroma in the cat. *J Small Anim Pract* 35:35–38, 1994.

55. Mills JHL, Lewis RJ: Adamantinoma—Histogenesis and differentiations from the periodontal fibromatous epulis and squamous cell carcinoma. *Can Vet J* 22:126–129, 1981.

56. Moore AS, Wood CA, Engler SJ, Bengtson AE. Radiation therapy for long-term control of odontogenic tumours and epulis in three cats. *J Feline Med Surg* 2(1):57-60, 2000.

57. Dubielzig RR, Adams WM, Brodey RS: Inductive fibroameloblastoma, and unusual dental tumor of young cats. *JAVMA* 174:720–722, 1979.

58. Dubielzig RR: Proliferative dental and gingival diseases of dogs and cats. *JAAHA* 18:577–584, 1982.

59. Brodey RS: Alimentary tract neoplasms in the cat: A clinicopathologic survey of 46 cases. *Am J Vet Res* 27:74–80, 1966.

60. Moore AS, Wood CA, Engler SJ, Bengston AE: Radiation therapy for long term control of odontogenic tumors and epulis in three cats. *J Feline Med Surg* 2:57–60, 2000.

61. Ohmachi T, Taniyama H, Nakade T, et al: Calcifying epithelial odontogenic tumours in small domesticated carnivores: Histological, immunohistochemical and electron microscopical studies. *J Comp Pathol* 114:305–314, 1996.

62. Breuer W, Geisel O, Linke RP, Hermanns W: Light microscopic, ultrastructural, and immunohistochemical examinations of two calcifying epithelial odontogenic tumors (CEOT) in a dog and a cat. *Vet Pathol* 31:415–420, 1994.

63. Langham RF, Bennett R, Koestner A: Amyloidosis associated with a calcifying ameloblastoma (calcifying epithelial odontoma) in a cat. *Vet Pathol* 21:549–550, 1984.

64. Abbott DP, Walsh K, Diters RW: Calcifying epithelial odontogenic tumours in three cats and a dog. *J Comp Pathol* 96:131–136, 1986.

65. Levene A: Sebaceous gland differentiation in tumours of the feline oral mucosa. *Vet Rec* 114:69, 1984.

66. Rest JR, Gumbrell RC, Heim P, Rushton-Taylor P: Oral fibropapillomas in young cats. *Vet Rec* 141:528, 1997.

67. Sironi G, Caniatti M, Scanziani E: Immunohistochemical detection of papillomavirus structural antigens in animal

hyperplastic and neoplastic epithelial lesions. *J Vet Med* 37:760–770, 1990.

68. Koestner A, Buerger L: Primary neoplasms of the salivary glands in animals compared to similar tumors in man. *Path Vet* 2:201–226, 1965.

69. Bosselut R, Samso A, Cattanei J: Cancer des glandes salivaires chez le chat. *Bull Algerien Carcinologie* 4:407–408, 1951.

70. Spangler WL, Culbertson MR: Salivary gland disease in dogs and cats: 245 cases (1985–1988). *JAVMA* 198:465–469, 1991.

71. Carberry CA, Flanders JA, Harvey HJ, Ryan AM: Salivary gland tumors in dogs and cats: a literature and case review. *JAAHA* 24:561–567, 1988.

72. Case MT, Simon J: Oncocytomas in a cat and a dog. *Vet Med Small Anim Clin* 61:41–43, 1966.

73. Wells GAH, Robinson M: Mixed tumour of salivary gland showing histological evidence of malignancy in a cat. *J Comp Pathol* 85:77–85, 1975.

74. Carpenter JL, Bernstein M: Malignant mixed (pleomorphic) mandibular salivary gland tumors in a cat. *JAAHA* 27:581–583, 1991.

75. Sozmen M, Brown PJ, Eveson JW: Salivary duct carcinoma in five cats. *J Comp Pathol* 121:311–319, 1999.

76. Burek KA, Munn RJ, Madewell BR: Metastatic adenocarcinoma of a minor salivary gland in a cat. *J Vet Med* 41:485–490, 1999.

77. Karbe E, Schiefer B: Primary salivary gland tumors in carnivores. *Can Vet J* 8:212–215, 1967.

78. Hammer A, Getzy D, Ogilvie G, Upton M, Klausner J, Kisseberth W, Klein M, Fineman L, Page R, Carr A, Holmberg D: Salivary gland neoplasia in the dog and cat: survival times and prognostic factors. *Proc.17th Annu Vet Cancer Soc*:87, 1997.

79. Cotchin E: Neoplasms in small animals. *Vet Rec* 63:67–72, 1951.

80. Gray H: Cancer of the oesophagus in the cat. *The Veterinary Record* 15:532–533, 1935.

81. Fernandes FH, Hawe RS, Loeb WF: Primary squamous cell carcinoma of the esophagus in a cat. *Compan Anim Pract* 16–22, 1987.

82. Vernon FF, Roudebush P: Primary esophageal carcinoma in a cat. *JAAHA* 16:547–550, 1980.

83. Happe RP, Gaag Ivd, Wolvekamp WThC, Van Toorenburg J: Esophageal squamous cell carcinoma in two cats. *Tijdschr. Diergeneesk.* 103:1080–1086, 1978.

84. Gualtieri M, Monzeglio MG, Di Giancamillo M: Oesophageal squamous cell carcinoma in two cats. *J Small Anim Pract* 40:79–83, 1999.

85. Dargent F, Gau M-L, Olivie J.: Primary oesophageal epidermoid carcinoma in a cat. *7th Annu Conference ESVIM*:119, 1997

86. Johnson K: Oesophageal carcinoma in a cat. *Aust Vet Pract* 6:228, 1976

87. MacDonald JM, Mullen HS, Moroff SD: Adenomatous polyps of the duodenum in cats: 18 cases (1985–1990). *JAVMA* 202:647–651, 1993.

88. Turk MAM, Gallina AM, Russell TS: Nonhematopoietic gastrointestinal neoplasia in cats: A retrospective study of 44 cases. *Vet Pathol* 18:614–620, 1981.

89. Cribb AE: Feline gastrointestinal adenocarcinoma: a review and retrospective study. *Can Vet J* 29:709–712, 1988.

90. Lingeman CH, Garner FM, Taylor DON: Spontaneous gastric adenocarcinomas of dogs: A review. *J Natl Cancer Inst* 47:137–153, 1971.

91. Patnaik AK, Liu S-K, Hurvitz AI, McClelland AJ: Nonhematopoietic neoplasms in cats. *J Natl Cancer Inst* 54:855–860, 1975.

92. Cotchin E: Neoplasia. In Wilkinson GT (ed): *Diseases of the Cat and Their Management.* Melbourne, Blackwell Scientific Publications, 1983.

93. Breese CE: What is your diagnosis? *JAVMA* 197:908–909, 1990.

94. Wright KN, Gomph RE, DeNovo Jr RC: Peritoneal effusion in cats: 65 cases (1981–1997). *JAVMA* 214:375–381, 1999.

95. Zikes CD, Spielman B, Shapiro W, et al: Gastric extramedullary plasmacytoma in a cat. *J Vet Intern Med* 12:381–383, 1998.

96. Bortnowski HB, Rosenthal RC: Gastrointestinal mast cell tumors and eosinophilia in two cats. *JAAHA* 28:271–275, 1992.

97. Olin FH, Lea RB, Kim C: Colonic adenoma in a cat. *JAVMA* 153:53–56, 1968.

98. Orr CM, Gruffydd-Jones TJ, Kelly DF: Ileal polyps in Siamese cats. *J Small Anim Pract* 21:669–674, 1980.

99. Penninck DG, Nyland TG, Kerr LY, Fisher PE: Ultrasonographic evaluation of gastrointestinal diseases in small animals. *Vet Radiol* 31:134–141, 1990.

100. Penninck DG, Crystal MA, Matz ME, Pearson SH: The technique of percutaneous ultrasound guided fine-needle aspiration biopsy and automated microcore biopsy in small animal gastrointestinal diseases. *Vet Radiol Ultrasound* 34:433–436, 1993.

101. Crystal MA, Penninck DG, Matz ME, et al: Use of ultrasound-guided fine-needle aspiration biopsy and automated core biopsy for the diagnosis of gastrointestinal diseases in small animals. *Vet Radiol* 34:438–444, 1993.

102. Birchard SJ, Couto CG, Johnson S: Nonlymphoid intestinal neoplasia in 32 dogs and 14 cats. *JAAHA* 22:533–537, 1986.

103. Rivers BJ, Walter PA, Feeney DA, Johnston GR: Ultrasonographic features of intestinal adenocarcinoma in five cats. *Vet Radiol Ultrasound* 38:300–306, 1997.

104. Loupal G, Pfeil C: Tumoren im darmtrakt der katze unter besonderer Berücksigtigung der nicht-hämatopoetischen Geschwiilste. *Berl Münch Teirärztl Wschr* 97:208–213, 1984.

105. Patnaik AK, Liu SK, Johnston GF: Feline intestinal adenocarcinoma: A clinicopathologic study of 22 cases. *Vet Pathol* 13:1–10, 1976.

106. Head KW, Else RW: Neoplasia and allied conditions of the canine and feline intestine. *Small Anim Intest Neopl* 190–208. 1981.

107. Kosovsky Je, Matthiesen DT, Patnaik AK: Small intestinal adenocarcinoma in cats: 32 cases (1978–1985). *JAVMA* 192:233–235, 1988.

108. Green ML, Smith JD, Kass PH. Surgical versus non-surgical treatment of feline small intestinal adenocarcinoma and the influence of metastasis on long-term survival in 18 cats (2000-2007). Can Vet J. 52(10):1101-1105, 2011.

109. Böhmer E, Matis U, Zedler W, Hänichen T: Dünndarmileus bei katze und hund–Katamnestische betrachtungen von 704 patienten. *Tierärztl Prax* 18:171–183, 1990.

110. Taylor PF, Kater JC: Adenocarcinoma of the intestine of the dog and cat. *Aust Vet* J 377–379. 1954.

111. Gerosa RM, de Esrada MMM: Colorectal resection in a cat with adenocarcinoma. *Feline Pract* 12:6–15, 1982.

112. Stewart C: Jejunal adenocarcinoma in a cat. *Aust Vet Pract* 27:131–136, 1997.

113. Palumbo NE, Perri SF: Adenocarcinoma of the ileum in a cat. *JAVMA* 164:607–608, 1974.

114. Theran P, Thornton GW: Case records of the Angell Memorial Animal Hospital. *JAVMA* 152:1017–1022, 1968.

115. Mayrhofer E: Enddarmneoplasma und chronische obstipation bei einem kater. *Wien Tierärztl Mschr* 71:103–104, 1984.

116. Patnaik AK, Johnson GF, Greene RW, et al: Surgical resection of intestinal adenocarcinoma in a cat, with survival of 28 months. *JAVMA* 178:479–481, 1981.

117. Weichselbaum RC, Feeney DA, Hayden DW: Comparison of upper gastrointestinal radiographic findings to histopathologic observations: A retrospective study of 41 dogs and cats with suspected small bowel infiltrative disease (1985 to 1990). *Vet Radiol Ultrasound* 35:418–426, 1994.

118. Slawienski MJ, Mauldin GE, Mauldin GN, Patnaik AK: Malignant colonic neoplasia in cats: 46 cases (1990–1996). *JAVMA* 211:878–881, 1997.

119. Mulligan RM: Spontaneous cat tumors. *Cancer Res* 11:271, 1951.

120. Alroy J, Leav I, DeLellis A, Weinstein RS: Distinctive intestinal mast cell neoplasms of domestic cats. *Lab Invest* 33:159–167, 1975.

121. Garner FM, Lingeman CH: Mast-cell neoplasms of the domestic cat. *Path Vet* 7:517–530, 1970.

122. Peaston AE, Griffey SM: Visceral mast cell tumour with eosinophilia and eosinophilic peritoneal and pleural effusions in a cat. *Aust Vet J* 71:215–217, 1994.

123. Rassnick KM, Williams LE, Kristal O et al: Lomustine for treatment of mast cell tumors in cats: 38 cases (1999-2005). J Am Vet Med Assoc 232(8):1200-1205, 2008.

124. Carakostas MC, Kennedy GA, Kittleson MD, Cook JE: Malignant foregut carcinoid tumor in a domestic cat. *Vet Pathol* 16:607–609, 1979.

125. Lahellec M, Joncourt L, Dhennin L: Étude clinique et histologique d'une tumeur carcinoïde du grêle chez un chat. *Bull Acad Vet* 45:363–365, 1972.

126. Patnaik AK, Lieberman PH, Johnson GF: Intestinal ganglioneuroma in a kitten—A case report and review of literature. *J Small Anim Pract* 19:735–742, 1978.

127. Barrand KR, Scudamore CL: Intestinal leiomyosarcoma in a cat. *J Small Anim Pract* 40:216–219, 1999.

128. Rowland PH, Linke RP: Immunohistochemical characterization of lambda light-chain-derived amyloid in one feline and five canine plasma cell tumors. *Vet Pathol* 31:390–393, 1994.

129. Hawkins EC, Feldman BF, Blanchard PC: Immunoglobulin A myeloma in a cat with pleural effusion and serum hyperviscosity. *JAVMA* 188:876–878, 1986.

Chapter 51

Feline tumors of liver, pancreas, and spleen

FELINE VISCERAL MAST CELL TUMORS

Clinical presentation

- Most common in older, non-purebred cats.
- Cats with visceral mast cell disease may present for nonspecific malaise, inappetence, weight loss, or vomiting, the latter of which is presumably due to gastroduodenal ulceration following the release of vasoactive amines (e.g., histamine, serotonin) that cause gastric parietal cell hyperplasia and increased gastric acid production.[5,8,9]
- The principle site for visceral mast cell tumor is the spleen.
- Moderately common.
- May be painful.

Staging and diagnosis

- Minimum data base (MDB): includes a CBC, biochemical profile, urinalysis, FIV/FeLV serology, T4 testing, aspirate or biopsy, three-view thoracic radiographs or computerized tomography of the chest.
- Ultrasonography and/or radiographs are practical and cost effective, however computerized tomography or magnetic resonance imaging of the tumor may be preferable in some cases.
  - While the spleen is the most common primary site for visceral MCT, the liver is involved in up to 90% of affected cats followed by visceral lymph nodes, bone marrow, lung, intestine, and kidney.[2,7]
    - Marrow, splenic and hepatic aspirates may be indicated.

Key point

The spleen is the most common primary site for visceral MCT, however liver, visceral lymph nodes, bone marrow, lung, intestine, and kidney metastases are seen in up to 90% of cats.

Treatment

This section is divided into three options:
- Comfort for those who want to improve quality of life.
- Comfort and control for those who want to improve quality of life while trying to provide some control of the tumor.
- Comfort and longer-term control for those who want to improve quality of life while trying to maximize the chance of controlling the tumor.

Key point

Surgery, CCNU and tyrosine kinase inhibitors have been shown to be beneficial in the management of cats with visceral mast cell tumors.

Comfort

- Therapy to enhance comfort (e.g.: prednisolone, Pepcid, diphenhydramine and if needed, tramadol, buprenorphine) and freedom from nausea, vomiting (e.g.: maropitant and/or metoclopramide), diarrhea (e.g.: metronidazole) and lack of appetite (e.g.: mirtazapine or cyproheptadine).

Comfort and control

Above mentioned therapy for comfort plus:
- Tyrosine kinase inhibitor such as toceranib or masitinib.
- CCNU has been used with success with an overall response rate of 50%. Median response duration was 168 days (range, 25 to 727 days). The most common toxicoses were neutropenia and thrombocytopenia.

Comfort and longer-term control

Above mentioned therapy for comfort plus:

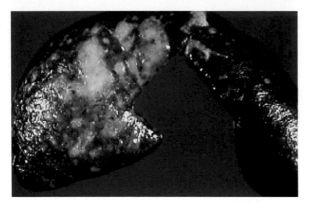

Figure 51-1: Cats with splenic mast cell tumors can do well after a splenectomy. The spleen often has a darker color with "white icing" over the surface. It is common to have concurrent involvement of the liver, lymph nodes and bone marrow. Systemic therapy with CCNU and/or a tyrosine kinase inhibitor postoperatively may be indicated.

- Splenectomy, even if there is concurrent disease in liver, lymph nodes and marrow, can result in improvement in quality of life and overall survival. Concern over the release of vasoactive amines due to surgical manipulation during splenectomy has led to the recommendation that cats be treated with corticosteroids and both H1 and H2-blocking antihistamines for 48 hours prior to surgery.
  - Postoperative adjuvant therapy with toceranib, masitinib and/or CCNU or vinblastine has been helpful.

FELINE HEMANGIOSARCOMA
Clinical presentation

- Moderately common, aggressive and invasive.
- Mesenteric hemangiosarcomas more common than those of spleen, liver, mediastinum, oral and nasal cavity.
- Hemangiosarcoma is the most often diagnosed neoplasm (60%) in cats, with the spleen as the most common location for neoplasia (37%).[25]
- Hemoabdomen is common.
- Clinical signs secondary to blood loss and ascites are common and include lethargy, anorexia, collapse and death.
- Not usually painful.

Staging and diagnosis

- Minimum data base (MDB): includes a CBC, biochemical profile, urinalysis, FIV/FeLV serology, T4 testing, surgical biopsy and three-view thoracic radiographs or computerized tomography of the chest; with a coagulation panel is ideal.
- Ultrasonography and/or radiographs are practical and cost effective, however computerized

tomography or magnetic resonance imaging of the tumor may be preferable in some cases.
- Ultrasonography is the imaging modality of choice, particularly in cats in which peritoneal effusion obscures radiographic details. The ultrasonographic appearance is most often that of multiple cavernous splenic nodules and in some cases, metastases to intraabdominal organs.
- In one study, 82% of cats were anemic, aspartate transaminase was increased in 53%, and metastatic lung disease was noted in 33% of affected cats.[26]

Treatment

This section is divided into two options:
- Comfort for those who want to improve quality of life.
- Comfort and control for those who want to improve quality of life while trying to provide some control of the tumor.

Comfort

- Therapy to enhance comfort (e.g.: NSAID, tramadol, buprenorphine) and freedom from nausea, vomiting (e.g.: maropitant and/or metoclopramide), diarrhea (e.g.: metronidazole) and lack of appetite (e.g.: mirtazapine or cyproheptadine). Transfusions and/or fluid therapy is often needed due to bleeding and volume depletion.

Comfort and control

Above mentioned therapy for comfort plus:
- Splenectomy. This surgical procedure has been reported in five cats.[21,23] Four of these cats died between 8 and 35 weeks after surgery, and one did not die and was alive 19 weeks after surgery.
- Adjuvant chemotherapy may be helpful. Doxorubicin is the most commonly mentioned in literature.

FELINE LYMPHANGIOMA AND LYMPHANGIOSARCOMA
Clinical presentation

- Rare.
- Similar biologic behavior to hemangiosarcoma.
- May be painful.
- Most often diagnosed on the skin, however it may involve the liver,[32] mediastinum,[33,34] abdominal serosa,[29] cranial mesentery,[34] oral cavity,[32] and tongue.[32]
- Chylous ascites or abdominal effusion may be found.

Staging and diagnosis

- Minimum data base (MDB): includes a CBC, biochemical profile, urinalysis, FIV/FeLV serology,

T4 testing, biopsy, three-view thoracic radiographs or computerized tomography of the chest.
- Ultrasonography and/or radiographs are practical and cost effective, however computerized tomography or magnetic resonance imaging of the tumor may be preferable in some cases.

Treatment

This section is divided into three options:
- Comfort for those who want to improve quality of life.
- Comfort and control for those who want to improve quality of life while trying to provide some control of the tumor.
- Comfort and longer-term control for those who want to improve quality of life while trying to maximize the chance of controlling the tumor.

Comfort

- Therapy to enhance comfort (e.g.: NSAID, tramadol, buprenorphine) and freedom from nausea, vomiting (e.g.: maropitant and/or metoclopramide), diarrhea (e.g.: metronidazole) and lack of appetite (e.g.: mirtazapine or cyproheptadine).

Comfort and control

Above mentioned therapy for comfort plus:
- Palliative radiation for localized disease, especially for those with extension into surrounding structures or regional metastases (e.g.: 2-5 dosages of radiation), to first enhance comfort, second, to reduce the rate of growth and third, to reduce the size of the tumor.

Comfort and longer-term control

Above mentioned therapy for comfort plus:
- Surgery.
- Definitive radiation if there is evidence of tumor extending beyond the surgical margins (e.g.: 16-19 dosages of radiation).
  - Doxorubicin may be helpful as an adjuvant treatment.

FELINE MYELOLIPOMA

Clinical presentation

- Uncommon benign liver tumor in older domestic cats; rarely affects the spleen.
- Tumors may be solitary and large or multiple.
- Usually asymptomatic, incidental finding.

Staging and diagnosis

- These tumors are benign, however they must be differentiated from malignant tumors that can and do metastasize
- Minimum data base (MDB): includes a CBC,

biochemical profile, urinalysis, FIV/FeLV serology, T4 testing, biopsy, three-view thoracic radiographs or computerized tomography of the chest.
- Ultrasonography is often the best diagnostic tool, however radiographs, computerized tomography, or magnetic resonance imaging of the tumor may be preferable in some cases.

Treatment

This section is divided into three options:
- Comfort for those who want to improve quality of life.
- Comfort and control for those who want to improve quality of life while trying to provide some control of the tumor.
- Comfort and longer-term control for those who want to improve quality of life while trying to maximize the chance of controlling the tumor.

Comfort

- Therapy to enhance comfort if needed (e.g.: NSAID, tramadol, buprenorphine) and freedom from nausea, vomiting (e.g.: maropitant and/or metoclopramide), diarrhea (e.g.: metronidazole) and lack of appetite (e.g.: mirtazapine or cyproheptadine).

Comfort and control

Above mentioned therapy for comfort plus:
- Palliative radiation for localized disease, especially for those with extension into surrounding structures or regional metastases (e.g.: 2-5 dosages of radiation), to first enhance comfort, second, to reduce the rate of growth and third, occasionally to reduce the size of the tumor.

Comfort and longer-term control

Above mentioned therapy for comfort plus:
- Splenectomy if indicated.

FELINE TUMORS OF THE LIVER PARENCHYMA

Clinical presentation

- Hepatoma and hepatocellular carcinoma may be part of a disease spectrum rather than distinct entities and may be seen at the same time.
- Uncommon in older cats.
- Nonspecific clinical signs including weakness due to a paraneoplastic syndrome causing hypoglycemia.
- Abdominal mass may be palpable.

Staging and diagnosis

- Minimum data base (MDB): includes a CBC, biochemical profile, urinalysis, FIV/FeLV serology, T4 testing, biopsy, three-view thoracic radiographs or computerized tomography of the chest.

- Ultrasonography and/or radiographs are practical and cost effective, however computerized tomography or magnetic resonance imaging of the tumor may be preferable in some cases.
  - Metastases, if they occur, are usually to regional lymph nodes.

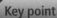

Key point

The routine access to ultrasound has increased the long-term cure and control rate of cats with liver tumors due to earlier detection and diagnosis.

Treatment

This section is divided into two options:
- Comfort for those who want to improve quality of life.
- Comfort and control for those who want to improve quality of life while trying to provide some control of the tumor.

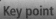

Key point

Resection of hepatocellular carcinoma has resulted in survival times in excess of two years post resection.

Comfort

- Therapy to enhance comfort (e.g.: NSAID, tramadol, buprenorphine) and freedom from nausea, vomiting (e.g.: maropitant and/or metoclopramide), diarrhea (e.g.: metronidazole) and lack of appetite (e.g.: mirtazapine or cyproheptadine).

Comfort and control

Above mentioned therapy for comfort plus:
- Surgery.
  - In one study, hepatocellular carcinoma was found equally in the left and right lobes, with survival time post resection of 2.4 years.[50]

FELINE TUMORS OF THE BILIARY SYSTEM

Clinical presentation

- Relatively uncommon.
- Spectrum of diseases from cholangiocarcinoma, bile duct or biliary adenocarcinoma, and biliary carcinoma.
- Can cause abdominal distension, anorexia, depression, vomiting, and weight loss.
- May be palpable.

Staging and diagnosis

- Minimum data base (MDB): includes a CBC, biochemical profile, urinalysis, FIV/FeLV serology,

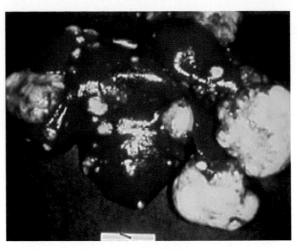

Figure 51-2: Primary and metastatic neoplasia of the liver in the cat is often associated with nonspecific clinical signs, elevated liver enzymes and occasionally, a palpable cranial abdominal mass. Radiographs of the chest and abdomen are good screening tests, however an ultrasound and ultrasound-guided biopsy or aspirate are often helpful at defining the specific diagnosis. If the liver malignancy is caused by a mast cell tumor or lymphoma, chemotherapy is often indicated. If it is a carcinoma or adenocarcinoma, then surgery may be helpful in some cases. If the disease is multifocal, as depicted here, surgery is not likely helpful for prolonging life significantly. Reprinted with permission from: Ogilvie GK, Moore AS. *Feline Oncology: A Comprehensive Guide for Compassionate Care.* Trenton NJ, Veterinary Learning Systems. 2002.

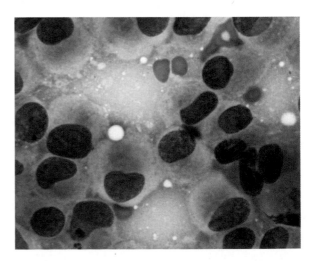

Figure 51-3: Aspirates of the liver mass may be diagnostic, as in this sample. Note large epithelial cells with abundant cytoplasm, diffuse cytoplasmic borders, tendency to clump, varying nuclear:cytoplasmic ratios and the occasional prominent nucleoli. While the cytology is suggestive of a carcinoma, cytology can occasionally be misleading. Therefore, whenever possible, a histologic biopsy should be obtained to confirm the diagnosis.

T4 testing, biopsy, three-view thoracic radiographs or computerized tomography of the chest.
- Ultrasonography and/or radiographs are practical and cost effective, however computerized tomography or magnetic resonance imaging of the tumor may be preferable in some cases.
  - The pattern of metastasis did not seem to differ among the three sites of origin; the most common sites of metastasis were the peritoneum, lungs, and regional lymph nodes,[2,25]

Treatment

This section is divided into two options:
- Comfort for those who want to improve quality of life.
- Comfort and control for those who want to improve quality of life while trying to provide some control of the tumor.

Comfort

- Therapy to enhance comfort (e.g.: NSAID, tramadol, buprenorphine) and freedom from nausea, vomiting (e.g.: maropitant and/or metoclopramide), diarrhea (e.g.: metronidazole) and lack of appetite (e.g.: mirtazapine or cyproheptadine).

Comfort and control

Above mentioned therapy for comfort plus:
- Surgery. Complete resection has been reported to result in median survival times exceeding two years.

FELINE CARCINOMA OF THE EXOCRINE PANCREAS

Clinical presentation

- Uncommon or unrecognized.
- Usually seen in older cats.
- Nonspecific clinical signs predominate including anorexia, severe weight loss, lethargy, and listlessness.
- May be painful.

Staging and diagnosis

- Minimum data base (MDB): includes a CBC, biochemical profile, urinalysis, FIV/FeLV serology, T4 testing, biopsy by ultrasound guidance or surgery and three-view thoracic radiographs or computerized tomography of the chest.
- Ultrasonography is the most practical imaging technique, however, radiographs, computerized tomography, or magnetic resonance imaging of the abdominal tumor are also effective.
  - Metastases to the liver, peritoneum, and regional lymph nodes are most commonly described,[62,71,74,75,77] however lung, spleen, diaphragm, GI tract, ovaries, kidneys, and pleura are all reported.[62,73,75,77,78]

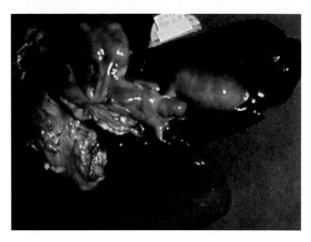

Figure 51-4: This necropsy specimen confirms the presence of a pancreatic carcinoma that involves almost the entire pancreas. Close inspection reveals thickening of the liver that is associated with hepatic metastases. The routine use of diagnostic ultrasound has resulted in an increase in the diagnoses of early stage pancreatic tumors, many that are low grade and associated with periods of anorexia and vomiting. The increase in the identification of these low grade tumors brings about the opportunity to increase the progression-free survival of cats with this condition by intervening surgically before the condition becomes inoperable. Reprinted with permission from: Ogilvie GK, Moore AS. *Feline Oncology: A Comprehensive Guide for Compassionate Care.* Trenton NJ, Veterinary Learning Systems. 2002.

Treatment

This section is divided into two options:
- Comfort for those who want to improve quality of life.
- Comfort and control for those who want to improve quality of life while trying to provide some control of the tumor.

Comfort

- Therapy to enhance comfort (e.g.: NSAID, tramadol, buprenorphine) and freedom from nausea, vomiting (e.g.: maropitant and/or metoclopramide), diarrhea (e.g.: metronidazole) and lack of appetite (e.g.: mirtazapine or cyproheptadine).

Comfort and control

Above mentioned therapy for comfort plus:
- Surgery. Is not an option if metastases are present but may be palliative if not. Gastrojejunostomy or enteral feeding (jejunostomy) tube placement is required.
  - Carboplatin and toceranib may be used adjuvantly.

References

1. Spangler WL, Culbertson MR: Prevalence and type of splenic diseases in cats: 455 cases (1985–1991). *JAVMA* 201:773–776, 1992.
2. Carpenter JL, Andrews LK, Holzworth J: Tumors and tumor-like lesions. In Holzworth J (ed): *Diseases of the Cat. Medicine and Surgery.* Philadelphia, WB Saunders, 1987, pp 407–596.
3. Kessler M, Fickenscher Y, von Bomhard D: Zum vorkommen primärer tumoren der milz bei der katze. *Kleintierpraxis* 43:601–608, 1998.
4. Confer AW, Langloss JM, Cashell IG: Long-term survival of two cats with mastocytosis. *JAVMA* 172:160–161, 1978.
5. Liska WD, MacEwen EG, Zaki FA, Gavery M: Feline systemic mastocytosis: A review and results of splenectomy in seven cases. *JAAHA* 15:589–579, 1979.
6. Madewell BR, Gunn CR, Gribble DH: Mast cell phagocytosis of red blood cells in a cat. *Vet Pathol* 20:638–640, 1983.
7. Goto N, Ozasa M, Takahashi R, Ishida K, Fujiwara K: Pathological observations of feline mast cell tumor. *Jpn J Vet Sci* 36:483–494, 1974.
8. Weller RE: Systemic mastocytosis and mastocytemia in a cat. *Mod Vet Pract* 59:41–43, 1978.
9. Kobayashi Y, Usuda H, Ochiai K, Itakura C: Malignant mesothelioma with metastases and mast cell leukaemia in a cat. *J Comp Pathol* 111:453–458, 1994.
10. Hasler UC, van den Ingh TSGAM: Malignant mastocytosis and duodenal ulceration in a cat. *Schweiz Arch Tierheilk* 120:263–268, 1978.
11. Lillie RD: Mast myelocyte leukemia in a cat. *Am J Pathol* 713–721, 1931.
12. Seawright AA, Grono LR: Malignant mast cell tumour in a cat with perforating duodenal ulcer. *J Path Bact* 87:107–111, 1964.
13. Crawford MA: Challenging cases in internal medicine: What's your diagnosis? *Vet Med* 84:1126–1143, 1989.
14. Wright KN, Gomph RE, DeNovo Jr RC: Peritoneal effusion in cats: 65 cases (1981–1997). *JAVMA* 214:375–381, 1999.
15. Schulman A: Splenic mastocytosis in a cat. *Calif Vet* 41:17–18, 1987.
16. Madewell BR, Munn RJ, Phillips LK: Ultrastructure of canine, feline and bovine mast cell neoplasms. *Am J Vet Res* 45:2066–2073, 1984.
17. Guerre R, Millet P, Groulade P: Systemic mastocytosis in a cat: remission after splenectomy. *J Small Anim Pract* 20:769–772, 1979.
18. Jeraj KP, O'Brien TD, Yano BL: Systemic mastocytoma associated with lymphosarcoma in an aged cat. *Can Vet J* 24:20–23, 1983.
19. Padrid PA, Mitchell RW, Ndukwu IM, et al: Cyproheptadine-induced attenuation of type-I immediate-hypersensitivity reactions of airway smooth muscle from immune-sensitized cats. *Am J Vet Res* 56:109–115, 1995.
20. Winter VH, Caarund C, Göltenboth R: Mastzellenleukose und duodenumkarzinom bei einem gepard (Azinonyx jubatus schräber). *Kleinterpraxis* 25:499–504, 1980.
21. Scavelli TD, Patnaik AK, Mehlaff CJ, Hayes AA: Hemangiosarcoma in the cat: retrospective evaluation of 31 surgical cases. *JAVMA* 187:817–819, 1985.
22. Patnaik AK, Liu S-K: Angiosarcoma in cats. *J Small Anim Pract* 18:191–198, 1977.
23. Kraje AC, Mears EA, Hahn KA, et al Unusual metastatic behavior and clinicopathologic findings in 8 cats with cutaneous or visceral hemangiosarcoma (1981–1997). *JAVMA* 214:670–672, 1999.
24. Johannes CM, Henry CJ, Turnquist SE et al: Hemangiosarcoma in cats: 53 cases (1992-2002). *J Am Vet Med Assoc* 231(12):1851-1856, 2007.
25. Culp WT, Weisse C, Kellogg ME, et al: Spontaneous hemoperitoneum in cats: 65 cases (1994-2006). *J Am Vet Med Assoc* 236(9):978-982, 2010.
26. Culp WT, Drobatz KJ, Glassman MM, et al. Feline visceral hemangiosarcoma. *J Vet Intern Med* 2008 22(1):148-152, 2008.
27. Lawrence HJ, Erb HN, Harvey HJ: Nonlymphomatous hepatobiliary masses in cats: 41 cases (1972 to 1991). *Vet Surg* 23:365–368, 1994.
28. MacEwen EG, Mooney S, Brown NO, Hayes AA: Management of feline neoplasms: surgery, immunotherapy and chemotherapy. In Holzworth J (ed): *Diseases of the Cat. Medicine and Surgery.* Philadelphia, WB Saunders, 1987, pp 597–606.
29. Gores BR, Berg J, Carpenter JL, Ullman SL: Chylous ascites in cats: Nine cases (1978–1993). *JAVMA* 205:1161–1164, 1994.
30. Mulligan RM: Spontaneous cat tumors. *Cancer Res* 11:271, 1951.
31. Ervin AM, Junge RE, Miller RE, Thornburg LP: Hemangiosarcoma in a cheetah (*Acinonyx Jubatus*). *J Zoo Anim Med* 19:143–145, 1988.
32. Lawler DF, Evans RH: Multiple hepatic cavernous lymphangiomas in an aged male cat. *J Comp Pathol* 109:83–87, 1993.
33. Stobie D, Carpenter JL: Lymphangiosarcoma of the mediastinum, mesentery and omentum in a cat with chylothorax. *JAAHA* 29:78–80, 1993.
34. Hinrichs U, Puhl S, Rutteman GR, et al: Lymphangiosarcomas in cats: A retrospective study of 12 cases. *Vet Pathol* 36:164–167, 1999.
35. Swayne DE, Mahaffey EA, Haynes SG: Lymphangiosarcoma and haemangiosarcoma in a cat. *J Comp Pathol* 100:91–96, 1989.
36. Ratcliffe HL: Incidence and nature of tumors in captive wild mammals and birds. *Am J Cancer* 17:116–135, 1933.
37. Gourley IM, Popp JA, Park RD: Myelolipomas of the liver in a domestic cat. *JAVMA* 158:2053–2057, 1971.
38. Tani K, Goryo M, Okada K: Hepatic myelolipoma in a cat. *J Fac Agric Iwate Univ* 22:177–180, 1996.
39. Schuh JCL: Hepatic nodular myelolipomatosis (myelolipomas) associated with a peritoneo-pericardial diaphragmatic hernia in a cat. *J Comp Pathol* 97:231–235, 1987.
40. Ikede BO, Downey RS: Multiple hepatic myelolipomas in a cat. *Can Vet J* 13:160–163, 1972.
41. McCaw DL, da Silva Curiel JMA, Shaw DP: Hepatic myelolipomas in a cat. *JAVMA* 197:243–244, 1990.
42. Lombard LS, Fortna HM, Garner FM, Brynjolfsson G: Myelolipomas of the liver in captive wild felidae. *Pathol Vet* 5:127–134, 1968.
43. Cardy RH, Bostrom RE: Multiple splenic myelolipomas in a cheetah (*Acinonyx jubatus*). *Vet Pathol* 51:556–558, 1978.
44. Wadsworth PF, Jones DM: Myelolipoma in the liver of a cheetah (*Acinonyx jubatus*). *J Zoo Anim Med* 11:75–76, 1980.
45. Munson L, Nesbit JW, Meltzer DGA, et al: Diseases in captive cheetahs (*Acinonyx jubatus jubatus*) in South Africa: A 20-year retrospective survey. *J Zoo Wildl Med* 30:342–347, 1999.
46. Walzner C: Noduläre lipomatose—"Myelolipome"—in der Mitz des gepards (*Acinonyx jubatus*). *Wien Tierärztl Mschr* 81:24, 1994.
47. Parihar NS, Charan K, Charkravarty IB: Lipomatosis in a hunting cheetah (*Acinonyx jubatus*). *Indian J Vet Pathol* 1:4–5, 1974.
48. Schmähl D, Habs M, Ivankovic S: Carcinogenesis of N-nitrosodiethylamine (DENA) in chickens and domestic cats. *Int J Cancer* 22:552–557, 1978.
49. Post G, Patnaik AK: Nonhematopoietic hepatic neoplasms in cats: 21 cases (1983–1988). *JAVMA* 201:1080–1082, 1992.
50. Goussev SA, Center SA, Randolph JF, et al: Clinical characteristics of hepatocellular carcinoma in 19 cats from a single institution (1980-2013). *JAAHA* 52(1):36-41.2016.
51. Thompson JC, Hickson PC, Johnstone AC, Jones BR: Observations on hypoglycemia associated with a hepatoma in a cat. *N Z Vet J* 43:186–189, 1995.
52. Rees CA, Goldschmidt MH: Cutaneous horn and squamous cell carcinoma in situ (Bowen's disease) in a cat. *JAAHA* 34:485–486, 1998.
53. Adler R, Wilson DW: Biliary cystadenoma of cats. *Vet Pathol* 32:415–418, 1995.
54. Trout NJ, Berg RJ, McMillan MC, et al: Surgical treatment of hepatobiliary cystadenomas in cats: Five cases (1988–1993). *JAVMA* 206:505–507, 1995.
55. Nyland TG, Koblik PD, Tellyer SE: Ultrasonographic evaluation of biliary cystadenomas in cats. *Vet Radiol Ultrasound* 40:300–306, 1999.
56. Hou PC: Primary carcinoma of bile duct of the liver of the cat (*Felis catus*) infested with *Chonorchis sinesis. J Path Bact* 87:239–244, 1964.
57. Peterson SL: Intrahepatic biliary cystadenoma in a cat. *Feline Pract* 14:29–32, 1984.
58. Feldman BF, Strafuss AC, Gabbert N: Bile duct carcinoma in the cat: three case reports. *Feline Pract* 1:33–39, 1976.
59. Sechet B, Regnier A, Diquelou A, et al: Tumeur hépatique primaire chez un chat: discussion a propos d'un cas de cholangiocarcinome. *Revue Méd Vét* 142:877–880, 1991.
60. Pastor J, Majo N, Arbona C, et al: Sclerosing adenocarcinoma of the extrahepatic bile duct in a cat. *Vet Rec* 140:367–368, 1997.
61. Chooi KF, Little PB: Immunoblastic lymphoma and cholangiocarcinoma in a cat. *Vet Rec* 120:578–579, 1987.
62. Pascal-Tenorio A, Olivry T, Gross TL, et al: Paraneoplastic alopecia associated with internal malignancies in the cat. *Vet Dermatol* 8:47–52, 1997.
63. Newell SM, Selcer BA, Girard E, et al: Correlations between ultrasonographic findings and specific hepatic diseases in cats: 72 cases (1985–1997). *JAVMA* 213:94–98, 1998.
64. Foley P, Miller L, Graham K, Bellamy J: Cholecystadenocarcinoma in a cat. *Can Vet J* 39:373–374, 1998.
65. Rehmtulla AJ: Occurrence of carcinoma of the bile ducts: A brief review. *Can Vet J* 15:289–292, 1974.
66. Minkus G, Hillemanns M: Botryoid-type embryonal rhabdomyosarcoma of liver in a young cat. *Vet Pathol* 34:618–621, 1997.
67. Lombard LS, Witte EJ: Frequency and types of tumors in

mammals and birds of the Philadelphia Zoological Garden. *Cancer* Res 19:127–141, 1959.

68. Hubbard GB, Schmidt RE, Fletcher KC: Neoplasia in zoo animals. *J Zoo Anim Med* 14:33–40, 1983.
69. Kennedy GA, Strafuss AC: Multiple neoplasia in an aged cougar. *J Zoo Anim Med* 7:24–26, 1976.
70. McClure HM, Chang J, Golarz MN: Cholangiocarcinoma in a Margay *(Felis wiedii)*. *Vet Pathol* 14:510–512, 1977.
71. Banner BF, Alroy J, Kipnis RM: Acinar cell carcinoma of the pancreas in a cat. *Vet Pathol* 16:543–547, 1979.
72. Godfrey DR: A case of feline paraneoplastic alopecia with secondary *Malassezia*-associated dermatitis. *J Small Anim Pract* 39:394–396, 1998.
73. Brooks DG, Campbell KL, Dennis JS, Dunstan RW: Pancreatic paraneoplastic alopecia in three cats. *JAAHA* 30:557–563, 1994.
74. Kipperman BS, Nelson RW, Griffey SM, Feldman EC: Diabetes mellitus and exocrine pancreatic neoplasia in two cats with hyperadrenocorticism. *JAAHA* 28:415–418, 1992.
75. Love NE, Jones C: What is your diagnosis? *JAVMA* 195:1285–1286, 1989.
76. Ditchfield J, Archibald J: Carcinoma of the pancreas in small animals. A report of two cases. *Small Anim Clin* 1:173–176, 1961.
77. Rowlatt U: Spontaneous epithelial tumours of the pancreas of mammals. *Br J Cancer* 21:82–107, 1967.
78. Tasker S, Griffon DJ, Nuttall TJ, Hill PB: Resolution of paraneoplastic alopecia following surgical removal of a pancreatic carcinoma in a cat. *J Small Anim Pract* 40:16–19, 1999.
79. McEwan NA: Nail disease in small animals. *Vet Dermatol Newsl* 11:18–19, 1987.
80. Rothwell TLW: Retractile mesenteritis in a cat. *Vet Rec* 130:492, 1992.
81. Kircher CH, Nielsen SW: Tumours of the pancreas. *Bull WHO* x53:195–202, 1992.
82. Swann HM, Sweet DC, Michel K: Complications associated with use of jejunostomy tubes in dogs and cats: 40 cases (1989–1994). *JAVMA* 210:1764–1767, 1997.
83. Van Der Riet FdStJ, McCully RM, Keen GA, Forder AA: Lymphosarcoma in a cat. *J South Afr Vet Assoc* 57–59, 1983.
84. Effron M, Griner L, Benirschke K: Nature and rate of neoplasia found in captive wild mammals, birds and reptiles at necropsy. *J Natl Cancer Inst* 59:185–198, 1977.

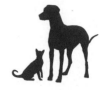

Chapter 52

Feline tumors of the urinary tract

FELINE RENAL TUMORS

Clinical presentation

- Relatively uncommon.
- Benign tumors are rare.
- Nephroblastomas are rare and typically seen in young cats.
- Renal lymphoma is relatively common. Other less common malignancies include transitional cell carcinoma (TCC) and renal cell carcinoma.
  - Azotemia may be present, particularly with bilateral tumors. Nonspecific signs of lethargy, anorexia, and weight loss are common.
- May be painful.

> **Key point**
> Cats with renal tumors often have nonspecific clinical signs often referable to renal insufficiency.

Staging and diagnosis

- Minimum data base (MDB): includes a CBC, biochemical profile, urinalysis, FIV/FeLV serology, T4 testing, biopsy or aspirate by ultrasound-guided or surgical approaches. Three-view thoracic radiographs or computerized tomography of the chest may be wise. Azotemia is common.
- Ultrasonography, computerized tomography, or magnetic resonance imaging of the abdomen may identify the local disease and assist in determining the presence of metastases.
  - Metastasis is very common for TCC, less so for renal carcinoma and nephroblastoma.
  - Lymphoma may cause dramatic lymphadenopathy that may include regional lymph nodes. An ultrasound-guided aspirate may be diagnostic.

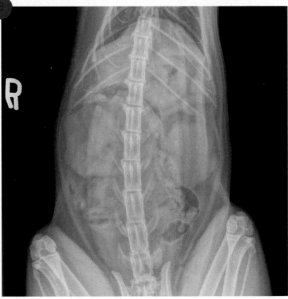

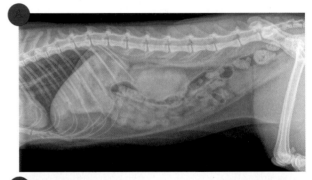

Figure 52-1: These radiographs confirm the presence of irregular kidneys. The differentials for this finding include neoplastic and nonneoplastic findings. Additional imaging, a biopsy or aspirate, blood work and a urinalysis are indicated as part of the diagnostic workup. Imaging courtesy of Lenore Anderson Mohammadian, DVM, MSpVM, Diplomate ACVR.

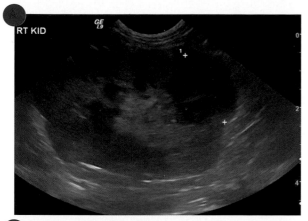

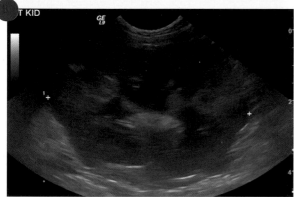

Figure 52-2: Ultrasound images of the right kidney of the same cat in figure 52-1. Note the altered echogenicity of the renal parenchyma. An ultrasound-guided aspirate was taken and blood work was secured that conformed a diagnosis of bilateral renal lymphoma and an elevated BUN and creatinine. Aggressive fluid therapy and treatment with the modified CHOP protocol resulted in complete remission and a resolution of azotemia within 3 weeks. Cats with renal lymphoma that are FeLV-negative can do well long-term with appropriate support and treatment. Imaging courtesy of Lenore Anderson Mohammadian, DVM, MSpVM, Diplomate ACVR.

Treatment

This section is divided into three options:
- Comfort for those who want to improve quality of life.
- Comfort and control for those who want to improve quality of life while trying to provide some control of the tumor.
- Comfort and longer-term control for those who want to improve quality of life while trying to maximize the chance of controlling the tumor.

Key point

Cats with renal lymphoma should be treated with combination chemotherapy, whereas those cats with renal carcinoma should be treated with surgery if renal function of the contralateral kidney is projected to be adequate.

Comfort

- Adequate hydration and supportive care is important to prevent or to treat azotemia. Therapy to enhance comfort (e.g.: prednisolone if the cat has renal lymphoma, tramadol, buprenorphine) and freedom from nausea, vomiting (e.g.: maropitant and/or metoclopramide), diarrhea (e.g.: metronidazole) and lack of appetite (e.g.: mirtazapine or cyproheptadine). Prednisolone can be quite helpful if renal lymphoma is the underlying cause.

Comfort and control

Above mentioned therapy for comfort plus:
- Palliative radiation is being explored, especially for those with extension into surrounding structures or regional metastases (e.g.: 2-5 dosages of radiation), to first enhance comfort, second, to reduce the rate of growth and third, occasionally to reduce the size of the tumor.
- If lymphoma is diagnosed, prednisolone with or without COP chemotherapy may be important.

Comfort and longer-term control

Above mentioned therapy for comfort plus:
- Renal lymphoma: CHOP chemotherapy with renal care if needed is indicated. Mitoxantrone should be substituted for doxorubicin if the patient is azotemic.
  - The overall estimated 1-year survival rate in all cats was 48.7%, and the 2-year survival rate was 39.9%.
- Nephrectomy may be helpful for carcinomas that involved one kidney and if the contralateral kidney has enough function to support the patient.
- Investigational: mitoxantrone or carboplatin for transitional cell carcinoma; doxorubicin or carboplatin for renal cell carcinoma; and vincristine, doxorubicin, and actinomycin D for nephroblastoma.

FELINE URINARY BLADDER TUMORS

Clinical presentation

- Increasing in prevalence, likely due to the common use of abdominal ultrasonography.
- Hematuria, pollakiuria, and stranguria are common clinical signs.
- Transitional cell carcinoma is the most common tumor type followed by leiomyoma and less commonly, leiomyosarcoma or squamous cell carcinoma.
- May be painful.
- Clinical signs similar to cystitis such as hematuria, pollakiuria and stranguria.[2,15,16,18–22]

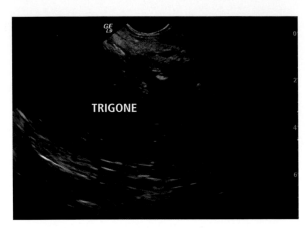

Figure 52-3: The more frequent use of diagnostic ultrasound in practice has dramatically increased the number and frequency of diagnoses of bladder tumors, specifically transitional cell carcinomas. These tumors should be biopsied to secure a specific diagnosis. Care should be taken not to "seed" the tumor along the biopsy tract. Imaging courtesy of Lenore Anderson Mohammadian, DVM, MSpVM, Diplomate ACVR.

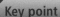

Key point

Many cats with transitional cell carcinoma of the bladder have clinical signs that are indistinguishable from those with lower urinary tract infections.

Staging and diagnosis

- Minimum data base (MDB): includes a CBC, biochemical profile, urinalysis, urine culture and sensitivity if indicated, FIV/FeLV serology, T4 testing, biopsy, three-view thoracic radiographs or computerized tomography of the chest.
- Ultrasonography and/or radiographs are practical and cost effective, however computerized tomography or magnetic resonance imaging of the tumor may be preferable in some cases.
- Tumors may appear to be apical rather than trigonal.
- Iliac lymph nodes and regional extension (and rarely lungs) are sites of metastasis for carcinomas.
- Metastasis appears to be rare for leiomyosarcomas.

Key point

A biopsy is necessary to definitively diagnose transitional cell carcinoma of the bladder. Every attempt should be made to prevent seeding tumor cells from a bladder tumor into the surrounding tissue via cystocentesis or surgery.

Treatment

This section is divided into three options:

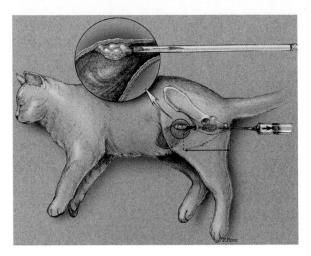

Figure 52-4: One minimally invasive way of obtaining a biopsy of a bladder mass is to insert an open ended urinary catheter up the urethra to the mass. Suction is applied with a syringe attached to the catheter while pulling the biopsy apparatus in and out to tear away pieces of the growth for submission for histopathology. Reprinted with permission from: Ogilvie GK, Moore AS. *Feline Oncology: A Comprehensive Guide for Compassionate Care*. Trenton NJ, Veterinary Learning Systems. 2002.

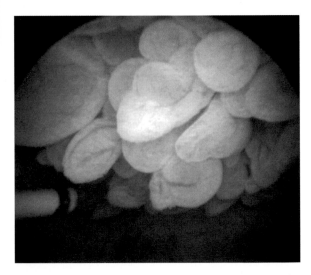

Figure 52-5: Cystoscopy can also be used to visualize the bladder for biopsy. This can be done in large cats through the urethra, or via a tiny stab incision through the bladder wall made during surgery. This cat had a benign polypoid condition of the bladder. Reprinted with permission from: Ogilvie GK, Moore AS. *Feline Oncology: A Comprehensive Guide for Compassionate Care*. Trenton NJ, Veterinary Learning Systems. 2002.

- Comfort for those who want to improve quality of life.
- Comfort and control for those who want to improve quality of life while trying to provide some control of the tumor.

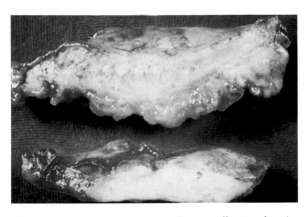

Figure 52-6: Surgery is generally not effective for the treatment of transitional cell carcinoma of the bladder, as the disease is often multifocal. Benign masses are more often localized and more successfully treated with resection.

- Comfort and longer-term control for those who want to improve quality of life while trying to maximize the chance of controlling the tumor.

Comfort

- Therapy to enhance comfort (e.g.: NSAID, tramadol, buprenorphine) and freedom from nausea, vomiting (e.g.: maropitant and/or metoclopramide), diarrhea (e.g.: metronidazole) and lack of appetite (e.g.: mirtazapine or cyproheptadine).
  - In one study involving cats with transitional cell carcinoma of the bladder, reduction of hematuria and/or dysuria was noted in 80% of cats treated with meloxicam, with a mean survival time of 311 days (range 10-1064); 1-year survival of 50%.[28]

Comfort and control

Above mentioned therapy for comfort plus:
- Palliative radiation, especially for those with extension into surrounding structures or regional metastases (e.g.: 2-5 dosages of radiation), to first enhance comfort, second, to reduce the rate of growth and third, occasionally to reduce the size of the tumor.
  - Carboplatin or mitoxantrone may be helpful as an adjuvant treatment.

Comfort and longer-term control

Above mentioned therapy for comfort plus:
- Surgery is the prime therapeutic modality, although tumors may recur even with a partial cystectomy.
- Radiation and/or mitoxantrone or carboplatin may be helpful in some cases.

References

1. Wimberly HC, Lewis RM: Transitional cell carcinoma in the domestic cat. *Vet Pathol* 16:223–228, 1979.
2. Carpenter JL, Andrews LK, Holzworth J: Tumors and tumor-like lesions. In Holzworth J (ed): *Diseases of the Cat. Medicine and Surgery.* Philadelphia, WB Saunders, 1987, pp 407–596.
3. Henry CJ, Turnquist SE, Smith A, et al: Primary renal tumors in cats: 19 cases (1992–1998). *J Feline Med Surg* 1:165–170, 1999.
4. Carlson RA, Badertscher RR: Feline renal pseudocyst with metastatic carcinoma of the contralateral kidney. *Feline Pract* 21:23–27, 1993.
5. Britt JO, Ryan CP, Howard EB: Sarcomatoid renal adenosarcoma in a cat. *Vet Pathol* 22:514–515, 1985.
6. Steinberg H, Thomson J: Bilateral renal carcinoma in a cat. *Vet Pathol* 31:704–705, 1994.
7. Biller DS, Bradley GA, Partington BP: Renal medullary rim sign: Ultrasonographic evidence of renal disease. *Vet Radiol Ultrasound* 33:286–290, 1992.
8. Yamazoe K, Ohashi F, Kadosawa T, et al: Computed tomography on renal masses in dogs and cats. *J Vet Med Sci* 56:813–816, 1994.
9. Walter PA, Johnston GR, Feeney DA, O'Brien TD: Applications of ultrasonography in the diagnosis of parenchymal kidney disease in cats: 24 cases (1981–1986). *JAVMA* 192:92–98, 1988.
10. Moon ML, Davenport DJ: What is your diagnosis? *JAVMA* 191:1491–1492, 1987.
11. Potkay S, Garman R: Nephroblastoma in a cat: The effects of nephrectomy and occlusion of the caudal vena cava. *J Small Anim Pract* 10:345–369, 1969.
12. Fitts RH: Bilateral feline embryonal sarcoma. *JAVMA* 136:616, 1960.
13. Nafe LA, Herron AJ, Burk RL: Hypertrophic osteopathy in a cat associated with renal papillary adenoma. *JAAHA* 17:659–662, 1981.
14. Clark WR, Wilson RB: Renal adenoma in a cat. *JAVMA* 193:1557–1559, 1988.
15. Kohno T, Matsuda H: Transitional-cell carcinoma of the urinary bladder in a cat. *Mod Vet Pract* 68:286–287, 1987.
16. Anderson WI: Transitional cell carcinoma encasing the distal ureter in a cat. *Mod Vet Pract* 67:824, 1986.
17. Buffington CAT, Chew DJ, Kendall MS, et al: Clinical evaluation of cats with nonobstructive urinary tract diseases. *JAVMA* 210:46–50, 1997.
18. Barrett RE, Nobel TA: Transitional cell carcinoma of the urethra in a cat. *Cornell Vet* 66:14–26, 1976.
19. Brearley MJ, Thatcher C, Cooper JE: Three cases of transitional cell carcinoma in the cat and a review of the literature. *Vet Rec* 118:91–94, 1986.
20. Dill Jr GS, McElyea Jr U, Stookey JL: Transitional cell carcinoma of the urinary bladder in a cat. *JAVMA* 160:743–745, 1972.
21. Schwarz PD, Greene RW, Patnaik AK: Urinary bladder tumors in the cat: A review of 27 cases. *JAAHA* 21:237–245, 1985.
22. Walker DB, Cowell RL, Clinkenbeard KD, Turgai J: Carcinoma in the urinary bladder of a cat: Cytologic findings and a review of the literature. *Vet Clin Pathol* 22:103–108, 1993.
23. Arnal C, Badiola JJ, García de Jalón JA, Juste R: Carcinoma de células de transición de la uretra en un gato. *Med Vet* 2:239–243, 1985.
24. Aumann M, Worth LT, Drobatz KJ: Uroperitoneum in cats: 26 cases (1986–1995). *JAAHA* 34:315–324, 1998.
25. Barrand KR: Rectal prolapse associated with urinary bladder neoplasia in a cat. *J Small Anim Pract* 40:222–223, 1999.
26. Sellon RK, Rottman JB, Jordan HL: Hypereosinophilia associated with transitional cell carcinoma in a cat. *JAVMA* 201:591–593, 1992.
27. Guptill L, Scott-Moncrieff CR, Janovitz EB: Response to high-dose radioactive iodine administration in cats with thyroid carcinoma that had previously undergone surgery. *JAVMA* 8:1055–1058, 1995.
28. Bommer NX, Hayes AM, Scase TJ, Gunn-Moore DA. Clinical features, survival times and COX-1 and COX-2 expression in cats with transitional cell carcinoma of the urinary bladder treated with meloxicam. *J Feline Med Surg.* 14(8):527-533, 2012.
29. Ogilvie GK, Moore AS, Obradovich JE, et al: Toxicoses and efficacy associated with the administration of mitoxantrone to cats with malignant tumors. *JAVMA* 202:1839–1844, 1993.
30. Dorn AS, Harris SG, Olmstead ML: Squamous cell carcinoma of the urinary bladder in a cat. *Feline Pract* 8:14–17, 1978.
31. Burk RL, Meierhenry EF, Schaubhut Jr CW: Leiomyosarcoma of the urinary bladder in a cat. *JAVMA* 167:749–751, 1975.
32. Sent U, Pothmann M, von Bomhard D: Felines urologisches Syndrom: Hervorgerufen durch ein leiomyosarkom der harnblase. *Kleintierpraxis* 42:663–668, 1997.
33. Speakman CF, Pechman RD, D'Andrea GH: Aortic thrombosis and unilateral hydronephrosis associated with leiomyosarcoma in a cat. *JAVMA* 182:62–63, 1983.
34. Swalec KM, Smeak DD, Baker AL: Urethral leiomyoma in a cat. *JAVMA* 195:961–1119, 1989.
35. Patnaik AK, Greene RW: Intravenous leiomyoma of the bladder in a cat. *JAVMA* 175:381–383, 1979.
36. Patnaik AK, Schwarz PD, Greene RW: A histopathologic study of twenty urinary bladder neoplasms in the cat. *J Small Anim Pract* 27:433–435, 1986.

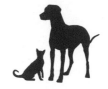

Chapter 53

Feline tumors of the endocrine system

FELINE THYROID ADENOMAS

Clinical presentation

- Moderately common, especially in older cats.
- Thyroid adenomas are quite common and often hyperfunctional, resulting in clinical signs of thyrotoxicosis. In contrast, adenocarcinomas are comparatively rare and often nonfunctional.
- A diet of canned food and an indoor lifestyle may increase the risk of developing hyperthyroidism due to a parathyroid adenoma.
- Thyrotoxic cats often steadily lose weight despite being polyphagic, can be either hyperactive or lethargic, and may develop clinical signs due to hypertrophic cardiomyopathy.
- Almost never painful.

> **Key point**
> This very common non-malignant condition is almost always associated with elevated thyroid hormone levels and clinical signs associated with thyrotoxicosis.

Staging and diagnosis

- Minimum data base (MDB): includes a CBC, biochemical profile, urinalysis, FIV/FeLV serology, T4 testing (T4 and T4 done by equilibrium dialysis, thyroid scintigraphy will help rule out a functional carcinoma., excisional biopsy and three-view thoracic radiographs or computerized tomography of the chest if an adenocarcinoma is suspected.
- Cardiac echocardiography, radiographs, computerized tomography, or magnetic resonance imaging of the chest, especially if a thyroid carcinoma is suspected.
- Advanced renal disease may be a confounding factor because when thyrotoxicosis is resolved, renal blood flow declines and renal values can worsen.
- Cardiomyopathy can complicate survival.

> **Key point**
> Thyroid scintigraphy and blood work is considered essential to stage cats with thyrotoxicosis.

Treatment

This section is divided into three options:
- Comfort for those who want to improve quality of life.
- Comfort and control for those who want to improve quality of life while trying to provide some control of the tumor.
- Comfort and longer-term control for those who want to improve quality of life while trying to maximize the chance of controlling the tumor.

> **Key point**
> Surgery, medical management and radioactive iodine-131 are all very effective treatments for cats with thyrotoxicosis.

Comfort

- Therapy to enhance comfort (e.g.: NSAID, tramadol, buprenorphine) and freedom from nausea, vomiting (e.g.: maropitant and/or metoclopramide), diarrhea (e.g.: metronidazole) and lack of appetite (e.g.: mirtazapine or cyproheptadine).
- Stabilize cardiac disease medically (could include short-term medical management of hyperthyroidism) prior to definitive treatment. Treatment of hyperthyroidism will worsen concurrent renal disease; consider methimazole, carbimazole or ipodate, as they are associated with high rate of control. Provide adequate nutrition to increase weight.

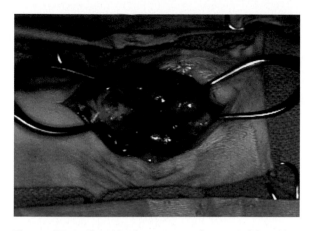

Figure 53-1: Thyroid adenomas can be treated by either medical management, radioactive iodine-131 or surgery. Surgery is generally quite effective, although hypocalcemia can delay or complicate recovery. Every attempt should be made to identify and re-implant the external parathyroid glands to prevent prolonged hypocalcemia.

Comfort and control

Above mentioned therapy for comfort plus:
- Intrathyroid injection of 95% ethanol may be effective for thyroid adenomas.
- Palliative radiation for thyroid carcinomas, especially for those with extension into surrounding structures or regional metastases (e.g.: 2-5 dosages of radiation), to first enhance comfort, second, to reduce the rate of growth and third, occasionally to reduce the size of the tumor.

Comfort and longer-term control

Above mentioned therapy for comfort plus:
- Extracapsular thyroidectomy. Bilateral disease is common; postoperative hypocalcemia due to removal of parathyroid tissue is usually transient but mandates monitoring and treating serum calcium.
- IV, SC or PO administration of ^{131}I is generally a very effective treatment and the treatment of choice if available.

FELINE THYROID ADENOCARCINOMA

Clinical presentation

- Moderately common.
- May be painful.

Staging and diagnosis

- Minimum data base (MDB): includes a CBC, biochemical profile, urinalysis, FIV/FeLV serology, T4 testing, biopsy, three-view thoracic radiographs or computerized tomography of the chest.

- Ultrasonography and/or radiographs are practical and cost effective, however computerized tomography or magnetic resonance imaging of the tumor may be preferable in some cases.

Treatment

This section is divided into three options:
- Comfort for those who want to improve quality of life.
- Comfort and control for those who want to improve quality of life while trying to provide some control of the tumor.
- Comfort and longer-term control for those who want to improve quality of life while trying to maximize the chance of controlling the tumor.

Comfort

- Therapy to enhance comfort (e.g.: NSAID, tramadol, buprenorphine) and freedom from nausea, vomiting (e.g.: maropitant and/or metoclopramide), diarrhea (e.g.: metronidazole) and lack of appetite (e.g.: mirtazapine or cyproheptadine).

Comfort and control

Above mentioned therapy for comfort plus:
- Palliative radiation, especially for those with extension into surrounding structures or regional metastases (e.g.: 2-5 dosages of radiation), to first enhance comfort, second, to reduce the rate of growth and third, occasionally to reduce the size of the tumor.

Comfort and longer-term control

Above mentioned therapy for comfort plus:
- Surgery.
- Definitive radiation if there is evidence of tumor extending beyond the surgical margins (e.g.: 16-19 dosages of radiation).
- IV, SC or PO administration of ^{131}I is generally a very effective treatment and the treatment of choice if available.
  - Some carcinomas will not uptake the ^{131}I, therefore surgery with or without definitive radiation may be indicated if there is evidence of tumor extending beyond the surgical margins (e.g.: 16-19 dosages of radiation).

FELINE THYROID CARCINOMA

Clinical presentation

- Relatively uncommon compared to thyroid adenomas.
- Almost always hyperfunctional and cause hyperthyroidism.
- Some are irregular in shape, multiple and

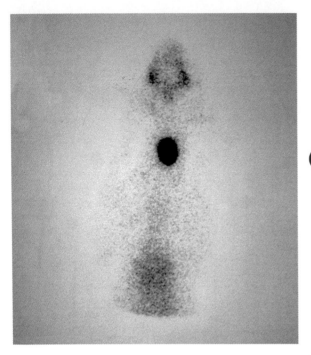

Figure 53-2: A nuclear ⁹⁹ᵐTcO₄– scan was done on this cat with a large peritracheal mass that was thought to be a thyroid malignancy and was adherent to surrounding tissues. The image shows intense uptake of the radiopharmaceutical without any evidence of metastases to surrounding tissues. The thyroid adenocarcinoma did uptake radioactive iodine 131, however this is not always true. The tumor resolved and the cat remained in remission for years. Reprinted with permission from: Ogilvie GK, Moore AS. *Feline Oncology: A Comprehensive Guide for Compassionate Care*. Trenton NJ, Veterinary Learning Systems. 2002.

encapsulated,[76] whereas others are large and may surround the trachea and esophagus and may cause dyspnea or dysphagia.[75]
- Functional papillary carcinoma predominate.[83]
- Rarely bilateral but often highly metastatic.[4,84]
- Usually not painful.
- The prevalence of severe hyperthyroidism, large thyroid tumors, multifocal disease, intrathoracic thyroid masses and suspected malignant disease all increase with disease duration in cats referred for radioiodine therapy.[85]

> **Key point**
> Thyroid carcinoma in the cat often presents as a large, irregular, lobulated mass in the peritracheal region.

Staging and diagnosis

- Minimum data base (MDB): includes a CBC, biochemical profile, urinalysis, FIV/FeLV serology, T4 testing, biopsy, three-view thoracic radiographs or computerized tomography of the chest. Since cardiomyopathy may be seen in thyrotoxic cats, an echocardiogram and ECG may be helpful.
- Ultrasonography, radiographs, computerized tomography, magnetic resonance imaging of the tumor.
- A nuclear ⁹⁹ᵐTcO₄– scan may show multiple cervical masses, extension of tumor into the thoracic inlet, mediastinal masses, or lung metastases.

> **Key point**
> Thoracic and regional lymph node metastases can occur in cats with thyroid carcinomas.

Treatment

This section is divided into two options:
- Comfort for those who want to improve quality of life.
- Comfort and control for those who want to improve quality of life while trying to provide some control of the tumor.

> **Key point**
> Surgery, external beam radiation or radioactive iodine-131 can be used to treat cats with thyroid carcinomas.

Comfort

- Therapy to enhance comfort (e.g.: NSAID, tramadol, buprenorphine) and freedom from nausea, vomiting (e.g.: maropitant and/or metoclopramide), diarrhea (e.g.: metronidazole), lack of appetite (e.g.: mirtazapine or cyproheptadine), clinical signs of thyrotoxicosis (e.g.: methimazole) and, if indicated, congestive heart failure (e.g.: atenolol, furosemide, enalapril).

Comfort and control

Above mentioned therapy for comfort plus:
- ¹³¹I therapy or palliative radiation, especially for those with extension into surrounding structures or regional metastases (e.g.: 2-5 dosages of radiation), to first enhance comfort, second, to reduce the rate of growth and third, occasionally to reduce the size of the tumor.
  - Survival generally ranges from 8 to 39 months (average, 19 months).[78,79]
  - Another group of investigators reported that single high-dose radioiodine therapy was successful in 6/8 cases of thyroid carcinoma, with complete resolution of hyperthyroidism, and was associated with prolonged survival times (181-2381 days).[76] They confirmed that the prognosis for feline thyroid carcinoma successfully treated with radioiodine is good, with extended survival times commonly achieved.

- Surgical excision, even if incomplete, may result in euthyroidism and clinical improvement.
  - Definitive radiation or ^{131}I may then be indicated if there is evidence of tumor extending beyond the surgical margins.

FELINE PANCREATIC ISLET CELL TUMORS

Clinical presentation

- Insulinomas are uncommon and are often known to cause hypoglycemia and subsequent neurologic signs such as nervousness,[94] inappetence,[95] episodic staggering, twitching of the leg, skin, and facial muscles[90, 91] and seizures.[90, 94]
- Gastrinomas are very rare and are associated with chronic vomiting due to the production of gastrin.

Staging and diagnosis

- Minimum data base (MDB): includes a CBC, biochemical profile, urinalysis, FIV/FeLV serology, T4 testing, biopsy, three-view thoracic radiographs or computerized tomography of the chest.
- Insulinomas.
  - Insulin: glucose ratio to rule in or out insulinomas.
  - Confirming presence Whipple's triad (i.e., hypoglycemia with neurologic signs that respond to glucose administration).
  - Glucagon tolerance test has been used to diagnose insulinoma,[90] but it is not recommended due to the risk of developing life-threatening clinical signs.
- Gastrinoma.
  - Gastrin levels to rule in or out a gastrinoma.
- Ultrasonography and/or radiographs are practical and cost effective, however computerized tomography or magnetic resonance imaging of the abdomen tumor that may be multiple.

Treatment

This section is divided into three options:
- Comfort for those who want to improve quality of life.
- Comfort and control for those who want to improve quality of life while trying to provide some control of the tumor.
- Comfort and longer-term control for those who want to improve quality of life while trying to maximize the chance of controlling the tumor.

Comfort

- Therapy to enhance comfort (e.g.: NSAID, tramadol, buprenorphine) and freedom from nausea, vomiting (e.g.: maropitant and/or metoclopramide), diarrhea (e.g.: metronidazole) and lack of appetite (e.g.: mirtazapine or cyproheptadine). Prednisolone may be helpful to raise glucose levels in those cats with

insulinomas. Many cats with insulinomas require the administration of glucose intravenously to maintain glucose homeostasis until more definitive therapy is employed. Gastrinomas may cause vomiting, which can be treated with maropitant citrate and/or metoclopramide.

Comfort and control

Above mentioned therapy for comfort plus:
- Medical palliation of signs of hypoglycemia using prednisolone may be successful. Diazoxide use not reported. H2 antihistamines may be effective to reduce gastric acid secretion associated with gastrinoma.

Comfort and longer-term control

Above mentioned therapy for comfort plus:
- Surgery to remove pancreatic mass or masses if localized.
- Tyrosine kinase inhibitors and/or gemcitabine are investigational but promising.

FELINE PARATHYROID TUMORS

Clinical presentation

- Uncommon.
- May be associated with a palpable parathyroid mass 2 to 6 cm in diameter.[101]
- May range histologically from hyperplasia to adenoma to parathyroid carcinoma.
- The tumors may be nonfunctional or may be functional and cause hypercalcemia.
- Clinical signs often non-specific, such as polyuria/polydipsia, lethargy, weight loss and anorexia.
- Not usually painful.

Staging and diagnosis

- Minimum data base (MDB): includes a CBC, biochemical profile including an ionized calcium, urinalysis, FIV/FeLV serology, T4 testing, biopsy, three-view thoracic radiographs or computerized tomography of the chest.
  - Productive parathyroid tumors may cause an elevated serum ionized calcium, low phosphorus and an elevated parathormone level.[99]
- Ultrasonography of the cervical region is practical, however computerized tomography or magnetic resonance imaging is a higher resolution diagnostic tool.

Key point

An elevated ionized calcium is often the first indication of a parathyroid tumor.

Treatment

This section is divided into two options:

- Comfort for those who want to improve quality of life.
- Comfort and control for those who want to improve quality of life while trying to provide some control of the tumor.

Comfort

- Therapy to enhance comfort (e.g.: NSAID, tramadol, buprenorphine) and freedom from nausea, vomiting (e.g.: maropitant and/or metoclopramide), diarrhea (e.g.: metronidazole) and lack of appetite (e.g.: mirtazapine or cyproheptadine). Fluid therapy (e.g.: 0.9% NaCl) may help induce calciuresis and reduce a hypercalcemic-induced nephropathy.

Comfort and control

Above mentioned therapy for comfort plus:

- Surgical excision of adenoma may be curative. Check other parathyroid glands, as multiple adenomas and concurrent adenocarcinomas are reported. Monitor serum calcium for hypocalcemia or return of hypercalcemia after surgery.
- Definitive radiation may be helpful at reducing regrowth of any residual disease.

FELINE PITUITARY TUMORS

Clinical presentation

- Relatively uncommon.
- Adenomas predominate that more arise from the anterior lobe of the pituitary that secrete growth hormone (GH) or thyroid stimulating hormone (TSH).
  - Most cats are presented due to insulin-resistant diabetes.
  - Some present with increased body mass with organomegaly causing an enlarging abdomen.[107,109,115]
  - Some cats are arthritic and have a large head and tongue, organomegaly, and a protruding lower jaw (prognathia inferior).
- Clinical signs associated with a space-occupying mass in the region of the pituitary gland (vision problems, anisocoria, pacing, aimless wandering, etc.) are uncommon as tumors are most often small.
- Other endocrine tumors may be present, fulfilling the criteria of multiple endocrine neoplasia (MEN).
  - In a series of 18 cats diagnosed at necropsy with pituitary tumors, 13 had thyroid adenomas and 13 had hyperplasia of the adrenal gland; 5 cats were diabetic and 5 had congestive heart failure thought to be due to excess growth hormone. One cat had a microscopic pheochromocytoma.

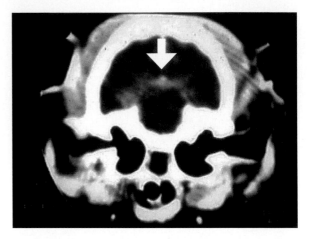

Figure 53-3: This cat with acromegaly, diabetes mellitus that is difficult to control, and mental dullness was imaged with a computerized tomography scan, which confirmed the presence of a pituitary macroadenoma. The cat was successfully treated with definitive radiation therapy and made a full recovery.

In another study of 14 cats, 6 had parathyroid hyperplasia.[107]
- Not usually painful.

> **Key point**
>
> While relatively uncommon, some cats with pituitary adenomas also have acromegaly that results in coarse, thickened facial features and diabetes mellitus that is difficult to regulate.

Staging and diagnosis

- Minimum data base (MDB): includes a CBC, biochemical profile, urinalysis, FIV/FeLV serology, T4 testing, biopsy, three-view thoracic radiographs or computerized tomography of the chest. An echocardiogram and ECG should be performed if cardiac disease is suspected.
- Computerized tomography or magnetic resonance imaging of the head and thus the tumor, the latter of which is usually quite small.
  - Acromegalic cats with CT or MRI evidence of a pituitary tumor often have frontal bone thickness greater than age-matched controls with and without a history of upper airway disease.[109] Evidence of soft tissue accumulation in the nasal cavity, sinuses, and pharynx may also be noted.
  - In one study, the CT findings of 16 cats with insulin-resistant diabetes were compared with findings in cats that had controlled diabetes; all resistant cats had a pituitary mass.[117]
- If acromegaly and arthritis is suspected, radiographs of the affected region may be helpful.[107,114]

Treatment

This section is divided into three options:

- Comfort for those who want to improve quality of life.
- Comfort and control for those who want to improve quality of life while trying to provide some control of the tumor.
- Comfort and longer-term control for those who want to improve quality of life while trying to maximize the chance of controlling the tumor.

Comfort

- Therapy to enhance comfort (e.g.: NSAID, tramadol, buprenorphine) and freedom from nausea, vomiting (e.g.: maropitant and/or metoclopramide), diarrhea (e.g.: metronidazole) and lack of appetite (e.g.: mirtazapine or cyproheptadine). All concurrent endocrine, neurologic and metabolic disease should be identified and treated. Steroids and/or mannitol may be helpful if the patient has increased intracranial pressure. Diabetes and cardiac disease, if present, must be treated.

Comfort and control

Above mentioned therapy for comfort plus:

- Palliative megavoltage radiation done after computerized tomography is used with radiation treatment planning (e.g.: 2-5 dosages of radiation) and can be helpful at limiting clinical signs by first enhancing comfort, second, reducing the rate of growth and third, occasionally reducing the size of the tumor.

Comfort and longer-term control

Above mentioned therapy for comfort plus:

- Surgery via transphenoidal hypophisectomy.[125] This surgical procedure requires unique training and expertise.
- Radiation therapy should be definitive and can be delivered by a standard linear accelerator or via highly precise, targeted stereotactic radiosurgery (e.g.: CyberKnife). Monitor serum profile and GH levels or perform a CT scan for macroadenomas.
- Somatostatin analogues may have effects that can reduce pituitary GH production, however the efficacy is unknown.
- Cryoablation of the tumor via transphenoidal approach has been done but is considered experimental.

FELINE HYPERADRENOCORTICISM

Clinical presentation

- Moderately common.
- Hyperadrenocorticism due to a pituitary adenoma that secretes ACTH is more common than hyperadrenocorticism due to an adrenal tumor.
- Most adrenal tumors are adenomas. Adrenal carcinomas have the potential to metastasize.
- Common signs are PU/PD due to insulin resistant diabetes mellitus, thin skin that tears easily, poor healing and, less commonly, CNS signs due to large pituitary tumors.
- Not usually painful.

> **Key point**
> Feline hyperadrenocorticism is often associated with PU/PD and unregulated diabetes mellitus.

Staging and diagnosis

- Minimum data base (MDB): includes a CBC, biochemical profile, urinalysis, FIV/FeLV serology, T4 testing, biopsy, three-view thoracic radiographs or computerized tomography of the chest.
- The diagnostic plan should include an ACTH response test, low and high dose dexamethasone suppression tests (0.015 and 1.0 mg/kg IV, respectively), and a determination of ACTH levels, if available, to help determine if there is a pituitary or adrenal-dependent hyperadrenocorticism.[108,118–123,126–131,134–145]
  - Low-dose dexamethasone suppression test results were shown in one study to be consistent with hyperadrenocorticism in 96% of cats, whereas ACTH stimulation testing was suggestive of hyperadrenocorticism in 56% of cats.[114]
- Ultrasonography and/or radiographs are practical and cost effective, however computerized tomography or magnetic resonance imaging of the brain or abdomen, or both to assess the tumor.
  - Investigators showed that the ultrasonographic appearance of the adrenal glands was consistent with the final clinical diagnosis 93% of cats with hyperadrenalcorticsm.[114]

> **Key point**
> Abdominal ultrasound is critical to identify abnormal adrenal gland size and shape, which is often associated with adrenal or pituitary-dependent hyperadrenocorticism.

Treatment

This section is divided into three options:

- Comfort for those who want to improve quality of life.
- Comfort and control for those who want to improve quality of life while trying to provide some control of the tumor.
- Comfort and longer-term control for those who want to improve quality of life while trying to maximize the chance of controlling the tumor.

Box 53-1. Testing for hyperadrenocorticism in cats* [108,118-123,126-131,134-145]

ACTH Response Test

The ACTH response test is a good screening test; results supported a diagnosis of hyperadrenocorticism in 14 of 18 cats.[126-128] The use of synthetic ACTH (cosyntropin or tetracosactrin) is preferred for this test. In normal cats, IV administration of 0.125 mg (125 µg) per cat should result in a 200% to 1400% increase in cortisol over baseline.[121,135-138]

IV administration gives greater stimulation and a longer duration of response (6 hours) than IM injection (2 hours), and IM injection of synthetic ACTH is painful.[139] A basal serum cortisol level should be obtained, and a second sample is collected 2 to 3 hours after IV administration of synthetic ACTH.[139] Lower doses of cosyntropin (1.25 or 12.5 µg/cat) will also cause a response, but the peak is earlier and short lived.[140] Likewise, dosages higher than 125 µg have no real advantage.[141] Cosyntropin can be diluted to a concentration of 5 µg/ml of saline and stored refrigerated for more than 4 months.[140]

ACTH gel (2.2 U/kg IM) has a similar effect.[142] ACTH gel induces an earlier peak that may return to baseline quickly.[136,142]

Dexamethasone suppression tests

Dexamethasone administered as an IV bolus should cause "negative feedback" suppression of ACTH secretion by the pituitary and a reduction in serum cortisol. Dexamethasone is chosen because it will not cross-react with cortisol measurements.

In dogs, the low dose dexamethasone suppression test (LDDST) is a good method of screening for hyperadrenocorticism. In cats, a dose of 0.01 mg/kg suppresses serum cortisol for 1 to 12 hours after administration, but levels return to baseline by 24 hours.[141,143,144] Samples are collected prior to dexamethasone administration and 6 to 10 hours afterward.[141] Lack of suppression does not confirm hyperadrenocorticism, as some normal cats will not experience a reduction in serum cortisol, possibly due to stress associated with concurrent diseases.[141,144] Despite limitations, this is still a preferred screening method.[108,119-121,123,126,127]

Some authors suggest that a dose of 0.015 mg/kg is more useful.[144] An even higher dose of dexamethasone (0.1 mg/kg), with samples collected on the same schedule, was not completely consistent in suppressing cortisol secretion in all normal cats.[141] This test, however, has been widely used to distinguish ATs from pituitary tumors. While suppression of cortisol secretion should occur with pituitary tumors, the autonomous secretion of cortisol by ATs should allow the cortisol to rise again after initial suppression ("escape").[118,126,127] This test is not always diagnostic in cats,[120,121] leading some authors to recommend a dexamethasone dose of 1.0 mg/kg (i.e., the high-dose dexamethasone suppression test [HDDST]) in cats.[131,134,142,145] This dose consistently causes cortisol suppression in all normal cats.[141,145]

Determination of ACTH and hormonal levels

ACTH levels can be measured, although samples need to be chilled immediately and handled carefully, and thus reducing the practicality of this test in many private practices. In normal cats, endogenous ACTH levels range from 10 to 60 pg/ml.[121,141] In cats with pituitary-dependent hyperadrenocorticism, ACTH levels have ranged from 90 to over 1000 pg/ml.[108,118,119,121,122,126,127] Cats with ATs should have low or normal serum ACTH levels.[130] Since pre- and postoperative hypocortisolemia and since hypersecretion of more than one adrenal hormone has occurred in cats with adrenal tumors, adrenal panels prior to surgery may be beneficial as part of the preoperative work-up.

Urinary cortisol

In cats, most cortisol is excreted in the bile. Therefore the ratio of urinary cortisol to urinary creatinine is quite low (13 x 10^{-6}),[129] making it a potentially useful screening test. In one study, all six cats with hyperadrenocorticism had a urinary cortisol: creatinine ratio above the reference range (median, 122 x 10^{-6}).[129]

---

* Adapted from and reprinted with permission from: Ogilvie GK, Moore AS. *Feline Oncology: A Comprehensive Guide for Compassionate Care*. Trenton NJ, Veterinary Learning Systems, 2001.

Comfort

- Therapy to enhance comfort (e.g.: NSAID, tramadol, buprenorphine) and freedom from nausea, vomiting (e.g.: maropitant and/or metoclopramide), diarrhea (e.g.: metronidazole) and lack of appetite (e.g.: mirtazapine or cyproheptadine). Management of diabetes and secondary infections is essential.

Comfort and control

Above mentioned therapy for comfort plus:

- Mitotane has been used in the past and is specifically toxic to the adrenal cortex and may improve symptoms and wound healing at doses ranging from 25 to 50 mg/kg/day in two divided doses. Some recommend starting at the lower dosage and still others suggest the concurrent administration of the mineralocorticoid fludrocortisone (0.01 mg/kg daily) and the glucocorticoid prednisolone (0.3 mg/kg daily).[19]
- Trilostane[152] (30 mg PO q24h) is generally considered the drug of choice and has been associated with a good response to therapy. ACTH stimulation testing recommended 3-4 hours post-administration at 1, 3, 6, 12 weeks and then every 6 months. Target cortisol concentration 1-2 mcg/dl.
- Palliative radiation for either adrenal or pituitary-induced hyperadrenocorticism has not been commonly used but has been suggested by some to first enhance comfort, second, to reduce the rate of growth and third, occasionally to reduce the size of the adrenal or pituitary tumor.

Comfort and longer-term control

Above mentioned therapy for comfort plus:

- Adrenalectomy is treatment of choice for both AT and PDH. Radiation is treatment for PDH with large tumor. Monitor adrenal function to avoid hypoadrenal crisis.

FELINE NON-CORTISOL SECRETING TUMORS

Clinical presentation

- Uncommon.
- Adrenal tumors may produce a number of hormones that may cause clinical signs that are nonspecific (weakness, blindness or gastrointestinal signs) or directly related to the hormonal abnormality induced by the tumor.
  - Aldosterone producing tumors may cause sodium retention and increased blood volume, which may cause hypertension, retinal hemorrhage, cardiac disease, weakness and depression.
  - Epinephrine secreting tumors such as pheochromocytomas and paragangliomas are rare and often incidental, whereas others are PU/PD, exhibit vomiting or diarrhea and listlessness.
  - Progesterone secreting tumors are rare and are associated with insulin resistance, in addition to alopecia, thinning of the skin, and poor wound healing.
- Not painful.

Staging and diagnosis

- Minimum data base (MDB): includes a CBC, biochemical profile, urinalysis, FIV/FeLV serology, T4 testing, biopsy, three-view thoracic radiographs or computerized tomography of the chest.
- Ultrasonography and/or radiographs are practical and cost effective, however computerized tomography or magnetic resonance imaging of the tumor may be preferable in some cases.

Treatment

This section is divided into three options:

- Comfort for those who want to improve quality of life.
- Comfort and control for those who want to improve quality of life while trying to provide some control of the tumor.
- Comfort and longer-term control for those who want to improve quality of life while trying to maximize the chance of controlling the tumor.

Comfort

- Therapy to enhance comfort (e.g.: NSAID, tramadol, buprenorphine) and freedom from nausea, vomiting (e.g.: maropitant and/or metoclopramide), diarrhea (e.g.: metronidazole) and lack of appetite (e.g.: mirtazapine or cyproheptadine). Symptomatic medical treatment with potassium chloride, amlodipine, and spironolactone for aldosterone-secreting tumors may be palliative. Presurgical stabilization is important for pheochromocytoma.

Comfort and control

Above mentioned therapy for comfort plus:

- Palliative radiation, especially for those with extension into surrounding structures or regional metastases (e.g.: 2-5 dosages of radiation), to first enhance comfort, second, to reduce the rate of growth and third, occasionally to reduce the size of the tumor.

Comfort and longer-term control

Above mentioned therapy for comfort plus:
- Adrenalectomy with supportive care postoperatively.
  - In one study[163] with cats with hypokalemia and an aldosterone secreting adrenal tumor, elevated concentrations of plasma aldosterone and adrenocortical neoplasia were documented in ten cats. Seven cases had adrenal adenomas and six had unilateral adrenal carcinomas. Three cases underwent medical treatment only with amlodipine, spironolactone and potassium gluconate, with two cats surviving 304 and 984 days. Ten cases underwent surgical adrenalectomy with cases remain alive between 240 and 1803 days.
  - In another study[164] of 10 cats that had surgery for an aldosterone secreting tumor that caused hypokalemia and hypertension, eight survived and were discharged from the hospital post adrenalectomy. The overall median survival was 1,297 days.

References

1. Holzworth J, Theran P, Carpenter JL, et al: Hyperthyroidism in the cat: Ten cases. *JAVMA* 176:345–353, 1980.
2. O'Brien SE, Riley JH, Hagemoser WA: Unilateral thyroid neoplasm in a cat. *Vet Rec* 107:199–200, 1980.
3. Jones BR, Johnstone AC: Hyperthyroidism in an aged cat. *N Z Vet J* 29:70–72, 1981.
4. Lucke VM: An histological study of thyroid abnormalities in the domestic cat. *J Small Anim Pract* 5:351–358, 1964.
5. Broussard JD, Peterson ME, Fox PR: Changes in clinical and laboratory findings in cats with hyperthyroidism from 1983–1993. *JAVMA* 206:302–305, 1995.
6. Miyamoto T, Kato M, Kuwamura M, et al: A first feline case of cardiomyopathy associated with hyperthyroidism due to thyroid adenoma in Japan. *Feline Pract* 26:6–9, 1998.
7. Peterson ME, Becker DV: Radioiodine treatment of 524 cats with hyperthyroidism. *JAVMA* 207:1422–1428, 1995.
8. Peterson ME, Livingston P, Brown RS: Lack of circulating thyroid stimulating immunoglobulins in cats with hyperthyroidism. *Vet Immunol Immunopathol* 16:277–282, 1987.
9. Kennedy RL: Autoantibodies in feline hyperthyroidism. *Res Vet Sci* 45:300–306, 1988.
10. Merryman JI, Buckles EL, Bowers G, et al: Overexpression of c-ras in hyperplasia and adenomas of the feline thyroid gland: An immunohistochemical analysis of 34 cases. *Vet Pathol* 36:117–124, 1999.
11. Scarlett JM, Moise NS, Rayl J: Feline hyperthyroidism: A descriptive and case control study. *Prev Vet Med* 6:295–309, 1988.
12. Kass PH, Peterson ME, Levy J, et al: Evaluation of environmental, nutritional, and host factors in cats with hyperthyroidism. *J Vet Intern Med* 13:323–329, 1999.
13. Jones BR, Hodge H, Davies E: The prevalence of feline immunodeficiency virus infection in hyperthyroid cats. *N Z Vet J* 23–24, 1995.
14. Hoenig M, Goldschmidt MH, Ferguson DC, et al: Toxic nodular goitre in the cat. *J Small Anim Pract* 23:1–12, 1982.
15. Joseph RJ, Peterson ME: Review and comparison of neuromuscular and central nervous system manifestations of hyperthyroidism in cats and humans. *Prog Vet Neurol* 3:114–119, 1998.
16. Kintzer PP, Peterson ME: Thyroid scintigraphy in small animals. *Semin Vet Med Surg Small Anim* 8:131–139, 1991.
17. Lenarduzzi RF, Jones L: Feline hyperthyroidism: Curing the condition, understanding the cause. *Vet Med* 81:242–244, 1986.
18. Rozanski EA, Stobie D: Laryngeal paralysis secondary to a cystic thyroid adenoma in a cat. *Feline Pract* 23:6–7, 1995.
19. Peterson ME, Kintzer PP, Cavanagh PG, et al: Feline hyperthyroidism: Pretreatment clinical and laboratory evaluation of 131 cases. *JAVMA* 183:103–110, 1983.
20. Aucoin DP, Rubin RL, Petereson ME, et al: Dose-dependent induction of anti-native DNA antibodies in cats by propylthiouracil. *Arthritis Rheum* 31:688–692, 1988.
21. Liu S-K, Peterson ME, Fox PR: Hypertrophic cardiomyopathy and hyperthyroidism in the cat. *JAVMA* 185:52–57, 1984.
22. Cowell RL, Cowell AK: Pseudochylous thoracic effusion and hyperthyroidism in a cat. *Mod Vet Pract* 80:309–312, 1985.
23. Fox PR, Petereson ME, Broussard JD: Electrocardiographic and radiographic changes in cats with hyperthyroidism: comparison of populations evaluated during 1992–1993 vs. 1979–1982. *JAAHA* 35:27–31, 1999.
24. Peterson ME, Graves TK, Cavanagh I: Serum thyroid hormone concentrations fluctuate in cats with hyperthyroidism. *J Vet Intern Med* 1:142–146, 1987.
25. Broome MR, Feldman EC, Turrel JM: Serial determination of thyroxine concentrations in hyperthyroid cats. *JAVMA* 192:49–51, 1988.
26. Chaitman J, Hess R, Senz R, et al: Thyroid adenomatous hyperplasia in euthyroid cats [abstract 67]. *J Vet Intern Med* 13:242, 1999.
27. Peterson ME, Gamble DA: Effect of nonthyroidal illness on serum thyroxine concentrations in cats: 494 cases (1988). *JAVMA* 197:1203–1208, 1990.
28. Graves TK, Peterson ME: Diagnosis of occult hyperthyroidism in cats. *Prob Vet Med* 2:683–692, 1990.
29. Peterson ME, Graves TK, Gamble DA: triiodothyronine (T3) suppression test. An aid in the diagnosis of mild hyperthyroidism in cats. *J Vet Intern Med* 4:233–238, 1990.
30. Refsal KR, Nachreiner RF, Stein BE, et al: Use of the triiodothyronine suppression test for diagnosis of hyperthyroidism in ill cats that have serum concentration of iodothyronines within normal range. *JAVMA* 199:1594–1601, 1991.
31. Hoenig M, Ferguson DC: Assessment of thyroid functional reserve in the cat by the thyrotropin-stimulation test. *Am J Vet Res* 44:1229–1232, 1983.
32. Tomsa K, Glaus TM, Kacl GM, et al: Thyrotropin-releasing hormone stimulation test to assess thyroid function in severely sick cats. *J Vet Intern Med* 15:89–93, 2001.
33. Moise NS, Dietze AE: Echocardiographic, electrocardiographic, and radiographic detection of cardiomegaly in hyperthyroid cats. *Am J Vet Res* 47:1487–1494, 1986.
34. Peterson ME, Keene B, Ferguson DC, et al: Electrocardiographic findings in 45 cats with hyperthyroidism. *JAVMA* 180:934–937, 1982.
35. Bond BR, Fox PR, Peterson ME, et al: Echocardiographic findings in 103 cats with hyperthyroidism. *JAVMA* 192:1546–1549, 1988.
36. Kobayashi DL, Peterson ME, Graves TK, et al: Hypertension in cats with chronic renal failure or hyperthyroidism. *J Vet Intern Med* 4:58–62, 1990.
37. Venzin I, Vannini R: Feline hyperthyreose. *Kleintierpraxis* 35:183–188, 1990.
38. DiBartola SP, Broome MR, Stein BS, et al: Effect of treatment of hyperthyroidism on renal function in cats. *JAVMA* 208:875–878, 1996.
39. Wisner ER, Théon AP, Nyland TG, et al: Ultrasonographic examination of the thyroid gland of hyperthyroid cats: comparison to 99mTcO4– scintigraphy. *Vet Radiol Ultrasound* 35:53–58, 1994.
40. Noxon JO, Thornburg LP, Dillender MJ, et al: An adenoma in ectopic thyroid tissue causing hyperthyroidism in a cat. *JAAHA* 19:369–372, 1983.
41. Peterson ME, Becker DV: Radionuclide thyroid imaging in 135 cats with hyperthyroidism. *Vet Radiol* 25:23–27, 1984.
42. Mooney CT, Thoday KL, Nicoll JJ, et al: Qualitative and quantitative thyroid imaging in feline hyperthyroidism using technetium-99M as pertechnetate. *Vet Radiol Ultrasound* 33:313–320, 1992.
43. Swalec KM, Birchard SJ: Recurrence of hyperthyroidism after thyroidectomy in cats. *JAAHA* 26:433–437, 1990.
44. Trepanier LA, Peterson ME: Pharmacokinetics of methimazole in normal cats and cats with hyperthyroidism. *Res Vet Sci* 50:69–74,1991.
45. Peterson ME: Propylthiouracil in the treatment of feline hyperthyroidism. *JAVMA* 179:485–487, 1981.
46. Peterson ME, Hurvitz AI, Leib MS, et al: Propylthiouracil-associated hemolytic anemia, thrombocytopenia and antinuclear antibodies in cats with hyperthyroidism. *JAVMA* 184:806, 1984.
47. Aucoin DP, Peterson ME, Hurvitz AI, et al: Propylthiouracil-induced immune-mediated disease in the cat. *J Pharm Exp Therap* 234:13–18, 1985.
48. Peterson ME, Kintzer PP, Hurvitz AI: Methimazole

treatment of 262 cats with hyperthyroidism. *J Vet Intern Med* 2:150,1988.

49. Reine NJ, Peterson ME, Hohenhaus AE: Effects of methimazole on hemostatic parameters in cats with hyperthyroidism [abstract 76]. *J Vet Intern Med* 13:245, 1999.

50. Mooney CT, Thoday KL, Doxey DL: Carbimazole therapy of feline hyperthyroidism. *J Small Anim Pract* 33:228–235, 1992.

51. Murray LAS, Peterson ME: Ipodate treatment of hyperthyroidism in cats. *JAVMA* 211:63–67, 1997.

52. Walker MC, Schaer M: Percutaneous ethanol treatment of hyperthyroidism in a cat. *Feline Pract* 26:10–12, 1998.

53. Wells AL, Long CD, Feldman EC, et al: Ultrasound guided percutaneous ethanol injection (PEI) for the treatment of 6 cats with bilateral hyperthyroidism [abstract 66]. *J Vet Intern Med* 13:242, 1999.

54. Goldstein RE, Long CD, Feldman EC, et al: Ultrasound guided percutaneous ethanol injection (PEI) for the treatment of 4 cats with unilateral hyperthyroidism [abstract 64]. *J Vet Intern Med* 13:241, 1999.

55. Jacobs G, Hutson C, Dougherty J, et al: Congestive heart failure associated with hyperthyroidism in cats. *JAVMA* 188:52–56, 1986.

56. Birchard SJ, Peterson ME, Jacobson A: Surgical treatment of feline hyperthyroidism: results of 85 cases. *JAAHA* 20:705–709, 1984.

57. Foster DJ, Thoday KL: Use of propranolol and potassium iodate in the presurgical management of hyperthyroid cats. *J Small Anim Pract* 40:307–315, 1999.

58. Flanders JA: Surgical treatment of hyperthyroid cats. *Mod Vet Pract* 67:711–715, 1986.

59. Flanders JA, Harvey HJ, Erb HN: Correspondence. *Vet Surg* 17:59, 1988.

60. Welches CD, Scavelli TD, Matthiesen DT, et al: Occurrence of problems after three techniques of bilateral thyroidectomy in cats. *Vet Surg* 18:392–396, 1989.

61. Liptak JM: Unilateral extracapsular thyroidectomy for a non-functional cystic thyroid adenoma. *Aust Vet Pract* 26:174–177, 1996.

62. Flanders JA: Surgical options for the treatment of hyperthyroidism in the cat. *J Feline Med Surg* 1:127–134, 1999.

63. Padgett SL, Tobias KM, Leathers CW, et al: Efficacy of parathyroid gland autotransplantation in maintaining serum calcium concentrations after bilateral thyroparathyroidectomy in cats. *JAAHA* 34:219–224, 1998.

64. Smith TA, Bruyette DS, Hoskinson JJ, et al: Radioiodine treatment outcome in hyperthyroid cats: Effect of prior methimazole treatment. *J Vet Intern Med* 9:183, 1995.

65. Meric SM, Rubin SI: Serum thyroxine concentrations following fixed-dose radioactive iodine treatment in hyperthyroid cats: 62 cases (1986–1989). *JAVMA* 197:621–623, 1990.

66. Craig A, Zuber M, Allan GS: A prospective study of 66 cases of feline hyperthyroidism treated with a fixed dose of intravenous [131]I. *Aust Vet Pract* 23:2–6, 1993.

67. Meric SM, Hawkins EC, Washabau RJ, et al: Serum thyroxine concentrations after radioactive iodine therapy in cats with hyperthyroidism. *JAVMA* 188:1038–1040, 1986.

68. Malik R, Lamb WA, Church DB: treatment of feline hyperthyroidism using orally administered radioiodine: a study of 40 consecutive cases. *Austr Vet J* 70:218–219, 1993.

69. Theon AP, VanVechten MK, Feldman E: A prospective randomized comparison of intravenous versus subcutaneous administration of radioiodine for treatment of feline hyperthyroidism: A study of 120 cats. *Am J Vet Res* 55:1734–1738, 1994.

70. Mooney CT: Radioactive iodine therapy for feline hyperthyroidism: Efficacy and administration routes. *J Small Anim Pract* 35:289–294, 1994.

71. Broome MR, Turrel JM, Hays MT: Predictive value of tracer studies for ^{131}I treatment in hyperthyroid cats. *Am J Vet Res* 49:193–197, 1988.

72. Turrel JM, Feldman EC, Hays M, et al: Radioactive iodine therapy in cats with hyperthyroidism. *JAVMA* 184:554–559, 1984.

73. Klausner JS, Johnston GR, Feeney DA, et al: Results of radioactive iodine therapy in 23 cats with hyperthyroidism. *Minn J Vet Med* 27:28–32, 1987.

74. Handelsman H, Broder LE, Slavik M, et al: Streptozotocin NSC-85998. Clinical brochure. *Invest Drug Branch Cancer Ther Eval Div Cancer treatment. National Cancer Inst*, pp 1–68, 1974.

75. Patnaik AK, Lieberman PH: Feline anaplastic giant cell adenocarcinoma of the thyroid. *Vet Pathol* 16:687–692, 1979.

76. Cowen PN, Jackson P: Thyroid carcinoma in a cat. *Vet Rec* 114:521–522, 1984.

77. King JM: Thyroid adenocarcinoma. *Vet Med* 89:1113, 1994.

78. Turrel JM, Feldman EC, Nelson RW, et al: Thyroid carcinoma causing hyperthyroidism in cats: 14 cases (1981–1986). *JAVMA* 193:359–364, 1988.

79. Guptill L, Scott-Moncrieff CR, Janovitz EB, et al: Response to high-dose radioactive iodine administration in cats with thyroid carcinoma that had previously undergone surgery. *JAVMA* 8:1055–1058, 1995.

80. Holzworth J, Husted P, Wind A: Arterial thrombosis and thyroid carcinoma in a cat. *Cornell Vet* 45:487–496, 1955.

81. Johnson KH, Osborne CA: Adenocarcinoma of the thyroid gland in a cat. *JAVMA* 156:906–912, 1970.

82. Clark ST, Meier H: A clinico-pathological study of thyroid disease in the dog and cat. *Zentralbl Veterinärmed* 5:17–32, 1958.

83. von Sandersleben J, Hänichen T: Tumours of the thyroid gland. *Bull WHO* 50:35–42, 1974.

84. Leav I, Schiller AL, Rijnber Rijnberk A, et al: Adenomas and carcinomas of the canine and feline thyroid. *Am J Pathol* 1976;83:61–93.

85. Peterson ME, Broome MR, :Rishniw M. Prevalence and degree of thyroid pathology in hyperthyroid cats increases with disease duration: a cross-sectional analysis of 2096 cats referred for radioiodine therapy. *J Feline Med Surg*. pii: 1098612X15572416, 2015.

86. Hibbert A, Gruffydd-Jones T, Barrett EL, et al: Feline thyroid carcinoma: diagnosis and response to high-dose radioactive iodine treatment. *J Feline Med Surg*. 11(2):116-24, 2009.

87. Naan EC, Kirpensteijn J, Kooistra HS, et al: Results of thyroidectomy in 101 cats with hyperthyroidism. *Vet Surg*. 35(3):287-293, 2006.

88. Li X, Steinburg H, Wallace C, et al: Functional thyroid follicular adenocarcinoma in a captive mountain lion *(Felis concolor)*. *Vet Pathol* 29:549–551, 1992.

89. Schmidt RE, Hubbard GB, Fletcher KC: Systematic survey of lesions from animals in a zoologic collection: IV. Endocrine glands. *J Zoo Anim Med* 17:24–28, 1986.

90. McMillan FD, Barr B, Feldman EC: Functional pancreatic islet cell tumor in a cat. *JAAHA* 21:741–746, 1985.

91. O'Brien TD, Norton F, Turner TM, et al: Pancreatic endocrine tumor in a cat: clinical, pathological, and immunohistochemical evaluation. *JAAHA* 26:453–457, 1990.

92. Priester WA: Pancreatic islet cell tumors in domestic animals. Data from 11 colleges of veterinary medicine in the United States and Canada. *J Natl Cancer Inst* 53:227–229, 1974.

93. Myers NCIII, Andrews GA, Chard-Bergstrom C: Chromogranin A plasma concentration and expression in pancreatic islet cell tumors of dogs and cats. *Am J Vet Res* 58:615–620, 1997.

94. Nielsen SW: Neoplastic diseases. In Catcott EJ (ed):*Feline Medicine and Surgery*. Santa Barbara, CA, American Veterinary Publications, 1964, pp 156–176.

95. Carpenter JL, Andrews LK, Holzworth J: Tumors and tumor-like lesions. In Holzworth J (ed): *Diseases of the Cat. Medicine and Surgery*. Philadelphia, .WB Saunders, 1987, pp 407–596.

96. Middleton DJ, Watson ADJ: Duodenal ulceration associated with gastrin-secreting pancreatic tumor in a cat. *JAVMA* 183:461–462, 1983.

97. van der Gaag I, van den Ingh TSGAM, Lamers CBHW, et al: Zollinger-Ellison syndrome in a cat. *Vet Q* 10:151–155, 1988.

98. Blunden AS, Wheeler SJ, Davies JV: Hyperparathyroidism in the cat of probable primary origin. *J Small Anim Pract* 27:791–798, 1986.

99. den Hertog E, Goossens MMC, van der Linden-Sipman JS, et al: Primary hyperparathyroidism in two cats. *Vet Q* 19:81–84, 1997.

100. Kallet AJ, Richter KP, Feldman EC, et al: Primary hyperparathyroidism in cats: Seven cases (1984–1989). *JAVMA* 199:1767–1771, 1991.

101. Marquez GA, Klausner JS, Osborne CA: Calcium oxalate urolithiasis in a cat with a functional parathyroid adenocarcinoma. *JAVMA* 206:817–819, 1995.

102. Sueda MT, Stefanacci JD: Ultrasound evaluation of the parathyroid glands in two hypercalcemic cats. *Vet Radiol Ultrasound* 41:448–451, 2000.

103. Doster AR, Armstrong DL, Bargar TW: Seminoma and parathyroid adenoma in a snow leopard (Panthera unica). *J Comp Pathol* 100:475–480, 1989.

104. Zaki FA, Liu S–K: Pituitary chromophobe adenoma in a cat. *Vet Pathol* 10:232–237, 1973.
105. Zaki F, Harris J, Budzilovich G: Cystic pituicytoma of the neurohypophysis in a Siamese cat. *J Comp Pathol* 85:467–471, 1975.
106. Davidson MG, Nasisse MP, Breitschwerdt EB, et al: Acute blindness associated with intracranial tumors in dogs and cats: eight cases (1984–1989). *JAVMA* 199:755–758, 1991.
107. Peterson ME, Taylor RS, Greco DS, et al: Acromegaly in 14 cats. *J Vet Intern Med* 4:192–201, 1990.
108. Goossens MMC, Feldman EC, Nelson RW, et al: Cobalt 60 irradiation of pituitary gland tumors in three cats with acromegaly. *JAVMA* 213:374–376, 1998.
109. Fischetti AJ, Gisselman K, Peterson ME. CT and MRI evaluation of skull bones and soft tissues in six cats with presumed acromegaly versus 12 unaffected cats. *Vet Radiol Ultrasound.* 53(5):535-539,2012.
110. Abrams-Ogg ACG, Holmberg DL, Stewart WA, et al: Acromegaly in a cat: Diagnosis by magnetic resonance imaging and treatment by cryohypophysectomy. *Can Vet J* 34:682–685, 1993.
111. Meij B, Voorhout G, van den Ingh TSGAM, et al: Transsphenoidal hypophysectomy for treatment of pituitary-dependent hyperadrenocorticism in 7 cats. *Vet Surg* 30:72–86, 2001.
112. Zaki FA, Hurvitz AI: Spontaneous neoplasms of the central nervous system of the cat. *J Small Anim Pract* 17:773–782, 1976.
113. Middleton DJ, Culvenor JA, Vasak E, et al: Growth hormone-producing pituitary adenoma, elevated serum somatomedin C concentrations and diabetes mellitus in a cat. *Can Vet J* 26:169–171, 1985.
114. Valentin SY, Cortright CC, Nelson RW, et al: Clinical findings, diagnostic test results, and treatment outcome in cats with spontaneous hyperadrenocorticism: 30 cases. *J Vet Intern Med.* 28(2):481-487, 2014.
115. Morrison SA, Randolf J, Lothrop CD: Hypersomatotropism and insulin-resistant diabetes mellitus in a cat. *JAVMA* 194:91–94, 1989.
116. Lichtensteiger CA, Wortman JA, Eigenmann JE: Functional pituitary acidophil adenoma in a cat with diabetes mellitus and acromegalic features. *Vet Pathol* 23:518–521, 1986.
117. Elliott DA, Feldman EC, Koblik PD, et al: Prevalence of pituitary tumors among diabetic cats with insulin resistance. *JAVMA* 216:1765–1768, 2000.
118. Furuzawa Y, Une Y, Nomura Y: Pituitary dependent hyperadrenocorticism in a cat. *J Vet Med Sci* 54:1201–1203, 1992.
119. Schwedes CS: Mitotane (o,p'-DDD) treatment in a cat with hyperadrenocorticism. *J Small Anim Pract* 38:520–524, 1997.
120. Zerbe CA, Nachreiner RF, Dunstan RW, et al: Hyperadrenocorticism in a cat. *JAVMA* 190:559–563, 1987.
121. Kipperman BS, Nelson RW, Griffey SM, et al: Diabetes mellitus and exocrine pancreatic neoplasia in two cats with hyperadrenocorticism. *JAAHA* 28:415–418, 1992.
122. Peterson ME, Steele P: Pituitary-dependent hyperadrenocorticism in a cat. *JAVMA* 189:680–683, 1986.
123. Immink WFGA, van Toor AJ, Vos JS, et al: Hyperadrenocorticism in four cats. *Vet Q* 14:81–85, 1992.
124. Usher DG: Hyperadrenocorticism in a cat. *Can Vet J* 32:326, 1991.
125. Meij BP, Auriemma E, Grinwis G, et al: Successful treatment of acromegaly in a diabetic cat with transsphenoidal hypophysectomy. *J Feline Med Surg* 12(5):406-410, 2010.
126. Duesberg CA, Nelson RW, Feldman EC, et al: Adrenalectomy for treatment of hyperadrenocorticism in cats: 10 cases (1988–1992). *JAVMA* 207:1066–1070, 1995.
127. Nelson RW, Feldman EC, Smith M.C: Hyperadrenocorticism in cats: Seven cases (1978–1987). *JAVMA* 193:245–250, 1988.
128. Watson PJ, Herrtage ME: Hyperadrenocorticism in six cats. *J Small Anim Pract* 39:175–184, 1998.
129. Goossens MMC, Meyer HP, Voorhout G, et al: Urinary excretion of glucocorticoids in the diagnosis of hyperadrenocorticism in cats. *Dom Anim Endocrin* 12:355–362, 1995.
130. Valentine RW: Feline hyperadrenocorticism: A rare case. *Feline Pract* 24:6–11, 1996.
131. Meijer JC, Lubberink AAME, Gruys E: Cushing's syndrome due to adrenocortical adenoma in a cat. *Tijdschr Diergeneesk* 103:1048–1051, 1978.
132. Jones CA, Refsal KR, Lerner RW: Adrenocortical adenocarcinoma in a cat. *JAAHA* 9:137–143, 1992.
133. Fox JG, Beatty JO: A case report of complicated diabetes mellitus in a cat. *JAAHA* 11:129–134, 1975.
134. Daley CA, Zerbe CA, Schick RO, et al: Use of metyrapone to treat pituitary-dependent hyperadrenocorticism in a cat with large cutaneous wounds. *JAVMA* 202:956–960, 1993.
135. Johnston SD, Mather EC: Feline plasma cortisol (hydrocortisone) measured by radioimmunoassay. *Am J Vet Res* 40:190–192, 1979.
136. Peterson ME, Kintzer PP, Foodman MS, et al: Adrenal function in the cat: comparison of the effects of cosyntropin (synthetic ACTH) and corticotropin gel stimulation. *Res Vet Sci* 37:331–333, 1984.
137. Sparkes AH, Adams DT, Douthwaite JA, et al: Assessment of adrenal function in cats: responses to intravenous synthetic ACTH. *J Small Anim Pract* 31:2–5, 1984.
138. Zimmer C, Hörauf A, Reusch C: Ultrasonographic examination of the adrenal gland and evaluation of the hypophyseal-adrenal axis in 20 cats. *J Small Anim Pract* 41:156–160, 2000.
139. Peterson ME, Kemppainen RJ: Comparison of intravenous and intramuscular routes of administering cosyntropin for corticotropin stimulation testing in cats. *Am J Vet Res* 53:1392–1395, 1992.
140. Peterson ME, Kemppainen RJ: Dose-response relation between plasma concentrations of corticotropin and cortisol after administration of incremental doses of cosyntropin for corticotropin stimulation testing in cats. *Am J Vet Res* 54:300–304, 1993.
141. Smith MC, Feldman EC: Plasma endogenous ACTH concentrations and plasma cortisol responses to synthetic ACTH and dexamethasone sodium phosphate in healthy cats. *Am J Vet Res* 48:1719–1724, 1987.
142. Zerbe CA, Refsal KR, Peterson ME, et al: Effect of nonadrenal illness on adrenal function in the cat. *Am J Vet Res* 48:451–454, 1987.
143. Medleau L, Cowan LA, Cornelius L.M: Adrenal function testing in the cat: The effect of low dose intravenous dexamethasone administration. *Res Vet Sci* 42:260–261, 1987.
144. Peterson ME, Graves TK: Effects of low dosages of intravenous dexamethasone on serum cortisol concentrations in the normal cat. *Res Vet Sci* 44:38–40, 1988.
145. Myers NC, Bruyette DS: Feline adrenocortical diseases: Part I–Hyperadrenocorticism. *Semin Vet Med Surg Small Anim* 9:137–143, 1994.
146. Howell MJ, Pickering CM: Calcium deposits in the adrenal glands of dogs and cats. *J Comp Pathol* 74:280–285, 1964.
147. Ross MA, Gainer JH, Innes JRM: Dystrophic calcification in the adrenal glands of monkeys, cats and dogs. *AMA Arch Pathol* 60:655–661, 1955.
148. Cartee RE, Bodner STF, Gray BW: Ultrasound examination of the feline adrenal gland. *J Diagn Med Sonog* 9:327–330, 1993.
149. Boord M, Griffin C: Progesterone secreting adrenal mass in a cat with clinical signs of hyperadrenocorticism. *JAVMA* 214:666–669,1999.
150. Willard MD, Nachreiner RF, Howard VC, et al: Effect of long-term administration of ketoconazole in cats. *Am J Vet Res* 47:2510–2513, 1986.
151. Duesberg C, Peterson ME: Adrenal disorders in cats. *Vet Clin North Am Small Anim Pract* 27:321–347, 1997.
152. Mellett Keith AM, Bruyette D, Stanley S. Trilostane therapy for treatment of spontaneous hyperadrenocorticism in cats: 15 cases (2004-2012). *J Vet Intern Med* 27(6):1471-1477, 2013.
153. Ahn A: Hyperaldosteronism in cats. *Semin Vet Med Surg Small Anim* 9:153–157, 1994.
154. Eger CE, Robinson WF, Huxtable CRR: Primary aldosteronism (Conn's syndrome) in a cat; a case report and review of comparative aspects. *J Small Anim Pract* 24:293–307, 1983.
155. Flood SM, Randolph JF, Gelzer ARM, et al: Primary hyperaldosteronism in two cats. *JAAHA* 35:411–416, 1999.
156. MacKay AD, Holt PE, Sparkes AH: Successful surgical treatment of a cat with primary aldosteronism. *J Feline Med Surg* 1:117–122, 1999.
157. Yu S, Morris JG: Plasma aldosterone concentration of cats. *Vet J* 155:63–68, 1998.
158. Patnaik AK, Erlandson RA, Lieberman PH, et al: Extra-adrenal pheochromocytoma (paraganglioma) in a cat. *JAVMA* 197:104–106, 1990.
159. Chun R, Jakovljevic S, Morrison WB, et al: Apocrine gland adenocarcinoma and pheochromocytoma in a cat. *JAAHA* 33:33–36, 1997.
160. Holzworth J, Coffin DL: Pancreatic insufficiency and diabetes mellitus in a cat. *Cornell Vet* 43:502–512, 1953.
161. Henry CL, Brewer WG, Montgomery RD, et al: Clinical vignette: adrenal pheochromocytoma. *J Vet Intern Med* 7:199–201, 1993.

162. Maher ER: Pheochromocytoma in the dog and cat: Diagnosis and management. *Semin Vet Med Surg Small Anim* 9:158–166, 1994.

163. Daniel G, Mahony OM, Markovich JE, et al: Clinical findings, diagnostics and outcome in 33 cats with adrenal neoplasia (2002-2013). *J Feline Med Surg.* pii: 1098612X15572035, 2015.

164. Lo AJ, Holt DE, Brown DC, et al: treatment of aldosterone-secreting adrenocortical tumors in cats by unilateral adrenalectomy: 10 cases (2002-2012). *J Vet Intern Med.* 28(1):137-143, 2014.

165. Rossmeisl JH, Scott-Moncrieff JCR, Siems J, et al: Hyperadrenocorticism and hyperprogesteronemia in a cat with an adrenocortical adenocarcinoma. *JAAHA* 36:512–517, 2000.

166. Becker TJ, Perry RL, Watson GL: Regression of hypertrophic osteopathy in a cat after surgical excision of an adrenocortical carcinoma. *JAAHA* 35:499–505, 1999.

167. Biller DS, Bradley GA, Partington BP: Renal medullary rim sign: ultrasonographic evidence of renal disease. *Vet Radiol Ultrasound* 33:286–290, 1992.

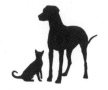

Chapter 54

Feline tumors of the reproductive system

FELINE TUMORS OF THE PROSTATE AND TESTICLE

Clinical presentation

- Uncommon.
- Often an incidental finding.
- Seminomas, interstitial cell tumors and teratomas predominate.[1-7]
- Prostatic tumors may cause dysuria and hematuria.
- Usually not painful.

Staging and diagnosis

- Minimum data base (MDB): includes a CBC, biochemical profile, urinalysis, FIV/FeLV serology, T4 testing, biopsy, three-view thoracic radiographs or computerized tomography of the chest.
- Ultrasonography, radiographs and abdominal ultrasound may be helpful to stage the patient, however metastases have rarely been seen except in teratomas.

Treatment

This section is divided into two options:
- Comfort for those who want to improve quality of life.
- Comfort and control for those who want to improve quality of life while trying to provide some control of the tumor.

Comfort

- Therapy to enhance comfort (e.g.: NSAID, tramadol, buprenorphine) and freedom from nausea, vomiting (e.g.: maropitant and/or metoclopramide), diarrhea (e.g.: metronidazole) and lack of appetite (e.g.: mirtazapine or cyproheptadine).

Comfort and control

Above mentioned therapy for comfort plus:
- Castration for testicular tumors.
- Radiation may be beneficial for prostatic tumors.
- Prostatectomy. One cat was treated by prostatectomy alone and lived 3 months before it was euthanized due to local metastasis that occluded the ureter and caused hydronephrosis.[12]
- Carboplatin or mitoxantrone have been used to treat cats with metastatic disease, however the efficacy remains unknown.

FELINE OVARIAN TUMORS

Clinical presentation

- Relatively uncommon.
- Large tumors may occur and cause signs related to size.
- Most often unilateral, however bilateral tumors have been documented.
- Granulosa cell tumors predominate followed by dysgerminomas, interstitial cell tumors, carcinomas, teratomas, sex-cord tumors, and a cystadenoma.
- Granulosa cell tumors may produce hormones and cause a persistent or irregular estrus, behavioral changes including aggressiveness, alopecia, anorexia and lethargy.
  - Abdominal distention may be noted and intra-abdominal or thoracic metastases have been noted.[14,15,18,19]
- Ovarian granulosa cell tumors and carcinomas appear to be highly malignant, while teratomas may be less likely to metastasize.
- May be painful.

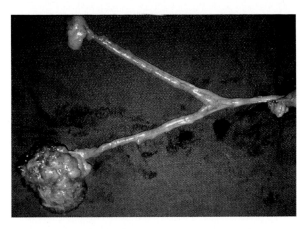

Figure 54-1: This ovarian tumor was removed from a cat that presented for a dermatologic problem. The ovarian mass was palpable on physical examination and visible on abdominal ultrasound. Resection resolved the cat's clinical signs. The histopathologic diagnosis was an ovarian carcinoma. Carboplatin was given adjuvantly and the cat did well long-term. Reprinted with permission from: Ogilvie GK, Moore AS. *Feline Oncology: A Comprehensive Guide for Compassionate Care*. Trenton NJ, Veterinary Learning Systems. 2002.

Staging and diagnosis

- Minimum data base (MDB): includes a CBC, biochemical profile, urinalysis, FIV/FeLV serology, T4 testing, biopsy, three-view thoracic radiographs or computerized tomography of the chest.
- Peritoneal metastases are most common, therefore ultrasonography and/or radiographs are practical and cost effective, however computerized tomography or magnetic resonance imaging of the abdomen, and thus the tumor, may be helpful to determine the extent of the disease.

> **Key point**
>
> Ovarian granulosa cell tumors and ovarian carcinomas may be quite malignant with a high metastatic rate, whereas teratomas are usually less aggressive.

Treatment

This section is divided into two options:
- Comfort for those who want to improve quality of life.
- Comfort and control for those who want to improve quality of life while trying to provide some control of the tumor.

Comfort

- Therapy to enhance comfort (e.g.: NSAID, tramadol, buprenorphine) and freedom from nausea, vomiting (e.g.: maropitant and/or

metoclopramide), diarrhea (e.g.: metronidazole) and lack of appetite (e.g.: mirtazapine or cyproheptadine).

Comfort and control

Above mentioned therapy for comfort plus:
- Surgery.
- Adjuvant carboplatin chemotherapy may be helpful when the tumor has metastasized or if it is malignant.

FELINE UTERINE TUMORS

Clinical presentation

- Relatively common.
- Adenomas or endometrial polyps, fibromas, leiomyomas, squamous cell carcinoma are more commonly seen than adenomyosis and lymphoma.
  - Adenoma may progress to adenocarcinoma, which can then metastasize.
  - Leiomyomas may be associated with cystic ovaries.
  - Carcinomas may metastasize and can cause a pyometra.
  - Adenomyosis is described as proliferation of ectopic endometrium within the myometrium that causes enlargement of the uterus.
- May be painful.

Staging and diagnosis

- Minimum data base (MDB): includes a CBC, biochemical profile, urinalysis, FIV/FeLV serology, T4 testing, biopsy, three-view thoracic radiographs or computerized tomography of the chest.
- Ultrasonography and/or radiographs are practical and cost effective, however computerized tomography or magnetic resonance imaging of the abdomen, and thus the tumor, may be helpful to determine the extent of the disease.
- If abdominal effusion is present, then fluid analysis and cytology is important.

Treatment

This section is divided into two options:
- Comfort for those who want to improve quality of life.
- Comfort and control for those who want to improve quality of life while trying to provide some control of the tumor.

Comfort

- Therapy to enhance comfort (e.g.: NSAID, tramadol, buprenorphine) and freedom from nausea, vomiting (e.g.: maropitant and/or metoclopramide), diarrhea (e.g.: metronidazole) and lack of appetite (e.g.: mirtazapine or cyproheptadine).

Comfort and control

Above mentioned therapy for comfort plus:
- Ovariohysterectomy is curative for benign tumors but only palliative for malignant tumors.
- Carboplatin or doxorubicin have been shown to help some patients with malignant tumors.

References

1. Ferreira da Silva J. Tertoma in a feline unilateral cryptorchid testis. *Vet Pathol.* 39(4):516, 2002.
2. Doxsee AL, Yager JA, Best SJ, Foster RA. Extratesticular interstitial and Sertoli cell tumors in previously neutered dogs and cats: a report of 17 cases. *Can Vet J* 47(8):763-766, 2006.
3. Meier H: Sertoli-cell tumor in the cat. Report of two cases. *North Am Vet* 37:979–981, 1956.
4. Joshua JO: Reproductive system. In *The Clinical Aspects of Some Diseases of Cats.* William Heinemann Medical Books Ltd, 1965, pp 119–140.
5. Sontas BH, Erdogan Ö, Apaydin Enginler SÖ, et al: Endometrial adenocarcinoma in two young queens. *J Small Anim Pract* 54(3):156-159, 2013.
6. Tucker AR, Smith JR. Prostatic squamous metaplasia in a cat with interstitial cell neoplasia in a retained testis. *Vet Pathol.* 45(6):905-909, 2008
7. Miller MA, Ramos-Vara JA, Dickerson MF, et al: Uterine neoplasia in 13 cats. *J Vet Diagn Invest.* 15(6):515-522, 2003
8. Michalska Z, Gucwinski A, Kocula K, R. Ied, H.D. S: Sertoli cell tumour in Bengal tiger (Panthera tigris tigris). *Akademie-Verlag, Erkrankungen der Zootiere Verhandlungsbericht des XIX Internationalen Symposiums uber die Erkrankungen der Zootiere* 18:305–307, 1977.
9. Karesh WB, Kunz LL: Bilateral testicular seminoma in a snow leopard. *JAVMA* 189:1201, 1986.
10. Hubbard BS, Vulgamoot JC, Liska WD: Prostatic adenocarcinoma in a cat. *JAVMA* 197:1493–1494, 1990.
11. Bigliardi E, Parmigiani E, Morini G: Neoplasia prostatica. *Summa* 16:79–80, 1999.
12. Tommasini M, Assin R, Lombardo S: Uretheral transposition in the colon of a cat affected by prostatic carcinoma [abstract 28]. *Vet Surg* 23:217, 1994.
13. Cotchin E: Neoplasia. In Wilkinson GT (ed): *Diseases of the Cat and Their Management.* Melbourne, Blackwell Scientific Publications, 1983.
14. Gelberg HB, McEntee K: Feline ovarian neoplasms. *Vet Pathol* 22:572–576, 1985.
15. Aliakbrai S, Ivoghli B: Granulosa cell tumor in a cat. *JAVMA* 174:1306–1308, 1979.
16. Azuma Y, Matsuo Y, Chen B-Y: Granulosa cell tumor in a cat with unilateral renal agenesis. *J Jpn Vet Med Assoc* 45:324–327, 1992.
17. Arbjerg J: Extra-ovarian granulosa cell tumor in a cat. *Feline Pract* 10:26–32, 1980.
18. Baker E: Malignant granulosa cell tumor in a cat. *JAVMA* 129:322–324, 1956.
19. Norris HJ, Garner FM, Taylor HB: Pathology of feline ovarian neoplasms. *J Pathol* 97:138–143, 1969.
20. Dehner LP, Norris HJ, Garner FM, Taylor HB: Comparative pathology of ovarian neoplasms. III. Germ cell tumours of canine, bovine, feline, rodent and human species. *J Comp Pathol* 8–0, 1970:
21. Gruys E, van Duk JE, Elsinghorst AM, van der Gaag I: Four canine ovarian teratomas and a nonovarian feline teratoma. *Vet Pathol* 13:455–459, 1976.
22. Andrews EJ, Stookey JL, Helland DR, Slaughter LJ: A histopathological study of canine and feline ovarian dysgerminomas. *Can J Comp Med* 38:85–89, 1974.
23. Basaraba RJ, Kraft SL, Andrews GA, Leipold HW, Small D: An ovarian teratoma in a cat. *Vet Pathol* 35:141–144, 1998.
24. Nielsen SW: Neoplastic diseases. In Catcott EJ (ed): *Feline Medicine and Surgery.* Santa Barbara, CA, American Veterinary Publications, 1964, pp 156–176.
25. Röcken H: Ovarialtumor und ovaraplasie bei einer katze. *Tierärztl Prax* 11:245–247, 1983.

26. Hofman W, Arbiter D, Scheele D: Sex cord stromal tumor of the cat: So-called androblastoma with Sertoli-Leydig cell pattern. *Brief Comm* 1998
27. Röcken H: Ein fibrothekom als faktor für einen verhaltensschaden bei einer katze. *Der Praktische Tierarzt* 4:344–346, 1984.
28. Karesh WB, Russell R: Ovarian dysgerminoma in a snow leopard (Panthera unicia). *J Zoo Anim Med* 19:223–225, 1988.
29. Schmidt RE, Hubbard GB, Fletcher KC: Systematic survey of lesion from animals in a zoologic collection: V. Reproductive system and mammary gland. *J Zoo Anim Med* 17:28–33, 1986.
30. Hubbard GB, Schmidt RE, Fletcher KC: Neoplasia in zoo animals. J Zoo Anim Med 14:33–40, 1983.
31. Bossart GD, Hubbell G: Ovarian papillary cystadenocarcinoma in a jaguar (Panthera onca). *J Zoo Anim Med* 14:73–76, 1983.
32. Munson L: A high prevalence of ovarian papillary cystadenocarcinomas in jaguars (Panthera onca). *Vet Pathol* 31:604, 1994.
33. Cotchin E: Spontaneous uterine cancer in animals. *Br J Cancer* 18:209–227, 1964.
34. Gelberg HB, McEntee K: Pathology of the canine and feline uterine tube. *Vet Pathol* 23:770–775, 1986.
35. Pack FD: Feline uterine adenomyosis. *Feline Pract* 10:45–47, 1986.
36. Gelberg HB, McEntee K: Hyperplastic endometrial polyps in the dog and cat. *Vet Pathol* 21:570–573, 1984.
37. Evans JG, Grant DI: A mixed mesodermal tumour in the uterus of a cat. *J Comp Pathol* 87:635–638, 1977.
38. Papparella S, Roperto F: Spontaneous uterine tumors in three cats. *Vet Pathol* 21:257–258, 1984.
39. Meier H: Carcinoma of the uterus in the cat: Two cases. *Cornell Vet* 46:188–200, 1956.
40. Puttannaiah GB, Seshadri SJ, Mohiyudeen S: A rare case of adenocarcinoma of uterus in a cat. *Curr Res Univ Agric Sci (Bangalore)* 4:156–158, 1975.
41. Belter LF, Crawford EM, Bates HR: Endometrial adenocarcinoma in a cat. *Pathol Vet* 5:429–431, 1968.
42. Berkin S, Tekeli Ö, Ünsüren H: Bir kedide uterusun mezensimal-mix tümörü. *A Ü Vet Fak Derg* 29:219–226, 1982.
43. Preiser H: Endometrial adenocarcinoma in a cat. *Pathol Vet* 1:485–490, 1964.
44. Minke JMHM, Hensen EJ, Misdorp W: Uterine carcinomas in mother cats after intrafetal inoculation of allogeneic tumor cells (K248 C and P). *Vet Immunol Immunopathol* 46:361–366, 1995.
45. O'Rouke MD, Geib LW: Endometrial adenocarcinoma in a cat. *Cornell Vet* 60:598–604, 1970.
46. Sorribas CE: Submucous uterine fibroma in a cat. *Mod Vet Pract.* 68:493, 1987.
47. Nava GA, Sbernardour U: Distocia materna nella gatta da leiomioma del corpo dell'utero. *Clin Vet Rassegna Polizia Sanitaria Higiene* 90:521–525, 1967.
48. Fukui K, Matsuda H: Uterine haemangioma in a cat. *Vet Rec* 113:375, 1983.
49. Lombard LS, Witte EJ: Frequency and types of tumors in mammals and birds of the Philadelphia Zoological Garden. *Cancer Res* 19:127–141, 1959.
50. Linnehan RM, Edwards JL: Endometrial adenocarcinoma in a Bengal tiger (Panthera tigris bengalensis) implanted with melengestrol acetate. *J Zoo Anim Med* 22:130–134, 1991.
51. Kollias GV, Calderwood-Mays MB, Short BG: Diabetes mellitus and abdominal adenocarcinoma in a jaguar receiving megestrol acetate. *JAVMA* 185:1383–1386, 1984.
52. Munson L, Stokes JE, Harrenstein LA: Uterine cancer in zoo felids on progestin contraceptives. *Vet Pathol* 32:578, 1995.
53. Frazier KS, Hines II ME, Ruiz C, et al: Immunohistochemical differentiation of multiple metastatic neoplasia in a jaguar (Panthera onca). *J Zoo Wildl Med* 25:286–293, 1994.
54. Winter H, Göltenboth R: Metastasierendes leiomyofibrosarkom bei einem nebelparder (Felis nebulosa Griff.). *Kleintierpraxis* 24:199–201, 1979.
55. Wolke RE: Vaginal leiomyoma as a cause of chronic constipation in the cat. *JAVMA* 143:1103–1105, 1963.
56. Patnaik AK: Histologic and immunohistochemical studies of granular cell tumors in seven dogs, three cats, one horse, and one bird. *Vet Pathol* 30:176–185, 1993.
57. Kollias GV, Bellah JR, Calderwood-Mays M, et l: Vaginal myxoma causing urethral and colonic obstruction in a tiger. *JAVMA* 187:1261–1262, 1985.

Chapter 55

Feline mammary neoplasias

FELINE MAMMARY FIBROADENOMATOSIS

(Synonyms include pericanalicular fibroadenoma, total fibroadenomatous change, benign mammary hypertrophy, mammary adenomatosis, fibroglandular hypertrophy, fibroepithelial hyperplasia, and fibroadenomatous hypertrophy)

Clinical presentation

- This uncommon condition is due to a very rapid proliferation of ectopic endometrium within the myometrium that causes enlargement of the uterus.
- Usually seen in young, intact females including some that are pregnant, or those cats of either sex treated with progestins.
- Younger cats usually have multiple affected glands with discoloration of overlying skin, whereas older cats often have hypertrophy of only one or two mammary glands, often in the inguinal region.
- May be painful.

Staging and diagnosis

- Minimum data base (MDB): includes a CBC, biochemical profile, urinalysis, FIV/FeLV serology, T4 testing, biopsy, three-view thoracic radiographs or computerized tomography of the chest. Cats with this condition may have a coagulopathy and may be best assessed with a coagulation profile.
- Ultrasonography and radiographic imaging of the tumor is not done commonly, but it could determine the extent of the disease.

Treatment

This section is divided into two options:

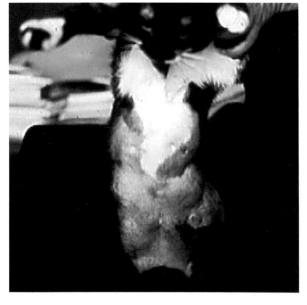

Figure 55-1: This young, intact female cat presented for dramatic enlargement of the mammary glands. A biopsy confirmed the presence of fibroepithelial hyperplasia. While some insist that this condition will resolve after an ovariohysterectomy or ovariectomy via a flank approach, others insist that the disorder of young, intact female cats will resolve on their own with time. Analgesics are often indicated, as they can be quite painful. Reprinted with permission from: Ogilvie GK, Moore AS. *Feline Oncology: A Comprehensive Guide for Compassionate Care.* Trenton NJ, Veterinary Learning Systems. 2002.

- Comfort for those who want to improve quality of life.
- Comfort and control for those who want to improve quality of life while trying to provide some control of the tumor.

Comfort

- Therapy to enhance comfort that is often present (e.g.: NSAID, tramadol, buprenorphine) and freedom from nausea, vomiting (e.g.: maropitant and/or metoclopramide), diarrhea (e.g.: metronidazole) and lack of appetite (e.g.: mirtazapine or cyproheptadine), although these are rarely seen.

Comfort and control

Above mentioned therapy for comfort plus:
- Ovariohysterectomy or ovariectomy is usually curative, however the rate of regression is slow. Some believe that these regress without therapy. Mastectomies are often associated with a high rate of complications and are not required to treat this condition.

FELINE BENIGN MAMMARY TUMORS

Clinical presentation

- Quite uncommon.
- Adenomas, intraductal papillomas and benign mixed mammary tumors have been described. Because they are often indistinguishable from the more common malignant mammary tumors, all mammary tumors should be assessed as if they were malignant.
- May be painful.

Staging and diagnosis

- Minimum data base (MDB): includes a CBC, biochemical profile, urinalysis, FIV/FeLV serology, T4 testing, biopsy, three-view thoracic radiographs or computerized tomography of the chest.
- Ultrasonography or radiographs to assess for intra-abdominal disease and to determine the extent of the local tumor may be helpful in some cases.
- Any solitary mammary tumor in a cat should be staged as if it were a malignant tumor before proceeding with surgical excision.

Treatment

This section is divided into two options:
- Comfort for those who want to improve quality of life.
- Comfort and control for those who want to improve quality of life while trying to provide some control of the tumor.

Comfort

- Therapy to enhance comfort (e.g.: NSAID, tramadol, buprenorphine) and freedom from nausea, vomiting (e.g.: maropitant and/or metoclopramide), diarrhea (e.g.: metronidazole) and lack of appetite (e.g.: mirtazapine or cyproheptadine).

Comfort and control

Above mentioned therapy for comfort plus:
- Mastectomy. If surgical excision is complete and the lesion is benign, no further treatment is necessary. Veterinary examinations should be scheduled every 6 months to check for recurrence or new, potentially malignant tumors.

FELINE MALIGNANT MAMMARY TUMORS

Clinical presentation

- Quite common in older unsprayed cats, or cats that were spayed late in life.
- Male cats uncommonly develop mammary tumors unless they are treated with progestins.
- Adenocarcinomas and solid carcinomas are the most common type, followed by mixed mammary tumors[6] and mammary sarcomas, the latter of which may be slow to metastasize.[19-22]
- Often large at the time of diagnosis, with one study confirming a median of 3 cm[3] with some tumors up to 13 cm[3].[24]
- Approximately half of the tumors are ulcerated at the time of presentation.[24,38,39]
- Axillary and inguinal lymph node metastasis is common, with even normal sized lymph nodes being infiltrated in approximately 27% of cats.[24]
- Ovariohysterectomy but not parity may prevent mammary tumor development, with one study suggesting that the relative risk for a spayed female developing mammary carcinoma was approximately half that of an intact cat.[17]
- Purebred cats, especially Siamese and Persian cats, may be at increased risk.[6,15,17, 2425,28,29]
- The post excisional survival period of affected cats is inversely proportional to tumor size, with cats with tumors greater than 3 cm in diameter had a 12-month median survival period, whereas those with tumors less than 3 cm in diameter had a 21-month survival period.
- Other prognostic factors for a favorable outcome include domestic shorthair breeds, increasing youth, absence of metastases, a well differentiated tumor (low mitotic count, nuclear and cellular pleomorphism, and tubule formation), lack of lymphovascular invasion, low AgNOR and Ki67 scores, and complete resection.
- May be painful.

Key point

Almost every tumor in the mammary gland of a cat must be considered as a malignant condition worthy of detailed staging and swift, definitive therapy.

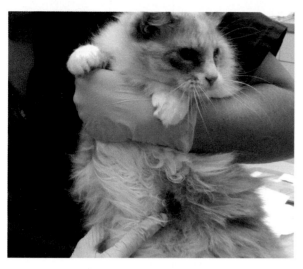

Figure 55-2: This 10 year old, intact female cat was presented on emergency for a raised, red, draining mass near a left first mammary gland. Chest radiographs and blood work were within normal limits and fine needle aspiration confirmed the presence of a carcinoma. The size of the tumor at the time of diagnosis can be very predictive of outcome.

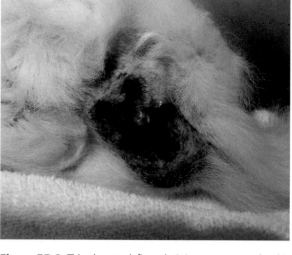

Figure 55-3: This ulcerated, firm, draining mammary gland is quite characteristic of a mammary adenocarcinoma. Cytology or a biopsy (excisional or incisional) can be used to confirm the diagnosis. A complete examination should be done in each case, to include careful palpation of all mammary glands and the regional axillary or inguinal lymph nodes.

Staging and diagnosis

- Minimum data base (MDB): includes a CBC, biochemical profile, urinalysis, FIV/FeLV serology, T4 testing, biopsy of regional lymph nodes and three-view thoracic radiographs or computerized tomography of the chest.
  - Necropsy revealed evidence of metastases in 120 of 129 cats that had undergone surgery to treat mammary carcinoma with axillary or inguinal lymph nodes affected in more than 80% of cats, while the sternal node was involved in 30% of cats. The majority of cats with sternal lymph node involvement also had pleural or pulmonary metastases.[43,44]
- Since metastases to the spleen, kidney, adrenal gland, peritoneal surfaces, and heart have been reported[6,15,16,38-40] abdominal ultrasonography, computerized tomography, or magnetic resonance imaging may be wise.

Key point

Chest radiographs and aspirates of any and all enlarged lymph nodes must be considered.

Treatment

This section is divided into three options:
- Comfort for those who want to improve quality of life.
- Comfort and control for those who want to improve quality of life while trying to provide some control of the tumor.

- Comfort and longer-term control for those who want to improve quality of life while trying to maximize the chance of controlling the tumor.

Comfort

- Therapy to enhance comfort (e.g.: NSAID, tramadol, buprenorphine) and freedom from nausea, vomiting (e.g.: maropitant and/or metoclopramide), diarrhea (e.g.: metronidazole) and lack of appetite (e.g.: mirtazapine or cyproheptadine).

Key point

Removal of the entire mammary chain that contains the tumor and the regional lymph nodes, if available, is recommended for cats with mammary tumors.

Comfort and control

Above mentioned therapy for comfort plus:
- Complete removal of the entire mammary chain with wide margins is the standard of care, however it is unlikely to be curative due to high rate of lymphatic invasion but may be palliative.[16]
  - The surgeon should submit the entire specimen for histologic review to ensure that complete margins have been obtained.[16]
  - When conservative surgery (removing only the affected gland and adjacent tissue) was compared with radical surgery (unilateral or bilateral mastectomy), there was no difference in survival between the two groups,[26,28] however

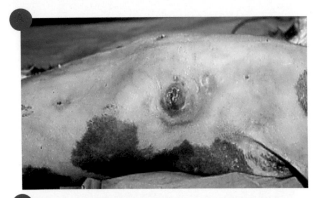

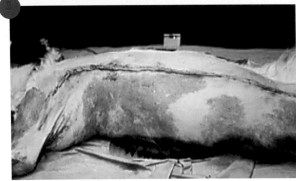

Figure 55-4: The patient with the mammary tumor is prepared for surgery by identifying all palpable tumor within the mammary tissue and by ensuring that there are no metastatic lesions in the lung, regional lymph nodes or elsewhere. If any one gland on one side is involved, that entire chain is removed. If there are tumors on the left and the right mammary chains, a unilateral mastectomy may need to be done to allow the skin to stretch adequately to allow a second radical mastectomy to be successfully performed several weeks later.

there was a marked difference in recurrence rates (0% and 43.4%, respectively). Given that recurrence is associated with a greater cost to the client due to additional therapy, including surgery, doing the more definitive radical surgery is definitely recommended.

- Survey data and histologic features for 108 carcinomas from 97 cats were analyzed with respect to overall survival and confirmed a median survival time of 31 months for cats with grade I tumors, 14 months for cats with grade II tumors, and 8 months for cats with grade III tumors.[27]
- Cats with World Health Organization stage II or III mammary carcinoma that were treated by radical full-chain mastectomy had no recurrence a median of 10.4 months after surgery; median survival time was 21.3 months.[55]

Comfort and longer term control

Above mentioned therapy for comfort and control plus:

- Chemotherapy, with most studies suggesting that doxorubicin may be the drug of choice, however mitoxantrone, carboplatin, cyclophosphamide, and paclitaxel may have efficacy. Radiation therapy unproven but may improve local control.
  - Twenty-six cats received five doses of doxorubicin (1 mg/kg IV every 3 weeks) following surgery, with the overall median survival being 25 to 41 weeks.[56] Cats with stage II disease that had not been previously treated with surgery appeared to be most benefitted, as they had the longest survival times (median 73 weeks).
  - In another study, 14 cats with measurable tumors were treated with doxorubicin (30 mg/m^2 IV every 2 weeks) for five treatments following biopsy. Nine cats had a partial response and 2 cats had some reduction in tumor size.[57] The cats lived 10 to 61 weeks (median, 31 weeks).
  - Doxorubicin (30 mg/m^2 IV every 3 weeks) was combined with cyclophosphamide (100 mg/m^2 daily for 4 days) to treat 14 cats with inoperable or metastatic mammary carcinomas. Three cats with lung metastases had a complete response to treatment for 26 to 49 weeks, and 2 cats had shorter partial responses (one for 7 and the other for 21 weeks).[25]
  - In yet another study evaluating the benefit of doxorubicin therapy, 37 cats treated with surgery alone were compared to 36 treated with surgery plus doxorubicin chemotherapy. While not statistically significant, the median disease-free survival in the surgery group was 372 days versus 676 days in the group of cats with surgery for the mammary cancer plus doxorubicin. The median survival times were 1,406 and 848 days, respectively. Cats that underwent a unilateral radical mastectomy had a survival time that was significantly longer for the surgery + chemotherapy compared to those who just had surgery (1,998 versus 414 days).[30]
  - Other investigators confirmed that the Kaplan-Meier median survival time of cats that received surgery and doxorubicin was 448 days, whereas the Kaplan-Meier median DFI was 255 days.[31]
  - Data from cats treated with mastectomy with or without carboplatin chemotherapy was assessed. Patients treated with surgery and chemotherapy presented a longer overall survival than those treated only with surgery.[32]

References

1. Nimmo JS, Plummer JM: Ultrastructural studies of fibro-adenomatous hyperplasia of mammary glands of 2 cats. *J Comp Pathol* 91:41–50, 1981.
2. Hayden DW, Johnson KH, Ghobrial HK: Ultrastructure of feline mammary hypertrophy. *Vet Pathol* 20:254–264, 1983.
3. Hinton M, Gaskell CJ: Non-neoplastic mammary hypertrophy in the cat associated either with pregnancy or with oral progesterone therapy. *Vet Rec* 100:277–280, 1977.
4. Hayden DW, Johnston SD, Kiang DT, et al: Feline mammary hypertrophy/fibroadenoma complex: clinical and hormonal aspects. *Am J Vet Res* 42:1699–1701, 1981.
5. Bostock DE: Canine and feline mammary neoplasms. *Br Vet J* 142:506–515, 1986.

6. Carpenter JL, Andrews LK, Holzworth J: Tumors and tumor-like lesions. In Holzworth J (ed): *Diseases of the Cat. Medicine and Surgery*. Philadelphia, WB Saunders, 1987, pp 407–596.
7. Bloom F, Allen HL: Feline mammary hypertrophy. *Vet Pathol* 11:561, 1974.
8. Allen HL: Feline mammary hypertrophy. *Vet Pathol* 10:501–508, 1973.
9. Graham TC, Wilson J: Mammary adenoma associated with pregnancy in the cat. *Vet Med Small Anim Clin* 67:82–84, 1972.
10. Seiler RJ, Kelly WR, Menrath VH, Barbero RD: Total fibroadenomatous change of the mammary glands of two spayed cats. *Feline Pract* 9:25–29, 1979.
11. Hayes AA, Mooney S: Feline mammary tumors. *Vet Clin North Am Small Anim Pract* 15:513–520, 1985.
12. Norris PJ, Blunden A: Fibro-adenoma of the mammary glands in a kitten. *Vet Rec* 104:233, 1979.
13. Preziosi R, Sarli G, Benazzi C, Marcato PS: Detection of proliferating cell nuclear antigen (PCNA) in canine and feline mammary tumors. *J Comp Pathol* 113:301–313, 1995.
14. Mandel M: Benign mammary hypertrophy. *Vet Med Small Anim Clin* 70:846–847, 1975.
15. Hayden DW, Nielsen SW: Feline mammary tumours. *J Small Anim Pract* 12:687–697, 1971.
16. Nielsen SW: The malignancy of mammary tumors in cats. *North Am Vet* 33:245–252, 1952.
17. Hayes Jr HM, Milne KL, Mandell CP: Epidemiological features of feline mammary carcinoma. *Vet Rec* 108:476–479, 1981.
18. Rutteman GR, Blankenstein MA, Minke J, Misdorp W: Steroid receptors in mammary tumours of the cat. *Acta Endocrinologica* 125:32–37, 1991.
19. Hayden DW, Ghobrial HK, Johnson KH, Buoen LC: Feline mammary sarcoma composed of cells resembling myofibroblasts. *Vet Pathol* 23:118–124, 1986.
20. Überreiter VO: Die tumoren der mamma bei hund und katze. *Wien Tierärztl Mschr* 8:481–503, 1968.
21. Überreiter VO: Die tumoren der mamma bei hund und katze. *Wien Tierärztl Mschr* 415–442, 1968.
22. Hampe JF, Misdorp W: Tumours and dysplasias of the mammary gland. *Bull WHO* 50:111–133, 1974.
23. Castagnaro M, Casalone C, Bozzetta E, et al: Tumour grading and the one-year post-surgical prognosis in feline mammary carcinomas. *J Comp Pathol* 119:263–275, 1998.
24. Weijer K, Hart AAM: Prognostic factors in feline mammary carcinoma. *J Natl Cancer Inst* 70:709–716, 1983.
25. Jeglum KA, deGuzman E, Young KM: Chemotherapy of advanced mammary adenocarcinoma in 14 cats. *JAVMA* 187:157–160, 1985.
26. Ito T, Kadosawa T, Mochizuki M, et al: Prognosis of malignant mammary tumor in 53 cats. *J Vet Med Sci* 58:723–726, 1996.
27. Mills SW, Musil KM, Davies JL, et al: Prognostic value of histologic grading for feline mammary carcinoma: a retrospective survival analysis. *Vet Pathol*. 52(2):238-349, 2015.
28. MacEwen EG, Hayes AA, Harvey HJ, et al: Prognostic factors for feline mammary tumors. *JAVMA* 185:201–204, 1984.
29. Feldman DG, Gross L: Electron microscopic study of spontaneous mammary carcinomas in cats and dogs: Virus-like particles in cat mammary carcinomas. *Cancer Res* 31:1261–1267, 1971.
30. McNeill CJ, Sorenmo KU, Shofer FS, et al: Evaluation of adjuvant doxorubicin-based chemotherapy for the treatment of feline mammary carcinoma. *J Vet Intern Med*. 23(1):123-129, 2009.
31. Novosad CA, Bergman PJ, O'Brien MG, et al: Retrospective evaluation of adjunctive doxorubicin for the treatment of feline mammarygland adenocarcinoma: 67 cases. *JAAHA* 42(2):110-120, 2006..
32. De Campos CB, Nunes FC, Lavalle GE, Cassali GD. Use of surgery and carboplatin in feline malignant mammary gland neoplasms with advanced clinical staging. *In Vivo* 28(5):863-866, 2014.
33. Misdorp W, Weijer K: Animal model: Feline mammary carcinoma. *Am J Pathol* 98:57–576, 1980.
34. Hernandez FJ, Chertack M, Gage PA: Feline mammary carcinoma and progestogens. *Feline Pract* 5:4–48, 1975.
35. Hamilton JM, Else RW, Forshaw P: Oestrogen receptors in feline mammary carcinomas. *Vet Rec* 99:47–479, 1976.
36. Elling H, Ungemach FR: Progesterone receptors in feline mammary cancer cytosol. *J Cancer Res Oncol* 100:32–327, 1981.
37. MacEwen EG, Hayes AA, Mooney S, et al: Evaluation of effect of levamisole on feline mammary cancer. *J Biol Resp Modif* 5:54–546, 1984.
38. Atasever A., Kul O: Metastase eines mammakarzinoms im zentralnervensystem bei einer katze. *Dtsch Tierärztk Wschr* 103:47–474, 1996.
39. Waters DJ, Honeckman A, Cooley DM, DeNicola D: Skeletal metastasis in feline mammary carcinoma: Case report and literature review. *JAAHA* 34:10–108, 1998.
40. Field EH: A contribution of the study of malignant growths in the lower animals. *JAMA* 23:98–985, 1894.
41. Silver IA: Symposium on mammary neoplasia in the dog and cat—I. The anatomy of the mammary gland of the dog and cat. *J Small Anim Pract* 7:68–696, 1966.
42. Wilcock BP, Peiffer Jr RJ, Davidson MG: The causes of glaucoma in cats. *Vet Pathol* 27:3–40, 1990.
43. Weijer K, Head KW, Misdorp W, Hampe JF: Feline malignant mammary tumors. I. Morphology and biology: Some comparisons with human and canine mammary carcinomas. *J Natl Cancer Inst* 49:169–1704, 1972.
44. Weijer K, Hampe JF, Misdorp W: Mammary carcinoma in the cat. A model in comparative cancer research. *Arch Chirurgicum Neerlandicum* 25:41–425, 1973.
45. Katsurada F, Okino T: Uber krebs bei katzen. *Jap J Cancer Res* 32:34–348, 1938.
46. Kas NP, van der Heul RO, Misdorp W: Metastatic bone neoplasms in dogs, cats and a lion (with some comparative remarks on the situation in man). *Zbl Vet Med (A)* 17:90–919, 1970.
47. DeVico G, Maiolino P: Prognostic value of nuclear morphometry in feline mammary carcinomas. *J Comp Pathol* 114:9–105, 1997.
48. Della Salda L, Sarli G, Benazzi C, Marcato PS: Giant cells in anaplastic mammary carcinoma of the dog and cat. *J Comp Pathol* 109:34–360, 1993.
49. Tateyama S, Shibata I, Yamaguchi R, et al: Participation of myofibroblasts in feline mammary carcinoma. *Jpn J Vet Sci* 50:104–1054, 1988.
50. Scanziani E, Mandelli G: Contributo allo studio della classificazione dei tumori mammari felini—Histologic classification of feline mammary tumors. *Alti-della Societa, Italiana-della Scienze Veterinarie* 39:55–554, 1986.
51. Ivanyi D, Minke JMHM, Hageman C, et al: Cytokeratins as markers of initial stages of squamous metaplasia in feline mammary carcinomas. *Am J Vet Res* 54:109–1102, 1993.
52. de las Mulas JM, del los Monteros AE, Bautista MJ, et al: Immunohistochemical distribution pattern of intermediate filament proteins and muscle actin in feline and human mammary carcinomas. *J Comp Pathol* 111:36–381, 1994.
53. De Vico G, Maiolino P, Restucci B: Silver-stained nucleolar (Ag-NOR) cluster size in feline mammary carcinomas: lack of correlation with histological appearance, mitotic activity, tumour stage, and degree of nuclear atypia. *J Comp Pathol* 113:6–73, 1995.
54. Castagnaro M, Casalone C, Ru G, et al: Argyrophilic nucleolar organiser regions (AgNORs) count as indicator of pos-surgical prognosis in feline mammary carcinomas. *Res Vet Sci* 64:97–100, 1998.
55. Fox LE, MacEwen EG, Kurzman ID, et al: L-MTP-PE treatment of feline mammary adenocarcinoma. *Proc 14th Annu Conf Vet Cancer Soc.*107–108, 1994.
56. Mauldin GE, Mooney SC, Patnaik AK, Mauldin GN: Adjuvant doxorubicin for feline mammary adenocarcinoma. *Proc 14th Annu Conf Vet Cancer Soc.*41, 1994.
57. Stolwijk JAM, Minke JMHM, Rutteman GR, et al: Feline mammary carcinomas as a model for human breast cancer. II. Comparison of in vivo and in vitro Adriamycin sensitivity. *Anticancer Res* 9:1045–1048, 1989.
58. Misdorp W: Incomplete surgery, local immunostimulation, and recurrence of some tumour types in dogs and cats. *Vet Q* 9:279–286, 1987.
59. Hruban Z, Carter WE, Meehan T, et al: Complex mammary carcinoma in a tiger (Panthera tigris*). J Zoo Anim Med* 19:226–230, 1988.
60. Harrenstien LA, Munson L, Seal US: Mammary cancer in captive wild felids and risk factors for its development: A retrospective study of the clinical behavior of 31 cases. *J Zoo Wildl Med* 27:468–476, 1996.
61. Frazier KS, Hines II ME, Ruiz C, et al: Immunohistochemical differentiation of multiple metastatic neoplasia in a jaguar (Panthera onca*). J Zoo Wildl Med* 25:286–293, 1994.
62. Gillette EL, Acland HM, Klein L: Ductular mammary carcinoma in a lioness. *JAVMA* 173:1099–1102, 1978.
63. Munson L, Stokes JE, Harrenstein LA: Uterine cancer in zoo felids on progestin contraceptives. *Vet Pathol* 32:578, 1995.
64. Chandra S, Laughlin DC: Virus-like particles in cystic mammary adenoma of a snow leopard. *Cancer Res* 35:3069–3074, 1975.

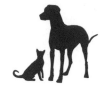

Chapter 56

Feline tumors of the respiratory tract

FELINE NASOPHARYNGEAL POLYPS

Clinical presentation

- Usually young cats (<2 years of age).
- Cough, gagging after eating, nasal signs, or otic discharge, sneezing, snuffling, and stertor; often mild but progressive. [1,3,6,8]
- Large polyps may cause ventral deviation of the soft palate.
- Rarely bilateral.
- Peripheral vestibular disease may be present.
- Rarely uncomfortable.

Staging and diagnosis

- MDB; otic and oral examination; skull radiographs including bullae; CT or MRI scan of the head, including the bullae if radiographs equivocal. Endoscopy of nasopharynx and otic examination with biopsy. One approach to more adequately visualize the polyp is to use a spay hook to pull the soft palate forward.
  - CT was shown by one set of investigators[9] to be an excellent imaging tool for the supportive diagnosis of nasopharyngeal polyps in cats. CT findings of a well-defined mass with strong rim enhancement, mass-associated stalk-like structure, and asymmetric tympanic bulla wall thickening with pathologic expansion of the tympanic bullae are highly indicative of an inflammatory polyp.

> **Key point**
> Staging should include an evaluation of bulla involvement via skull radiographs or CT imaging. Involvement of the bullae provides reasoning to surgically address this involvement with a bulla osteotomy.

Treatment

Initial

- The polyp is grasped and pulled via gentle, uniform traction.
- A bulla osteotomy, drainage and bacteriologic culture and sensitivity sampling should be performed if there are signs or images confirming tympanic bulla involvement.[3,7,10]
  - One study in cats confirmed that cats that have a ventral bulla osteotomy for removal of inflammatory polyps or masses is unlikely to affect hearing as measured via air-conducted brainstem auditory evoked response. They also showed that cats developed short-term Horner's syndrome.[10]
- A lateral ear resection may be required when polyps involve the otic canal.[4]
- Most cats are cured with appropriate therapy.
  - Regrowth following surgery was noted in only 6 of 31 cats in one series.[3]

FELINE INTRA-NASAL TUMORS

Clinical presentation

- Moderately common.
- Benign nasal tumors include adenomas, fibromas, fibropapillomas, chondromas are quite rare.
- Malignant nasal tumors include the more common adenocarcinoma, undifferentiated carcinoma, squamous cell carcinoma and lymphoma (discussed below). Sarcomas are uncommon.
- Nasal discharge, epiphora, facial deformity and epistaxis are less common than snuffling, and sneezing. Seizures due to intracranial invasion are rare.
- May be painful.

Staging and diagnosis

- Minimum data base (MDB): includes a CBC, biochemical profile, urinalysis, FIV/FeLV serology, T4 testing, transnostril biopsy, needle aspirate of regional lymph nodes and three-view thoracic radiographs or computerized tomography of the chest. Titers for cryptococcus may be helpful in ruling out this differential.
- Skull radiographs are less valuable than computerized tomography or magnetic resonance imaging of the skull, and thus the tumor.
- Obtaining a biopsy through the nostril via curettage, biopsy cup, endoscopic biopsy or high pressure saline nasal lavage is recommended. Obtaining a biopsy through the skin is not encouraged, as radiation dosage to the skin at the region of the incision would be high, resulting in increased morbidity.

Treatment

This section is divided into three options:
- Comfort for those who want to improve quality of life.
- Comfort and control for those who want to improve quality of life while trying to provide some control of the tumor.
- Comfort and longer-term control for those who want to improve quality of life while trying to maximize the chance of controlling the tumor.

Comfort

- Therapy to enhance comfort (e.g.: NSAID, tramadol, buprenorphine) and freedom from nausea, vomiting (e.g.: maropitant and/or metoclopramide), diarrhea (e.g.: metronidazole) and lack of appetite (e.g.: mirtazapine or cyproheptadine).

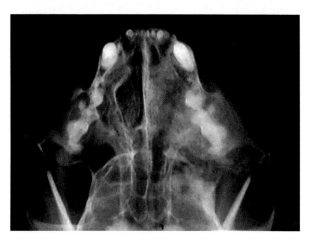

Figure 56-1: While CT or MRI are the diagnostic methods of choice for nasal or skull tumors, radiographs are practical and cost effective. This image shows a highly destructive lesion of the left nasal cavity and the surrounding structures. A biopsy or an aspirate are required to determine the underlying cause of this destructive disease (infectious, inflammatory, neoplastic or other causes). Imaging courtesy of Lenore Anderson Mohammadian, DVM, MSpVM, Diplomate ACVR.

Comfort and control

Above mentioned therapy for comfort plus:
- Radiation, either definitive or palliative.
  - Radiation therapy markedly improved the prognosis for most cats. Surgical debulking of the tumor followed by orthovoltage radiation to doses of 25 to 50 Gy was used to treat six cats with nasal carcinoma.[21] No recurrence was seen in four cats. One was still alive 26 months after treatment and another died without evidence of tumor 40 months after treatment.
  - The median overall survival time and progression-free survival in 65 cats with tumors treated with palliative hypofractionated radiation therapy were 432 days and 229 days, respectively.[19] No significant difference between overall survival time of cats with nasal lymphoma and that of cats with other tumors was observed.

Comfort and longer-term control

Above mentioned therapy for comfort plus:
- Chemotherapy. Carboplatin likely to be the most effective.

FELINE OLFACTORY NEUROBLASTOMA

Clinical presentation

- Quite uncommon.
- Sneezing, dyspnea, unilateral nasal discharge, wheezing, and cough have been described.[28,29]

- Many cats in the past have been FeLV-positive.
- Responses to therapy are generally short-term.
- May be painful.

Staging and diagnosis

- Minimum data base (MDB): includes a CBC, biochemical profile, urinalysis, FIV/FeLV serology, T4 testing, biopsy, three-view thoracic radiographs or computerized tomography of the chest.
- Radiographs may be of some help, however computerized tomography or magnetic resonance imaging of the head, and thus the tumor, is important.

Treatment

This section is divided into three options:
- Comfort for those who want to improve quality of life.
- Comfort and control for those who want to improve quality of life while trying to provide some control of the tumor.
- Comfort and longer-term control for those who want to improve quality of life while trying to maximize the chance of controlling the tumor.

Comfort

- Therapy to enhance comfort (e.g.: NSAID, tramadol, buprenorphine) and freedom from nausea, vomiting (e.g.: maropitant and/or metoclopramide), diarrhea (e.g.: metronidazole) and lack of appetite (e.g.: mirtazapine or cyproheptadine).

Comfort and control

Above mentioned therapy for comfort plus:
- Palliative radiation, especially for those with extension into surrounding structures or regional metastases (e.g.: 2-5 dosages of radiation), to first enhance comfort, second, to reduce the rate of growth and third, occasionally to reduce the size of the tumor.

Comfort and longer-term control

Above mentioned therapy for comfort plus:
- Definitive radiation therapy.

FELINE NASAL LYMPHOMA

Clinical presentation

- Moderately common.
- In a survey investigating the causes of nasopharyngeal disease in cats, lymphoma, seen in 26 of 53 (49%) cats, was the most common diagnosis.[31]
- Most common clinical signs include nasal discharge, dyspnea, epistaxis, stertor, facial

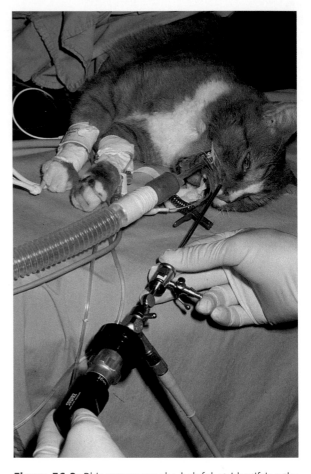

Figure 56-2: Rhinoscopy may be helpful at identifying the location of an intranasal disease or disorder and to obtain specific biopsies, aspirates or cultures.

deformity, anorexia, epiphora, exophthalmos, and sneezing.[34]
- Rarely involves tissues outside the nasal cavity, including the retropharyngeal tissue, chest or abdomen, however that should be considered during staging.
- Usually not painful.

Staging and diagnosis

- Minimum data base (MDB): includes a CBC, biochemical profile, urinalysis, bone marrow aspirate, abdominal ultrasound, FIV/FeLV serology, T4 testing, biopsy, three-view thoracic radiographs or computerized tomography of the chest.
- Skull radiographs may be helpful, however computerized tomography or magnetic resonance imaging of the head, and thus the tumor, is preferable.
- Obtaining a biopsy through the nostril via curettage, biopsy cup, endoscopic biopsy or

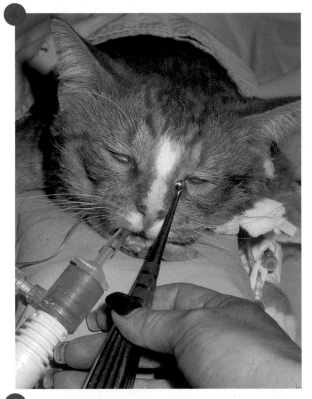

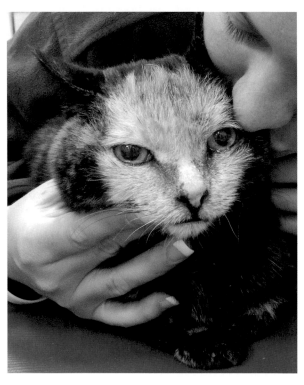

Figure 56-4: Cats with localized intranasal lymphoma respond well to radiation therapy and/or chemotherapy. If radiation is employed, the skin and hair color may be changed in the irradiated field, as depicted here.

brushings or high pressure saline nasal lavage is recommended. Obtaining a biopsy through the skin is not encouraged, as radiation dosage to the skin at the region of the incision would be high, resulting in increased morbidity.

Key point

Cats with nasal lymphoma should be staged to determine if the disease has spread to the liver, spleen, lymph nodes and marrow.

Treatment

This section is divided into two options:
- Comfort for those who want to improve quality of life.
- Comfort and control for those who want to improve quality of life while trying to provide some control of the tumor.

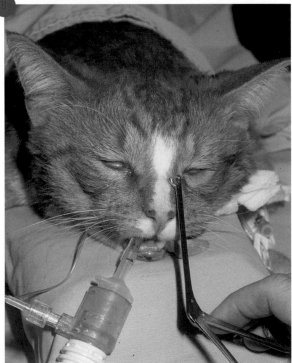

Figure 56-3: Once the location of the intranasal disease or disorder has been identified, a biopsy can be obtained with a curette or a cup biopsy instrument. Regardless of the method used, to reduce the risk of damaging the brain, the biopsy instrument is never advanced beyond the level of the medial canthus of the eye.

Key point

Most cats with nasal lymphoma respond quite well to radiation therapy and/or systemic chemotherapy.

Comfort

- Therapy to enhance comfort (e.g.: NSAID OR prednisolone, tramadol, buprenorphine) and freedom from nausea, vomiting (e.g.: maropitant and/or metoclopramide), diarrhea (e.g.: metronidazole) and lack of appetite (e.g.: mirtazapine or cyproheptadine).

Comfort and control

Above mentioned therapy for comfort plus:
- Radiation therapy or chemotherapy alone or in combination is equally effective for nasal disease, but chemotherapy is needed for cats with systemic disease. Long survivals possible in FeLV-negative cats.
  - Coarse fractionated radiation therapy may have the same efficacy as conventional fractionation in the treatment of feline nasal lymphoma.[38]
  - The median overall survival time and progression-free survival in 65 cats with tumors treated with palliative hypofractionated radiation therapy was 432 days and 229 days, respectively. No significant difference between overall survival time of cats with nasal lymphoma and that of cats with other tumors was observed.[19]
  - The records of 19 cats treated for stage I nasal lymphoma with megavoltage radiation therapy (median dose = 42 Gy) and combination chemotherapy given over 6 months were reviewed to confirm a median progression-free interval for all cats being 945 days (31 months).[21]
  - Cats with nasal lymphoma achieving a complete remission in response to combination chemotherapy had a survival time of 749 days.[24]

FELINE LARYNGEAL TUMORS

Clinical presentation

- Uncommon.
- Lymphoma, SCC, and adenocarcinoma predominate.
  - Lymphoma should always be considered a systemic disease and should be evaluated as such.
  - SCC may appear as an annular constriction that is invasive deep into laryngeal tissues and the surrounding pharynx in most cats.[14,42,46]
  - Cats with laryngeal adenocarcinoma may have clinical evidence of metastases to the cervical lymph nodes, lungs, spleen, and adrenal glands.[48]
- Dyspnea progressing to respiratory distress with or without dysphonia.
- May be painful.

Staging and diagnosis

- Minimum data base (MDB): includes a CBC, biochemical profile, urinalysis, FIV/FeLV serology, T4 testing, laryngeal ultrasonography or endoscopy, abdominal ultrasonography, bone marrow aspirate, lymph node evaluation, biopsy of the tumor, and three-view thoracic radiographs or computerized tomography of the chest.
  - Ultrasound-guided biopsy may be less invasive than the intraluminal route to confirm a diagnosis of laryngeal neoplasia.[44]
- Radiographs or ultrasound of the cervical region may not be as helpful as computerized tomography or magnetic resonance imaging of that region.

Treatment

This section is divided into three options:
- Comfort for those who want to improve quality of life.
- Comfort and control for those who want to improve quality of life while trying to provide some control of the tumor.
- Comfort and longer-term control for those who want to improve quality of life while trying to maximize the chance of controlling the tumor.

Comfort

- Therapy to enhance comfort (e.g.: NSAID or prednisolone, tramadol, buprenorphine) and freedom from nausea, vomiting (e.g.: maropitant and/or metoclopramide), diarrhea (e.g.: metronidazole) and lack of appetite (e.g.: mirtazapine or cyproheptadine).
- A tracheostomy may be necessary prior to definitive treatment if the cat is in acute respiratory distress.

Comfort and control

Above mentioned therapy for comfort plus:
- Palliative radiation, especially for those with extension into surrounding structures or regional metastases (e.g.: 2-5 dosages of radiation), to first enhance comfort, second, to reduce the rate of growth and third, occasionally to reduce the size of the tumor.

Comfort and longer-term control

Above mentioned therapy for comfort plus:
- Multimodal approach for cats with squamous cell carcinoma of the larynx including medical treatment (thalidomide, piroxicam and bleomycin), radiation therapy (accelerated, hypofractionated protocol) and surgery has been reported.[26] Treatment was well tolerated, with 3 cats alive and in complete remission at data analysis closure after 759, 458 and 362 days. Cats treated with surgery to provide immediate ability to breathe followed by chemotherapy and radiation therapy can be quite effective.

FELINE TRACHEAL TUMORS

Clinical presentation

- Uncommon.
- Lymphoma, squamous cell carcinoma most common, followed by oncocytomas or basal cell carcinomas.

- Coughing, dyspnea, cyanosis, increased respiratory sounds most prominent on inspiration. May be painful.

Staging and diagnosis

- Minimum data base (MDB): includes a CBC, biochemical profile, urinalysis, FIV/FeLV serology, T4 testing, biopsy via fiber optic tracheoscopy or trans-tracheal aspirates and three-view thoracic radiographs or preferably, computerized tomography of the chest.
- Radiographs or ultrasonography of trachea is good, however computerized tomography, or magnetic resonance imaging of the trachea, and thus the tumor, is preferable.

Treatment

This section is divided into three options:
- Comfort for those who want to improve quality of life.
- Comfort and control for those who want to improve quality of life while trying to provide some control of the tumor.
- Comfort and longer-term control for those who want to improve quality of life while trying to maximize the chance of controlling the tumor.

Comfort

- Therapy to enhance comfort (e.g.: NSAID or prednisolone if lymphoma, tramadol, buprenorphine) and freedom from nausea, vomiting (e.g.: maropitant and/or metoclopramide), diarrhea (e.g.: metronidazole) and lack of appetite (e.g.: mirtazapine or cyproheptadine).

Comfort and control

Above mentioned therapy for comfort plus:
- Palliative radiation, especially for those with extension into surrounding structures or regional metastases (e.g.: 2-5 dosages of radiation), to first enhance comfort, second, to reduce the rate of growth and third, occasionally to reduce the size of the tumor. This is most effective for the treatment of lymphoma.

Comfort and longer-term control

Above mentioned therapy for comfort plus:
- Tumor removal by tracheal resection and anastomosis.
  - Thoracotomy and tracheostomy were performed in three cats. One cat had an extensive infiltrative tumor and was euthanized.[52] Tracheal resection was performed in the other two in which a 2.5[51] or 3[53] cm length of trachea needed to be resected. There was no follow-up beyond surgical recovery in one cat,[51] but the other had no evidence of disease 1 year after surgery.

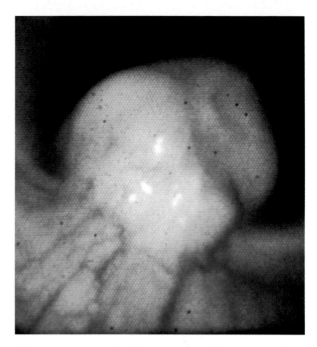

Figure 56-5: Tracheal tumors are often best imaged during tracheoscopy and/or CT imaging. A key aspect of imaging is to determine how extensive the mass is to ensure it can be cured with tracheal resection and anastomosis. An alternative to surgery is radiation therapy or endoscopic guided stenting or laser therapy.

- Definitive radiation may be helpful if there is evidence of tumor extending beyond the surgical margins or if the tumor is lymphoma (e.g.: 16-19 dosages of radiation).
- Multiagent CHOP chemotherapy may be helpful if the tumor is lymphoma. Carboplatin and/or doxorubicin chemotherapy may be helpful if the tumor is a carcinoma.

FELINE LUNG TUMORS

Clinical presentation

- Carcinomas are relatively common, followed by the rare occurrence of sarcomas and benign tumors such as adenoma[60,61] and adenomatosis.[62]
- Most affected cats are older with vague clinical signs such as anorexia, lethargy, weight loss, vomiting, and ataxia.[60,63,66]
- Metastases to the digits causing swelling, permanent exsheathment of multiple nails, paronychia, or cellulitis with loose claws is the cause of lameness in some cats,[64,70,72-76] while metastases to muscles may cause lameness in others.[69,77,78]
  - In a series of 64 cats with digital carcinomas, 56 had metastases from a pulmonary tumor and only 8 had a primary nailbed SCC.[80]
- Only half of the cats have clinical signs related to the respiratory tract.

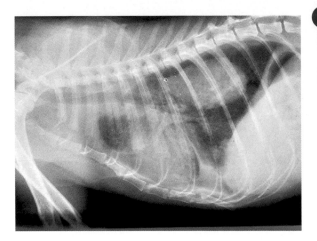

Figure 56-6: Radiograph of a cat with a primary lung tumor with evidence of a small amount of pleural effusion. Removal of the tumor and treatment with intracavitary chemotherapy such as carboplatin or mitoxantrone may be helpful. In general, the presence of pleural effusion is not a positive clinical finding.

- Paraneoplastic syndromes such as hypertrophic osteopathy, neurologic abnormalities and skin lesions are rare.

Staging and diagnosis

- Minimum data base (MDB): includes a CBC, biochemical profile, urinalysis, FIV/FeLV serology, T4 testing, and three-view thoracic radiographs or computerized tomography of the chest.
- Preoperative diagnosis may also be obtained by ultrasound-guided fine-needle aspiration, blind aspiration,[60] fluoroscopic-guided,[86] and by CT may be the most accurate for small or less peripheral lesions.[87]
- Pleural effusion is seen in up to one-third of cats[60,66] and may be severe.[14,60,61,63,66,70] In a series of 82 cats with pleural effusion of all causes, pulmonary carcinoma was confirmed to be the cause in 5 cats.[85] Cytologic examination of the effusion may be diagnostic for carcinoma and should thus be performed.
- Ultrasonography, radiographs or computerized tomography to assess for intra-abdominal disease or extent of the local tumor may be helpful in some cases.
- Any solitary lung tumor in a cat should be staged as if it were a malignant tumor before proceeding with surgical excision.

Treatment

This section is divided into three options:
- Comfort for those who want to improve quality of life.
- Comfort and control for those who want to improve quality of life while trying to provide some control of the tumor.
- Comfort and longer-term control for those who

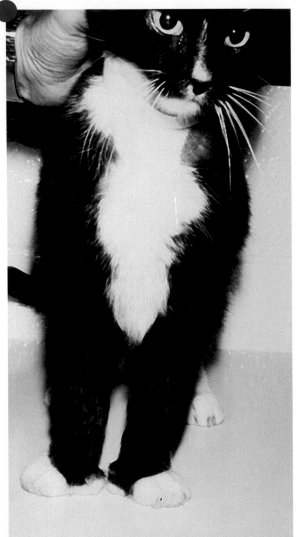

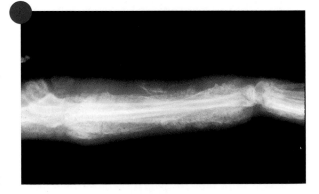

Figure 56-7: The cat in A had a primary lung tumor and thickened painful extremities. The radiograph from this cat (B) confirmed the presence of periosteal new bone growth that is generally perpendicular to the long axis of the bone. This radiograph is highly suggestive of a paraneoplastic syndrome called hypertrophic osteopathy. Treatment of the underlying disorder and analgesics are often helpful.

want to improve quality of life while trying to maximize the chance of controlling the tumor.

Comfort

- Therapy to enhance comfort (e.g.: NSAID or prednisolone if lymphoma, tramadol, buprenorphine) and freedom from nausea, vomiting (e.g.: maropitant and/or metoclopramide), diarrhea (e.g.: metronidazole) and lack of appetite (e.g.: mirtazapine or cyproheptadine).

Comfort and control

Above mentioned therapy for comfort plus:

- Palliative radiation, especially for those with extension into surrounding structures or regional metastases (e.g.: 2-5 dosages of radiation), to first enhance comfort, second, to reduce the rate of growth and third, occasionally to reduce the size of the tumor. The use of stereotactic surgery enhances the accuracy of this type of therapy.

Comfort and longer-term control

Above mentioned therapy for comfort plus:

- Lung lobectomy.
  - Primary lung tumors were surgically removed from 21 cats in one study.[91] Eighteen cats died due to metastatic disease between 2 weeks and 51 months after surgery; their median survival was approximately 4 months.
  - The survival time of 20 cats that had their primary lung tumors removed revealed that the presence of clinical signs at the time of diagnosis, pleural effusion, evidence of metastasis at the time of surgery, and moderately and poorly differentiated tumors on histopathology were factors that were significantly correlated with reduced survival times. Of the cats that survived to the time of suture removal, the median survival time was 64 days.[92]

References

1. Bedford PGC, Coulson A, Sharp NJH, Longstaffe JA: Nasopharyngeal polyps in the cat. *Vet Rec* 109:551–553, 1981.
2. Stanton ME, Wheaton LG, Render JA, Blevins WE: Pharyngeal polyps in two feline siblings. *JAVMA* 186:1311–1313, 1985.
3. Kapatkin A, Matthiesen DT, Noone K, et al: Results of surgical treatment for nasopharyngeal inflammatory polyps in 31 cats. *Vet Surg* 18:59, 1989.
4. Harvey CE, Goldschmidt MH: Inflammatory polypoid growths in the ear canal of cats. *J Small Anim Pract* 19:669–677, 1978.
5. Lane JG, Orr CM, Lucke VM, Gruffydd-Jones TJ: Nasopharyngeal polyps arising in the middle ear of the cat. *J Small Anim Pract* 22:511–522, 1981.
6. Elkins AD: Resolving respiratory distress created by a nasopharyngeal polyp. *Vet Med* 82:1234–1235, 1987.
7. Trevor PB, Martin RA: Tympanic bulla osteotomy for treatment of middle-ear disease in cats: 19 cases (1984–1991). *JAVMA* 202:123–128, 1993.
8. Baker G: Nasopharyngeal polyps in cats. *Vet Rec* 111:43, 1982.
9. Oliveira CR, O'Brien RT, Matheson JS, Carrera I. Computed tomographic features of feline nasopharyngeal polyps. *Vet Radiol Ultrasound.* 53(4):406-411, 2012.
10. Anders BB, Hoelzler MG, Scavelli TD et al: Analysis of auditory and neurologic effects associated with ventral bulla osteotomy for removal of inflammatory polyps or nasopharyngeal masses in cats. *J Am Vet Med Assoc.* 233(4):580-585, 2008.
11. Williams JM, White RAS: Total ear canal ablation combined with lateral bulla osteotomy in the cat. *J Small Anim Pract* 33:225–227, 1992.
12. Caniatti M, Roccabianca P, Ghisleni G, et al: Evaluation of brush cytology in the diagnosis of chronic intranasal disease in cats. *J Small Anim Pract* 39:73–77, 1998.
13. Madewell BR, Priester WA, Gillette EL, Snyder SP: Neoplasms of the nasal passages and paranasal sinuses in domesticated animals as reported by 13 veterinary colleges. *Am J Vet Res* 37:851–856, 1976.
14. Carpenter JL, Andrews LK, Holzworth J: Tumors and tumor-like lesions. In Holzworth J (ed): *Diseases of the Cat. Medicine and Surgery.* Philadelphia, WB Saunders, 1987, pp 407–596.
15. Cox NR, Brawner WR, Powers RD, Wright JC: Tumors of the nose and paranasal sinuses in cats: 32 cases with comparison to a national database (1977 through 1987). *JAAHA* 27:339–347, 1991.
16. Gilger BC, McLaughlin SA, Whitley RD, Wright JC: Orbital neoplasms in cats: 21 cases (1974–1990). *JAVMA* 201:1083–1086, 1992.
17. Galloway PE, Kyles A, Henderson JP: Nasal polyps in a cat. *J Small Anim Pract* 38:78–80, 1997.
18. Peiffer Jr RL, Spencer C, Popp JA: Nasal squamous cell carcinoma with periocular extension and metastasis in a cat. *Feline Pract* 8:43–46, 1978.
19. Fujiwara-Igarashi A, Fujimori T, Oka M et al: Evaluation of outcomes and radiation complications in 65 cats with nasal tumours treated with palliative hypofractionated radiotherapy. *Vet J.* 202(3):455-461, 2014.
20. Theon AP, Peaston AE, Madewell BR, Dungworth DL: Irradiation of nonlymphoproliferative neoplasms of the nasal cavity and paranasal sinuses in 16 cats. *JAVMA* 204:78–83, 1994.
21. Sfiligoi G, Théon AP, Kent MS. Response of nineteen cats with nasal lymphoma to radiation therapy and chemotherapy. 48(4):388-393, *Vet Radiol Ultrasound.* 2007.
22. Straw RC, Withrow SJ, Gillette EL, McChesney AE: Use of radiotherapy for the treatment of intranasal tumors in cats: Six cases (1980–1985). *JAVMA* 189:927–929, 1986.
23. Ogilvie GK, Moore AS, Obradovich JE, et al: Toxicoses and efficacy associated with the administration of mitoxantrone to cats with malignant tumors. *JAVMA* 202:1839–1844, 1993.
24. Taylor SS, Goodfellow MR, Browne WJ et al: Feline extranodal lymphoma: response to chemotherapy and survival in 110 cats. *J Small Anim Pract.* 50(11):584-592, 2009.
25. Lord PF, Kapp DS, Schwartz A, Morrow DT: Osteogenic sarcoma of the nasal cavity in a cat: Postoperative control with high dose-per-fraction radiation therapy and metronidazole. *Vet Radiol* 23:23–26, 1982.
26. Marconato L, Buchholz J, Keller M, et al: Multimodal therapeutic approach and interdisciplinary challenge for the treatment of unresectable head and neck squamous cell carcinoma in six cats: a pilot study. *Vet Comp Oncol.* 11(2):101-112, 2013.
27. Scavelli TD, Patnaik AK, Mehlaff CJ, Hayes AA: Hemangiosarcoma in the cat: retrospective evaluation of 31 surgical cases. *JAVMA* 187:817–819, 1985.
28. Cox NR, Power RD: Olfactory neuroblastomas in two cats. *Vet Pathol* 26:341–343, 1989.
29. Schrenzel MD, Higgins RJ, Hinrichs SH, ET AL: Type C retroviral expression in spontaneous feline olfactory neuroblastomas. *Acta Neuropathol* 80:547–553, 1990.
30. Cotter SM, Essex M, Hardy Jr WD: Serological studies of normal and leukemic cats in a multiple-case leukemia cluster. *Cancer Res* 34:1061–1069, 1974.
31. Allen HS, Broussard J, Noone K: Nasopharyngeal diseases in cats: A retrospective study of 53 cases (1991–1998). *JAAHA* 35:457–461, 1999.
32. Legendre AM, Carrig CB, Howard DR, Dade AW: Nasal tumor in a cat. *JAVMA* 167:481–483, 1975.
33. Saik JE, Toll SL, Diters RW, Goldschmidt MH: Canine and feline laryngeal neoplasia: A 10 year survey. *JAAHA* 22:359–365, 1986.
34. Haney SM, Beaver L, Turrel J, et al: Survival analysis of 97 cats with nasal lymphoma: a multi-institutional retrospective study (1986-2006). *J Vet Intern Med.* 23(2):287-294, 2009.
35. Van Der Riet FdStJ, McCully RM, Keen GA, Forder AA: Lymphosarcoma in a cat. *J South Afr Vet Assoc* 57–59, 1983.
36. Vail DM, Moore AS, Ogilvie GK, Volk LM: Feline lymphoma (145 cases): Proliferation indices, cluster of differentiation 3 immunoreactivity, and their association with prognosis in 90 cats. *J Vet Intern Med* 12:349–354, 1998.
37. Elmslie RE, Ogilvie GK, Gillette EL, McChesney-Gillette S: Radiotherapy with and without chemotherapy for localized lymphoma in 10 cats. *Vet Radiol* 32:277–280, 1991.
38. North SM, Meleo K, Mooney S, Mauldin GN: Radiation therapy

in the treatment of nasal lymphoma in cats. *Proc 14th Annu Conf Vet Cancer Soc*:21, 1994.

39. Gibbs C: Radiographic examination of the pharynx, larynx and soft-tissue structures of the neck in dogs and cats. *Vet Annu* 26:227–241, 1986.

40. Tasker S, Foster DJ, Corcoran BM, et al: Obstructive inflammatory laryngeal diseases in three cats. *J Feline Med Surg* 1:53–59, 1999.

41. Harvey CE, O'Brien JA: Surgical treatments of miscellaneous laryngeal conditions in dogs and cats. *JAAHA* 18:557–562, 1982.

42. Carlisle CH, Biery DN, Thrall DE: Tracheal and laryngeal tumors in the dog and cat: literature review and 13 additional patients. *Vet Radiol* 32:229–235, 1991.

43. Patterson DF, Meier H: Surgical intervention in intestinal lymphosarcoma in two cats. *JAVMA* 127:495–498, 1955.

44. Rudorf H, Brown P: Ultrasonography of laryngeal masses in six cats and one dog. *Vet Radiol Ultrasound* 39:430–434, 1998.

45. O'Handley P, Stickle R: What is your diagnosis? *JAVMA* 191:1492–1493, 1987.

46. Wheeldon EB, Amis TC: Laryngeal carcinoma in a cat. *JAVMA* 186:80–81, 1985.

47. Collet MP: Cancer primitif du larynx chez une chatte. *Bull Soc Sci Vet Lyon* 38:219–226, 1935.

48. Lieberman LL: Feline adenocarcinoma of the larynx with metastasis to the adrenal gland. *JAVMA* 125:153–154, 1954.

49. Vasseur PB, Patnaik AK: Laryngeal adenocarcinoma in a cat. *JAAHA* 17:639–641, 1981.

50. Paul-Murphy J, Lloyd K, Turrel JM, et al: Management of a Schwannoma in the larynx of a lion. *JAVMA* 189:1202–1203, 1986.

51. Cain GR, Manley P: Tracheal adenocarcinoma in a cat. *JAVMA* 182:614–616, 1983.

52. Beaumont PR: Intratracheal neoplasia in two cats. *J Small Anim Pract* 23:29–35, 1982.

53. Zimmermann U, Müller F, Pfleghaar S: Zwei fälle von histogenetisch unterschiedlichen trachealtumoren bei katzen. *Kleintierpraxis* 37:409–412, 1992.

54. Schneider PR, Smith CW, Feller DL: Histiocytic lymphosarcoma of the trachea in a cat. *JAAHA* 15:485–487, 1979.

55. Glock R: Primary pulmonary adenomas of the feline. *Iowa State Vet* 23:155–156, 1961.

56. Veith LA: Squamous cell carcinoma of the trachea in a cat. *Feline Pract* 4:30–32, 1974.

57. Neer TM, Zeman D: Tracheal adenocarcinoma in a cat and review of the literature. *JAAHA* 23:377–380, 1987.

58. Lobetti RG, Williams MC: Anaplastic tracheal squamous cell carcinoma in a cat. *Tydskr S Afr Vet Ver* 63:132–133, 1992.

59. Kim DY, Kim JR, Taylor HW, Lee YS: Primary extranodal lymphosarcoma of the trachea in a cat. *J.Vet Med Sci.* 58:703–706, 1996.

60. Hahn KA, McEntee MF: Primary lung tumors in cats: 86 cases (1979–1994). *JAVMA* 211:1257–1260, 1997.

61. Barr F, Gruffydd-Jones TJ, Brown PJ, Gibbs C: Primary lung tumours in the cat. *J Small Anim Pract* 28:1115–1125, 1987.

62. Moulton JE, von Tscharner C, Schneider R: Classification of lung carcinomas in the dog and cat. *Vet Pathol* 18:513–528, 1981.

63. Koblik PD: Radiographic appearance of primary lung tumors in cats. *Vet Radiol* 27:66–73, 1986.

64. Brown PJ, Hoare CM, Rochlitz I: Multiple squamous cell carcinoma of the digits in two cats. *J Small Anim Pract* 26:323–328, 1985.

65. Carr SH: Secondary hypertrophic pulmonary osteoarthropathy in a cat. *Feline Pract* 1:25–26, 1971.

66. Mehlhaff CJ, Mooney S: Primary pulmonary neoplasia in the dog and cat. *Vet Clin North Am Small Anim Pract* 15:1061–1068, 1985.

67. Carpenter RH, Hansen JF: Diffuse pulmonary bronchiolo-alveolar adenocarcinoma in a cat. *Calif Vet* 4:11–14, 1982.

68. Gottfried SD, Popovitch CA, Goldschmidt MH, Schelling C: Metastatic digital carcinoma in the cat: A retrospective study of 36 cats (1992–1998). *JAAHA* 36:501–509, 2000.

69. Goldfinch N, Argyle DJ. Feline lung-digit syndrome: unusual metastatic patterns of primary lung tumours in cats. *J Feline Med Surg.* 2012 Mar;14(3):202-208, 2012.

70. Moore AS, Middleton DJ: Pulmonary adenocarcinoma in three cats with non-respiratory signs only. *J Small Anim Pract* 23:501–509, 1982.

71. Teunissen VGHB, Stokhof AA: Tumoren in der Brusthöhle. *Kleintierpraxis* 26:501–506, 1981.

72. Loser C, Lawrenz B, Werner H-G, et al: Primäre lungentumore mit metastasierung in die phalangen bei der katze. *Jahrgang* 43:425–442, 1998.

73. Pollack M, Martin RA, Diters RW: Metastatic squamous cell carcinoma in multiple digits of a cat: case report. *JAAHA* 20:835–839, 1984.

74. Scott-Moncrieff JC, Elliott GS, Radovsky A, Blevins WE: Pulmonary squamous cell carcinoma with multiple digital metastases in a cat. *J Small Anim Pract* 30:696–699, 1989.

75. May C, Newsholme SJ: Metastasis of feline pulmonary carcinoma presenting as multiple digital swelling. *J Small Anim Pract* 30:302–310, 1989.

76. Jacobs TM, Tomlinson MJ: The lung-digit syndrome in a cat. *Feline Pract* 25:31–36, 1997.

77. Schmitz JA, Bailey DE, Bailey RB: Bronchogenic carcinoma in a cat presenting as rear leg lameness. *Feline Pract* 8:18–22, 1978.

78. Chauvet AE, Shelton GD: Neuromuscular weakness as a primary clinical sign associated with metastatic neoplasia in two cats. *Feline Pract* 25:6–9, 1997.

79. Meschter CL: Disseminated sweat gland adenocarcinoma with acronecrosis in a cat. *Cornell Vet* 81:195–203, 1991.

80. van der Linde-Sipman JS, van den Ingh ThSGAM: Primary and metastatic carcinomas in the digits of cats. *Vet Q* 22:141–145, 2000.

81. Roberg J: Hypertrophic pulmonary osteoarthropathy. *Feline Pract* 7:18–22, 1977.

82. Hamilton HB, Severin GA, Nold J: Pulmonary squamous cell carcinoma with intraocular metastasis in a cat. *JAVMA* 185:307–309, 1984.

83. Gionfriddo JR, Fix AS, Niyo Y, et al: Ocular manifestations of a metastatic pulmonary adenocarcinoma in a cat. *JAVMA* 197:372–374, 1990.

84. Dorn AS, Harris SG, Olmstead ML: Squamous cell carcinoma of the urinary bladder in a cat. *Feline Pract* 8:14–17, 1978.

85. Davies C, Forrester SD: Pleural effusion in cats: 82 cases (1987–1995). *J Small Anim Pract* 37:217–224, 1996.

86. McMillan MC, Kleine LJ, Carpenter JL: Fluoroscopically guided percutaneous fine-needle aspiration biopsy of thoracic lesions in dogs and cats. *Vet Radiol* 29:194–197, 1988.

87. Tidwell AS, Johnson KL: Computed tomography-guided percutaneous biopsy in the dog and cat: Description of technique and preliminary evaluation in 14 patients. *Vet Radiol Ultrasound* 35:445–446, 1994.

88. Gustafsson P, Wolfe D: Bone-metastasizing lung carcinoma in a cat. *Cornell Vet* 58:425–430, 1968.

89. Gram WD, Wheaton LG, Snyder PW, et al: Feline hypertrophic osteopathy associated with pulmonary carcinoma. *JAAHA* 26:425–428, 1990.

90. LaRue SM, Withrow SJ, Wykes PM: Lung resection using surgical staples in dogs and cats. *Vet Surg* 16:238–240, 1987.

91. Hahn KA, McEntee MF: Prognosis factors for survival in cats after removal of a primary lung tumor: 21 cases (1979–1994). *Vet Surg* 27:307–311, 1998.

92. Maritato KC, Schertel ER, Kennedy SC, et al: Outcome and prognostic indicators in 20 cats with surgically treated primary lung tumors. *J Feline Med Surg.* 16(12):979-984, 2014.

Chapter 57

Feline cardiovascular tumors

FELINE CHEMODECTOMA

Clinical presentation

- Rare condition.
- Usually not painful.
- Cats with carotid body tumors may present with as a palpable neck mass.
- Heart base or aortic body tumors sometimes present with pericardial or pleural effusions causing dyspnea.

Staging and diagnosis

- Minimum data base (MDB): includes a CBC, biochemical profile, urinalysis, bone marrow aspirate, abdominal ultrasound, FIV/FeLV serology, T4 testing, biopsy, three-view thoracic radiographs or preferably, computerized tomography of the chest.
- Radiographs or ultrasound of the tumor itself may be helpful, however computerized tomography or magnetic resonance imaging is preferable.

Treatment

This section is divided into three options:
- Comfort for those who want to improve quality of life.
- Comfort and control for those who want to improve quality of life while trying to provide some control of the tumor.
- Comfort and longer-term control for those who want to improve quality of life while trying to maximize the chance of controlling the tumor.

Comfort

- Therapy to enhance comfort (e.g.: NSAID or prednisolone if lymphoma, tramadol, buprenorphine) and freedom from nausea, vomiting (e.g.: maropitant and/or metoclopramide),

diarrhea (e.g.: metronidazole) and lack of appetite (e.g.: mirtazapine or cyproheptadine). Thoracocentesis or pericardiocentesis may provide transient improvement in quality of life.

Comfort and control

Above mentioned therapy for comfort plus:
- Palliative radiation (e.g.: 2-5 dosages of radiation) to first enhance comfort, second, to reduce the rate of growth and third, occasionally to reduce the size of the tumor.

Comfort and longer-term control

Above mentioned therapy for comfort plus:
- Surgery is rarely curative, but it may downsize the tumor and/or improve quality of life.
- Stereotactic radiosurgery is being explored as an option to provide longer-term control of the local tumor.

FELINE CARDIAC LYMPHOMA

Clinical presentation

- The heart is commonly involved by infiltration in cats with multicentric lymphoma; however, such infiltration is rarely of clinical significance.
- Clinical signs may result from pericardial or pleural effusion and include breathing issues, weakness, lethargy, syncope, etc.
- May be uncomfortable.

Staging and diagnosis

- Minimum data base (MDB): includes a CBC, biochemical profile, urinalysis, FIV/FeLV serology, T4 testing, biopsy, three-view thoracic radiographs or computerized tomography of the chest.
- Ultrasonography, radiographs, and computerized tomography imaging of the chest, and thus the

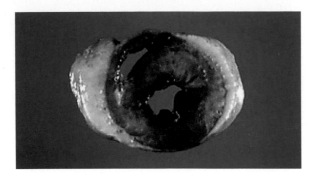

Figure 57-1: Lymphoma involving the epicardium of the heart of a cat that presented with pleural effusion and with an echocardiogram that confirmed a restrictive cardiomyopathy. The best treatment for this type of condition is a modified CHOP protocol with or without thoracic palliative radiation.

tumor, may be helpful. Pericardiocentesis or aspiration of pleural or abdominal effusion may aid in making a diagnosis.

Treatment

This section is divided into three options:
- Comfort for those who want to improve quality of life.
- Comfort and control for those who want to improve quality of life while trying to provide some control of the tumor.
- Comfort and longer-term control for those who want to improve quality of life while trying to maximize the chance of controlling the tumor.

Comfort

- Therapy to provide some benefit for the lymphoma by prescribing prednisolone plus therapy to enhance comfort and freedom from nausea, vomiting (e.g.: maropitant and/or metoclopramide), diarrhea (e.g.: metronidazole) and lack of appetite (e.g.: mirtazapine, cyproheptadine). Therapy including furosemide and enalapril to treat any evidence of heart disease.

Comfort and control (first remission)

Above mentioned therapy for comfort plus:
- CCNU (lomustine) at 60 mg/m² body surface area PO q3 weeks for 5 treatments. Note that treatment delays may be required due to neutropenia and/or thrombocytopenia.
- COP protocol (cyclophosphamide, vincristine and prednisolone) has been shown to be helpful for cats with lymphoma.

- Palliative radiation (e.g.: 2-5 dosages of radiation) to first enhance comfort, second, to reduce the rate of growth and third, occasionally to reduce the size of the tumor.

Comfort and longer-term control (first remission)

Above mentioned therapy for comfort plus:
- CHOP chemotherapy to include cyclophosphamide, vincristine, prednisolone, doxorubicin and, in some cases, L-asparaginase.

References

1. Scavelli TD, Patnaik AK, Mehlaff CJ, et al: Hemangiosarcoma in the cat: retrospective evaluation of 31 surgical cases. *JAVMA* 187:817–819, 1985.
2. Patnaik AK, Liu S-K: Angiosarcoma in cats. *J Small Anim Pract* 18:191–198, 1977.
3. Kraje AC, Mears EA, Hahn KA, et al: Unusual metastatic behavior and clinicopathologic findings in 8 cats with cutaneous or visceral hemangiosarcoma (1981–1997). *JAVMA* 1999;214:670–672.
4. Rush JE, Keene BW, Fox PR: Pericardial disease in the cat: A retrospective evaluation of 66 cases. *JAAHA* 26:39–46, 1990.
5. Ryan CP, Walder EJ: Feline fibrosarcoma of the heart. *Calif Vet* 8:12–14, 1980.
6. Campbell MD, Gelberg HB: Endocardial ossifying myxoma of the right atrium in a cat. *Vet Pathol* 37:460–462, 2000.
7. Venco L, Kramer L, Sola LB, et al: Primary cardiac rhabdomyosarcoma in a cat. *JAAHA* 37:159–163, 2001.
8. Tilley LP, Bond B, Patnaik AK, et al: Cardiovascular tumors in the cat. *JAAHA* 17:1009–1021, 1981.
9. Carpenter JL, Andrews LK, Holzworth J: Tumors and tumor-like lesions. In Holzworth J (ed): *Diseases of the Cat. Medicine and Surgery.* Philadelphia, WB Saunders 1987, pp 407–596.
10. Yates WDG, Lester SJ, Mills JHL: Chemoreceptor tumors diagnosed at the Western College of Veterinary Medicine 1967–1979. *Can Vet J* 21:124–129, 1980.
11. Nielsen SW: Neoplastic diseases. In Catcott EJ (ed): *Feline Medicine and Surgery.* Santa Barbara, CA, American Veterinay Publications, 1964, pp 156–176.
12. Collins DR: Thoracic tumor in a cat. *Vet Med Small Anim Clin* 59:459, 1964.
13. Lusk Jr RH, Ettinger SJ, Barr EA: Ultrasound diagnosis of a feline heart tumor. *Calif Vet* 41:9–10, 1987.
14. Fossum TW, Dru Forrester S, Swenson CL, et al: Chylothorax in cats: 37 cases (1969–1989). *JAVMA* 198:672–678, 1991.
15. Tillson DM, Fingland RB, Andrews GA: Chemodectoma in a cat. *JAAHA* 30:586—590, 1994.
16. Paola JP, Hammer AS, Smeak DD, et al: Aortic body tumor causing pleural effusion in a cat. *JAAHA* 30:281–285, 1994.
17. Buergelt CD, Das KM: Aortic body tumor in a cat, a case report. *Pathol Vet* 5:84–90, 1968.
18. George C, Steinberg H: An aortic body carcinoma with multifocal thoracic metastases in a cat. *J Comp Pathol* 101:467–469, 1989.
19. Willis R, Williams AE, Schwarz T, et al: Aortic body chemodectoma causing pulmonary oedema in a cat. *J Small Anim Pract* 42:20–23, 2001.
20. Tidwell AS, Johnson KL: Computed tomography-guided percutaneous biopsy: Criteria for accurate needle tip identification. *Vet Radiol Ultrasound* 35:440–444, 1994.
21. Tidwell AS, Johnson KL: Computed tomography-guided percutaneous biopsy in the dog and cat: Description of technique and preliminary evaluation in 14 patients. *Vet Radiol Ultrasound* 35:445–446, 1994.
22. Brummer DG, Moise NS: Infiltrative cardiomyopathy responsive to combination chemotherapy in a cat with lymphoma. *JAVMA* 195:1116–1119, 1989.
23. Meurs KM, Miller MW, Mackie JR, et al: Syncope associated with cardiac lymphoma in a cat. *JAAHA* 30:583–585, 1994.
24. Machida N, Yamaga Y, Kagota K, et al: Paroxysmal atrial tachycardia in a cat. *J Jpn Vet Med Assoc* 44:1030–1033, 1991.

Chapter 58

Feline thymoma, mesothelioma, and histiocytosis

FELINE THYMOMA

Clinical presentation

- Relatively uncommon mediastinal epithelial malignancy of the thymus that rarely, if ever, spreads.
- Vomiting, regurgitation, coughing and choking have been described.
- Acute or chronic dyspnea associated with a non-compressible cranial thorax and a caudally displaced heart.
- Paraneoplastic syndromes include myasthenia gravis, a dermatologic disorder and hypertrophic osteopathy.
  - Signs referable to myasthenia gravis including weakness, lethargy, dysphonia, inability to stand and megaesophagus.
  - Dermatologic condition may be seen in cats with a nonpruritic, seborrheic alopecia that involvs the ventral neck, abdomen, thorax, medial limbs, and paws, some of which can have a hair coat color change from orange to white.[23,24]
- Usually not painful.

> **Key point**
> Most cats with mediastinal thymomas present with a gradual onset of weight loss, anorexia and, later in the course of the disease, dyspnea.

Staging and diagnosis

- Minimum data base (MDB): includes a CBC, biochemical profile, urinalysis, FIV/FeLV serology, T4 testing, and three-view thoracic radiographs or computerized tomography of the chest. A biopsy or aspirate should be done via ultrasonographic, radiographic or CT-guided techniques.

- Ultrasonography and/or radiographs are practical and cost effective, however computerized tomography or magnetic resonance imaging of the tumor can be used to obtain a biopsy or aspirate of the mediastinal mass. On ultrasound, the mass is usually cystic with multiple variably sized cysts or occasionally one very large cyst.[3]
- Acetylcholesterase antibody titers (AchRAb) and skin biopsy may be indicated in some cats.
  - A serum AchRAb titer above 0.30 nmol/L is diagnostic for myasthenia gravis,[27,30] although cats with titers below 10 nmol/L may not show muscular weakness at diagnosis. Early diagnosis will allow appropriate treatment prior to surgery and will improve the chances for an uncomplicated outcome.[4,10,14]

> **Key point**
> Chest radiographs or thoracic CT and either an aspirate or a biopsy of the mediastinal mass is ideal to confirm the suspicion of a thymoma.

Treatment

This section is divided into three options:
- Comfort for those who want to improve quality of life.
- Comfort and control for those who want to improve quality of life while trying to provide some control of the tumor.
- Comfort and longer-term control for those who want to improve quality of life while trying to maximize the chance of controlling the tumor.

> **Key point**
> Most cats with a mediastinal thymoma respond very well to surgical removal or radiation therapy.

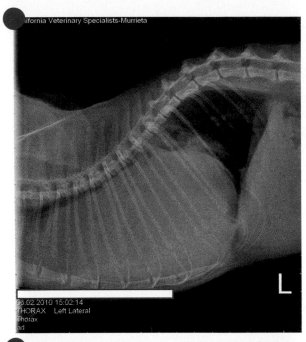

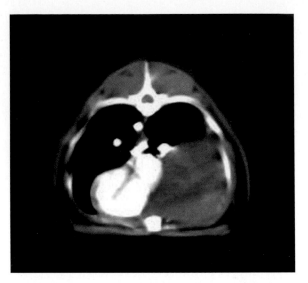

Figure 58-2: Computerized tomography of the chest that contains the thymoma that is deviating the heart. The CT confirms that the tumor is not invading or originating from the lung and that it is localized to the mediastinum. Imaging courtesy of Lenore Anderson Mohammadian, DVM, MSpVM, Diplomate ACVR.

Comfort

- Therapy to enhance comfort (e.g.: NSAID or prednisolone, tramadol, buprenorphine) and freedom from nausea, vomiting (e.g.: maropitant and/or metoclopramide), diarrhea (e.g.: metronidazole) and lack of appetite (e.g.: mirtazapine or cyproheptadine). Prednisolone may reduce the normal lymphocyte population within the malignant epithelial cells.

Comfort and control

Above mentioned therapy for comfort plus:
- Palliative radiation, especially for those with extension into surrounding structures or regional metastases (e.g.: 2-5 dosages of radiation), to first enhance comfort, second, to reduce the rate of growth and third, occasionally to reduce the size of the tumor.
- Combination chemotherapy (COP or preferably, CHOP) has been successful at resulting in control of some thymomas, especially those with a rich lymphocytic component.

Comfort and longer-term control

Above mentioned therapy for comfort plus:
- Surgery. Surgical resection often by a median sternotomy approach is usually successful and often curative.[10]
  - Cats treated with excision of the tumor alone resulted in a median overall survival time of

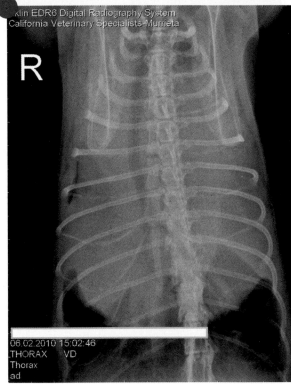

Figure 58-1: Radiographs from a cat with a large, non-compressible mass in the chest that was aspirated and found to contain an admixture of small lymphocytes, mast cells, and a few epithelial cells. The radiographs confirm a large mass within the anterior chest. An ultrasound-guided biopsy was performed to confirm the presence of a thymoma. Resection (see figure 58-3) was successful. Imaging courtesy of Lenore Anderson Mohammadian, DVM, MSpVM, Diplomate ACVR.

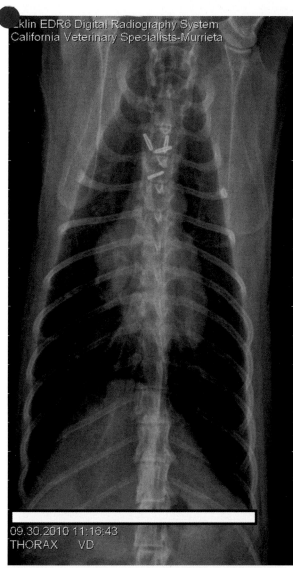

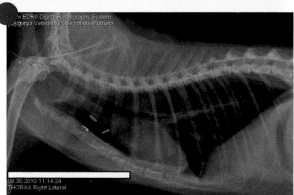

Figure 58-3: Postoperative thoracic radiographs from the same patient with a thymoma imaged in figure 58-1. Feline thymomas are generally resectable, with many being cured with surgery. Another alternative treatment is radiation therapy. Imaging courtesy of Lenore Anderson Mohammadian, DVM, MSpVM, Diplomate ACVR.

1,825 days, with a 1-year survival rate of 89% and a 3-year survival rate of 74%.[7]

- Definitive radiation alone or if there is evidence of tumor extending beyond the surgical margins (e.g.: 16-19 dosages of radiation).
  - A retrospective study was performed on seven cats with various stages of thymoma treated with radiation alone or as an adjunctive therapy, with a median survival time of 720 days (range, 485 to 1,825+ days), although complete remissions are rare.[9]

FELINE MESOTHELIOMA

Clinical presentation

- Rare cause of effusion in any of the body cavities in cats.[35-37]
- Emaciation, lethargy, anorexia, dyspnea, discomfort from effusion in the chest or abdomen.
- May be painful.

Staging and diagnosis

- Minimum data base (MDB): includes a CBC, biochemical profile, urinalysis, FIV/FeLV serology, T4 testing, biopsy of any masses seen or cytology of body cavity effusion, three-view thoracic radiographs or computerized tomography of the chest.
- It is often impossible to distinguish cytologically between reactive and malignant mesothelial cells.
- Ultrasonography and/or radiographs are practical and cost effective, however computerized tomography or magnetic resonance imaging of the region where effusion may be identified may be preferable.

Treatment

This section is divided into two options:
- Comfort for those who want to improve quality of life.
- Comfort and control for those who want to improve quality of life while trying to provide some control of the tumor.

Comfort

- Therapy to enhance comfort (e.g.: NSAID, tramadol, buprenorphine) and freedom from nausea, vomiting (e.g.: maropitant and/or metoclopramide), diarrhea (e.g.: metronidazole) and lack of appetite (e.g.: mirtazapine or cyproheptadine). Serial removal of fluid in the chest or abdomen as needed for comfort is palliative.

Comfort and control

Above mentioned therapy for comfort plus:
- Palliative radiation of the involved cavity may be helpful.
- Intracavitary carboplatin or mitoxantrone may be palliative.

FELINE MALIGNANT HISTIOCYTOSIS

Clinical presentation

- Very rare tumor.
- Nonspecific signs of listlessness, inappetence, and weight loss.
- Organomegaly may be noted on physical examination.
- Begins as localized lesions, which rapidly disseminate to many organs. Primary sites include spleen, lung, skin, brain (meninges), lymph node, bone marrow, and synovial tissues of limbs.[44]
- An indolent localized form originates in the skin of cats.[44]

Staging and diagnosis

- Minimum data base (MDB): includes a CBC, biochemical profile, urinalysis, FIV/FeLV serology, T4 testing, and three-view thoracic radiographs or computerized tomography of the chest. A biopsy or aspirate should be done via ultrasonographic, radiographic or CT-guided techniques.
- Ultrasonography and/or radiographs are practical and cost effective, however computerized tomography or magnetic resonance imaging of the tumor can be used to obtain a biopsy or aspirate of the mediastinal mass. On ultrasound the mass is usually cystic with multiple variably sized cysts or occasionally one very large cyst.[3]
- Acetylcholesterase antibody titers (AchRAb) and skin biopsy may be indicated in some cats.

Treatment

This section is divided into three options:
- Comfort for those who want to improve quality of life.
- Comfort and control for those who want to improve quality of life while trying to provide some control of the tumor.
- Comfort and longer-term control for those who want to improve quality of life while trying to maximize the chance of controlling the tumor.

Comfort

- Therapy to enhance comfort (e.g.: NSAID or prednisolone, tramadol, buprenorphine) and freedom from nausea, vomiting (e.g.: maropitant and/or metoclopramide), diarrhea (e.g.: metronidazole) and lack of appetite (e.g.: mirtazapine or cyproheptadine). Prednisolone may be palliative.

Comfort and control

Above mentioned therapy for comfort plus:
- Palliative radiation, especially for those with extension into surrounding structures or regional metastases (e.g.: 2-5 dosages of radiation), to first enhance comfort, second, to reduce the rate of growth and third, occasionally to reduce the size of the tumor.
- Combination chemotherapy (COP or preferably, CHOP) may be palliative in some cases. The true value of chemotherapy has yet to be defined.

Comfort and longer-term control

Above mentioned therapy for comfort plus:
- Surgery. Surgical resection is rarely curative since most, but not all, cases are multicentric.
- Definitive radiation alone for the rare localized form of the disease or if there is evidence of tumor extending beyond the surgical margins (e.g.: 16-19 dosages of radiation).

References

1. Carpenter JL, Holzworth J: Thymoma in 11 cats. *JAVMA* 181:240–251, 1982.
2. Martin RA, Evans EW, August JR, Franklin JE: Surgical treatment of a thymoma in a cat. *JAAHA* 22:347–354, 1986.
3. Galloway PEJ, Barr FJ, Holt PE, et al: Cystic thymoma in a cat with cholesterol-rich fluid and an unusual ultrasonographic appearance. *J Small Anim Pract* 38:220–224, 1997.
4. Scott-Moncrieff JC, Cook Jr JR, Lantz GC: Acquired myasthenia gravis in a cat with thymoma. *JAVMA* 196:1291–1293, 1990.
5. Day MJ: Review of thymic pathology in 30 cats and 36 dogs. *J Small Anim Pract* 38:393–403, 1997.
6. Forster-van Hufte MA, Curtis CF, White RN: Resolution of exfoliative dermatitis and *Malassezia pachydermatis* overgrowth in a cat after surgical thymoma resection. *J Small Anim Pract* 38:451–454, 1997.
7. Zitz JC, Birchard SJ, Couto GC, et al: Results of excision of thymoma in cats and dogs: 20 cases (1984-2005). *J Am Vet Med Assoc.* 232(8):1186-1192, 2008.
8. Carpenter JL, Andrews LK, Holzworth J: Tumors and tumor-like lesions. In Holzworth J (ed): *Diseases of the Cat. Medicine and Surgery.* Philadelphia, WB Saunders, 1987, pp 407–596.
9. Smith AN, Wright JC, Brawner WR Jr, et al: Radiation therapy in the treatment of canine and feline thymomas: a retrospective study (1985-1999). *JAAHA* 37(5):489-496, 2001.
10. Gores BR, Berg J, Carpenter JL, Aronsohn MG: Surgical treatment of thymoma in cats: 12 cases (1987–1992). *JAVMA* 204:1782–1785, 1994.
11. Richards CD: Hypertrophic osteoarthropathy in a cat. *Feline Pract* 7:41–43, 1977.
12. Carpenter JL, Valentine BA: Brief communications and case reports. Squamous cell carcinoma arising in two feline thymomas. *Vet Pathol* 29:541–543, 1992.
13. Mettler F: Thymome bei hund und katze. *Schweiz Arch Tierheilk* 117:577–584, 1975.
14. van Oosterhout ICAM, Teske E, Vos JH, Koeman JP: Myasthenia gravis en een thymoom bij een kat. *Tijdschr Diergeneesk* 114:499–505, 1989.
15. Willard MD, Tvedten H, Walshaw R, Aronson E: Thymoma in a cat. *JAVMA* 176:451–453, 1980.
16. Kobayashi Y, Yoshida K, Sawashima K, et al: Thymoma in a cat. *J Jpn Vet Med Assoc* 46:582–584, 1993.
17. Dubielzig RR, DeLaney RG: A thymoma in a cat. *Vet Med Small Anim Clin* 75:1270–1272, 1980.
18. Malik R, Gabor L, Hunt GB, et al: Benign cranial mediastinal lesionas in three cats. *Aust Vet J* 75:183–187, 1997.
19. Middleton DJ, Ratcliffe RC, Xu FN: Thymoma with distant metastases in a cat. *Vet Pathol* 22:512–514, 1985.
20. Mackey L: Clear-cell thymoma and thymic hyperplasia in a cat. *J Comp Pathol* 85:367–371, 1975.
21. Gorman PD: What is your diagnosis? *JAVMA* 202:993–994, 1993.
22. Hauser B, Mettler F: Malignant thymoma in a cat. *J Comp Pathol* 94:311–313, 1984.
23. Scott DW, Yager JA, Johnston KM: Exfoliative dermatitis in association with thymoma in three cats. *Feline Pract* 23:8–13, 1995.
24. Godfrey DR: Dermatosis and associated systemic signs in a cat with thymoma and recently treated with an imidacloprid preparation. *J Small Anim Pract* 40:333–337, 1999.

25. Bonnard P, Dralez F: A propos d'un cas de thymome chez un chat. *Le Point Veterinaire* 23:1089–1094, 1992.

26. O'Dair HA, Holt PE, Pearson GR, Gruffydd-Jones TJ: Acquired immune-mediated myasthenia gravis in a cat associated with a cystic thymus. *J Small Anim Pract* 32:198–202, 1991.

27. Shelton GD, Ho M, Kass PH: Risk factors for acquired myasthenia gravis in cats: 105 cases (1986–1998*). J Am Vet Med Assoc* 216:55–57, 2000.

28. Rae CA, Jacobs RM, Couto CG: A comparison between the cytological and histological characteristics in thirteen canine and feline thymomas. *Can Vet J* 30:497–500, 1989.

29. Vos JH, Stolwijk J, Ramaekers FCS, et al: The use of keratin antisera in the characterization of a feline thymoma. *J Comp Pathol* 102:71–77, 1990.

30. Ducoté JM, Dewey CW, Coates JR: Clinical forms of acquired myasthenia gravis in cats. *Compend Contin Educ Pract Vet* 21:440–447, 1999.

31. Anilkumar TV, Voigt RP, Quigley PJ, et al: Squamous cell carcinoma of the feline thymus with widespread apoptosis. *Res Vet Sci* 56:208–215, 1994.

32. Ellison GW, Garner MM, Ackerman N: Idiopathic mediastinal cyst in a cat. *Vet Radiol Ultrasound* 35:347–349, 1994.

33. Sugiyama M, Ohashi S, Mitani S, et al: A feline case of malignant mesothelioma in the pleura. *Bull Nippon Vet Zootech Coll* 26:3–8, 1977.

34. Kobayashi Y, Usuda H, Ochiai K, Itakura C: Malignant mesothelioma with metastases and mast cell leukaemia in a cat. *J Comp Pathol* 111:453–458, 1994.

35. Raflo CP, Nuernberger SP: Abdominal mesothelioma in a cat. *Vet Pathol* 15:781–783, 1978.

36. Andrews EJ: Pleural mesthelioma in a cat. *J Comp Pathol* 83:259–263, 1973.

37. Akiyama K, Akiyama R, Suzuki Y: A case of feline peritoneal mesothelioma with psammoma bodies. *Jpn J Vet Sci* 44:975–979, 1982.

38. Umphlet RC, Bertoy RW: Abdominal mesothelioma in a cat. *Modern Vet Pract* 69:71–73, 1988.

39. Paola JP, Hammer AS, Smeak DD, Merryman JI: Aortic body tumor causing pleural effusion in a cat. *JAAHA* 30:281–285, 1994.

40. Schaer M, Meyer D: Benign peritoneal mesothelioma, hyperthyroidism, nonsuppurative hepatitis, and chronic disseminated intravascular coagulation in a cat: A case report. *JAAHA* 24:195–202, 1988.

41. Tilley LP, Owens JM, Wilkins RJ, Patnaik AK: Pericardial mesothelioma with effusion in a cat. *JAAHA* 11:60–65, 1975.

42. Suzuki Y, Sugimura M, Atoji Y, Akiyama K: Lymphatic metastasis in a case of feline peritoneal mesothelioma. *Jpn J Vet Sci* 47:511–516, 1985.

43. Rao AT, Acharjyo LN: Pleural mesothelioma in a tigress. *Indian J Vet Pathol* 18:174–175, 1994.

44. Moore PF. A review of histiocytic diseases of dogs and cats. *Vet Pathol* 51(1):167-184, 2014.45.Court EA, Earnest-Koons KA, Barr SC, Gould II WJ: Malignant histiocytosis in a cat. *JAVMA* 203:1300–1302, 1993.

46. Walton RM, Brown DE, Burkhard MJ, et al: Malignant histiocytosis in a domestic cat: Cytomorphologic and immunohistochemical features. *Vet Clin Pathol* 26:56–60, 1997.

47. Freeman L, Stevens J, Loughman C, Tompkins M: Clinical vignette: Malignant histiocytosis in a cat. *J Vet Intern Med* 9:171–173, 1995.

48. Kraje AC, Patton CS, Edwards DF: Malignant histiocytosis in 3 cats. *J Vet Intern Med* 15:252–256, 2001.

49. Gafner F, Bestetti GE: Feline maligne histiozytose und lysozymnachweis. *Schweiz Arch Tierheilk* 130:349–356, 1988.

50. Fritz D, Georges C, Hopfner CL: Malignant histiocytosis in a cat. *Feline Pract* 27:6–8, 1999.

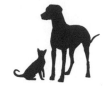

Chapter 59

Feline tumors of skin and surrounding structures

FELINE BENIGN SKIN TUMORS

Clinical presentation

- Hair matrix tumors are rare.
- Papillomas are rare and tend to be viral-induced.
- Benign plasmacytomas are rare and must be distinguished from the malignant variant that present similar to multiple myeloma.
- Lipomas may occur anywhere on body but are uncommon.
- Dilated pore of Winer and trichoepithelioma are characterized by a cystic structure similar to an epidermal inclusion cyst that is derived from the follicular sheath and may present initially as a raised lesion that may "open-up" to leave a crater-like lesion.
- Benign skin tumors are usually not usually painful.

> **Key point**
> Basal cell carcinomas are the most common melanocytic-containing tumor of cats.

Staging and diagnosis

- Minimum data base (MDB): includes a CBC, biochemical profile, urinalysis, FIV/FeLV serology, T4 testing, and three-view thoracic radiographs or computerized tomography of the chest.
- If the malignant form of plasma cell tumor is suspected, it should be staged as a multiple myeloma, including serum electrophoresis and bone marrow aspirate.
- Ultrasonography and/or radiographs are practical and cost effective.

Treatment

This section is divided into two options:

- Comfort for those who want to improve quality of life.
- Comfort and control for those who want to improve quality of life while trying to provide some control of the tumor.

> **Key point**
> Resection and/or cryotherapy of a benign basal cell tumor is usually curative.

Comfort

- Therapy to enhance comfort (e.g.: NSAID, tramadol, buprenorphine) and freedom from nausea, vomiting (e.g.: maropitant and/or metoclopramide), diarrhea (e.g.: metronidazole) and lack of appetite (e.g.: mirtazapine or cyproheptadine).

Comfort and control

Above mentioned therapy for comfort plus:
- Complete excision.

FELINE BENIGN BASAL CELL TUMORS

Clinical presentation

- The most common skin tumor of cats.
- Accounts for 25-30% of all skin tumors.
- Basal cell tumors are most common melanocytic tumor in cats, and that they are the most common benign skin tumor despite the other terms (e.g., basal cell carcinoma, basosquamous carcinoma, basal cell epithelioma).
  - Must be distinguished from *basal cell carcinoma* and *basosquamous carcinoma*, which are invasive, less common malignant variants,[22] some of which were recently reclassified on the basis of their lineage as trichoblastoma.[9]

- Often solitary and small, however some have been 7 cm in size.
- May be painful.

Staging and diagnosis

- Minimum data base (MDB): includes a CBC, biochemical profile, urinalysis, FIV/FeLV serology, T4 testing, biopsy, three-view thoracic radiographs or computerized tomography of the chest.

Treatment

This section is divided into two options:
- Comfort for those who want to improve quality of life.
- Comfort and control for those who want to improve quality of life while trying to provide some control of the tumor.

Comfort

- Therapy to enhance comfort (e.g.: NSAID, tramadol, buprenorphine) and freedom from nausea, vomiting (e.g.: maropitant and/or metoclopramide), diarrhea (e.g.: metronidazole) and lack of appetite (e.g.: mirtazapine or cyproheptadine).

Comfort and control

- Surgery should be curative.

FELINE MALIGNANT BASAL CELL TUMORS

Clinical presentation

- Invasive, nonpigmented, solid tumors usually located on the head and neck that may metastasize to regional lymph node and elsewhere.
- May be painful.

Staging and diagnosis

- Minimum data base (MDB): includes a CBC, biochemical profile, urinalysis, FIV/FeLV serology, T4 testing, biopsy, three-view thoracic radiographs or computerized tomography of the chest.
- Ultrasonography and/or radiographs are practical and cost effective, however computerized tomography or magnetic resonance imaging of the tumor may be preferable in some cases.

Treatment

This section is divided into three options:
- Comfort for those who want to improve quality of life.
- Comfort and control for those who want to improve quality of life while trying to provide some control of the tumor.
- Comfort and longer-term control for those who want to improve quality of life while trying to maximize the chance of controlling the tumor.

Comfort

- Therapy to enhance comfort (e.g.: NSAID, tramadol, buprenorphine) and freedom from nausea, vomiting (e.g.: maropitant and/or metoclopramide), diarrhea (e.g.: metronidazole) and lack of appetite (e.g.: mirtazapine or cyproheptadine).

Comfort and control

Above mentioned therapy for comfort plus:
- Palliative radiation, especially for those with extension into surrounding structures or regional metastases (e.g.: 2-5 dosages of radiation), to first enhance comfort, second, to reduce the rate of growth and third, occasionally to reduce the size of the tumor.

Comfort and longer-term control

Above mentioned therapy for comfort plus:
- Surgery.
- Definitive radiation if there is evidence of tumor extending beyond the surgical margins (e.g.: 16-19 dosages of radiation).
- Doxorubicin and carboplatin are the chemotherapeutic agents most likely to delay or prevent metastasis.

FELINE BENIGN GLANDULAR TUMORS

Clinical presentation

- Uncommon.
- Apocrine gland adenomas have a predilection for the head, with nearly 60% of these tumors occurring at this site, with fewer occurring on the back, neck, abdomen, perineum, and hind leg.[1-3,25]
- Sebaceous gland hyperplasia may be difficult to differentiate from sebaceous adenoma, but both are rare.
- May be painful.

Staging and diagnosis

- Minimum data base (MDB): includes a CBC, biochemical profile, urinalysis, FIV/FeLV serology, T4 testing, biopsy, three-view thoracic radiographs or computerized tomography of the chest.

Treatment

This section is divided into two options:
- Comfort for those who want to improve quality of life.
- Comfort and control for those who want to improve quality of life while trying to be curative of the tumor.

Comfort

- Therapy to enhance comfort (e.g.: NSAID, tramadol, buprenorphine) and freedom from nausea, vomiting (e.g.: maropitant and/or metoclopramide), diarrhea (e.g.: metronidazole) and lack of appetite (e.g.: mirtazapine or cyproheptadine).

Comfort and control

Above mentioned therapy for comfort plus:
• Surgery should be curative.

FELINE MALIGNANT GLANDULAR TUMORS

Clinical presentation

• Apocrine adenocarcinomas may be ulcerated and are found most commonly on the head, followed by the legs, pinnae, axilla, rump, thigh, thoracic wall and perineum.[1,3,25]
• May metastasize to regional lymph nodes and elsewhere.
• May be painful.

Staging and diagnosis

• Minimum data base (MDB): includes a CBC, biochemical profile, urinalysis, FIV/FeLV serology, T4 testing, biopsy, three-view thoracic radiographs or computerized tomography of the chest.
• Ultrasonography and/or radiographs are practical and cost effective, however computerized tomography or magnetic resonance imaging of the tumor may be preferable in some cases.

Treatment

This section is divided into three options:
• Comfort for those who want to improve quality of life.
• Comfort and control for those who want to improve quality of life while trying to provide some control of the tumor.
• Comfort and longer-term control for those who want to improve quality of life while trying to maximize the chance of controlling the tumor.

Comfort

• Therapy to enhance comfort (e.g.: NSAID, tramadol, buprenorphine) and freedom from nausea, vomiting (e.g.: maropitant and/or metoclopramide), diarrhea (e.g.: metronidazole) and lack of appetite (e.g.: mirtazapine or cyproheptadine).

Comfort and control

Above mentioned therapy for comfort plus:
• Palliative radiation, especially for those with extension into surrounding structures or regional metastases (e.g.: 2-5 dosages of radiation), to first enhance comfort, second, to reduce the rate of growth and third, occasionally to reduce the size of the tumor.

Comfort and longer-term control

Above mentioned therapy for comfort plus:
• Surgery.
• Definitive radiation if there is evidence of tumor extending beyond the surgical margins (e.g.: 16-19 dosages of radiation).

FELINE CUTANEOUS MELANOMA

Clinical presentation

• Moderately common and must be distinguished from pigmented basal cell tumors or lentigo simplex.
• Approximately 80% of cutaneous melanomas in cats are black in color and may be seen as masses that are nodular or papilloma-like in some cats and sessile, pedunculated, or crateriform in others.[31]
• May occur on the head, in particular on the pinna and at the base of the ear, however they have been diagnosed on the trunk, limbs, digits, tail and perineum.[2,3,28-30,33]
• Cutaneous melanomas of the epithelioid type were malignant in 80% of cases, spindloid tumors were malignant in 29% of cases, and round cell tumors were malignant about half of the time.[30]
• Most often site of metastasis is the regional lymph node.
• Usually not painful.

> **Key point**
> Eighty percent of cutaneous melanomas are pigmented.

Staging and diagnosis

• Minimum data base (MDB): includes a CBC, biochemical profile, urinalysis, FIV/FeLV serology, T4 testing, biopsy, three-view thoracic radiographs or computerized tomography of the chest.
• Ultrasonography and/or radiographs are practical and cost effective, however computerized tomography or magnetic resonance imaging of the tumor may be preferable in some cases.

Treatment

This section is divided into three options:
• Comfort for those who want to improve quality of life.
• Comfort and control for those who want to improve quality of life while trying to provide some control of the tumor.
• Comfort and longer-term control for those who want to improve quality of life while trying to maximize the chance of controlling the tumor.

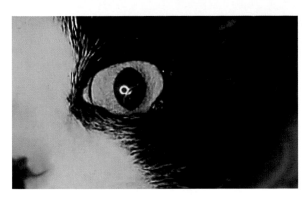

Figure 59-1: Basal cell carcinomas can be pigmented, as can cutaneous melanomas. The eyelid tumor depicted here is a melanoma that was diagnosed by cytology. The tumor was treated successfully with cryotherapy. Three rapid freezes were followed each by a slow thaw. Reprinted with permission from: Ogilvie GK, Moore AS. Feline Oncology: A Comprehensive Guide for Compassionate Care. Trenton NJ, Veterinary Learning Systems. 2002.

Comfort

- Therapy to enhance comfort (e.g.: NSAID, tramadol, buprenorphine) and freedom from nausea, vomiting (e.g.: maropitant and/or metoclopramide), diarrhea (e.g.: metronidazole) and lack of appetite (e.g.: mirtazapine or cyproheptadine).

Comfort and control

Above mentioned therapy for comfort plus:
- Palliative or coarse fractionated radiation, especially for those that are not amenable to localized therapy or that have with extension into surrounding structures or regional metastases (e.g.: 2-5 dosages of radiation), to first enhance comfort, second, to reduce the rate of growth and third, occasionally to reduce the size of the tumor.
- Cryotherapy may be of value if the tumor is small.

Comfort and longer-term control

Above mentioned therapy for comfort plus:
- Surgery.
- Definitive radiation if there is evidence of tumor extending beyond the surgical margins (e.g.: 16-19 dosages of radiation).
- Use of a DNA, xenogeneic melanoma vaccine that was originally developed for the dog has been used to delay or prevent recurrence or spread in the cat.

FELINE CUTANEOUS MAST CELL TUMORS

Clinical presentation

- Moderately common, representing up to 20% of all skin tumors.

- May be single, multiple, or diffuse (miliary), with most also described as hairless, firm, and between 2 and 5 cm in diameter.[2,38]
- Cats that have multiple tumors do not always develop systemic disease,[37] whereas cats with solitary tumors may later develop multiple cutaneous tumors without evidence of systemic disease.
- Approximately half of the tumors appear on the skin of the head and neck.[2,3]
- Tumors contain vasoactive substances such as histamine and serotonin that may cause some to be pruritic and erythematous,[2] which may lead to self-trauma and secondary ulceration.[37,40,42,45,49,52]
- May be painful.

Staging and diagnosis

- Minimum data base (MDB): includes a CBC, biochemical profile, urinalysis, FIV/FeLV serology, T4 testing, bone marrow aspirate, biopsy and three-view thoracic radiographs or computerized tomography of the chest.
  - Cytology may confirm the presence of very fine granules within the cytoplasm, however some mast cell tumors do not stain well.
  - Histiocytic MCTs in Siamese cats may regress spontaneously.
  - Histologic biopsies confirm the diagnosis, although grading did not correlate with recurrence or survival.[37]
- Ultrasonography and/or radiographs are practical and cost effective, however computerized tomography or magnetic resonance imaging of the tumor may be preferable in some cases. Aspirates of liver, spleen and lymph nodes may be indicated.

> **Key point**
> Cutaneous mast cell tumors may be single or multiple and occasionally associated with splenomegaly and bone marrow involvement.

Treatment

This section is divided into three options:
- Comfort for those who want to improve quality of life.
- Comfort and control for those who want to improve quality of life while trying to provide some control of the tumor.
- Comfort and longer-term control for those who want to improve quality of life while trying to maximize the chance of controlling the tumor.

Comfort

- Therapy to enhance comfort (e.g.: NSAID or more likely prednisolone, tramadol, buprenorphine)

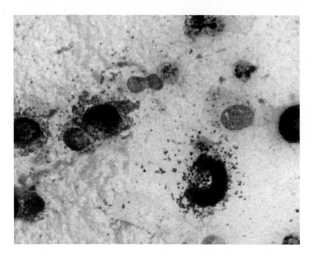

Figure 59-2: Mast cell tumors are composed of cells with granules that are metachromatic in color. Grading from either cytology or histopathology has not been shown to be predictive of outcome.

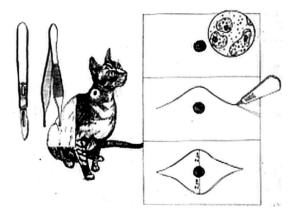

Figure 59-3: Surgery is usually quite effective at resolving feline mast cell tumors. Every attempt should be made to obtain wide and deep margins. Mast cell tumors in cats tend to be more focal than those of the dog. An elliptical incision is made to allow adequate resection. Reprinted with permission from: Ogilvie GK, Moore AS. Feline Oncology: A Comprehensive Guide for Compassionate Care. Trenton NJ, Veterinary Learning Systems. 2002.

and freedom from nausea, vomiting (e.g.: maropitant and/or metoclopramide), diarrhea (e.g.: metronidazole) and lack of appetite (e.g.: mirtazapine or cyproheptadine).

- Treatment with prednisolone and cimetidine was not successful in reducing the number or size of cutaneous lesions in cats with systemic mast cell disease.[43]

Comfort and control

Above mentioned therapy for comfort plus:

- Tyrosine kinase inhibitor such as toceranib.
- CCNU may be effective.
  - In one study involving 38 cats with mast cell tumors, 7 cats had a complete response and 12 had a partial response, for an overall response rate of 50% and a median response duration of 168 days (range, 25 to 727 days).[8]

Comfort and longer-term control

Above mentioned therapy for comfort plus:

- Surgical resection may be curative. Many tumors are only minimally invasive, but it is prudent to obtain wide margins if anatomically possible.
  - Thirty cats had cutaneous mast cell tumors excised, 20 with incomplete margins. Only 2 of these 20 tumors recurred and did so within a year of surgery. Sixteen of the cats were followed for more than 3 years, and no cat died due to mast cell disease.[39]
  - Forty two cats with dermal tumors had their dermal mast cell tumors excised, with no tumor recurrence 1 year after surgery in 34 cats.
- If surgery is incomplete, then definitive radiation may be of value for treating some patients with invasive mast cell tumors that may not respond to additional surgery.

FELINE SQUAMOUS CELL CARCINOMA

Clinical presentation

- Approximately 20% of all skin tumors in the USA and Europe, whereas it is the most common skin tumor in cats from Australia and New Zealand, accounting for approximately 50% of all skin tumors.[6]
- Most common in cats that lack skin pigment and in those cats with limited hair coverage.
- White cats are at least five times more likely to develop cutaneous SCC than any other color cat.[22]
- In studies involving over 600 cats, the overall incidence of cutaneous SCC varies but the proportion involving the face is between 80% and 90%.[1,3,6,22]
- Multiple cutaneous SCC of other body sites has been termed *multicentric SCC in situ*, or *Bowen's disease.*
- Cutaneous SCC may often start as epidermal dysplasia following chronic sunlight exposure[67] that progresses to squamous cell carcinoma in situ and will eventually form an invasive cutaneous tumor.
- Metastases are uncommon until late in the course of the disease. Most common sites include pulmonary and lymph nodes.
- May be painful.

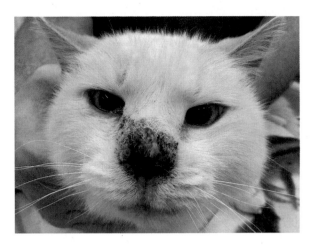

Figure 59-4: Outdoor cats with thin and/or white hair coat are predisposed to developing solar-induced squamous cell carcinoma. These locally invasive tumors often occur on the nose (depicted here), ears and eyelids. Clients should be warned that where there is one squamous cell carcinoma, there are often many others. Diagnosis is made by biopsy. Early resection, treatment with cryotherapy, imiquimod cream or photodynamic therapy with elimination of solar exposure can be helpful.

Key point

This tumor is often seen in white cats and in areas with limited hair coverage.

Staging and diagnosis

- Minimum data base (MDB): includes a CBC, biochemical profile, urinalysis, FIV/FeLV serology, T4 testing, bone marrow aspirate biopsy and three-view thoracic radiographs or computerized tomography of the chest.
- Ultrasonography and/or radiographs are practical and cost effective, however computerized tomography or magnetic resonance imaging of the tumor may be preferable in some cases.

Key point

Cutaneous squamous cell carcinomas rarely metastasize.

Treatment

This section is divided into three options:
- Comfort for those who want to improve quality of life.
- Comfort and control for those who want to improve quality of life while trying to provide some control of the tumor.
- Comfort and longer-term control for those who want to improve quality of life while trying to maximize the chance of controlling the tumor.

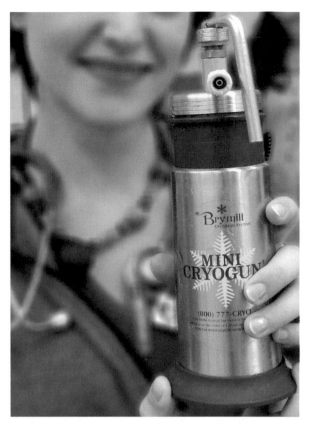

Figure 59-5: Cryotherapy can be used to treat well-defined skin tumors that are smaller than 1.5 cm in diameter. Larger tumors may not freeze uniformly. Liquid nitrogen is added to the cryogun depicted here. Various adapters are added to allow the liquid nitrogen to be applied to the tumor in a spray or via a contact applicator. Three separate quick freezes separated by a slow period of thawing is generally very helpful.

Key point

Surgical excision or cryotherapy may be quite effective if applied appropriately.

Comfort

- Therapy to enhance comfort (e.g.: NSAID, tramadol, buprenorphine) and freedom from nausea, vomiting (e.g.: maropitant and/or metoclopramide), diarrhea (e.g.: metronidazole) and lack of appetite (e.g.: mirtazapine or cyproheptadine). Precancerous actinic keratosis, or tumors that have not invaded beyond the basement membrane (T_{is}), may respond to retinoic acid derivatives/carotenoids. Etretinate or analogs such as acitretin and Soriatane® have been used at a dose of 10 mg/cat/day and anecdotally appears to result in regression of actinic keratoses and in situ lesions.

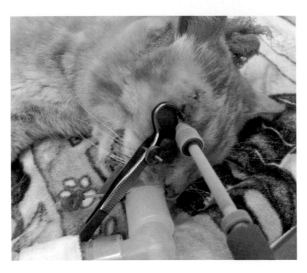

Figure 59-6: This eyelid squamous cell carcinoma is being frozen with a contact probe attached to the cryogun. The Chalazion clamp is in place to slow the rate of thaw.

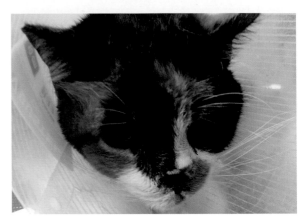

Figure 59-8: This cat had a surgical procedure to remove the nasal planum that was destroyed by a squamous cell carcinoma. Reprinted with permission from: Ogilvie GK, Moore AS. Feline Oncology: A Comprehensive Guide for Compassionate Care. Trenton NJ, Veterinary Learning Systems. 2002.

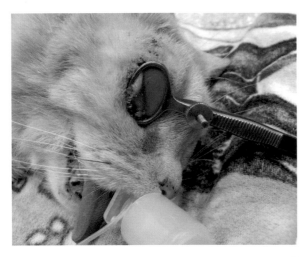

Figure 59-7: Eyelid tumors such as this squamous cell carcinoma can be best frozen by limiting the blood flow to the area. In this case, a Chalazion clamp is applied to the eyelid, slowing the rate of thaw of the liquid nitrogen induced freeze.

Comfort and control

Above mentioned therapy for comfort plus:
- Photodynamic therapy and cryotherapy have both been shown to benefit focal, accessible skin tumors less than 1 cm in diameter.
  - Photodynamic therapy requires specific equipment including a laser of a unique wave length and a photosensitizer.
  - Liquid nitrogen was used in one study to treat 163 SCC lesions on 102 cats. A cryoprobe was used to monitor the temperature of the tissue, which was frozen to –25°C to –40°C twice with

an intervening thaw cycle.[22] Complete resolution was seen in all (50) pinna lesions and all (23) eyelid lesions treated in this manner. Complete resolution was seen in 73 of 90 nasal planum lesions (81%).
- Imiquimod cream 5% has antiviral effects against for genital warts and has been shown to be effective to treat superficial, small squamous cell carcinomas by modulating the immune system locally. A small amount of the cream is rubbed into the region immediately around the tumor daily for up to six weeks.
  - Imiquimod 5%, a novel immune response modifier that has been reported as a successful treatment for Bowen's disease in humans, was used to treat cutaneous squamous cell carcinoma in 12 cats. Most cats (75%) developed new lesions that also responded to imiquimod 5% cream in all cats treated. Five cats (41%) had side effects suspected to be associated with the use of imiquimod 5% cream, including local erythema (25%), increased liver enzymes, neutropenia (8%), and partial anorexia and vomiting (8%). Kaplan-Meier median survival time probabilities for cats in this study was 1189 days.

Comfort and longer-term control

Above mentioned therapy for comfort plus:
- Surgery.
  - Surgical excision of the nasal planum (21 cats) or the pinna (18 cats) resulted in complete surgical margins in all but 7 cats. The tumor recurred in 2 of these cats in which surgical margins were incomplete.[60] The median disease-free interval for all 39 cats was 20 months, which was longer than for cryosurgery (8.5 months) in the same study.

- Radiation
  - Radiation therapy with a strontium-90 handheld source delivers a very high dose of radiation that penetrates only 3 to 5 mm below the skin surface. Strontium-90 was used to treat small (T_{is} and T_1) lesions of the nasal plane in 25 cats.[72] One year after treatment, 22 cats (89%) were tumor free; the median progression-free survival time was 34 months.
  - Standard orthovoltage or megavoltage radiation therapy has been shown to also be quite effective at the local control of cutaneous squamous cell carcinoma.
    - Ninety cats with SCC of the nasal planum received orthovoltage radiation (40 Gy in 10 fractions). Those cats with T_1 lesions had a mean progression-free survival of 53.2 months, which was significantly better than cats with T_3 or T_4 lesions (18.8 and 15.3 months, respectively).[63]

FELINE MULTICENTRIC SCC IN SITU (BOWEN'S DISEASE)

Clinical presentation

- Relatively uncommon.
- Sunlight does not seem to be a factor in tumor development.
- Lesions are usually not pruritic, however they are pigmented to ulcerated, small (5 mm to 3 cm in diameter) and can be plaque-like or papillated, partially alopecic, and crusted.
- While the lesions are often multiple and develop over time, they do not commonly metastasize.
- Lesions may occur throughout the body, including the head, neck, thighs, shoulders, ventral abdomen and paws.[86–88]
- May be painful.

Staging and diagnosis

- Minimum data base (MDB): includes a CBC, biochemical profile, urinalysis, FIV/FeLV serology, T4 testing, biopsy, three-view thoracic radiographs or computerized tomography of the chest.
- Ultrasonography and/or radiographs are practical and cost effective, however computerized tomography or magnetic resonance imaging of the tumor may be preferable in some cases.

Treatment

This section is divided into three options:
- Comfort for those who want to improve quality of life.
- Comfort and control for those who want to improve quality of life while trying to provide some control of the tumor.
- Comfort and longer-term control for those who want to improve quality of life while trying to maximize the chance of controlling the tumor.

Comfort

- Therapy to enhance comfort (e.g.: NSAID, tramadol, buprenorphine) and freedom from nausea, vomiting (e.g.: maropitant and/or metoclopramide), diarrhea (e.g.: metronidazole) and lack of appetite (e.g.: mirtazapine or cyproheptadine). Precancerous actinic keratosis, or tumors that have not invaded beyond the basement membrane (T_{is}) may respond to retinoic acid derivatives/carotenoids. Etretinate or analogs such as acitretin and Soriatane® have been used at a dose of 10 mg/cat/day and anecdotally appear to result in regression of actinic keratoses and in situ lesions.

Comfort and control

Above mentioned therapy for comfort plus:
- Photodynamic therapy and cryotherapy have both been shown to benefit focal, accessible skin tumors less than 1 cm in diameter.
  - Photodynamic therapy requires specific equipment including a laser of a unique wave length and a photosensitizer.
  - Cryotherapy uses liquid nitrogen to do three quick freezes and three slow thaws.
- Imiquimod cream 5% has antiviral effects against genital warts and has been shown to be effective to treat superficial, small squamous cell carcinomas by modulating the immune system locally.[19] A small amount of the cream is rubbed into the region immediately around the tumor daily for up to six weeks.

Comfort and longer-term control

Above mentioned therapy for comfort plus:
- Surgery.
- Radiation
  - Radiation therapy with a strontium-90 handheld source delivers a very high dose of radiation that penetrates only 3 to 5 mm below the skin surface.
  - Standard orthovoltage or megavoltage radiation therapy has been shown to also be quite effective at the local control of cutaneous squamous cell carcinoma.

FELINE CUTANEOUS HEMANGIOMA

Clinical presentation

- In cats, these tumors commonly occur on the skin.
- Bleeding from the tumor and bruising around the lesion are the most common clinical finding.
- Identification of metastases is not common but may be found in the lung, lymph nodes, liver and spleen.
- Cats with poorly pigmented skin may be predisposed. Possibly actinically induced.
- Usually not painful.

Staging and diagnosis

- Minimum data base (MDB): includes a CBC, biochemical profile, urinalysis, FIV/FeLV serology, T4 testing, biopsy, three-view thoracic radiographs or computerized tomography of the chest.
- Ultrasonography and/or radiographs are practical and cost effective, however computerized tomography or magnetic resonance imaging of the tumor may be preferable in some cases.

Treatment

This section is divided into three options:
- Comfort for those who want to improve quality of life.
- Comfort and control for those who want to improve quality of life while trying to provide some control of the tumor.
- Comfort and longer-term control for those who want to improve quality of life while trying to maximize the chance of controlling the tumor.

Comfort

- Therapy to enhance comfort (e.g.: NSAID, tramadol, buprenorphine) and freedom from nausea, vomiting (e.g.: maropitant and/or metoclopramide), diarrhea (e.g.: metronidazole) and lack of appetite (e.g.: mirtazapine or cyproheptadine).

Comfort and control

Above mentioned therapy for comfort plus:
- Palliative radiation, especially for those with extension into surrounding structures or regional metastases (e.g.: 2-5 dosages of radiation), to first enhance comfort, second, to reduce the rate of growth and third, occasionally to reduce the size of the tumor.

Comfort and longer-term control

Above mentioned therapy for comfort plus:
- Surgery. In one survey, median survival was 40 weeks, with 5 cats alive 18 to 112 weeks after surgery.[92]
- Radiation may also be effective for controlling local disease.
- Chemotherapy is as of yet unproven, however it is believed that doxorubicin is likely the drug of choice.

FELINE CUTANEOUS HEMANGIOSARCOMA

Clinical presentation

- Affects older cats; may be more common in males.
- Possibly actinically induced. Cats with poorly pigmented skin may be predisposed.

- Sarcomas are often ulcerated or cause subcutaneous bleeding.

Staging and diagnosis

- MDB and abdominal ultrasonography; evaluate regional lymph nodes. Lungs are the most common site for metastasis, but widespread metastasis is often seen.

Treatment

Initial

- Surgical excision needs to be wide.

Adjunctive

- Incomplete excision may require radiation therapy (no published efficacy).
- Metastatic rate is high, so chemotherapy warranted; doxorubicin, ifosfamide, and carboplatin are potentially active drugs.

Supportive

- Analgesia as needed; anti-inflammatories may be palliative.

FELINE CUTANEOUS LYMPHANGIOSARCOMA/ LYMPHANGIOMA

Clinical presentation

- Rare tumor of the skin and subcutis.
- Metastases to the lung, muscles and regional lymph nodes is possible.
- May be painful.

Staging and diagnosis

- Minimum data base (MDB): includes a CBC, biochemical profile, urinalysis, FIV/FeLV serology, T4 testing, biopsy, three-view thoracic radiographs or computerized tomography of the chest.
- Ultrasonography and/or radiographs are practical and cost effective, however computerized tomography or magnetic resonance imaging of the tumor may be preferable in some cases.

Treatment

This section is divided into three options:
- Comfort for those who want to improve quality of life.
- Comfort and control for those who want to improve quality of life while trying to provide some control of the tumor.
- Comfort and longer-term control for those who want to improve quality of life while trying to maximize the chance of controlling the tumor.

Comfort

- Therapy to enhance comfort (e.g.: NSAID, tramadol, buprenorphine) and freedom from nausea, vomiting (e.g.: maropitant and/or metoclopramide), diarrhea (e.g.: metronidazole) and lack of appetite (e.g.: mirtazapine or cyproheptadine).

Comfort and control

Above mentioned therapy for comfort plus:
- Palliative radiation, especially for those with extension into surrounding structures or regional metastases (e.g.: 2-5 dosages of radiation), to first enhance comfort, second, to reduce the rate of growth and third, occasionally to reduce the size of the tumor.

Comfort and longer-term control

Above mentioned therapy for comfort plus:
- Surgery.
- Definitive radiation if there is evidence of tumor extending beyond the surgical margins (e.g.: 16-19 dosages of radiation).

FELINE CUTANEOUS LYMPHOMA

Clinical presentation

- Moderately common.
- Lymphoma affecting the skin of cats can be epidermotropic (known as mycosis fungoides), while the other is not restricted to this site and may infiltrate more deeply.
- Presents as singular or multiple painful, 1 mm-3 cm diameter cutaneous plaques that are often erythematous and may be seen with generalized scaliness, or crusting due to epidermal exfoliation.[101,103-106, 109,110,113]
- While many cats are FeLV and FIV-negative, FeLV antigens have been found in the tumor via immunohistochemistry.

Staging and diagnosis

- Minimum data base (MDB): includes a CBC, biochemical profile, urinalysis, FIV/FeLV serology, T4 testing, biopsy, three-view thoracic radiographs or computerized tomography of the chest.
  - Biopsy is required for definitive diagnosis of cutaneous lymphoma. Histopathologic findings of epidermotrophism and accumulation of atypical pleomorphic lymphocytes in Pautrier's microabscesses is pathognomonic for the variant of cutaneous lymphoma known as mycosis fungoides.[105,106,109-112]
    - Mycosis fungoides is assumed to be a T-cell variant of cutaneous lymphoma.

- Some cutaneous lymphomas have been shown to be of B-cell derivation.[113]
- Ultrasonography and/or radiographs are practical and cost effective, however computerized tomography or magnetic resonance imaging of the tumor may be preferable in some cases.

Treatment

This section is divided into three options:
- Comfort for those who want to improve quality of life.
- Comfort and control for those who want to improve quality of life while trying to provide some control of the tumor.
- Comfort and longer-term control for those who want to improve quality of life while trying to maximize the chance of controlling the tumor.

Comfort

- Therapy to enhance comfort (e.g.: NSAID or prednisolone, tramadol, buprenorphine) and freedom from nausea, vomiting (e.g.: maropitant and/or metoclopramide), diarrhea (e.g.: metronidazole) and lack of appetite (e.g.: mirtazapine or cyproheptadine). Neither oral nor topical prednisolone appears to be successful in inducing remission,[101,106,112] although some reduction in pruritus may occur. Retinoids such as Accutane, isotretinoin or acitretin may be helpful in some cats.[110]

Comfort and control

Above mentioned therapy for comfort plus:
- Palliative external beam radiation, especially for those with localized lesions or extension into surrounding structures or regional metastases (e.g.: 2-5 dosages of radiation), with the goal to first enhance comfort, second, to reduce the rate of growth and third, occasionally to reduce the size of the tumor.[105] Multiple lesions treated with strontium-90 plesiotherapy has been reported to cause complete regression.114

Comfort and longer-term control

Above mentioned therapy for comfort plus:
- Surgery or definitive radiation for localized lesions, however it is reasonable to suspect that additional lesions will occur. Enhancing control with chemotherapy is logical.
- Chemotherapy. CCNU as a single agent, COP or a CHOP protocol with or without CCNU may improve quality of life for cats with cutaneous lymphoma.[115,116]
  - Chemotherapy with vincristine, cyclophosphamide, and prednisolone has caused a dramatic short-term improvement in lesions.[105,107]

References

1. Miller MA, Nelson SL, Turk JR, et al: Cutaneous neoplasia in 340 cats. *Vet Pathol* 28:389–395, 1991.
2. Carpenter JL, Andrews LK, Holzworth J: Tumors and tumor-like lesions. In Holzworth J (ed): *Diseases of the Cat. Medicine and Surgery*. Philadelphia, WB Saunders, 1987, pp 407–596.
3. Goldschmidt MH, Shofer FS: *Skin Tumors of the Dog and Cat*. New York, Pergamon Press, 1992.
4. Bostock DE: Neoplasms of the skin and subcutaneous tissues in dogs and cats. Br *Vet J* 142:1–19, 1986.
5. Litster AL, Sorenmo KU. Characterisation of the signalment, clinical and survival characteristics of 41 cats with mast cell neoplasia. *J Feline Med Surg*. 8(3):177-183, 2006..
6. Burrows AK, Lee EA, Shaw SE, et al: Skin neoplasms of cats in Perth. *Aust Vet Pract* 24:11–15, 1994.
7. Luther PB, Scott DW, Buerger RG: The dilated pore of Winer—An overlooked cutaneous lesion of cats. *J Comp Pathol* 101:375–379, 1989.
8. Rassnick KM, Williams LE, Kristal O, et al: Lomustine for treatment of mast cell tumors in cats: 38 cases (1999-2005). *J Am Vet Med Assoc*. 232(8):1200-12005, 2008.
9. Abramo F, Pratesi F, Cantile C, et al: Survey of canine and feline follicular tumours and tumour-like lesions in central Italy. *J Small Anim Pract* 40:479–481, 1999.
10. Finnie JW, Leong ASY, Milios J: Multiple piloleiomyomas in a cat. *J Comp Pathol* 113:201–204, 1995.
11. Lozano-Alarcón F, Lewis II TP, Clark EG, et al: Persistent papillomavirus infection in a cat. *JAAHA* 32:392–396, 1996.
12. Carney HC, England JJ, Hodgin EC, et al: Papillomavirus infection of aged Persian cats. *J Vet Diagn Invest* 2:294–299, 1990.
13. Gumbrell RC, Rest JR, Bredelius K, Batchelor DJ, Williamson J: Dermal fibropapillomas in cats. *Vet Rec* 142:376, 1998.
14. Breuer W, Colbatzky F, Platz S, Hermanns W: Immunoglobulin-producing tumours in dogs and cats. *J Comp Pathol* 109:203–216, 1993.
15. Kyriazidou A, Brown PJ, Lucke VM: Immunohistochemical staining of neoplastic and inflammatory plasma cell lesions in feline tissues. *J Comp Pathol* 100:337–341, 1989.
16. Lucke VM: Primary cutaneous plasmacytomas in the dog and cat. *J Small Anim Pract* 28:49–55, 1987.
17. Carothers MA, Johnson GC, DiBartola SP, et al: Extramedullary plasmacytoma and immunoglobulin-associated amyloidosis in a cat. *JAVMA* 195:1593–1597, 1989.
18. Cotchin E: Skin tumours of cats. *Res Vet Sci* 2:353–361, 1961.
19. Gill VL, Bergman PJ, Baer KE, et al: Use of imiquimod 5% cream (Aldara) in cats with multicentric squamous cell carcinoma in situ: 12 cases (2002-2005). *Vet Comp Oncol*. 6(1):55-64, 2008.
20. Esplin DG: Infiltrating lipoma in a cat. *Feline Pract* 14:24–25, 1984.
21. Diters RW, Walsh KM: Feline basal cell tumors: A review of 124 cases. *Vet Pathol* 21:51–56, 1984.
22. Clarke RE: Cryosurgical treatment of feline cutaneous squamous cell carcinoma. *Aust Vet Pract* 21:148, 1991.
23. Fehrer SL, Lin SH: Multicentric basal cell tumors in a cat. *JAVMA* 189:1469–1470, 1986.
24. Withrow SJ, Straw RC: Resection of the nasal planum in nine cats and five dogs. *JAAHA* 26:219–222, 1990.
25. Kalaher KM, Anderson WI, Scott DW: Neoplasms of the apocrine sweat glands in 44 dogs and 10 cats. *Vet Rec* 127:400–403, 1990.
26. van der Linde-Sipman JS, van den Ingh ThSGAM: Primary and metastatic carcinomas in the digits of cats. *Vet Q* 22:141–145, 2000.
27. Macy DW: Darier's sign associated with a cutaneous mast cell tumour in a cat with multiple neoplasms. *J Small Anim Pract* 29:597–602, 1988.
28. Patnaik AK, Mooney S: Feline melanoma: A comparative study of ocular, oral, and dermal neoplasms. *Vet Pathol* 25:105–112, 1988.
29. Miller Jr WH, Scott DW, Anderson WI: Feline cutaneous melanocytic neoplasms: A retrospective analysis of 43 cases (1979–1991). *Vet Dermatol* 4:19–26, 1993.
30. van der Linde-Sipman JS, De Wit MML, van Garderen E, et al: Cutaneous malignant melanomas in 57 cats: identification of (amelanotic) signet-ring and balloon cell types and verification of their origin by immunohistochemistry, electron microscopy, and in situ hybridization. *Vet Pathol* 34:31–38, 1997.
31. Goldschmidt MH, Liu SMS, Shofer FS: Feline dermal melanoma: A retrospective study. *Vet Derm* 2:285–291, 1992.
32. Howard-Martin MO, Qualls Jr CW: Metastatic melanoma in a cat. *Feline Pract* 16:6–8, 1986.
33. Day MJ, Lucke VM: Melanocytic neoplasia in the cat. *J Small Anim Pract* 36:207–213, 1995.
34. Scott DW: Lentigo simplex in orange cats. *Comp Anim Pract* 23–25, 1987.
35. Roels S, Tilmant K, Ducatelle R: PCNA and Ki67 proliferation markers as criteria for prediction of clinical behaviour of melanocytic tumours in cats and dogs. *J Comp Pathol* 121:13–24, 1999.
36. Wood CA, Moore AS, Frimberger AE, et al: Phase I evaluation of carboplatin in tumor bearing cats. *Proc 16th Annu Conf Vet Cancer Soc*:39–40, 1996.
37. Buerger RG, Scott DW: Cutaneous mast cell neoplasia in cats: 14 cases (1975–1985). *JAVMA* 190:1440–1444, 1987.
38. Wilcock BP, Yager JA, Zink MC: The morphology and behavior of feline cutaneous mastocytomas. *Vet Pathol* 23:320–324, 1986.
39. Molander-McCrary H, Henry CJ, Potter K, et al: Cutaneous mast cell tumors in cats: 32 cases (1991–1994). *JAAHA* 34:281–284, 1998.
40. Head KW: Cutaneous mast-cell tumours in the dog, cat and ox. *Br J Dermatol* 70:389–408, 1957.
41. Chastain CB, Turk MA, O'Brien D: Benign cutaneous mastocytomas in two litters of Siamese kittens. *JAVMA* 193:959–960, 1988.
42. Crafts GA, Pulley LT: Generalized cutaneous mast cell tumor in a cat. *Feline Pract* 5:57–58, 1975.
43. Cohen SJ, Koch F: Cutaneous mastocytosis with metastases in a domestic cat. *Feline Pract* 10:41–43, 1980.
44. Goto N, Ozasa M, Takahashi R, et al: Pathological observations of feline mast cell tumor. *Jpn J Vet Sci* 36:483–494, 1974.
45. Bell A, Mason K, Mitchell G, Miller R: Visceral and cutaneous mast cell neoplasia in a cat. *Aust Vet Pract* 24:86–91, 1994.
46. Madewell BR, Gunn CR, Gribble DH: Mast cell phagocytosis of red blood cells in a cat. *Vet Pathol* 20:638–640, 1983.
47. Garner FM, Lingeman CH: Mast-cell neoplasms of the domestic cat. *Pathol Vet* 7:517–530, 1970.
48. Anderson WI: Efficacy of topical 5-fluorouracil and triamcinolone acetonide in feline cutaneous mast cell tumors. *Feline Pract* 15:34–35, 1985.
49. Meier H: Feline mastocytoma: Two cases. *Cornell Vet* 47:220–226, 1957.
50. Holzinger EA: Feline cutaneous mastocytomas. *Cornell Vet* 63:87–93, 1973.
51. Scott DW: Epidermal mast cells in the cat. *Vet Dermatol* 1:65–69, 1990.
52. Monlux WS: Mastocytoma in a feline—A case report. *Southwestern Vet* 6:153–154, 1953.
53. Padrid PA, Mitchell RW, Ndukwu IM, et al: Cyproheptadine-induced attenuation of type-I immediate-hypersensitivity reactions of airway smooth muscle from immune-sensitized cats. *Am J Vet Res* 56:109–115, 1995.
54. Brown CA, Chalmers SA: Diffuse cutaneous mastocytosis in a cat. *Vet Pathol* 27:366–369, 1990.
55. Barr MC, Butt MT, Anderson KL, et al: Spinal lymphosarcoma and disseminated mastocytoma associated with feline immunodeficiency virus infection in a cat. *JAVMA* 202:1978–1980, 1993.
56. Cheli R, Addis F, Mortellaro CM, et al: Hematoporphyrin derivative photochemotherapy of spontaneous animal tumors: clinical results with optimized drug dose. *Cancer Lett* 23:61–66, 1984.
57. Seiler RJ, Punita I: Neoplasia of domestic mammals: Review of cases diagnosed at Universiti Pertanian Malaysia. *Kajian Veterinar* 11:80–84, 1979.
58. Bostock DE: The prognosis in cats bearing squamous cell carcinoma. *J Small Anim Pract* 13:119–125, 1972.
59. Frimberger AE, Moore AS, Cincotta L, Cotter SM, Foley JW: Photodynamic therapy of naturally occurring tumors in animals using a novel benzophenothiazine photosensitizer. *Clin Cancer Res* 4:2207–2218, 1998.
60. Lana SE, Ogilvie GK, Withrow SJ, et al: Feline cutaneous squamous cell carcinoma of the nasal planum and pinnae: 61 cases. *JAAHA* 33:329–332, 1997.
61. Dorn CR, Taylor DON, Schneider R: Sunlight exposure and risk of developing cutaneous and oral squamous cell carcinomas in white cats. *J Natl Cancer Inst* 46:1073–1078, 1971.
62. Ciampi L: Su deu casi di cancroide cutaneo nei gatti bianchi. *La Nuova Veterinaria* 15:342–349, 1949.
63. Thèon AP, Madewell BR, Shearn VI, Moulton JE: Prognostic factors associated with radiotherapy of squamous cell carcinoma of the nasal planum in cats. *JAVMA* 206:991–996, 1995.
64. Teifke JP, Löhr CV: Immunohistochemical detection of P53 overexpression in paraffin wax-embedded squamous cell carcinomas of cattle, horses, cats and dogs. *J Comp Pathol* 114:205–210, 1996.
65. Carlisle CH, Gould S: Response of squamous cell carcinoma of the nose of the cat to treatment with X-rays. *Vet Radiol* 23:186–192, 1982.
66. Hutson CA, Rideout BA, Pedersen NC: Neoplasia associated with feline immunodeficiency virus infection in cats of Southern California. *JAVMA* 199:1357–1362, 1991.
67. Evans EG, Madewell BR, Stannard AA: A trial of 13-cis-retinoic acid for treatment of squamous cell carcinoma and preneoplastic lesions of the head in cats. *Am J Vet Res* 46:2553–2557, 1985.

68. Peaston AE, Leach MW, Higgins RJ: Photodynamic therapy for nasal and aural squamous cell carcinoma in cats. *JAVMA* 202:1261–1265, 1993.

69. Buhles WC, Theilen GH: Preliminary evaluation of bleomycin in feline and canine squamous cell carcinoma. *Am J Vet Res* 34:289–291, 1973.

70. Thèon AP, Van Vechten MK, Madewell BR: Intratumoral administration of carboplatin for treatment of squamous cell carcinomas of the nasal plane in cats. *Am J Vet Res* 57:205–210, 1996.

71. Cox NR, Brawner WR, Powers RD, Wright JC: Tumors of the nose and paranasal sinuses in cats: 32 cases with comparison to a national database (1977 through 1987). *JAAHA* 27:339–347, 1991.

72. VanVechten MK, Thèon AP: Strontium-90 plesiotherapy for treatment of early squamous cell carcinomas of the nasal planum in 25 cats. *Proc 13th Annu Conf Vet Cancer Soc*:107–108, 1993.

73. Kaser-Hotz B, Egger B, Ruslander D,et al: Radiation therapy of feline facial squamous cell carcinoma with 72 MeV protons. *Proc 7th Europ Soc Vet Intern Med*:113, 1997.

74. Owen LM: *TNM Classification of Tumors in Domestic Animals*. Geneva, World Health Organization, 1980, pp 46–47.

75. Irving RA, Daz RS, Eales L: Porphyrin values and treatment of feline solar dermatitis. *Am J Vet Res* 43:2067–2069, 1982.

76. Leach MW, Peaston AE: Adverse drug reaction attributable to aluminum phthalocyanine tetrasulphonate administration in domestic cats. *Vet Pathol* 31:283–287, 1994.

77. Stell AJ, Langmack K, Dobson JM: treatment of superficial squamous cell carcinoma of the nasal planum in cats using photodynamic therapy [abstract]. *42nd BSAVA Congress*, 1999.

78. Shelley BA, Bartels KE, Ely RW, Clark DM: Use of the neodymium:yttrium-aluminum-garnet laser for treatment of squamous cell carcinoma of the nasal planum in a cat. *JAVMA* 201:756–758, 1992.

79. Thèon AP, Peaston AE: Pre-operative irradiation of facial tumors in cats [abstract 54]. *J Vet Intern Med* 6:122, 1992.

80. Knapp DW, Richardson RC, BeNicola DB, et.al.: Cisplatin toxicity in cats. *J Vet Intern Med* 1:29–35, 1987.

81. Harvey HJ, MacEwen EG, Hayes AA: Neurotoxicosis associated with use of 5-fluorouracil in five dogs and one cat. *JAVMA* 171:277–278, 1977.

82. Henness AM, Theilen GH, Madewell BR, Crow SE: Neurotoxicosis associated with use of 5-fluorouracil. *JAVMA* 171:692, 1977.

83. Theilen GH: Adverse effect from use of 5-fluorouracil. *JAVMA* 191:276, 1987.

84. Orenberg EK, Luck EE, Brown DM, Kitchell BE: Implant delivery system: Intralesinal delivery of chemotherapeutic agents for treatment of spontaneous skin tumors in veterinary patients. *Clin Dermatol* 9:561–568, 1992.

85. Rogers KS: Feline cutaneous squamous cell carcinoma. *Feline Pract* 22:7–9, 1994.

86. Baer KE, Helton K: Multicentric squamous cell carcinoma in situ resembling Bowen's disease in cats. *Vet Pathol* 30:535–543, 1993.

87. Miller Jr WH, Affolter V, Scott DW, Suter MM: Multicentric squamous cell carcinomas *in situ* resembling Bowen's disease in five cats. *Vet Dermatol* 3:177–182, 1992.

88. Turrel JM, Gross TL: Multicentric squamous cell carcinoma in situ (Bowen's disease) of cats. *Proc 11th Annu Conf Vet Cancer Soc*:84, 1991.

89. Gross TL, Clark EG, Hargis AM, et al: Giant cell dermatosis in FeLV-positive cats. *Vet Dermatol* 4:117–122, 1994.

90. LeClerc SM, Clark EG, Haines DM: Papillomavirus infection in association with feline cutaneous squamous cell carcinoma in situ. *Proc Am Assoc Vet Derm/Am Coll Vet Derm* 13:125–126, 1997.

91. Rees CA, Goldschmidt MH: Cutaneous horn and squamous cell carcinoma in situ (Bowen's disease) in a cat. *JAAHA* 34:485–486, 1998.

92. Scavelli TD, Patnaik AK, Mehlaff CJ, Hayes AA: Hemangiosarcoma in the cat: Retrospective evaluation of 31 surgical cases. *JAVMA* 187:817–819, 1985.

93. Miller MA, Ramos JA, Kreeger JM: Cutaneous vascular neoplasia in 15 cats: Clinical, morphologic, and immunohistochemical studies. *Vet Pathol* 29:329–336, 1992.

94. Kraje AC, Mears EA, Hahn KA, et al: Unusual metastatic behavior and clinicopathologic findings in 8 cats with cutaneous or visceral hemangiosarcoma (1981–1997). *JAVMA* 214:670–672, 1999.

95. Lawler DF, Evans RH: Multiple hepatic cavernous lymphangiomas in an aged male cat. *J Comp Pathol* 109:83–87, 1993.

96. Hinrichs U, Puhl S, Rutteman GR, et al: Lymphangiosarcomas in cats: A retrospective study of 12 cases. *Vet Pathol* 36:164–167, 1999.

97. Swayne DE, Mahaffey EA, Haynes SG: Lymphangiosarcoma and haemangiosarcoma in a cat. *J Comp Pathol* 100:91–96, 1989.

98. Patnaik AK, Liu S-K: Angiosarcoma in cats. *J Small Anim Pract* 18:191–198, 1977.

99. Walsh KM, Abbott DP: Lymphangiosarcoma in two cats. *J Comp Pathol* 94:611–613, 1984.

100. Walton DK, Berg RJ: Cutaneous lymphangiosarcoma in a cat. *Feline Pract* 13:21–26, 1983.

101. Caciolo PL, Nesbitt GH, Patnaik AK, Hayes AA: Cutaneous lymphosarcoma in the cat: A report of nine cases. *JAAHA* 20:491–496, 1984.

102. Dallman MJ, Noxon JO, Stogsdill P: Feline lymphosarcoma with cutaneous and muscle lesions. *JAVMA* 181:166–168, 1982.

103. Dust A, Norris AM, Valli VEO: Cutaneous lymphosarcoma with IgG monoclonal gammapathy, serum hyperviscosity and hypercalcemia in a cat. *Can Vet J* 23:235–239, 1982.

104. Rosenkrantz WS, Griffin CE, Barr RJ: Clinical evaluation of cyclosporine in animal models with cutaneous immune-mediated disease and epitheliotropic lymphoma. *JAAHA* 25:377–384, 1989.

105. Baker JL, Scott DW: Mycosis fungoides in two cats. *JAAHA* 25:97–101, 1989.

106. Kottkamp C, Walter JH, Löblich-Beardi B, Opitz M: Das kutane lymphosarkom der katze. *Kleintierpraxis* 41:357–366, 1996.

107. Legendre AM, Becker PU: Feline skin lymphoma: Characterization of tumor and identification of tumor-stimulating serum factor(s). *Am J Vet Res* 40:1805–1807, 1979.

108. Sent U, Pothmann M: A case of cutaneous lymphosarcoma associated with mycosis fungoides in a cat. *Feline Pract* 24:6–9, 1996.

109. Schick RO, Murphy GF, Goldschmidt MH: Cutaneous lymphosarcoma and leukemia in a cat. *JAVMA* 203:1155–1158, 1993.

110. Plant JD: Would you have diagnosed cutaneous epitheliotropic lymphoma in these two cats. *Vet Med* 86:801–806, 1991.

111. Caciolo PL, Hayes AA, Patnaik AK, et al: A case of mycosis fungoides in a cat and literature review. *JAAHA* 19:505–512, 1983.

112. Tobey JC, Houston DM, Breur GJ, et al: Cutaneous T-cell lymphoma in a cat. *JAVMA* 204:606–609, 1994.

113. Day MJ: Immunophenotypic characterization of cutaneous lymphoid neoplasia in the dog and cat. *J Comp Pathol* 112:79–96, 1995.

114. Foster SF, Charles JA, Swinney GR, Malik R: Multiple crusted cutaneous plaques in a cat. *Aust Vet J* 77:360, 1999.

115. Burr HD, Keating JH, Clifford CA, Burgess KE. Cutaneous lymphoma of the tarsus in cats: 23 cases (2000-2012). *J Am Vet Med Assoc.* 244(12):1429-1434, 2014.

116. Komori S, Nakamura S, Takahashi K, Tagawa M. Use of lomustine to treat cutaneous nonepitheliotropic lymphoma in a cat. *J Am Vet Med Assoc.* 226(2):237-239, 2005.

117. Vail DM, Moore AS, Ogilvie GK, Volk LM: Feline lymphoma (145 cases): Proliferation indices, cluster of differentiation 3 immunoreactivity, and their association with prognosis in 90 cats. *J Vet Intern Med* 12:349–354, 1998.

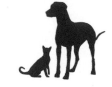

Chapter 60

Feline soft tissue sarcomas

Clinical presentation

- Moderately common, with injection site sarcomas more likely to appear in the subcutis, while non-injection site tumors occur more frequently in the dermis.[43]
- Highly locally invasive with a relatively low probability of metastases.[7]
- Firm dermal mass anywhere on body, however they appear to occur more common at injection sites including vaccinations.[44,47] Injection site sarcomas have also arisen at the site of antibiotic administration, SC fluid administration,[44,49-51] long-acting corticosteroid injection,[48] or lufenuron injection (Program® 6 month injectable).[52]
  - The distribution of tumors appears to be moving away from the intrascapular region due to recent adoption of vaccination guidelines to vaccinate in the extremities or tail.[7]
- Ulceration may occur in large tumors.
- Incidence peaks at 3 and 8 years of age.[7]
  - Injection site sarcomas usually occur in younger cats; increased risk with increased number of vaccinations at one site.[7]
- The virus FeSV may cause multiple tumors in young FeLV-positive cats.[7]
- Approximately 75% of injection sarcomas have been found to contain *p53* and *c-kit* oncogene,[61] whereas approximately one-third of tumors contained both *p53* and *mdm-2*, suggesting these factors and others result in an increased risk of developing the disease.[7]
- Fibrosarcoma is the most common soft tissue sarcoma, followed by osteosarcoma, malignant fibrous histiocytoma (histiocytic sarcoma), giant cell tumor, myofibroblastic sarcoma, rhabdomyosarcoma, leiomyosarcoma, chondrosarcoma, undifferentiated sarcoma, neurofibrosarcoma/nerve sheath tumor, and liposarcoma.
- Tumors are dermal in origin and may vary in size

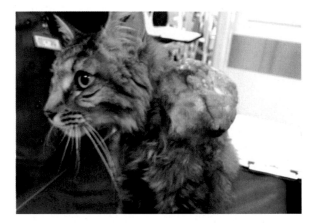

Figure 60-1: Soft tissue sarcomas can occur anywhere on the body. Injection site sarcomas tend to occur in the site of previous injections, including the intrascapular region. They have a relatively low risk of metastases but are highly invasive into surrounding tissues. Surgery, if done, must be extraordinarily wide and deep. Follow up radiation therapy is often recommended to delay or prevent local recurrence.

from 0.3 to 15 cm in diameter[7] and are typically not well demarcated or ulcerated.
- Metastasis appears to be uncommon (<28%), regardless of the subtype of soft tissue sarcoma, but may be identified in lungs, skin, spleen, kidney, and lymph node.
- May be painful.

Key point

Injection-site sarcomas occur in sites of prior injection, usually within the subcutis, whereas non-injection site sarcomas often occur in the dermis.

Staging and diagnosis

- Minimum data base (MDB): includes a CBC, biochemical profile, urinalysis, FIV/FeLV serology, T4 testing, pre-operative biopsy, three-view thoracic radiographs or computerized tomography of the chest.
  - Histologic grade was associated with distant metastasis, with cats having grade 3 tumors being significantly more likely to develop metastasis than cats with grade 1 and 2 tumors.[75]
- Ultrasonography and/or radiographs are practical and cost effective, however computerized tomography or magnetic resonance imaging of the tumor has dramatically enhance the ability to determine the extent of the disease and the presence of metastases.

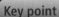

Key point

Distant metastatic disease occurs in less than 30% of cats with soft tissue sarcomas, however the primary tumor is essentially always highly locally invasive.

Treatment

This section is divided into three options:
- Comfort for those who want to improve quality of life.
- Comfort and control for those who want to improve quality of life while trying to provide some control of the tumor.
- Comfort and longer-term control for those who want to improve quality of life while trying to maximize the chance of controlling the tumor.

Key point

Extensive surgery, radiation therapy, immunotherapy and chemotherapy are often required to provide long-term control of this disease.

Comfort

- Therapy to enhance comfort (e.g.: NSAID, tramadol, buprenorphine) and freedom from nausea, vomiting (e.g.: maropitant and/or metoclopramide), diarrhea (e.g.: metronidazole) and lack of appetite (e.g.: mirtazapine or cyproheptadine).

Comfort and control

Above mentioned therapy for comfort plus:
- Palliative radiation, especially for those with extension into surrounding structures or regional metastases (e.g.: 2-5 dosages of radiation), to first enhance comfort, second, to reduce the rate of growth and third, occasionally to reduce the size of the tumor.

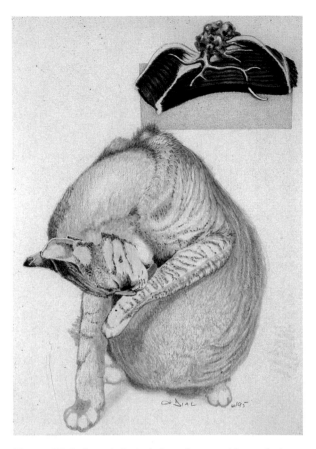

Figure 60-2: An artist's depiction of a cat with a soft tissue sarcoma. The anatomic cross section depicts the local invasion that extends out from the palpable site like tendrils. Surgery is only effective if the palpable site is removed along with the tendrils. Reprinted with permission from: Ogilvie GK, Moore AS. Feline Oncology: A Comprehensive Guide for Compassionate Care. Trenton NJ, Veterinary Learning Systems. 2002.

Comfort and longer-term control

Above mentioned therapy for comfort plus:
- Extraordinarily wide and deep surgical excision.
  - In a study of 84 cats surgically treated for soft tissue sarcoma, 60 cats (70%) had tumor recurrence an average of 3.5 months later.[7]
  - A similar recurrence rate of over 80% was seen in another study in which the median tumor-free period following surgical excision was 4 months.[31]
  - Tumors that involve the limb often recur after an attempted local excision, but the likelihood of long-term control following amputation is high.[4,16,19,27,28,30]
  - Radical excision of injection site sarcomas resulted in an overall median survival time of 901 days. Median survival time of cats with and without metastasis was 388 and 1,528 days, respectively. The metastasis rate similar to rates reported previously; the local recurrence rate

appeared to be substantially less than rates reported after less aggressive surgeries, with or without adjuvant treatment.[11]

- Definitive radiation if there is evidence of tumor extending beyond the surgical margins (e.g.: 16-19 dosages of radiation), or stereotactic body radiation therapy in 2-3 dosages.
  - Cats treated with brachytherapy using iridium-192 (^{192}Ir) implants after surgery resulted in recurrence rate in one study was 70%, with a median survival of 8 months,[24] whereas in the other group of cats, 50% of tumors recurred and the median disease-free interval was 12.5 months.[31]
  - In a study of 31 cats treated with orthovoltage radiation to a dose of 51 to 60 Gy following incomplete surgical excision, median tumor-free interval was 18 months and median survival was 22 months.[38]
  - High-dose radiation therapy (57 Gy) was used to treat 25 cats with soft tissue sarcomas and resulted in a median survival time for all cats of 700 days.[39]
  - A study was done evaluate outcomes of stereotactic body radiation therapy (SBRT) in 11 cats with injection-site sarcomas (ISS). Eight of 11 cats either had a partial or complete response, with a median progression-free interval and overall survival time of 242 days and 301 days, respectively.[17]
  - Seventy-three cats with vaccine-associated sarcoma given postsurgical curative (n = 46, most with clean margins) or coarse fractionated radiotherapy (n = 27, most with either macroscopic disease or dirty margins). The former animals displayed a median survival of 43 months and a median progression free interval (PFI) of 37 months and the latter reached a median survival of 24 months and a median PFI of 10 months.[20]
- Chemotherapy may delay or prevent recurrence or metastases.
  - Twenty-one cats with primary or recurrent soft tissue sarcomas received 3 cycles of neoadjuvant epirubicin (25 mg/m^{-2}) chemotherapy followed by a surgical resection of tumor and surrounding musculature.[29] This was followed by a further 3 cycles of adjuvant epirubicin chemotherapy. The cases were then evaluated, with a median follow-up time of 1072 days. Three cats had recurrences 264, 664 and 1573 after surgery. A median survival time could not be calculated as over 80% of the study population remained alive or were censored due to death from other causes.
  - Sixty-nine cats were treated for injection-site sarcomas and were divided into two subgroups: those subjected to four doxorubicin cycles combined with radical surgical excision 10 days after the second chemotherapy cycle (group A, 49 cats), or those treated with surgery alone (group B, 20 cats). In group A, 28 cats were alive at the end of the follow-up period. In this group, the

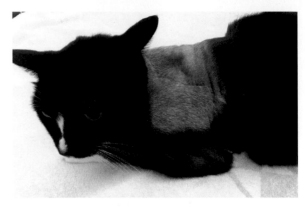

Figure 60-3: This cat had her soft tissue sarcoma resected with wide and deep margins followed by radiation, which caused skin and hair color changes. The cat remained tumor free for three years.

recurrence rate was 40.8%, while lung metastasis occurred in 12% of cats. In group B, eight animals were alive at the end of the follow-up period, while the rates of recurrence and metastasis were 35% and 10%. These data suggest that doxorubicin was not effective in this group.[32]
  - Twenty-eight cats with injection-site sarcomas were treated with various dosages of CCNU, with a median progression-free survival and median duration of response of 60.5 and 82.5 days, respectively.[35]
  - A study was done to determine whether the addition of doxorubicin chemotherapy affected the outcome of cats with incompletely excised, nonvisceral soft tissue sarcomas undergoing postoperative radiotherapy. Median disease-free interval with concurrent radiotherapy and doxorubicin chemotherapy (15.4 months) was significantly longer than the median disease-free interval with radiotherapy alone (5.7 months).[36]
- Immunotherapy may contribute to longer survival in cats treated with local therapies for fibrosarcoma.
  - Tenogeneic cells (Vero hIL-2) that secrete human recombinant interleukin-2 (hrIL-2) were infiltrated around feline soft tissue sarcomas at the time of surgical resection and implantation of ^{192}Ir seeds for brachyradiotherapy.[24] This infiltration was repeated 5 days later and another five times over the next 2 months. Of 16 cats treated by this protocol, two had local recurrence and three had metastases, with an overall median survival of 16 months. In comparison, 11 of 16 cats that did not receive Vero hIL-2 cells had tumor recurrence and a median survival of 8 months.
  - A canarypox feline IL-2 therapy has been developed and is marketed for the treatment of soft tissue sarcomas in cats that are concurrently being treated with either surgery or radiation therapy. Results are promising.

References

1. de las Mulas JM, de los Monteros AE, Carrasco L, et al: Immunohistochemical distribution pattern of intermediate filament proteins in 50 feline neoplasms. *Vet Pathol* 32:692–701, 1995.
2. Moore AS, Madewell BR, Lund JK: Immunohistochemical evaluation of intermediate filament expression in canine and feline neoplasms. *Am J Vet Res* 50:88–92, 1989.
3. Jones SA, Strafuss AC: Scanning electron microscopy of nerve sheath neoplasms. *Am J Vet Res* 39:1069–1072, 1978.
4. Jones BR, Alley MR, Johnstone AC, et al: Nerve sheath tumours in the dog and cat. *N Z Vet J* 43:190–196, 1995.
5. Silva ALA, Serakides R: Schwannoma tipo Antoni A em gato. *Arq Bras Med Vet Zootec* 47:257–259, 1995.
6. Hartmann K, Day MJ, Thiry E, et al: Feline injection-site sarcoma: ABCD guidelines on prevention and management. *J Feline Med Surg.* 17(7):606-613, 2015.
7. Ladlow J. Injection site-associated sarcoma in the cat: treatment recommendations and results to date. *J Feline Med Surg.* 15(5):409-418, 2013.
8. Roth L: Rhabdomyoma of the ear pinna in four cats. *J Comp Pathol* 103:237–240, 1990.
9. Kalat M, Mayr B, Schleger W, et al: Trisomy D2 in a feline neurofibroma. *Res Vet Sci* 48:256, 1990.
10. Kalat M, Mayr B, Schleger W, et al: Chromosomal hyperdiploidy in a feline sarcoma. *Res Vet Sci* 51:227–228, 1991.
11. Phelps HA, Kuntz CA, Milner RJ, et al: Radical excision with five-centimeter margins for treatment of feline injection-site sarcomas: 91 cases (1998-2002). *J Am Vet Med Assoc.* 1;239(1):97-106. 2011.
12. Mayr B, Schaffner G, Kurzbauer R, et al: Mutations in tumour suppressor gene p53 in two feline fibrosarcomas. *Br Vet J* 151:707–713, 1995.
13. Mayr B, Reifinger M, Alton K, Schaffner G: Novel p53 tumour suppressor mutations in cases of spindle cell sarcoma, pleomorphic sarcoma and fibrosarcoma in cats. *Vet Res Comm* 22:249–255, 1998.
14. Kanjilal S, Banerji N, Fifer A, et al: p53 tumor suppressor gene alterations in vaccine-associated feline sarcoma. *Proc. 9th Annu Conf Vet Cancer Soc*:48, 1999.
15. Hershey AE, Dubielzieg RR, Helfand SC: Overexpression of p53 in feline vaccine-associated sarcomas. *Proc. 9th Annu Conf Vet Cancer Soc*:32, 1999.
16. Cook JL, Turk JR, Tomlinson JL, et al: Fibrosarcoma in the distal radius and carpus of a four-year-old Persian. *JAAHA* 34:31–33, 1998.
17. Nolan MW, Griffin LR, Custis JT, LaRue SM. Stereotactic body radiation therapy for treatment of injection-site sarcomas in cats: 11 cases (2008-2012). *J Am Vet Med Assoc.* 243(4):526-531, 2013.
18. Trout NJ, Pavletic MM, Kraus KH: Partial scapulectomy in the management of sarcomas in three dogs and two cats. *Vet Surg* 1998.
19. Brown NO, Patnaik AK, Mooney SC, et al: Soft tissue sarcomas in the cat. *JAVMA* 173:744–779, 1978.
20. Eckstein C, Guscetti F, Roos M, et al: A retrospective analysis of radiation therapy for the treatment of feline vaccine-associated sarcoma. *Vet Comp Oncol.* 7(1):54-68, 2009.
21. Ruben JMS: Neurofibrosarcoma in a 19-year-old cat. *Vet Rec* 113:135, 1983.
22. Levy MS, Mauldin G, Kapatkin AS, Patnaik AK: Nonlymphoid vertebral canal tumors in cats: 11 cases (1987–1995). *JAVMA* 210:663–664, 1997.
23. Watrous BJ, Lipscomb TP, Heidel JR, Normal LM: Malignant peripheral nerve sheath tumor in a cat. *Vet Radiol Ultrasound* 40:638–640, 1999.
24. Quintin-Colonna F, Devauchelle P, Fradelizi D, et al: Gene therapy of spontaneous canine melanoma and feline fibrosarcoma by intratumoral administration of histoincompatible cells expressing human interleukin-2. *Gene Therap* 3:1104–1112, 1996.
25. Davidson EB, Gregory CR, Kass PH: Surgical excision of soft tissue fibrosarcomas in cats. *Vet Surg* 26:265–269, 1997.
26. Cronin K, Page RL, Spodnick G, et al: Radiation therapy and surgery for fibrosarcoma in 33 cats. *Vet Radiol Ultrasound* 39:51–56, 1998.
27. Brown NO, Hayes AA, Mooney S,: Combined modality therapy in the treatment of solid tumors in cats. *JAAHA* 16:719–722, 1980.
28. Hershey AE, Sorenmo KU, Hendrick MJ, et al: Prognosis for presumed feline vaccine-associated sarcoma after excision: 61 cases (1986–1996). *JAVMA* 216:58–61, 2000.
29. Bray J, Polton G. Neoadjuvant and adjuvant chemotherapy combined with anatomical resection of feline injection-site sarcoma: results in 21 cats. *Vet Comp Oncol* doi: 10.1111/vco.12083, 2014.
30. Bostock DE, Dye MT: Prognosis after surgical excision of fibrosarcomas in cats. *JAVMA* 175:727–728, 1979.
31. Devauchelle P: Interest and limits of brachytherapy (interstitial radiotherapy) as adjuvant treatment of feline soft tissue sarcomas. *Proc ESVIM* #7:44, 1997.
32. Martano M, Morello E, Ughetto M, et al: Surgery alone versus surgery and doxorubicin for the treatment of feline injection-site sarcomas: a report on 69 cases. *Vet J* 170(1):84-90, 2005.
33. Straw RC, Withrow SJ, Powers BE: Partial or total hemipelvectomy in the management of sarcomas in nine dogs and two cats. *Vet Surg* 21:183–188, 1992.
34. Bowmann KLT, Birchard SJ, Bright RM: Complications associated with the implantation of polypropylene mesh in dogs and cats: A retrospective study of 21 cases (1984–1996). *JAAHA* 34:225–233, 1998.
35. Saba CF, Vail DM, Thamm DH. Phase II clinical evaluation of lomustine chemotherapy for feline vaccine-associated sarcoma. *Vet Comp Oncol* 10(4):283-291, 2012.
36. Hahn KA, Endicott MM, King GK, et al: Evaluation of radiotherapy alone or in combination with doxorubicin chemotherapy for the treatment of cats with incompletely excised soft tissue sarcomas: 71 cases (1989-1999). *J Am Vet Med Assoc.* 231(5):742-745, 2007.
37. Hilmas DE, Gillette EL: Radiotherapy of spontaneous fibrous connective-tissue sarcomas in animals. *J Natl Cancer Inst* 56:365–368, 1976.
38. Bongiovanni S, Bengtson AE, Gliatto JM, et al: Prognostic indicators associated with adjuvant radiotherapy for cats with soft tissue sarcoma. *Proc 19th Annu Conf Vet Cancer Soc*:44, 1999.
39. Bregazzi VS, LaRue SM, McNiel E, et al: treatment with a combination of doxorubicin, surgery, and radiation versus surgery and radiation alone for cats with vaccine-associated sarcomas: 25 cases (1995–2000). *JAVMA* 218:547–550, 2001.
40. Kleiter M, Leschnik M: Postoperative chemotherapie zur behandlung eines zweifach rezidivierten vakzine-assoziierten fibrosarkoms. *Kleintierpraxis* 43:295–302, 1998.
41. Mir LM, Devauchelle P, Quintin-Colonna F, et al: First clinical trial of cat soft-tissue sarcomas treatment by electrochemotherapy. *Br J Cancer* 76:1617–1622, 1997.
42. King GK, Yates KM, Greenlee PG, et al: The effect of acemannan immunostimulant in combination with surgery and radiation therapy on spontaneous canine and feline fibrosarcomas. *JAAHA* 31:439–447, 1995.
43. Doddy FD, Glickman LT, Glickman NW, Janovitz EB: Feline fibrosarcomas at vaccination sites and non-vaccination sites. *J Comp Pathol* 114:165–174, 1996.
44. Kass PH, Barnes Jr WG, Spangler WL, et al: Epidemiologic evidence for a causal relation between vaccination and fibrosarcoma tumorigenesis in cats. *JAVMA* 203:396–405, 1993.
45. Hendrick MJ, Shofer FS, Goldschmidt MH, et al: Comparison of fibrosarcomas that developed at vaccination sites and at non-vaccination sites in cats: 239 cases (1991–1992). *JAVMA* 205:1425–1429, 1994.
46. Hendrick MJ, Brooks JJ: Postvaccinal sarcomas in the cat: Histology and immunohistochemistry. *Vet Pathol* 31:126–129, 1994.
47. Esplin DG, McGill LD, Meininger AC, Wilson SR: Postvaccination sarcomas in cats. *JAVMA* 202:1245–1247, 1993.
48. Lester S, Clemett T, Burt A: Vaccine site-associated sarcomas in cats: Clinical experience and a laboratory review (1982–1993). *JAAHA* 32:91–95, 1996.
49. Burton G, Mason KV: Do postvaccinal sarcomas occur in Australian cats? *Aust Vet J* 75:102–106, 1997.
50. Macy DW: Current understanding of vaccination site-associated sarcomas in the cat. *J Feline Med Surg* 1:15–21, 1999.
51. Gagnon A-C: Drug injection-associated fibrosarcoma in a cat. *Feline Pract* 28:18–21, 2000.
52. Esplin DG, Bigelow M, McGill LD, Wilson SR: Fibrosarcoma at the site of a lufenuron injection in a cat. *Vet Cancer Soc Newsl* 23:8–9, 1999.
53. Coyne MJ, Postorino Reeves NC, Rosen DK: Estimated prevalence of injection-site sarcomas in cats during 1992. *JAVMA* 210:249–251, 1997.
54. Macy DW, Hendrick MJ: The potential role of inflammation in the development of postvaccinal sarcomas in cats. *Vet Clin North Am Small Anim Pract* 26:103–109, 1996.
55. Hendrick M, Goldschmidt MH, Shofer F, et al: Postvaccinal sarcomas in the cat: epidemiology and electron probe microanalytical identification of aluminum. *Cancer Res* 52:5391–5394, 1992.

56. Dubielzieg RR, Hawkins KL, Miller PE: Myofibroblastic sarcoma originating at the site of rabies vaccination in a cat. *J Vet Diagn Invest* 5:637–638, 1993.

57. Peiffer RL, Monticello T, Bouldin TW: Primary ocular sarcomas in the cat. *J Small Anim Pract* 29:105–116, 1988.

58. Dubielzig RR, Everitt J, Shadduck JA, Albert DM: Clinical and morphologic features of post-traumatic ocular sarcomas in cats. *Vet Pathol* 27:62–65, 1990.

59. Hardy Jr WD: The feline sarcoma viruses. *JAAHA* 17:981–997, 1981.

60. Ellis JA, Jackson ML, Bartsch RC, et al: Use of immunohistochemistry and polymerase chain reaction for detection of oncornaviruses in formalin-fixed, paraffin-embedded fibrosarcomas from cats. *JAVMA* 209:767–771, 1996.

61. Goad MEP, Lopez MK, Goad DL: Expression of tumor suppressor genes and oncogenes in feline injection-site associated sarcomas [abstract 129]. *J Vet Intern Med* 13:258, 1999.

62. Esplin DG, Campbell R: Widespread metastasis of a fibrosarcoma associated with a vaccination site in a cat. *Feline Practi* 23:13–16, 1995.

63. Rudmann DG, Van Alstine WG, Doddy F, et al: Pulmonary and mediastinal metastases of a vaccination-site sarcoma in a cat. *Vet Pathol* 33:466–469, 1996.

64. Sandler I, Teeger M, Best S: Metastatic vaccine associated fibrosarcoma in a 10-year-old cat. *Can Vet J* 38:374, 1997.

65. Briscoe C, Lipscomb T, McKinney LA: Pulmonary metastasis of a feline postvaccinal fibrosarcoma. *Vet Pathol* 32:564, 1995.

66. Fulton LM, Bromberg NM, Goldschmidt MH: Soft tissue fibrosarcoma with intraocular metastasis in a cat. *Prog Vet Comp Ophthalmol* 1:129–132, 1991.

67. Esplin DG, Jaffe MH, McGill LD: Metastasizing liposarcoma associated with a vaccination site in a cat. *Feline Pract* 24:20–23,1996.

68. Snyder SP, Theilen GH: Transmissible feline fibrosarcoma. *Nature* 221:1074–1075, 1969.

69. Aldrich CD, Pedersen NC: Persistent viremia after regression of primary virus-induced feline fibrosarcomas. *Am J Vet Res* 35:1383–1387, 1974.

70. Essex M, Klein G, Snyder SP, Harrold JB: Correlation between humoral antibody and regression of tumours induced by feline sarcoma virus. *Nature* 233:195–196, 1971.

71. Irgens K, Wyers M, Moraillon A, et al: Isolement d'un virus sarcomatogene felin a partir d'un firbrosarcome spontane du Chat: Etude de pouvoir sacomtagene in vivo. *C R Acad Sci Paris* 276:1783–1786, 1973.

72. Hardy WD Jr: Oncogenic viruses of cats: The feline leukemia and sarcoma viruses. In Holzworth J (ed): *Diseases of the Cat. Medicine and Surgery*. Philadelphia, WB Saunders, 1987, pp 246–268.

73. Effron M, Griner L, Benirschke K: Nature and rate of neoplasia found in captive wild mammals, birds and reptiles at necropsy. *J Natl Cancer Inst* 59:185–198, 1977.

74. Saunders G: Disseminated leiomyosarcoma in a Bengal tiger. *JAVMA* 185:1387–1388, 1984.

75. Romanelli G, Marconato L, Olivero D, et al: Analysis of prognostic factors associated with injection-site sarcomas in cats: 57 cases (2001-2007). *J Am Vet Med Assoc.* 232(8):1193-1199, 2008.

Body surface area conversion chart

Weight (kg) to body surface area (m²) - Dogs

kg	m²	kg	m²	kg	m²	kg	m²	kg	m²
0.5	0.064	10.0	0.469	20.0	0.744	30.0	0.975	40.0	1.181
1.0	0.101	11.0	0.500	21.0	0.759	31.0	0.997	41.0	1.201
2.0	0.160	12.0	0.529	22.0	0.785	32.0	1.018	42.0	1.220
3.0	0.210	13.0	0.553	23.0	0.817	33.0	1.029	43.0	1.240
4.0	0.255	14.0	0.581	24.0	0.840	34.0	1.060	44.0	1.259
5.0	0.295	15.0	0.608	25.0	0.864	35.0	1.081	45.0	1.278
6.0	0.333	16.0	0.641	26.0	0.886	36.0	1.101	46.0	1.297
7.0	0.370	17.0	0.668	27.0	0.909	37.0	1.121	47.0	1.302
8.0	0.404	18.0	0.694	28.0	0.931	38.0	1.142	48.0	1.334
9.0	0.437	19.0	0.719	29.0	0.953	39.0	1.162	49.0	1.352
								50.0	1.371

Weight (kg) to body surface area (m²) - Cats

kg	m²	kg	m²	kg	m²	kg	m²	kg	m²
0.1	0.022	1.4	0.125	3.6	0.235	5.8	0.323	8.0	0.400
0.2	0.034	1.6	0.137	3.8	0.244	6.0	0.330	8.2	0.407
0.3	0.045	1.8	0.148	4.0	0.252	6.2	0.337	8.4	0.413
0.4	0.054	2.0	0.159	4.2	0.260	6.4	0.345	8.6	0.420
0.5	0.063	2.2	0.169	4.4	0.269	6.6	0.352	8.8	0.426
0.6	0.071	2.4	0.179	4.6	0.277	6.8	0.360	9.0	0.433
0.7	0.079	2.6	0.189	4.8	0.285	7.0	0.366	9.2	0.439
0.8	0.086	2.8	0.199	5.0	0.292	7.2	0.373	9.4	0.445
0.9	0.093	3.0	0.208	5.2	0.300	7.4	0.380	9.6	0.452
1.0	0.100	3.2	0.217	5.4	0.307	7.6	0.387	9.8	0.458
1.2	0.113	3.4	0.226	5.6	0.315	7.8	0.393	10.0	0.464

ABRIDGED FORMULARY FOR THE CANINE & FELINE CANCER PATIENT

Acepromazine

Use: Preanesthetic, sedative.
How Supplied: Injectable: 10 mg/ml, 50 ml vial. Oral: 10 and 25 mg tablets.
Canine Dose: 0.062-0.25 mg/kg (0.03-0.11 mg/lb) parenteral. Maximum IV dose: 3 mg/dog. 1.1-2.2 mg/kg (0.5-1.0 mg/lb) oral.
Feline Dose: 0.025-0.05 mg/kg IV, SQ, IM (use with butorphanol for painful procedures).

Actinomycin D

Use: Antineoplastic agent.
How Supplied: Injectable: 0.5 mg vial.
Canine Dose: 0.5-0.9 mg/m² IV slow infusion (>20 min.) q1-3wk.

Feline Dose: 0.5-0.9 mg/m² IV slow infusion (>20 min.) q3wk.

Alimentation, oral

Use: Nutritional Supplement.
How Supplied: Oral liquid: 8 oz cans, 1.06 calories/ml.
Feline Dose: Calculate animal's daily caloric requirement (DCR). Day 1: Give 0.25 DCR. Day 2: Give 0.5 DCR. Day 3 and beyond: Give total DCR divided into frequent feedings (four to seven meals/day) or by constant infusion.

Amoxicillin

Use: Broad-spectrum antibiotic.
How Supplied: Injectable: 250 mg/ml, 25 g vial. Oral: 50, 100, 200, and 400 mg tablets. 50 mg/ml suspension, 15 ml bottle.
Canine Dose: 11-22 mg/kg (5-10 mg/lb) PO bid to tid
Feline Dose: 11 mg/kg (5 mg/lb) PO, SQ, IM bid

Amoxicillin-clavulanic acid

Use: Broad-spectrum antibiotic (effective against many penicillinase-producing pathogens)
How Supplied: Oral: Fixed combination with four parts amoxicillin and one part clavulanic acid as the potassium salt. 62.5, 125, 250, and 375 mg tablets of drug combination. 62.5 mg/ml suspension, 15 ml bottle
Canine Dose: 13.75 mg/kg (6.25 mg/lb) of combination PO bid.
Feline Dose: 13.75 mg/kg (6.25 mg/lb) of combination PO bid.

Ampicillin sodium

Use: Broad-spectrum antibiotic.
How Supplied: Injectable: 1 g vial.
Canine Dose: 22 mg/kg (10 mg/lb) IM, IV tid.
Feline Dose: 22 mg/kg (10 mg/lb) IM, IV, SQ tid.
Note: Approximately 6% loss of potency/8 h when mixed to 100 mg/ml and stored in a refrigerator.

L-asparaginase

Use: Antineoplastic agent.
How Supplied: Injectable: 10,000 U/vial.
Canine Dose: 10,000-20,000 U/m² or 400 U/kg IM weekly.
Feline Dose: 10,000 U/m² IM, SQ q1-3wk.
Note: Watch for anaphylaxis!

Aspirin

Use: Analgesic, antipyretic, antiprostaglandin.
How Supplied: Oral: 80 and 325 mg tablets, 1 lb powder.
Canine Dose: 10-25 mg/kg PO q12hr for analgesia.
Feline Dose: 10 mg/kg (4.5 mg/lb) PO q48-72h prn for analgesia.

Atipamezole HCL

Use: Alpha₂ adrenergic antagonist; antagonizes agonists such as medetomidine, dexmedetomidine, and xylazine.
How Supplied: Injectable: 5 mg/ml, 10 ml multidose vial.
Canine Dose: Inject same volume as used for medetomidine/dexmedetomidine IM. The range of doses is 0.32 mg/kg for small animals (8.5 lbs), 0.23 mg/kg for medium-sized animals (24 lbs), and up to 0.14 mg/kg for large-sized animals (100 lbs).
Feline Dose: Inject same volume as used for medetomidine/dexmedetomidine IM.

Atropine

Use: Anticholinergic, mydriatic, cycloplegia
How Supplied: Injectable: 0.5 mg/ml (small animal) in 100 ml vial. Ophthalmic Ointment: 1% ophthalmic ointment in 3.5 g tubes. Ophthalmic Solution: 1% ophthalmic solution in 15 ml bottles
Canine/Feline Dose: 0.04 mg/kg (0.02 mg/lb) IV, SQ, IM.

Azathioprine

Use: Immunosuppressive, antimetabolite.
How Supplied: Oral: 50 mg tablet.
Canine Dose: 2.2 mg/kg/day for 4 days, then 1 mg/kg PO eod.
Feline Dose: 0.3-1.0 mg/kg PO eod.
Note: Not recommended for use in cats by some authors because of potential for fatal toxicity and difficulty in accurate dosing.

Bleomycin

Use: Antineoplastic agent.
How Supplied: Injectable: 15 U vial (1 U = 1 mg).
Canine Dose: 0.3-0.5 U/kg weekly IM or SQ to total cumulative dose of 125-200 U/m²; IV push over at least 10 minutes.
Feline Dose: 0.3-0.5 U/kg weekly IM or SQ to total cumulative dose of 125-200 U/m²; IV push over at least 10 minutes.

Bupivicaine

Use: Long-acting local anesthetic.
How Supplied: Injectable: 0.75%, 30 ml single-dose vial.
Canine Dose: This dose in your formulary: 0.005-0.02 mg/kg IM, IV, SQ q6-12h 7 mg/kg (maximum) per site.
Feline Dose: 1-2 mg/4.5 kg for local blocks and/or intrapleural infusion.

Buprenorphine

Use: Opioid partial agonist
How Supplied: Injectable: 0.3 mg/ml, 1 ml ampule

Canine Dose: 0.007-0.02 mg/kg IM, SQ.
Feline Dose: 0.005-0.01 mg/kg IM, IV, SQ q4-12h.
Note: Schedule V Controlled Substance.

Busulfan

Use: Antineoplastic Agent.
How Supplied: Oral: 2 mg tablet.
Feline Dose:.2 mg/m² PO sid.

Butorphanol

Use: Central-acting analgesic; narcotic agonist/antagonist.
How Supplied: Injectable: 10 mg/ml, 50 ml vial. Oral: 5 mg tablets.
Canine Dose: 0.1 mg/kg (0.045 mg/lb) IV. 0.1-0.4 mg/kg (0.045-0.18 mg/lb) SQ, IM q6-12h. 0.55 mg/kg (0.25 mg/lb) PO q 6-12h.
Feline Dose: 0.1-0.4 mg/kg IM, IV, SQ q1-4h for analgesia. 0.8 mg/kg IV q2h for somatic pain. 0.4 mg/kg IM q8h for nausea and vomiting.
Note: Butorphanol possesses antagonist properties and will reverse the effects of narcotics. Therefore, do not give butorphanol within 12 hours of any preoperative or intraoperative narcotics. Schedule IV Controlled Substance.

Calcium gluconate/ borogluconate

Use: Hypocalcemia.
How Supplied: Injectable: 10% solution, 10 ml ampule. 23% solution, 500 ml vial. 26% with Mg, P, and dextrose in 500 ml vials (NorcalciphosTM).
Canine Dose: 10-30 ml 10%.
Feline Dose: 1-1.5 ml/kg 10% solution IV (slowly over 10-20 minutes).

Carboplatin

Use: Antineoplastic Agent.
How Supplied: Injectable: 50, 150, and 450 mg vials
Canine Dose: 250-300 mg/m², depending on size of patient.
Feline Dose: 200-220 mg/m² IV q3wk.
Note: Dilute with 5% dextrose in water to 10 mg/ml .

Carprofen

Use: Analgesic, anti-inflammatory.
How Supplied: Oral: 25, 75, and 100 mg tablets. Injectable: 50 mg/ml, 20 ml vial.
Canine Dose: 2.2 mg/kg (1 mg/lb) PO bid. 2.2 mg/kg SQ bid, 4.4 mg/kg SQ sid.

Cefadroxil

Use: First-generation cephalosporin antibiotic.
How Supplied: Oral: 50 and 100 mg tablets.
Canine Dose: 11-22 mg/kg (5-10 mg/lb) PO bid.
Feline Dose: 11-22 mg/kg (5-10 mg/lb) PO bid.

Cefazolin

Use: First-generation cephalosporin antibiotic.
How Supplied: Injectable: 250 mg, 500 mg, and 1 g vials.
Canine Dose: 22 mg/kg (10 mg/lb) IV, IM, SQ q8h.
Feline Dose: 22 mg/kg (10 mg/lb) IV, IM, SQ q8h.
Note: For surgical prophylaxis, give within 30 minutes of surgery and repeat every 2.5 hours.

Cefoxitin

Use: Second-generation cephalosporin antibiotic.
How Supplied: Injectable: 1 g vial.
Canine Dose: 22 mg/kg (10 mg/lb) tid.
Feline Dose: 22 mg/kg (10 mg/lb) slow IV tid.

Cephalexin

Use: First-generation cephalosporin antibiotic.
How Supplied: Oral: 25 mg/ml suspension in 15 ml and 100 ml bottles. 250 and 500 mg capsules
Canine Dose: 11-22 mg/kg (5-10 mg/lb) PO tid.
Feline Dose: 11-22 mg/kg (5-10 mg/lb) PO tid.

Chlorambucil

Use: Antineoplastic agent.
How Supplied: Oral: 2 mg coated tablet.
Canine Dose: 0.2 mg/kg or 6 mg/m² sid or eod.
Feline Dose: 6 mg/m² sid (or equivalent thereof in one week's time).

Chlorpheniramine

Use: Antihistamine.
How Supplied: Oral: 4 mg tablet.
Canine Dose: 4-8 mg PO bid to tid.
Feline Dose: 2-4 mg PO sid to bid.

Chlorpromazine

Use: Tranquilizer, antiemetic.
How Supplied: Injectable: 25 mg/ml, 2 ml ampule.
Canine Dose: Antiemetic: 0.11 mg/kg (0.05 mg/lb) IM, IV q8h. Tranquilization: 1-2 mg/kg (0.5-0.9 mg/lb) IM, IV q8h.
Feline Dose: 0.5 mg/kg IM or SQ q6-8h.

Cimetidine

Use: H2-receptor antagonist.
How Supplied: Injectable: 150 mg/ml in 2 and 8 ml vials. Oral: 100, 200, and 300 mg tablets.
Canine Dose: 4 mg/kg (1.8 mg/lb) PO, IV q6h. 5.5 mg/kg (2.5 mg/lb) IV tid.
Feline Dose: 2.5 mg/kg (1.14 mg/lb) PO or IV slow push bid.

Cisapride

Use: Cholinergic enhancer, GI-emptying adjunct.
How Supplied: Oral: 10 mg tablet.

Canine Dose: 0.1-0.5 mg/kg PO (30 minutes before meals) up to tid.
Feline Dose: 0.1-0.5 mg/kg PO (30 minutes before meals) up to tid.

Cisplatin

Use: Antineoplastic agent.
How Supplied: Injectable: 1 mg/ml in 10, 50, and 100 ml vials.
Canine Dose: Follow oncology protocol (50-70 mg/m^2 IV with diuresis).
Feline Dose: Intralesional use only.
Note: Not for IV use in cats – FATAL.

Clindamycin

Use: Antibiotic.
How Supplied: Oral: 25, 75, and 150 mg capsules. 25 mg/ml solution, 20 ml bottle.
Canine Dose: 5.5-11.0 mg/kg (2.5-5.0 mg/lb) PO bid.
Feline Dose: 12.5 mg/kg (5.7 mg/lb) PO bid for 28 days for toxoplasmosis.

Codeine/acetominophen

Use: Analgesic.
How Supplied: Oral: Tablets contain 60 mg codeine and 300 mg acetaminophen.
Canine Dose: 0.5-2.0 mg/kg (of codeine) PO q6-8h.
Note: Schedule III Controlled Substance.

Cyclophosphamide

Use: Antineoplastic agent.
How Supplied: Oral: 25 and 50 mg tablets. Injectable: 100 mg, 200 mg, 500 mg, 1 g, and 2 g vials (reconstituted with 20 ml of D5W to make 10 mg/ml).
Canine Dose: 50 mg/m^2 once daily 3-4 days per week or q3wk, or 250 mg/m^2 PO or 200 mg/m^2 IV once every three weeks (give with furosemide to reduce the risk of cystitis).
Feline Dose: 250 mg/m^2 IV, PO q3wk for 4-8 treatments. Or 50 mg/m^2 PO, IV sid on days 3, 4, 5, and 6 following doxorubicin administration.

Cyproheptadine

Use: Appetite stimulant, antidepressant, antiemetic.
How Supplied: Oral: 4 mg (scored) tablet.
Canine Dose: 0.5 mg/kg PO tid.
Feline Dose: 1-2 mg/cat PO sid-bid.

Cytarabine

Use: Antineoplastic agent.
How Supplied: Injectable: 100 mg, 500 mg, 1 g, and 2 g vials (reconstituted to 20 mg/ml).
Canine Dose: Low dose: 10 mg/m^2 sid or bid SQ or IM. High dose: 60 mg/m^2 sid for 4 days q3wks SQ, IM, or IV. For granulomatous meningoencephalitis: 200 mg/m^2 as a constant rate infusion over 48 hours or 50 mg/m^2 SQ bid for 2 consecutive days – repeat dosage schedule every 3 weeks.
Feline Dose: 60-100 mg/m^2 IV constant rate infusion daily for 2-4 days; if no toxicity, increase to 150 mg/m^2 daily for 4 days. Or 10 mg/m^2 SQ sid-bid

Dacarbazine

Use: Antineoplastic agent.
How Supplied: Injectable: 100 and 200 mg vials.
Canine Dose: 800 mg/m^2 every 3-4 weeks or 20 mg/m^2 daily for five consecutive days every three weeks.
Note: Give dolasetron as a prophylactic antiemetic.

Desmopressin (DDAVP)

Use: ADH derivative, increases factor VIII activity.
How Supplied: Injectable: 0.01% solution.
Canine Dose: 1 µg/kg (0.44 µg/lb) SQ 20-30 minutes before collecting blood or performing surgery.

Dexamethasone

Use: Corticosteroid therapy.
How Supplied: Injectable: 2 mg/ml, 100 ml vial.
Oral: 0.25 and 4 mg tablets. 0.1% Ophthalmic ointment with neomycin (3.5 mg/g) and polymyxin B (10,000 U/g) in 3.5 g tubes. 0.1% Ophthalmic suspension, 15 ml bottle. 0.1 % Ophthalmic suspension with neomycin (3.5 mg/ml) and polymyxin B (10,000 U/ml), 5 ml bottle.
Feline Dose: 0.28-2.2 mg/kg (0.125-1.0 mg/lb) PO, IM. Screening dose: 0.1 mg/kg IV. Suppression dose: 1.0 mg/kg IV. Antiemetic: 1 mg/cat IV.

Dexmedetomidine

Use: Alpha$_2$ adrenergic agonist; small animal sedative, anesthetic.
How Supplied: 0.5 mg/ml (500 mcg/ml), 10 ml multidose vial.
Canine Dose: Sedation and anesthesia: 375 mcg/m^2 IV, 500 mcg/m^2 IM. The mcg/kg dosage decreases as body weight increases. Preanesthetic: 125-375 mcg/m^2 IM, depending on duration and severity of the procedure and anesthetic regimen.
Feline Dose: Sedation, anesthesia, preanesthetic: 40 mcg/kg IM. The expected sedative and analgesic effects are reached within 15 minutes and maintained for up to 60 minutes.

Dextrazone

Use: Cardioprotectant.
How Supplied: 500 mg vial with dilutent.
Canine Dose: 30 mg for every 1 mg of doxorubicin

Diazepam

Use: Tranquilizer, anticonvulsant, appetite stimulant.
How Supplied: Injectable: 5 mg/ml, 2 and 10 ml vials.

Canine Dose: 1 mg/kg (0.5 mg/lb) IM. 1 mg/kg IV to effect (increase in 5 mg increments). 0.2 mg/kg/hr constant rate infusion starting dose. 1-2 mg/kg per rectum to effect up to maximum dose of 40 mg.

Feline Dose: Anesthetic induction: 0.1-1 mg/kg IV (use with butorphanol for painful procedures). Appetite stimulant: 0.05-0.1 mg/kg IV. Premedication: 0.2 mg/kg IV sid to bid.

Note: Schedule IV Controlled Substance.

Dimenhydrinate

Use: Antihistamine, antiemetic.

How Supplied: Injectable: 50 mg/ml, 1 and 10 ml vials. Oral: 50 mg tablet. 12.5 mg/4 ml in 90 ml, pts and gals; 12.5 mg/5 ml in 120 ml bottle; 15.62 mg/5 ml in 480 ml bottle.

Canine Dose: Antiemetic: 4-8 mg/kg PO tid. Antihistamine: 4-8 mg/kg PO bid to tid.

Feline Dose: Antiemetic: 8 mg/kg PO tid. Antihistamine: 4 mg/cat PO tid.

Diphenhydramine

Use: Antihistamine, antiemetic.

How Supplied: Oral: 12.5 mg tablet, 25 and 50 mg capsules. 12.5 mg/ml oral elixir in 4 and 16 oz bottles. Injectable: 50 mg/ml, 1 and 10 ml vials. 10 mg/ml, 10 and 30 ml vials. Topical: 2% conditioner, 8 oz bottle.

Canine Dose: 2-4 mg/kg IM, IV, PO q6-8h.

Feline Dose: 2-4 mg/kg PO, IM tid.

Dolasetron mesylate

Use: Antiemetic.

How Supplied: Injectable: 20 mg/ml single-use 0.625 ml ampule, 0.625 ml fill in 2 ml, single-use 5 ml vials, and 25 ml multi-dose vial. Oral: 50 and 100 mg tablets.

Canine Dose: 0.6-1 mg/kg PO or IV slowly.

Feline Dose: 0.6-1 mg/kg IV slowly.

Doxorubicin

Use: Antineoplastic agent.

How Supplied: Injectable: 2 mg/ml in 10, 20, 50, 150, and 200 mg vials.

Canine Dose: 30 mg/m^2 IV (1 mg/kg for dogs <10 kg) repeated every 21 days to an accumulated dosage of 180 mg/m^2.

Feline Dose: 1-1.1 mg/kg or 20-25 mg/m^2 IV slow infusion (over 30 min) q3wk. Maximum cumulative dose: 180-240 mg/m^2 over lifetime.

Note: Dilute with NaCl solution prior to IV administration and give SLOWLY.

Doxycycline

Use: Long-acting broad-spectrum tetracycline, metalloproteinase inhibitor.

How Supplied: Oral: 100 mg tablet and 10 mg/ml suspension, 16 oz bottle.

Canine Dose: 5 mg/kg (2.3 mg/lb) PO sid to bid.

Feline Dose: 5 mg/kg (2.3 mg/lb) PO sid to bid.

Edrophonium chloride

Use: Cholinergic (anticholinesterase) agent.

How Supplied: Injectable: 10 mg/ml, 1 ml ampule, 10 and 15 ml vials.

Canine Dose: need correct dose, 5 in plumb.

Feline Dose: need correct dose, 4 in plumb.

Note: Have atropine and endotracheal tube readily available in case of overdose.

Enrofloxacin

Use: Broad-spectrum antibacterial (Fluoroquinolone).

How Supplied: Injectable: 22.7 mg/ml, 20 ml vial. Oral: 22.7, 68, 136 mg tablets.

Canine Dose: 5 mg/kg (1.13 mg/lb) PO, IM sid. Dose may be increased to 20 mg/kg sid depending on infection and/or situation. Daily dose may be divided and given bid.

Feline Dose: 5 mg/kg (1.13 mg/lb) PO, IM sid. Dose may be increased to 20 mg/kg sid depending on infection and/or situation. Daily dose may be divided and given bid.

Note: Per manufacturer, dosages greater than 5 mg/kg sid in cats may be associated with blindness, temporary blindness, partial blindness, and mydriasis.

Epoetin alfa

Use: Stimulation of RBC production.

How Supplied: Injectable: 4000 U/ml, 1 ml vial.

Canine Dose: 100 U/kg SQ three times weekly (initially). May be decreased to twice weekly or increased in 50 U/kg increments depending on response.

Feline Dose: 100 U/kg SQ three times weekly (initially). May be decreased to twice weekly or increased in 50 U/kg increments depending on response.

Note: Antibody development to erythropoietin may cause anemia.

Erythromycin

Use: Macrolide antibiotic.

How Supplied: Oral: 250mg tablet.

Feline Dose: 11-22 mg/kg (5-10 mg/lb) PO tid with a small amount of food.

Etomidate

Use: Anesthetic, hypnotic.

How Supplied: Injectable: 2 mg/ml, 20 ml vial.

Canine Dose: 1 mg/kg IV.

Feline Dose: 1 mg/kg IV.

Etretinate

Use: Antineoplastic agent.

How Supplied: Oral: 10 and 25 mg capsules.
Feline Dose: 10 mg/cat PO sid.

Famotidine

Use: H$_2$-receptor antagonist.
How Supplied: Injectable: 10 mg/ml, 20 ml vial. Oral: 10 and 20 mg tablets.
Canine Dose: 0.5-1 mg/kg PO, SQ, IV sid-bid.
Feline Dose: 0.5 mg/kg PO, SQ, IV sid-bid.

Fatty acids

Use: Fatty acid supplement.
How Supplied: Oral: capsules – small, medium, and large animal sizes. Liquid: 60 ml bottle.
Canine Dose: 100-200 mg/kg PO.
Feline Dose: Capsules (small animal size for patients <30 lb): 1-2/day PO. Liquid: 0.5 ml/10 lb/day PO.

Fentanyl

Use: Narcotic analgesic.
How Supplied: Injectable: 0.05 mg/ml (50 mcg/ml), 2, 5, 10, and 20 ml ampules; 30 ml and 50 ml vials; preservative free in 2, 5, 10, and 20 ml ampules. Transdermal: 1.25 mg (12.5 mcg/hr), 2.5 mg (25 mcg/hr), 5 mg (50 mcg/hr), 7.5 mg (75 mcg/hr), and 10 mg (100 mcg/hr).
Canine Dose: 4 mcg/kg (1.9 mcg/lb) IV. 2-4 mcg/kg/hr constant rate infusion. 4-10 mcg/kg (1.8-4.5 mcg/lb) SQ, IM. Total dose not to exceed 500 mcg (0.5 mg) per dog. 12.5-25 mcg/hr transdermal patch for dogs <5 kg. 25 mcg/hr transdermal patch for 5-10 kg dogs. 50 mcg/hr transdermal patch for 10-20 kg dogs. 75 mcg/hr transdermal patch for 20-30 kg dogs. 100 mcg/hr transdermal patch for dogs >30 kg.
Feline Dose: 1-3 mcg/kg IV, followed by a CRI at 1-4 mcg/kg/hr. 12 mcg/hr transdermal patch (for a 4-5 kg cat); replace q3-5d
Note: Schedule II Controlled Substance.

5-Fluorouacil

Use: Antineoplastic agent.
How Supplied: Injectable: 500 mg, 5 g ampules or vials. Topical: 1% or 2 % ointment or solution.
Canine Dose: 5-10 mg/kg IV weekly. Topical: Apply small amount weekly prn for tumor dissolution.
Note: Contraindicated in cats.

Furosemide

Use: Diuretic.
How Supplied: Injectable: 50 mg/ml, 100 ml vial. Oral: 12.5 and 50 mg tablets; 10 mg/ml solution in 60 ml bottle.
Canine Dose: 2.5-5 mg/kg sid-bid PO, IV, IM.
Feline Dose: 1-2 mg/kg (0.45-0.9 mg/lb) IM, IV sid-bid. 2.2 mg/kg (1 mg/lb) PO sid-bid.

Gemcitabine

Use: Antineoplastic Agent.
How Supplied: Injectable: 200 mg and 1 g vials.
Canine Dose: 250-300 mg/m^2 IV weekly for 4 weeks with a 1 week "rest" before reinitiating the treatment cycle.
Note: Toxicity and probably efficacy depend on the rate that the drug is infused. Preliminary studies suggest that the drug should be infused over a 30-90 minute period.

Gentamicin

Use: Aminoglycoside antibiotic.
How Supplied: Injectable: 100 mg/ml, 100 ml vial. 0.3% Ophthalmic ointment, 3.5 g tube. 0.3% Ophthalmic solution, 5 ml bottle. 0.3% Gentamicin with 0.1% betamethasone ophthalmic solution, 5 ml bottle. 0.3% Gentamicin with 0.1% betamethasone otic solution, 7.5 ml bottle.
Canine Dose: 6.6 mg/kg IM, IV, SQ as a single daily dose or may be divided bid or tid.
Feline Dose: 2.2-4.4 mg/kg IV, IM, SQ tid.
Note: If given IV, administer slowly.

Glycopyrrolate

Use: Anticholinergic agent.
How Supplied: Injectable: 0.2 mg/ml, 20 ml vial.
Canine Dose: 11 mcg/kg (5 mcg/lb) IM, IV, SQ.

Halothane

Use: Inhalant anesthetic.
How Supplied: Liquid for anesthesia, 250 ml bottle. Dose: 3% (induction); 0.5%-1.5% maintenance. Deliver via endotracheal tube and standard anesthetic delivery system with oxygen as needed for surgical plane of anesthesia.

Heparin sodium

Use: Anticoagulant in vivo and in vitro.
How Supplied: Injectable: 1000 U/ml, 10 ml vial
Canine Dose: 2 U/ml intraocular irrigation. 1-2 U/ml for heparinized saline. 300 U/kg IV bolus, 600 U/kg/day constant-rate infusion.
Feline Dose: 2 U/ml intraocular irrigation. 1-2 U/ml for heparinized saline. 200 U/kg IV bolus.

Hetastarch

Use: Plasma volume expansion.
How Supplied: Injectable: 6% in normal saline, 500 ml bag.
Feline Dose: 10-15 ml/kg/day IV.

Hydrocodone/homatropine

Use: Antitussive.
How Supplied: Oral: Hydrocodone 5 mg/homatropine 1.5 mg tablet.

Canine Dose: 0.22 mg/kg (of hydrocodone) PO bid-tid.
Note: Calculate dose considering 5mg/tablet. Schedule III Controlled Substance

Hydrocortisone

Use: Corticosteroid therapy.
How Supplied: 1 % Ophthalmic ointment with neomycin, polymyxin B, and bacitracin, 3.5 g tube. 1% Otic formulation with Burow's Solution, 1 oz bottle. 1% Topical conditioner, 8 oz bottle. 1% Astringent spray, 4 oz bottle.

Hydroxyurea

Use: Antineoplastic agent.
How Supplied: Oral: 500 mg capsule.
Canine Dose: 80 mg/kg PO q3d (reformulate).
Feline Dose: 80 mg/kg PO q3d.

Idrarubicin

Use: Antineoplastic agent.
How Supplied: Oral: 2 mg tablet. Injectable: 5 and 10 mg vials.
Feline Dose: 2 mg/cat/day PO, IV for 3 consecutive days q3wk.

Ifosfamide

Use: Antineoplastic agent.
How Supplied: Injectable: 1 g vial.
Canine Dose: 350 (dogs <10 kg) to 375 mg/m² q3wk.
Note: Must give with IV saline diuresis and mesna (included in package).

Insulin

Use: Diabetes mellitus, hyperkalemia.
How Supplied: Injectable: 100 U/ml, 10 ml vial (plain crystalline, regular, Lente, NPH, and Ultra-Lente).
Feline Dose: 0.5-1.0 U/kg (0.23-0.45 U/lb) of regular insulin SQ q12-24h, then adjust dosage to clinical response.

Iron dextran

Use: Hematinic.
How Supplied: Injectable: 100 mg iron/ml, 100 ml vial.
Feline Dose: 11-22 mg/kg (5-10 mg/lb) IM.

Isoflurane

Use: Inhalant anesthetic.
How Supplied: Liquid for anesthesia, 100 ml bottle.

Isotretinoin

Use: Antineoplastic agent for mycosis fungoides.
How Supplied: 10, 20, 40 mg capsules.
Canine Dose: 1-3 mg/kg/day.

Kaolin/pectin

Use: Antidiarrheal.
How Supplied: Oral suspension, 6 oz bottle.
Canine Dose: 1-2 ml/kg PO q2-6h.
Feline Dose: 1-2 ml/kg PO q2-6h.

Ketamine

Use: Neuroleptanalgesia.
How Supplied: Injectable: 100 mg/ml, 10 ml vial.
Canine Dose: 10-21 mg/kg (4.5-9.5 mg/lb) IM. 2.2-4.4 mg/kg (1-2 mg/lb) IV.
Feline Dose: Anesthesia/analgesia: 6-10 mg/kg (2.7-4.5 mg/lb) IV. Restraint: 11 mg/kg (5 mg/lb) IM. Anesthesia: 22-33 mg/kg (10-15 mg/lb) IM. Anti-anxiety: 0.5-1.0 mg/kg IM q30min.

Ketoprofen

Use: Anti-inflammatory agent.
How Supplied: Injectable: 100 mg/ml, 100 ml vial.
Canine Dose: 1 mg/kg single postsurgical dose IV, IM
Feline Dose: 1-2 mg/kg IV, IM, SQ single postsurgical dose.

L-asparaginase

Use: Antineoplastic agent.
How Supplied: Injectable: 10,000 U vial.
Canine Dose: 10,000-20,000 U/m² or 400 U/kg IM weekly.
Feline Dose: 10,000 U/m² or 400 U/kg IM q7-21d.
Note: Anaphylaxis can occur.

Lidocaine

Use: Local and topical anesthetic, antiarrhythmic.
How Supplied: Injectable: 2% solution, 100 ml vial. Oral Topical Solution: 2% (viscous), 100 ml bottle.
Canine Dose: 2-5 mg/kg IV bolus administered over 2-3 min. 50-120 µg/kg/min constant-rate infusion. NOTE: Use caution. Start CRI at 60 µg/kg/min and increase by 10 µg increments every 2 hours if no or minimal response is noted.
Feline Dose: 0.5 mg/kg 3 hours prior to bupivacaine for local anesthesia.

Lomustine (CCNU)

Use: Antineoplastic agent.
How Supplied: Oral: 10, 40, and 100 mg capsules.
Canine Dose: Initial: 60-90 mg/m² PO q4-6wk.
Feline Dose: Initial: 60 mg/m² PO q5-8wk. Slowly increase dose to 80 mg/m² PO if toxicity is minimal.

Maropitant citrate

Use: Neurokinin receptor antagonist, antiemetic.
How Supplied: Injectable: 10 mg/ml, 20 ml vial. Oral: 16, 24, 60, and 160 mg in blister packs (4 tablets per pack; carton of 10).

Canine Dose: 1 mg/kg SQ q24hr or 2 mg/kg PO q24hr for up to 5 consecutive days.
Feline Dose: 1-2 mg/kg SQ q24hr or 2 mg/kg PO q24hr for up to 5 consecutive days.
Note: Used extra-label in cats.

Mechlorethamine HCL

Use: Antineoplastic agent.
How Supplied: 10 mg powder for injection.
Canine Dose: 3 mg/m² IV as part of MOPP protocol.
Feline Dose: 5 mg/m² IV or intracavitary prn.

Meclizine

Use: Antiemetic (related to labyrinthitis).
How Supplied: Oral: 12.5 and 25 mg tablets.
Canine Dose: 25 mg/dog PO sid.
Feline Dose: 6.25-12.5 mg/cat PO sid.

Medetomidine

Use: Small animal sedative, analgesic.
How Supplied: Injectable: 1 mg/ml 10 ml vial.
Canine Dose: 0.75 mg/m² IV or 1 mg/m² IM.
Feline Dose: 5-20 µg/kg IM or 0.001-0.01 mg/kg IM, SQ, IV over 0.5-2 hr for anesthesia.
Note: Combine with butorphanol for painful procedures.

Megesterol acetate

Use: Appetite stimulant, feline dermatopathies.
How Supplied: Oral: 5 and 20 mg tablets.
Canine Dose: 0.5 mg/kg daily for 3 days, then every 2-3 days thereafter to enhance appetite.
Feline Dose: 2.5-5 mg total daily dose for 5 days, then once or twice/week for maintenance (lowest frequency possible) or 2.5-5 mg total dose qod until appetite improves. 0.25-0.5 mg/kg daily for 3-5 days, then every 48-72 hours thereafter.

Melphalan

Use: Antineoplastic agent.
How Supplied: Oral: 2 mg tablet. Injectable: 500 mg vial.
Canine Dose: 0.1 mg/kg sid for 10 days, then reduce to eod.
Feline Dose: 0.1 mg/kg sid for 10 days, then 0.05 mg/kg/day. Or 2 mg/m² sid for 7 to 10 days, then no therapy for 2-3 weeks. Usually results in 2 mg PO qod with or without prednisone at 20 mg/m² PO qod.

Meperidine

Use: Opioid agonist.
How Supplied: Injectable: 50 mg/ml, 30 ml vial.
Canine Dose: 3-5 mg/kg IM, SQ.
Feline Dose: 2-5 mg/kg IM, SQ q2h.
Note: Schedule II Controlled Substance.

6-Mercaptopurine

Use: Antineoplastic agent, immunosuppressant.
How Supplied: Oral: 50 mg tablet.
Canine Dose: 50 mg/m² PO sid to effect, then every other day or as needed.
Feline Dose: 50 mg/m² PO sid.

Mesna

Use: Uroprotectant for cyclophosphamide and ifosfamide to prevent hemorrhagic cystitis.
How Supplied: Solution of 100 mg/ml.
Canine Dose: 60% of the daily ifosfamide mg dosage IV.

Methimazole

Use: Antithyroid agent.
How Supplied: Oral: 5 mg tablet.
Feline Dose: 5 mg/cat tid for 2 weeks, reduce to 5 mg/cat bid if euthyroid.

Methotrexate

Use: Antineoplastic agent.
How Supplied: Oral: 2.5 mg tablet. Injectable: 5 mg, 20 mg, 50 mg, 100 mg, 200 mg, 250 mg, and 1 g vials.
Canine Dose: 2.5 mg/m² PO, IV, IM, SQ sid.
Feline Dose: 2.5 mg/m² PO, IV, IM, SQ sid.

Methylprednisolone

Use: Corticosteroid therapy.
How Supplied: Injectable: 20 mg/ml, 10 ml vial; 40 mg/ml, 5 ml vial.
Feline Dose: 5.5 mg/kg (2.5 mg/lb) to maximum of 20 mg IM, SQ.

Metoclopramide

Use: Antiemetic, GI disorders.
How Supplied: Injectable: 5 mg/ml, 20 ml vial.
Oral: 5 mg and 10 mg tablets, 1 mg/ml solution.
Canine Dose: 1-2 mg/kg/day constant rate infusion IV. 0.2-0.4 mg/kg (0.1-0.2 mg/lb) tid, 30 min before meals PO.
Feline Dose: 1-2 mg/kg/day constant rate infusion IV. 0.2-0.4 mg/kg (0.1-0.2 mg/lb) IM, SQ tid. 0.4-0.6 mg/kg PO q4h.

Metronidazole

Use: Amoebiasis, giardiasis, trichomoniasis, balantidiasis, anaerobic infections.
How Supplied: Oral: 250 mg and 500 mg tablets. 25 mg/ml suspension (compounded).
Canine Dose: 32 mg/kg (15 mg/lb) bid for 8 days for giardiasis. 10-15 mg/kg tid for 5 days for Clostridium perfringens infection.
Feline Dose: 15-25 mg/kg PO q12-24hr daily for 5-7 days for giardiasis.

Note: CAUTION!!! Avoid overdosing, especially in larger dogs. Deaths have been reported at the 32 mg/kg dose in larger dogs.

Misoprostal

Use: Prevention of NSAID-induced gastric ulcers.
How Supplied: 100 µg (scored) tablet.
Canine Dose: 2-4 µg/kg PO tid-qid.
Note: Pregnant women should handle the drug with caution.

Mitoxantrone

Use: Antineoplastic agent.
How Supplied: Injectable: 2 mg/ml concentrate to be diluted for IV administration.
Canine Dose: 5.5 mg/m^2 IV every three weeks.
Feline Dose: 6.5 mg/m^2 IV every three weeks.
Note: Give IV over at least 3 minutes.

Morphine

Use: Analgesic.
How Supplied: Injectable: 1 mg/ml. 1 mg/ml, 10 ml single-dose ampule (for epidural use only). 15 mg/ml, 1 ml and 20 ml vials.
Canine Dose: Epidural: 0.1 mg/kg (use preservative-free formulation). 0.5-2 mg/kg (0.25-1 mg/lb) IM, SQ. 0.05-0.1 mg/kg (0.025-0.045 mg/lb) for pulmonary edema. 1.1-2.2 mg/kg SQ as an emetic
Feline Dose: 0.05-0.2 mg/kg IV q1-4h. 0.05-0.2 mg/kg IM, SQ q2-6h.
Note: Schedule II Controlled Substance.

Nalbuphine

Use: Narcotic agonist-antagonist.
How Supplied: Injectable: 20 mg/ml 10 ml multiple-dose vial.
Canine Dose: Premedication: 0.5-1 mg/kg SQ, IM
Feline Dose: Premedication: 0.2-0.4 mg/kg SQ, IM

Naloxone

Use: Narcotic antagonist.
How Supplied: Injectable: 400 µg/ml, 1 ml and 10 ml vials. 0.4 mg/ml, 10 ml vial.
Canine Dose: 15 µg/kg (6.8 µg/lb) – Usually 400 µg IM, IV, SQ.
Feline Dose: 0.05-0.1 mg/kg IV.
Note: The half-life of naloxone is shorter than most other narcotics. If it is used for reversal, animals must be watched carefully for returning signs of narcotic activity.

Nystatin

Use: Candidiasis.
How Supplied: Oral: 100,000 U/ml suspension in 5 ml and 60 ml bottles. Cream: 100,000 U/g with neomycin, thiostrepton, and triamcinolone in water-washable base, 7.5 g tube. Ointment: 100,000 U/g with neomycin, thiostrepton, and triamcinolone in oil base, 7.5 ml tube.
Canine Dose: 100,000 U PO q6h.
Feline Dose: 100,000 U PO q6h.

Omeprazole

Use: Antisecretory compound, ulcer management
How Supplied: Oral: 20 mg sustained-release capsule.
Canine Dose: 0.7 mg/kg PO sid (approximately one capsule per dog).
Feline Dose: 0.7 mg/kg PO sid.

Ondansetron

Use: Prevention of nausea and vomiting associated with chemotherapy, surgery, etc.
How Supplied: Injectable: 4 mg/ml, 2 ml vial. Oral: 4 mg tablet.
Canine Dose: 0.1 mg/kg IV 15 min before and 4 hr after chemotherapy.
Feline Dose: 0.1 mg/kg IV 15 min before and 4 hr after chemotherapy.
Note: Give slowly IV (over 2-5 min) or dilute.

Oxacillin sodium

Use: Treatment of penicillinase-producing *Staphylococcus* spp.
How Supplied: Oral: 250 mg capsule.
Canine Dose: 12-24 mg/kg (5.5-11 mg/lb) PO tid.
Feline Dose: 12-24 mg/kg (5.5-11 mg/lb) PO tid.

Oxymorphone

Use: Narcotic analgesic.
How Supplied: Injectable: 1.5 mg/ml, 1 ml ampule, 10 ml vial.
Canine Dose: 0.11-0.22 mg/kg (0.05-0.1 mg/lb) IM, IV, SQ (maximum dose: 4.5 mg/dog).
Feline Dose: 0.05-0.1 mg/kg IM, SQ q2-6h. 0.02-0.05 mg/kg IV q2-4h.
Note: Schedule II Controlled Substance.

Paclitaxel

Use: Antineoplastic agent.
How Supplied: Injectable: 50 mg/5 ml, 5 ml vial.
Canine Dose: 130 mg/m^2 IV q3wk slow infusion *after* dexamethasone, diphenhydramine, and cimetidine therapy.
Feline Dose: 5 mg/kg IV q3wk (investigational).
Note: Dilute with 0.9% NaCl to a concentration of 0.6-0.7 mg/ml.

Pamidronate

Use: Treatment of hypercalcemia.
How Supplied: Injectable: 30 and 90 mg vials.
Canine Dose: 1-2 mg/kg IV over 2 hours – 3 hours after and 1 hour before a saline diuresis at 18.3 ml/kg/hr.

Parenteral fluids

Use: Caloric, electrolyte, and fluid replacement.

How Supplied: Injectable: 2.5% dextrose + 0.45% NaCl in 1000 ml bag. 5% dextrose solution in 1000 ml bag (~ 4 calories/g dextrose). 50% dextrose in 500 ml vial. Extracellular Replacement Fluid (ECF), 2 L bottle, 20 L carboys (contains 140 mEq/l Na, 5 mEq/l K, 115 mEq/l Cl, and 30 mEq/l). Lactated Ringer's Solution: 250 and 1000 ml bags (contains 131 mEq/l Na, 4 mEq/l K, 3 mEq Ca 110mEq/l Cl, and 28 mEq/l lactate). Normal Saline: 250 and 1000 ml bottles and 150, 250, 500, 1000, and 3000 ml bags (contains 155 mEq/l of both Na and Cl). Normosol®-R: 1000, 3000, and 5000 ml bags (contains 140 mEq/l Na, 5 mEq/l K, 3 mEq/l Mg, 98 mEq/l Cl, 27 mEq/l acetate, and 23 mEq/l gluconate). Plasma-Lyte®: 1000 ml bag (same as Normosol®-R except for pH). 5% Sodium bicarbonate solution (~ 0.6 mEq/ml): 500 ml bottle. 5% NaCl: 500 ml bag.

Penicillin g potassium

Use: Gram-positive infections.

How Supplied: Injectable: 1 million, 5 million, and 20 million U vials. (Contains 1.68 mEq of potassium/million U).

Canine Dose: 20,000-40,000 U/kg IV q4-6h.

Feline Dose: 22,000 U/kg (10,000 U/lb) SQ, IM, IV q4-6h (minimum dose).

Note: Half-life is approximately 30 min.

Pentobarbitol, sodium

Use: Sedative, anticonvulsant, IV anesthetic, euthanasia.

How Supplied: Injectable: 50 mg/ml, 50 ml vial. Euthanasia Solution: 400 mg/ml, 250 ml vial.

Canine Dose: Approximately 25-30 mg/kg IV for anesthesia. 3-15 mg/kg given slowly IV until effect for anticonvulsant. 88 mg/kg (40 mg/lb) IV for euthanasia.

Feline Dose: Approximately 25-30 mg/kg IV for anesthesia. 3-15 mg/kg given slowly IV until effect for anticonvulsant. 88 mg/kg (40 mg/lb) IV for euthanasia.

Note: Schedule II Controlled Substance.

Phenobarbitol

Use: Sedative, anticonvulsant.

How Supplied: Injectable: 130 mg/ml (sodium salt) 1 ml vial. Oral: 15, 30, 60, 100 mg tablets.

Canine Dose: 2 mg/kg PO bid to start; base increases in dose on serum levels. One time loading dose: 6-20 mg/kg IV.

Feline Dose: 2 mg/kg PO bid to start; base increases in dose on serum levels. One time loading dose: 6-20 mg/kg IV.

Note: Diazepam (IV or rectally) may be given concurrently, since IV phenobarbitol requires 20-30 minutes to exert an anticonvulsant effect. Schedule IV Controlled Substance.

Piroxicam

Use: Analgesic, anti-inflammatory, antineoplastic agent.

How Supplied: Oral: 10 mg and 20 mg capsules (2.5 mg and 5 mg capsules commonly compounded).

Canine Dose: 0.3 mg/kg PO sid for 3-5 days, then q24-48h thereafter.

Feline Dose: Analgesia: 0.3 mg/kg PO sid for 4 days, then 0.3 mg/kg PO q48h. Antineoplastic: 0.3 mg/kg PO q48h.

Note: Use cautiously – nephrotoxicity, GI ulceration common – may compound nephrotoxicity of chemotherapeutics.

Potassium bromide

Use: Anticonvulsant.

How Supplied: Oral: 250 mg/ml.

Canine Dose: 10-30 mg/kg (4.5-13.6 mg/lb) PO bid.

Note: Steady state is reached more rapidly if an oral loading dose (400-600 mg/kg) of sodium bromide is given in divided multiple doses over a 48-hour period.

Potassium gluconate

Use: Oral potassium supplement.

How Supplied: Oral: 2 mEq (468 mg) tablet. Oral Powder: 2 mEq (468 mg) potassium gluconate/0.25 teaspoon (0.65 g), 4 oz bottle.

Feline Dose: 2.5-7.0 mEq/cat/day divided according to number of feedings.

Prednisolone

Use: Corticosteroid therapy.

How Supplied: Injectable: 50 mg/ml acetate suspension, 30 ml vial. Oral: 5 mg tablet. 1% Ophthalmic suspension, 10 ml bottle.

Canine Dose: 0.5-2.2 mg/kg (0.23-1 mg/lb) IM, PO.

Feline Dose: 0.5-2.2 mg/kg (0.23-1 mg/lb) IM, PO q 24-48h.

Prednisolone sodium phosphate

Use: Corticosteroid therapy.

How Supplied: Injectable: 20 mg/ml (14.8 mg of prednisolone base per ml), 50 ml vial.

Canine Dose: 0.5-2.2 mg/kg (0.23-1 mg/lb) IV.

Feline Dose: 0.5-2.2 mg/kg (0.23-1 mg/lb) IV q 24-48h.

Prednisone

Use: Corticosteroid therapy, antineoplastic agent.

How Supplied: Oral: 5, 10, 20, and 50 mg tablets, 1 mg/ml oral solution. Injectable: 10 and 40 mg/ml vials.

Canine Dose: 0.5-2.2 mg/kg (0.23-1 mg/lb) PO.

Feline Dose: 0.5-2.2 mg/kg (0.23-1 mg/lb) PO sid. Antineoplastic Dose: 30-40 mg/m^2 IM, PO sid or eod for 21 days, then 1 mg/kg PO sid for 4 weeks, and 1 mg/kg eod thereafter.

Procarbazine

Use: Antineoplastic agent.
How Supplied: May need to be compounded.
Canine Dose: 50 mg/m^2 PO sid for 14 days as part of MOPP protocol.
Feline Dose: 10 mg/cat/day for 14 days as part of the MOPP protocol.

Prochlorperazine

(Compazine®, Darbazine®)
Use: Antiemetic.
How Supplied: Injectable: 5 mg/ml, 2 ml ampule.
Feline Dose: Compazine®: 0.1-0.5 mg/kg IM, SQ q6-8h. Darbazine®: 0.5-0.8 mg/kg IM, SQ q12h.

Propofol

Use: Anesthesia.
How Supplied: Injectable: 10 mg/ml, 20 ml ampule.
Canine Dose: 4-6 mg/kg IV, titrated to effect.
Feline Dose: 2-6 mg/kg IV, given slowly to effect.

Propanolol

Use: Beta-blocker.
How Supplied: Injectable: 1 mg/ml, 1 ml ampule.
Canine Dose: 0.04-0.06 mg/kg (0.02-0.03 mg/lb) IV, slowly.

Ranitidine

Use: H$_2$-receptor antagonist.
How Supplied: Injectable: 25 mg/ml, 6 ml vial. Oral: 15 mg/ml syrup, 480 ml bottle; 75, 150, and 300 mg tablets.
Canine Dose: 2 mg/kg PO, SQ, IV bid-tid.
Feline Dose: 3.5 mg/kg PO bid; 2.5 mg/kg IV bid.

Streptozocin-streptozoticin

Use: Antineoplastic agent for insulinoma.
How Supplied: Injectable: 100 mg/ml, 1 g vial.
Canine Dose: 500 mg/m^2 IV every 2-3 weeks – 0.9% saline is given IV at 18.3 ml/kg/hr for 3 hours, then streptozocin is administered at 500 mg/m^2 over two hours with the saline diuresis continuing. After streptozocin infusion is completed, continue saline diuresis for another two hours. Butorphanol 0.4 mg/kg IM is given at the end of the streptozocin portion of the infusion as an antiemetic, although ondansetron or dolasetron may be more effective.

Sucralfate

Use: Duodenal ulcer treatment.
How Supplied: Oral: 100 mg/ml solution, 480 ml bottle; 1 g tablet.
Canine Dose: 0.5 g/small dog, 1 g/large dog PO tid 1 hour prior to feeding.
Feline Dose: 0.25 g/cat PO tid 1 hr prior to feeding.

Sulfasalazine

Use: Sulfonamide.
How Supplied: Oral: 500 mg tablet.
Canine Dose: 12.5 mg/kg (5.7 mg/lb) PO qid for 2 weeks. With improvement, may reduce dose to 6.25 mg/kg (2.85 mg/lb) qid for 2 weeks.

Tiletamine and zolazepam

Use: Combination dissociative anesthetic/tranquilizer.
How Supplied: Injectable: 5 ml vial (Tiletamine – equivalent to 250 mg free base; Zolazepam – equivalent to 250 mg free base). When 5 ml of sterile diluent is added a concentration of 50 mg/ml of each drug (100 mg/ml combined) is produced.
Canine Dose: 6.6-9.9 mg/kg IM for diagnostic purposes. 9.9-13.2 mg/kg IM for minor procedures of short duration. If supplemental doses are needed, give doses less than the initial dose and total dose should not exceed 26.4 mg/kg. Atropine (0.04 mg/kg) should be used concurrently to control hypersalivation.
Feline Dose: 9.7-11.9 mg/kg IM for minor procedures of short duration. 10.6-12.5 mg/kg IM for mild to moderate levels of anesthesia. If supplemental doses are needed, give doses less than the initial dose and total dose should not exceed 72 mg/kg. Atropine (0.04 mg/kg) should be used concurrently to control hypersalivation.
Note: Schedule III Controlled Substance.

Tramadol

Use: Opiate agonist.
How Supplied: Oral: 50 mg tablet.
Canine Dose: 1-4 mg/kg PO q6h.
Feline Dose: 4 mg/kg PO bid.

Triamcinolone

Use: Corticosteroid therapy.
How Supplied: Injectable: 2 mg/ml, 25 ml vial. 6 mg/ml and 40 mg/ml, 5 ml vials.
Canine Dose: 0.11-0.22 mg/kg.
Feline Dose: 0.1-0.2 mg/kg (0.045-0.09 mg/lb) IM, SQ sid.

N,N',N"-triethylenethiophosphoramide

Use: Antineoplastic agent.
How Supplied: Injectable: 15 mg vial.
Feline Dose: Maximum systemic dosage: 9 mg/m^2 IM, SQ q3wk. Bladder installation: 30 mg/m^2 once q3-4wk, remove 1 hr later.

Trimethoprim-sulfamethoxazole

Use: Antibacterial.
How Supplied: Combination product containing one